Thieme

Diagnostic Imaging of Congenital Heart Defects

Diagnosis and Image-Guided Treatment

Matthias Gutberlet, MD, PhD, EBCR
Professor of Cardiac Imaging
Chair, Department of Diagnostic and Interventional Radiology
Heart Center Leipzig
University Leipzig
Leipzig, Germany

1011 illustrations

Thieme
Stuttgart • New York • Delhi • Rio de Janeiro

Library of Congress Cataloging-in-Publication Data
is available from the publisher.

This book is an authorized translation of the 1st German edition published and copyrighted 2017 by Georg Thieme Verlag, Stuttgart. Title of the German edition: Bildgebende Diagnostik angeborener Herzfehler mit bildgestützter Therapie

Translator: Capri Beene, Akron, OH, USA
Illustrator: Martin Hoffmann, Neu-Ulm, Germany

Important note: Medicine is an ever-changing science undergoing continual development. Research and clinical experience are continually expanding our knowledge, in particular our knowledge of proper treatment and drug therapy. Insofar as this book mentions any dosage or application, readers may rest assured that the authors, editors, and publishers have made every effort to ensure that such references are in accordance with **the state of knowledge at the time of production of the book.**

Nevertheless, this does not involve, imply, or express any guarantee or responsibility on the part of the publishers in respect to any dosage instructions and forms of applications stated in the book. **Every user is requested to examine carefully** the manufacturers' leaflets accompanying each drug and to check, if necessary in consultation with a physician or specialist, whether the dosage schedules mentioned therein or the contraindications stated by the manufacturers differ from the statements made in the present book. Such examination is particularly important with drugs that are either rarely used or have been newly released on the market. Every dosage schedule or every form of application used is entirely at the user's own risk and responsibility. The authors and publishers request every user to report to the publishers any discrepancies or inaccuracies noticed. If errors in this work are found after publication, errata will be posted at www.thieme.com on the product description page.

Some of the product names, patents, and registered designs referred to in this book are in fact registered trademarks or proprietary names even though specific reference to this fact is not always made in the text. Therefore, the appearance of a name without designation as proprietary is not to be construed as a representation by the publisher that it is in the public domain.

Georg Thieme Verlag KG
Rüdigerstrasse 14, 70469 Stuttgart, Germany
+49 [0]711 8931 421, customerservice@thieme.de

Thieme Publishers New York
333 Seventh Avenue, New York, NY 10001 USA
+1 800 782 3488, customerservice@thieme.com

Thieme Publishers Delhi
A-12, Second Floor, Sector-2, Noida-201301
Uttar Pradesh, India
+91 120 45 566 00, customerservice@thieme.in

Thieme Publishers Rio,
Thieme Publicações Ltda.
Edifício Rodolpho de Paoli, 25º andar
Av. Nilo Peçanha, 50 – Sala 2508
Rio de Janeiro 20020-906 Brasil
+55 21 3172 2297/ +55 21 3172 1896

Cover design: Thieme Publishing Group
Typesetting by DiTech Process Solutions

Printed in Germany by CPI Books 5 4 3 2 1

ISBN 978-3-13-240251-5

Also available as an e-book:
eISBN 978-3-13-240364-2

MIX
Papier aus verantwortungsvollen Quellen
FSC® C083411

Dedicated to my wife Petra Matouschek.

Contents

Foreword

Diagnostic Imaging of Congenital Heart Defects addresses the full scope of imaging diagnostic techniques for congenital heart defects, supplemented by detailed graphics and excellent images of heart defects, ranging from simple to complex, including the most common congenital cardiomyopathies.

Although congenital heart defects were hardly the focus of physicians a decade ago due to extremely low survival rates, nowadays the treatment of these types of defects has become a matter of interdisciplinary cooperation among pediatric and adult cardiologists, heart surgeons, intensive care physicians, anesthetists, and radiologists.

Imaging techniques play a decisive role in diagnosing innate, congenital heart defects, identifying subsequent illnesses or residual findings, and in facilitating treatment. It is this interdisciplinarity, in particular, that has helped imaging techniques achieve such high-quality standards.

Congenital heart defects are characterized by their enormous variety. This is reflected by the 70 different ICD-10 codes (International Statistical Classification of Diseases and Related Health Problems [WHO]) and 206 IPCC-Codes (International Pediatric and Congenital Cardiac Code of the International Society for Nomenclature of Pediatric and Congenital Heart Disease [ISNPCHD]; www.ipccc.net). Accurate imaging requires extensive prior knowledge of and familiarity with the pathoanatomy of congenital heart defects.

Generally speaking, patients with congenital heart defects must undergo multiple corrective or palliative procedures during the course of their lives. Growth and degeneration can also lead to structural changes in the heart. The success of treatments, as well as morphological and functional changes, can only be identified in a timely manner via accurate imaging. In order to implement most efficiently and assess the various imaging techniques in everyday routines, one requires adequate knowledge of the various treatment methods within the field of congenital heart defects.

Parallel to the development of various treatment methods, there is an increasing demand for knowledge regarding the embryological development and genetic basis of congenital heart defects. It has been proven crucial that relationships and differences between heart defects can be expressed using an unambiguous nomenclature, particularly for research purposes. The "International Society for Nomenclature of Paediatric and Congenital Heart Disease" has dedicated itself to this task. Thus, the common, colloquial designations for the types of transposition of the great arteries (*D-TGA* and *L-TGA*) do not adequately describe these heart defects in unambiguous terms, which must more accurately be termed *complete transposition with intact ventricular septum or congenitally corrected transposition.*

This book provides an excellent overview of multimodal imaging diagnostics for congenital heart defects, from diagnosis to treatment. In the initial days, an awareness of cardiac imaging applied primarily to acquired diseases, and thus to the left ventricle.

Assessment methods in adult cardiology, however, do not possess a 1:1 correspondence to congenital heart defects, which focus on the right ventricle and pulmonary circulation. This issue is being addressed by the idea of competence networks, particularly by *Kompetenznetz Angeborene Herzfehler e.V.* (Competence Network for Congenital Heart Defects). In addition, an intense effort is being expended to standardize and implement imaging methods for congenital heart defects in a reasonable manner. The results of these efforts are detailed in this book, which contain significant contributions by a multidisciplinary team of authors and scientists in the competence network for congenital heart defects.

I thank everyone who has contributed to the success of this interdisciplinary work and believe that this book will enrich the previous literature on congenital heart defects considerably.

Ulrike Bauer, MD
Managing Director,
Kompetenznetz Angeborene Herzfehler e.V.

Preface

Diagnostic Imaging of Congenital Heart Defects encompasses a broad spectrum, sometimes, extremely rare and complex illnesses. This kind of book always brings a sort of balance between conveying the solid fundamentals and the specialized knowledge. This is particularly difficult if the book cannot and does not wish to be an actual textbook on the topic of congenital heart defects. For this reason, it was crucial to strike a balance between an atlas-like preparation and presentation of extensive photographic material from various modalities and a short, content-related description of the various clinical pictures with hospitals, diagnostics, and treatment.

In cases of congenital heart defects, the derivations from embryology are also a factor, which we have included at the very beginning. In addition, we have included a brief introduction to the technology of the various available modalities, though without any claim that this list is complete. We were obligated to make a deliberate selection, which, from the authors' and publisher's perspective, is necessary in order to understand how to choose the most appropriate and least invasive diagnostic procedures possible. Regardless, space was devoted to newer procedures whose clinical benefits may not yet have been fully proven.

Despite the many authors and their various backgrounds, we attempted to create a book with a unified structure intended to simplify flow and readability. The Note boxes, references to other chapters in the book, and Clinical Correlation references aim to do just that. A unified nomenclature is of great importance with congenital heart defects, especially in light of quality assurance aspects. Categorization may be less precise in everyday clinical practice without compromising adequate patient care. The chapters are written by practitioners including all area of imaging diagnostics based on everyday clinical practices.

We believe that despite all limitations, we have created a comprehensive book including all aspects of imaging diagnostics and imaging-supported treatment, and we hope that you enjoy studying this work and using it as a reference.

The publisher, editor, and authors are grateful for any feedback and look forward to a lively dialogue with the readers, including suggestions to improve the book for any subsequent editions.

Matthias Gutberlet, MD, PhD, EBCR

Acknowledgments

Interdisciplinary cooperation is a valuable commodity in medicine. Regular interdisciplinary exchanges must take place, especially within subspecialties with continual advancements. No single person can convey the entirety of knowledge within a specialty—much less a medical specialty or subspecialty.

This is especially true for relatively rare illnesses such as congenital heart defects. For this reason, we strove to assemble an interdisciplinary team of authors for each of the individual chapters and subchapters in this book. Various experts from the disciplines of anatomy, cardiac and pediatric cardiac surgery, cardiology and pediatric cardiology, as well as physics, radiology and even electrophysiology from the United States, Germany, Austria, Switzerland, and the Czech Republic were involved in this book's creation. I would like to extend my profound and sincere thanks to all of them for their tireless effort, advice, and, above all, for their dedication.

None of this would have been possible without the support of Thieme Publishers, under the direction of Stephan Konnry and his coworkers. The editors and authors also extend special thanks to Mrs. Apoorva—the book's project manager—for her patience even when the deadlines for completion were delayed significantly. A special thank you to Thieme's graphic design department, who went to great lengths to implement and visualize the author's most complex requests.

Interdisciplinary concepts, as I have become familiar with them during cooperation in clinical settings and in scientific projects within the congenital heart defects competence network, contributed enormously to this book. To this end, I would personally like to extend heartfelt thanks to Peter Lange, MD, PhD, founder of the competence network and my clinical teacher. Furthermore, I would like to thank the Competence Network of Congenital Heart Defects and its Managing Director, Dr. Ulrike Bauer, for their continuous support.

The editors and authors would also like to thank all the coworkers of the hospitals and institutions, especially the hospitals belonging to the Leipzig Heart Center, who could not be listed explicitly here, primarily for making these excellent images available to us.

I hope that you will find this read enjoyable and informative.

Matthias Gutberlet, MD, PhD, EBCR

Contributors

Editor-in-Chief

Matthias Gutberlet, MD, PhD, EBCR
Professor of Cardiac Imaging
Chair, Department of Diagnostic and Interventional Radiology
Heart Center Leipzig
University Leipzig
Leipzig, Germany

Contributing Authors

Hashim Abdul-Khaliq, MD
University Professor
Clinic for Pediatric Cardiology
Saarland University Hospital
Homburg, Germany

Farhad Bakhtiary, MD
Associate Professor
Department of Cardiac Imaging
Leipzig Heart Center
University Hospital Leipzig
Leipzig, Germany

Philipp Beerbaum, MD
University Professor
Department of Pediatric Cardiology
Intensive Care Clinic
Hannover Medical School
Hannover, Germany

Petra Böttler, MD
Pediatric Practice
Freiburg, Germany

Jens Bremerich, MD, EBCR
Associate Professor
Department of Medical Radiology
University Hospital of Basel
Basel, Switzerland

Arno Bücker, MD, MSc
University Professor
Department of Diagnostic and Interventional Radiology Clinic
Saarland University Hospital
Homburg, Germany

Ingo Dähnert, MD
University Professor
Clinic of Pediatric Cardiology
Leipzig Heart Center
University Hospital Leipzig
Leipzig, Germany

Joachim G. Eichhorn, MD
Associate Professor
Clinic of Pediatric and Adolescent
Leverkusen Hospital
Leverkusen, Germany

Florentine Gräfe, MD
Senior Physician
Clinic of Pediatric Cardiology
Leipzig Heart Center
University Hospital Leipzig
Leipzig, Germany

Gerald F. Greil, MD, PhD
University Professor
Department of Pediatrics
Children's Medical Center
UT Southwestern Medical Center
Texas, USA

Matthias Grothoff, MD, EBCR
Associate Professor
Department of Diagnostic and Interventional Radiology
University Hospital Leipzig
Leipzig Heart Center
Leipzig, Germany

Jan Janoušek, MD, PhD
Chief
Children's Heart Centre
2nd Faculty of Medicine
Charles University
Motol University Hospital
Prague, Czech Republic

Willi A. Kalender, MD
University Professor
Institute of Medical Physics
University of Erlangen-Nuremberg
Erlangen, Germany

Christian Kellenberger, MD
Associate Professor
Department of Pediatric Radiology
Children's Hospital Zurich - Eleonore Foundation
Zürich, Switzerland

Martin Kostelka, MD
University Professor
Clinic of Cardiac Surgery
Leipzig Heart Center
University Hospital Leipzig
Leipzig, Germany

Titus Kühne, MD
Associate Professor
Department of Congenital Heart Disease
German Heart Institute Berlin
Pediatric Cardiology
Berlin, Germany

Eberhard Künzel, MD
Department of Diagnostic and Interventional Radiology
Leipzig Heart Center
University Hospital Leipzig
Leipzig, Germany

Heiner Latus, MD
Department of Congenital Heart Disease
German Heart Institute Berlin
Munich, Germany

Lukas Lehmkuhl, MD, EBCR
Associate Professor
Department of Diagnostic and Interventional Radiology
Leipzig Heart Center
University Hospital Leipzig
Leipzig, Germany

Joachim Lotz, MD
University Professor
Institute for Diagnostic and Interventional Radiology
University of Göttingen
Göttingen, Germany

Philipp Lurz, MD
Associate Professor
Department of Congenital and Genetic Heart Defects
University Hospital Leipzig
Leipzig Heart Center
Leipzig, Germany

Marcus Makowski, MD
Associate Professor
Department of Radiology
Charité – Universitätsmedizin Berlin
Berlin, Germany

Friedrich Wilhelm Mohr, MD
University Professor
University Hospital Leipzig
Leipzig Heart Center
Department of Cardiac Surgery
Leipzig, Germany

Nicole Nagdyman, MD
Associate Professor
German Heart Center Munich
Department of Pediatric Cardiology
Munich, Germany

Axel Rentzsch, MD
Saarland University Hospital
Pediatric Cardiology Clinic
Homburg, Germany

Samir Sarikouch, MD
Associate Professor
Department of Cardiothoracic, Transplant, and Vascular Surgery
Hannover Medical School
Hannover, Germany

Achim A. Schmaltz, MD
University Professor
Department of Pediatric Cardiology
Essen University Hospital
Essen, Germany

Wolfgang Schmidt, MD†
University Professor
Department of Anatomy
University Hospital Leipzig
Leipzig, Germany

Erich Sorantin, MD
University Professor
Department of Radiology
Medical University of Graz
Graz, Austria

Michael Steinmetz, MD
Pediatrician
Pediatric Cardiology and Intensive Care Clinic
University Medical Center Göttingen
Heart Center
Göttingen, Germany

1 Cardiogenesis and Classification of Congenital Heart Defects

Eberhard Kuenzel, Wolfgang Schmidt†

1.1 Cardiogenesis

A firm basis of knowledge regarding the regular morphogenesis of the heart and cardiac-adjacent vascular system (normogenesis) and of chronological sequence (▸ Table 1.1) makes it easier to obtain a basic understanding of complex congenital heart defects. The determination periods for pathogenesis are important with regard to the formal genesis of congenital defects (▸ Table 1.2). A multitude of different pathogenetic mechanisms can cause identical malformations during these periods.

Table 1.1 Temporal determination of individual structures during cardiogenesis (selection).

Structure	Ovulatory age (Days)	Crown-rump length (mm)	Carnegie stage[1]
Cardiogenic plate	19	1.5	9
Cardiac tube	19–26	1.5–4.5	9–11
Cardiac loop	22–30	2–5	10–12
Septum primum	28–44	4–14	13–17
Septum secundum	42–60	11–31	17–23
Interventricular septum	28–51	4–18	13–19
Specific conduction system	28–51	4–18	13–19
Coronary arteries	37–51	8–18	16–19
Aortic arch and pulmonary arteries	26–44	3–14	12–17

Table 1.2 Temporal determination of cardiovascular malformations (selection).[2]

Malformation	Acronym	Ovulatory age (Day)	Carnegie stage[1]
Dextrocardia		22–26	10–11
Anomalous pulmonary venous connection/return	APVC/APVR	26–38	12–15
Ostium primum defect	ASD I	30–42	13–17
Ostium secundum defect	ASD II	35–60	15–23
Persistent atrioventricular canal		32–48	14–18
Interventricular septal defects	VSD	32–48	14–18
Double outlet left ventricle	DOLV	28–42	13–16
Double outlet right ventricle	DORV	28–38	13–15
Ventricular hypoplasia		42–60	17–23
Stenosis of the atrioventricular valves		42–60	17–23
Stenosis of the semilunar valves		35–60	15–23
Transposition of the great arteries	TGA	35–42	15–16
Tetralogy of Fallot	TOF	42–51	17–20
Aortopulmonary window (aortopulmonary septal defect)	APSD	35–42	15–16

1.1.1 Precordial Phase (Weeks 1 and 2 of Development Post Ovulation)

During the precordial phase (▶ Fig. 1.1a), a primitive circulatory system is formed to ensure that the embryo is supplied with nutrients. Once it reaches a thickness of 0.1 mm, the embryo can no longer be supplied with nutrients via diffusion alone. The embryonic blood islands fuse gradually into a primitive reticular capillary system. At the start of week 3 of development, the angioblasts migrating from the yolk sac group together and then form simple endothelial tubes. These tubes transform subsequently into organ-type, final vessel patterns under the influence of humoral and hemodynamic factors via proliferation, differentiation, and regression.

1.1.2 Cardiac Phase (Weeks 3–8 of Development Post Ovulation)

True cardiogenesis begins in the embryo, now approximately 1.5 mm long, with the formation of the horseshoe-shaped cardiogenic plate (▶ Table 1.1). During the blastoderm's development and the massive growth of the dorsal neural tube, the cardiogenic zone is displaced caudal-ventrally. Afterward, the ventral thoracic wall closes over the pericardial cavity above the ectoderm. A single, three-layer cardiac tube forms from the fusion of the extraembryonic and intraembryonic vessel plexus (▶ Fig. 1.1b). This structure, now approximately 1 mm long, consists of an inner endocardial lining, an external myoepicardial layer, and an intermediate gelatinous matrix area (cardiac jelly). The initially elongated cardiac tube then connects dorsally to the serous-lined epicardial cavity via a wide mesocardium. Vascular poles for the cranial artery and caudal vein are already distinguishable during this stage. The venous vascular poles situated in the transverse septum provide drainage for both the extraembryonic and intraembryonic venous branches. The cardiogenic plate formed on day 22 p.o., now actively contracting, pumps the blood along the cranial arterial vascular pole into the paired dorsal aortae. These aortic arteries are likewise connected to the placenta via the umbilical arteries.

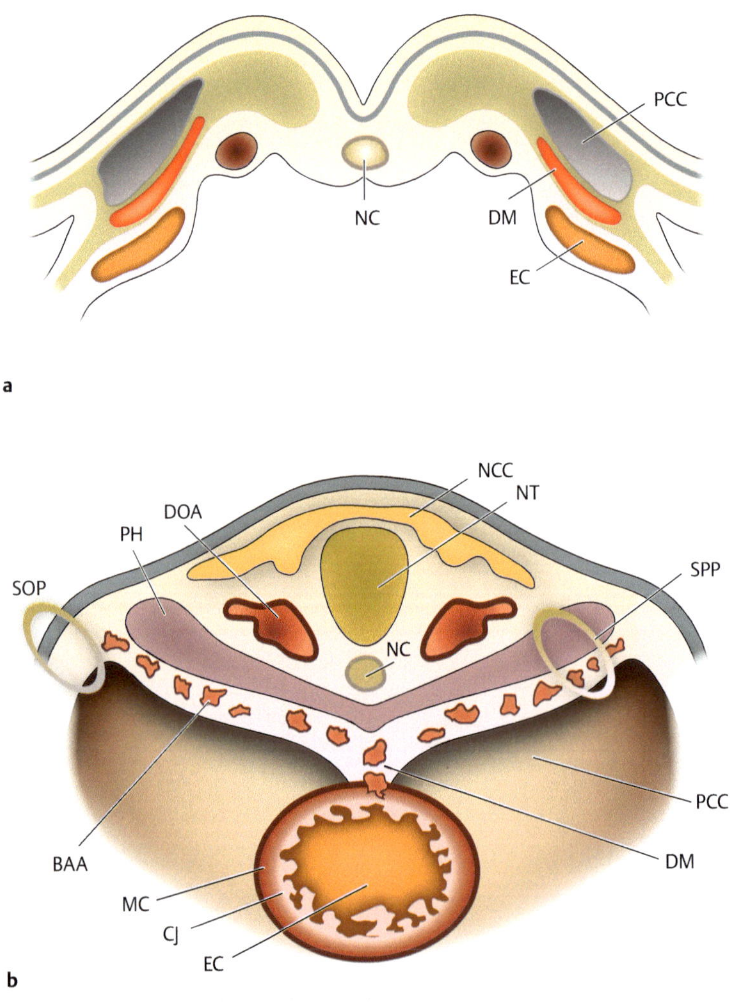

Fig. 1.1 Initial phases of cardiogenesis. Schematic depiction.
BAA = branchial arch arteries (epithelial progenitor cells of the pharyngeal arch arteries)
CJ = cardiac jelly
DM = dorsal mesocardium
DOA = dorsal aorta
EC = endocardial cushion
MC = myocardium
NC = notochord (dorsal cord)
NCC = migrating neural crest cells
NT = neural tube
PCC = pericardial cavity
PH = pharynx
SOP = somatopleura
SPP = splanchnic pleura

a Precordial phase: Cluster of angiogenetic progenitor cells form the primitive vascular system of the blastoderm via confluent blood islands and endothelial tubes.

b Cardiac phase: Development of the cardiogenic plate into a single cardiac tube.

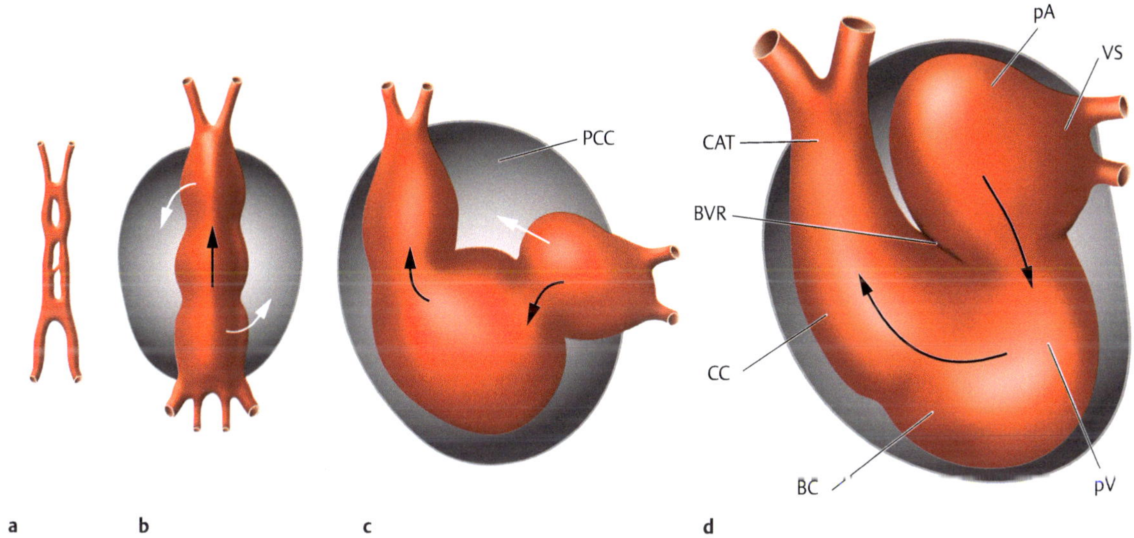

Fig. 1.2 Cardiac looping process. Schematic depiction. Developmental stages from the primitive cardiac tube to the final heart after loop formation (cardiac looping), with segmentation and derivatives. The black arrows within the heart each indicate the direction of blood flow from the venous to the arterial portal, while the other arrows indicate the direction of cardiac rotation or invagination. Normogenesis corresponding to dextrorotation (D-loop) is depicted here.

BC = bulbus cordis
BVR = bulboventricular ridge (initial asymmetry ca. day 23 p.o.)
CAT = common arterial trunk (truncus arteriosus)
CC = conus cordis
PCC = pericardial cavity
pA = primitive atrium (primitive right atrium)
pV = primitive ventricle (primitive right ventricle)
VS = venous sinus (venous sinus)
a Stage 1 (front view).
b Stage 2 (front view).
c Stage 3 (side view).
d Stage 4 (side view).

This transformation of the elongated cardiac tube into an arched cardiac tube occurs on approximately day 21 (▶ Fig. 1.2). In contrast to previous morphogenesis occurring exclusively in symmetry, asymmetric lateralization takes place for the first time in the form of cardiac looping, which lasts only about 24 hours. This usually occurs autonomously and independently of hemodynamic factors. Once the cardiac tube has been relatively fixed at the vascular poles, the stretched "systemic arterial" portion of the cardiac tube deviates ventral-caudally and then toward the right. The inferior "systemic venous" inflow portion of the cardiac tube deviates dorsally and then to the left during the course of this primary dextrorotation (d-loop) of the central section with rightward convexity. As of day 23 p.o., already defined sections of the cardiac tube and the sulci dividing them can be distinguished (▶ Fig. 1.2), namely, the venous sinus, atrium commune or primitive atrium, primitive ventricle, bulbus cordis, conus cordis, and truncus arteriosus.

Significant bulging of the individual cardiac tube segments, which demarcates additional external furrows and folds, occurs between days 26 and 30. They will later be of importance during septation, the development of the valve system, and differentiation of the conduction system. The technical conditions that allow final separation of the pulmonary and systemic circulation vascular beds by means of complex internal septation of a primary singular, tubular lumens are achieved during the cardiac plate's displacement from the neck region to the superior thoracic area (descensus cordis), as necessitated by growth.

Since the cavum is not yet smooth in structure at the start of tube formation (cardiac looping), initial trabeculation then develops adjacent to the interventricular foramen (▶ Fig. 1.3). Subsequently, the primitive ventricle that will later form the majority of the morphologic left ventricle is completely trabeculated. The morphologic right ventricle develops from the proximal, curved section of the bulbus cordis. The joint outflow tract for both ventricles is formed from the distal, elongated section of the bulbus. The truncus arteriosus is formed from the roots of the major arteries.

Clinical Relevance

Any disruptions occurring during formation of the cardiac loop (cardiac looping) can lead to various malformations, including *ventricular inversion* or *congenitally corrected TGA, DORV*, or *auricular juxtaposition*.

Cardiogenesis is not fully completed until after birth, upon the functional closure of the foramen ovale and obliteration of the ductus arteriosus.

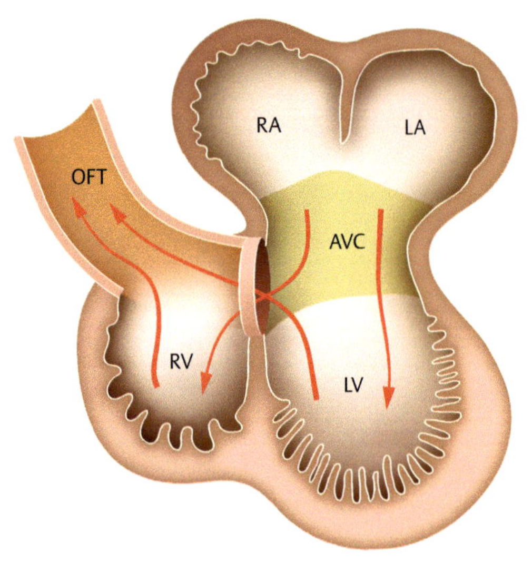

Fig. 1.3 Main blood flow paths at the time of cardiac loop formation. Schematic depiction. Formation of the outflow segment occurs primarily via the development of the ventricular loop (later the right ventricle); a direct outflow tract does, however, already exist between the developing left ventricle and the arterial segment. Coronary section, ventral view.
AVC = atrioventricular channel
LA = left atrium
LV = left ventricle
OFT = outflow tract
RA = right atrium
RV = right ventricle

Morphogenesis of the Atrial Region

The final atrium gains its structure via four complex mechanisms:

- Incorporation of the venous sinus,
- Formation of the systemic vein junction region,
- Development of the atrial sinus valves and the valve apparatus of the foramen ovale, and
- Atrial compartmentalization via development of the interatrial septa.

The smooth-walled venous sinus is integrated into the final atrial segment during days 28–30 p.o. In addition to a main section draining into the atrial segment, a left and right sinus horn—each incorporating the paired cardinal, umbilical, and vitelline veins—can be differentiated on the venous sinus (▶ Fig. 1.4). Once the primary portal circulatory system has developed, the lower hollow veins directly adjacent to the heart first develop from the right hepatic vein, and the upper hollow veins from the right sinus horn. The atrial segment is separated from the venous sinus on day 26 p.o., with the development of a crescent-shaped, left-facing sinoatrial septum. This causes functional separation of the presumptive left atrium from the right atrium, whose broad connection to the venous sinus remains in place. Hence, all cardiopetal veins are connected exclusively to the final right atrium. Within the scope of progressive atrialization of the central venous sinus section, venous valves (▶ Fig. 1.5 and ▶ Fig. 1.6) and the venous sinus septum—from which the valve of the inferior vena cava (Eustachian valve) and the coronary sinus valve (Thebesian valve) are later derived—are distinguishable (▶ Fig. 1.5). While the smooth-walled, dorsally situated areas are formed by integrating the primary veins of the venous sinus on the left and the primary pulmonary veins on the right, the muscular trabeculated auricles are remnants of the primitive atrium.

Note

Mobile, threadlike, or reticulated remnants of the right sinus vein valve that generally extend from the crista terminalis to the junction of the inferior vena cava in the coronary sinus within the right atrium are known as “Chiari networks.”

Morphogenesis of the Pulmonary Veins

The pulmonary buds are initially supplied with blood via the visceral vessels. Pulmonary venous drainage into the left and right superior cardinal veins occurs via the pulmonary plexus and the splanchnic veins. Only after the primitive (or primary) pulmonary vein stem has sprouted from the posterior wall of the left atrium (day 28–30 p.o.; ▶ Fig. 1.6) do the first anastomoses appear between the pulmonary and peribronchial capillary plexus and the twice-divided pulmonary venous stem. First the primary pulmonary vein stem, then the four distinct pulmonary veins formed by its two divisions are incorporated into the posterior wall of the left atrium by means of relative growth movements. Thus, the smooth, thin posterior wall of the morphologic left atrium develops from the primary pulmonary veins, though not the retroposed trabeculated portion of the atrium.

Clinical Relevance

- Supracardiac and cardiac TAPVR are the result of failed induction originating in the cardinal venous system. In contrast, infracardiac TAPVR is defined as arrested development with persistence of the embryonic state, accompanied by complete drainage of the splanchnic venous system.
- Incomplete integration of the primary pulmonary vein into the posterior wall of the left atrium leads to persistence of a fibromuscular septum for subcompartmentation of the left atrium, known as *left triatrial heart*.

Compartmentation of the Atrial Region

During invagination of the atrial wall, two valve-like structures—the sinoatrial valves—that fuse cranially to

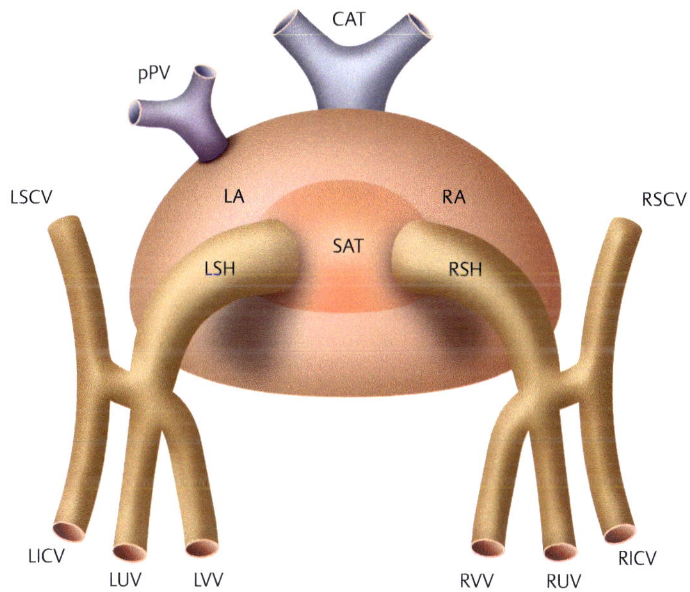

Fig. 1.4 Primitive venous system in primary bilateral symmetrical configuration. Schematic depiction. Drainage into the primitive atrium of the developing heart via the ipsilateral sinus horn. Dorsal view.

CAT = common arterial trunk (truncus arteriosus)
LA = left atrium
LICV = left inferior cardinal vein
LSCV = left superior cardinal vein
LSH = left sinus horn
LUV = left umbilical vein
LVV = left vitelline vein
pPV = primitive pulmonary vein
RA = right atrium
RICV = right inferior cardinal vein
RSCV = right superior cardinal vein
RSH = right sinus horn
RUV = right umbilical vein
RVV = right vitelline vein
SAT = sinoatrial transition

the septum spurium and later regresses, are demarcated on the sinoatrial transition. True septation becomes externally visible upon development of a constriction—the atrioventricular sulcus, which is located along the bend between the bulbus cordis and truncus arteriosus. Nearly simultaneously, the interatrial sulcus forms on the posterior-cranial circumference of the primitive atrium, corresponding luminally to the septum primum, which is also semicircular. The free, concave lower margin of the septum primum that primarily provides vertical separation between the common atrium comprises the upper margin of the foramen, or ostium primum. As of approximately day 35 p.o., there is visible evidence of multiple, successively confluent perforations from which the foramen or ostium secundum emerges.

The fusion of portions of the lower margin of the septum primum with the endocardial cushion located on the plane of the later atrioventricular valves causes the ostium primum to decrease in size before finally disappearing between days 37 and 42 p.o. In the meantime, the ostium secundum ensures the hemodynamically crucial horizontal connection of the atria, which is subsequently modified by the development of the septum secundum located further to the right. The septum secundum also emerges between the septum primum and the venous sinus valve as a development of the anterior cranial atrial roof and grows in the direction of the base of the heart or endocardial cushion. The foramen ovale, whose functional closure and subsequent postnatal obliteration marks the end of final separation of the atria, forms by connecting the free margins of the septum primum to those of the septum secundum. The foramen ovale valve extending from the septum primum is first pressed into the limbus extending from the septum secundum as a result of postnatal pressure increases in the left atrium (▶ Fig. 1.7) thereby completing the fossa ovalis.

Clinical Relevance

- ASD II, the most common form of ASD, likely results from disproportionate apoptosis during the fenestration and total regression of the septum primum, and generally results in an extensive ASD.
- ASD I is characterized by the presence of an ASD in cases of intact ventricular septum and actually corresponds to a partial atrioventricular septal defect.

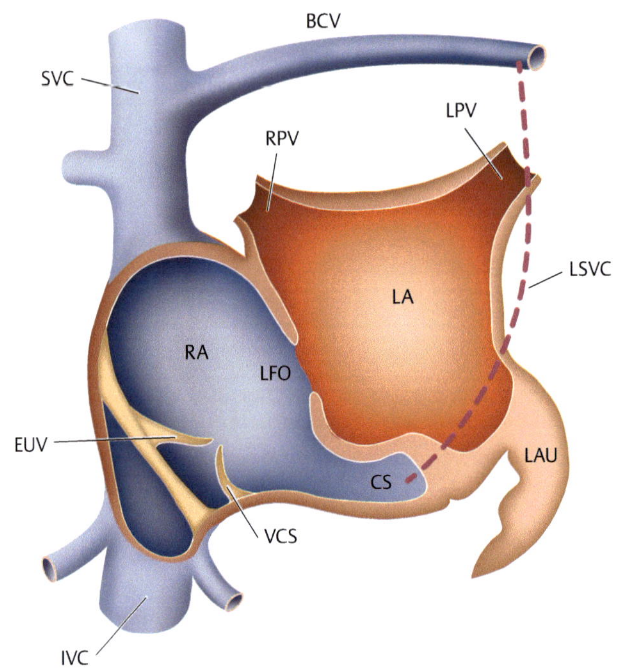

Fig. 1.5 Final heart-adjacent venous system. Schematic depiction. Regression of the left sinus horn and the left cardinal venous system, and right displacement of the ostia. A persistent left superior vena cava (SVC) (dotted line) with the usual junction to the coronary sinus in the right atrium results from incomplete regression to the oblique vein of the left atrium (oblique Ligament of Marshall). Ventral view.

BCV = brachiocephalic vein
CS = coronary sinus
EUV = Eustachian valve (valve of the inferior vena cava)
IVC = inferior vena cava
LA = left atrium
LAU = left auricle
LFO = limbus of fossa ovalis
LPV = left pulmonary vein
LSVC = left superior vena cava
RA = right atrium
RPV = right pulmonary vein
SVC = superior vena cava
VCS = valve of the coronary sinus (Thebesian valve)

Development of the Heart-Adjacent and Body Venous System

The venous system is much more variable than the arterial system due to the development of a heterogeneous capillary network from which the final vascular beds form initially based on regional preference.

The sinus horns, bilaterally symmetrical from this point onward, can then be perceived as the proximal portion of the non-fused early embryonic endocardial tubes that feed into the venous sinus (▶ Fig. 1.8a).

Fundamentally, a distinction can be made on both sides between three main venous systems:

- Umbilical veins,
- Vitelline veins, and
- Cardinal veins.

All three systems drain their blood via the ipsilateral sinus horn into the common venous sinus functioning as a sinoatrial transition (▶ Fig. 1.4). In doing so, the umbilical veins transport the oxygen- and nutrient-rich chorionic villi and placental villi blood from the umbilical cord, while the vitelline veins transport the blood from the vitelline, visceral, and portal venous systems and the supracardinal and infracardinal veins transport blood from the embryo's superior and inferior body segments. The umbilical veins quickly connect to the capillary plexus and sinusoids of the disproportionately fast-developing liver, so that their blood henceforth flows directly to the venous sinus via intrahepatic anastomoses. After involution of the extrahepatic portion of the umbilical veins, their blood can only reach the venous portal of the heart transhepatically, along with the vitelline venous blood. After involution of the left sinus horn, this blood reaches the venous portal posthepatically, via the right vitelline vein. Conversely, a shunt system essential to embryonic fetal circulation develops, namely the venous sinus that transports oxygen-rich umbilical venous blood directly to the heart by circumventing the hepatic vascular bed. Finally, the right umbilical vein completely regresses so that placental blood can reach the left umbilical vein only via the liver (▶ Fig. 1.8b). The left umbilical vein and the venous duct are obliterated postnatally to become the venous ligament of the liver.

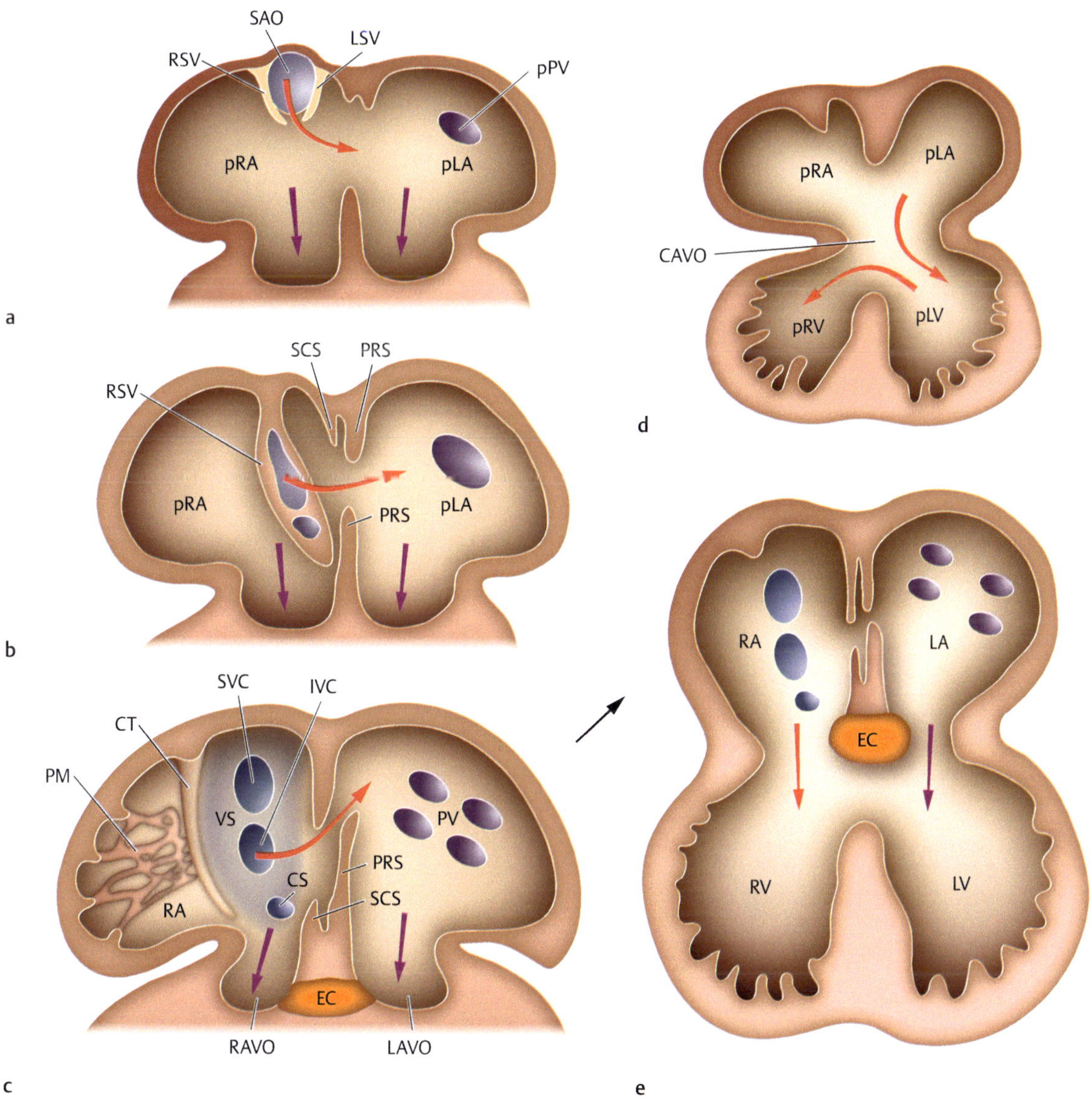

Fig. 1.6 Morphogenesis of the sinoatrial transition and septation of the primitive atrium. Schematic depiction. Developmental stages of morphogenesis with development of the final, separated atria with associated venous ostia after the integration of heart-adjacent veins and the sinus wall. Open coronal, ventral view. The arrows indicate blood flow.

CAVO = common atrioventricular ostium
CS = coronary sinus
CT = crista terminalis
EC = endocardial cushion
IVC = inferior vena cava
LAVO = left atrioventricular ostium
LSV = left sinus valve
LV = left ventricle
pLA = primitive left atrium
pLV = primitive left ventricle
PM = pectinate muscles
pPV = primitive pulmonary vein
pRA = primitive right atrium
PRS = primary septum
pRV = primitive right ventricle
PV = pulmonary veins
RA = right atrium
RAVO = right atrioventricular ostium
RSV = right sinus valve
RV = right ventricle
SAO = sinoatrial ostium
SCS = secondary septum
SVC = superior vena cava
VS = venous sinus

a Stage 1.
b Stage 2.
c Stage 3.
d Fig. with ventricle. Stage before 1–3
e Fig. with ventricle. Stage 3.

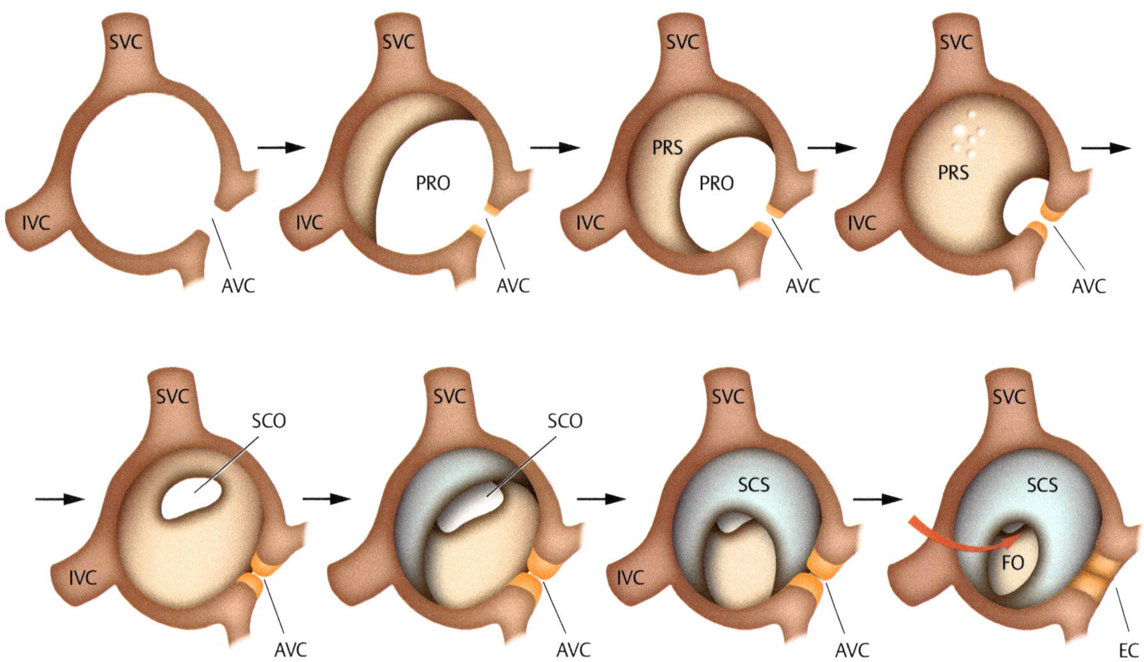

Fig. 1.7 Development of septation in the common atrium. Schematic depiction. Depiction of the successive development of lens-like septa and formation of the final fossa ovalis via the development of the ostium primum and ostium secundum. Concurrent compartmentation of the common atrioventricular canal via coordinated merging of the endocardial cushions. Right lateral view.
AVC = atrioventricular channel
EC = endocardial cushion
FO = foramen ovale
IVC = inferior vena cava
PRO = primary ostium
PRS = primary septum
SCO = secondary ostium
SCS = secondary septum
SVC = superior vena cava

Clinical Relevance

- In cases of atypical obliteration of the right inferior cardinal venous system followed by a missing hepatic segment of the inferior vena cava, the hepatic veins drain directly into the right atrium. Alternatively, the systemic venous blood in the lower half of the body is transferred into the superior vena cava via the azygos and hemiazygos system or transverse anastomoses. This is known as azygos continuation syndrome.
- Persistence of the left anterior cardinal vein, the common cardinal vein, and the left sinus horn leads to persistent left superior vena cava, which follow the course of the ligament of Marshall and the oblique left atrial vein, and generally drain into the right atrium via an enlarged coronary sinus (▶ Fig. 1.5). In addition, the dilated coronary sinus is not fully separated from the left atrium, corresponding to a *coronary sinus atrial septal defect.* A normal superior vena cava (right) may be present, hypoplastic, or even completely absent.

Morphogenesis of the Atrioventricular Valves

After the atrioventricular septa merge between days 38 and 42 p.o., slit-like ostia, which later form the presumptive tricuspid and mitral valves, persist between the lateral boundaries and the wall of the atrioventricular canal. Endocardial padding (known as endocardial cushions; ▶ Fig. 1.9)—luminal protrusions within the atrioventricular transition—takes on a key role here.

The final structures of the atrioventricular valve apparatus—cuspids, tendinous cords, and papillary muscles—form primarily via the directed development of excavations of the endocardial surface near the base of the heart. Myofibrils within the endocardial reticulum begin to differentiate after day 60 p.o. They develop in the subendocardial mesenchyme and settle in the endocardial cushions near the base of the heart (ventricle inlet) from which the atrioventricular valves form in a significantly less aggregate manner than in the apex. The vast majority of myogenic elements in the trabecular meshwork near the apex of the ventricular apparatus form the foundation for the later papillary

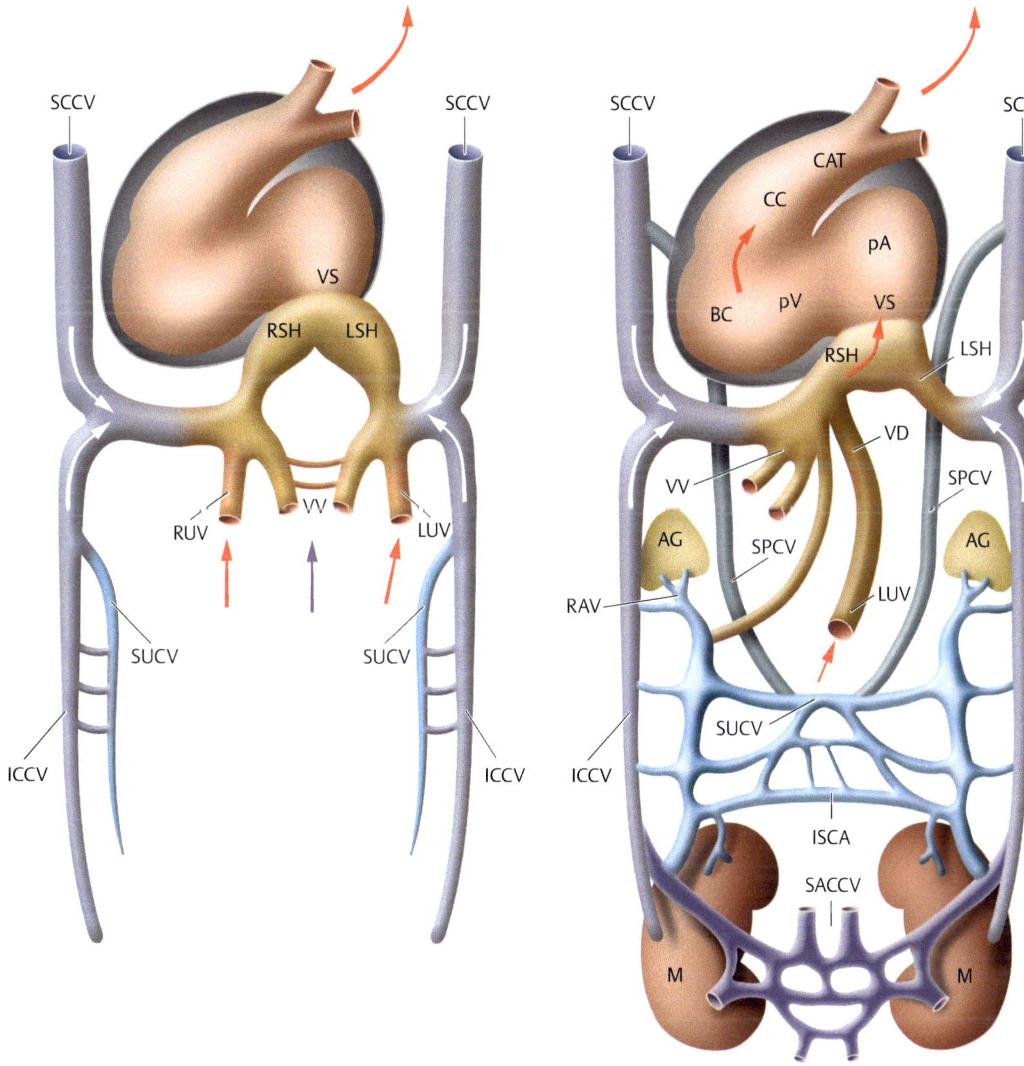

a b

Fig. 1.8 Morphogenesis of the primary symmetrical venous system. Schematic depiction of the cardinal venous system and the supracardinal, subcardinal, and sacrocardinal veins, including numerous anastomoses. Right lateralization within the scope of cardiac development. The arrows indicate the direction of blood flow.

AG = adrenal gland
BC = bulbus cordis
CAT = common arterial trunk (truncus arteriosus)
CC = conus cordis
ICCV = inferior common cardinal vein
ISCA = intersubcardinal anastomoses
LSH = left sinus horn
LUV = left umbilical vein
M = metanephros
pA = primitive atrium
pV = primitive ventricle
RAV = right adrenal vein
RSH = right sinus horn
RUV = right umbilical vein
SACCV = sacrocardinal vein
SCCV = superior common cardinal vein
SCSCA = subsacrocardinal anastomosis
SPCV = supracardinal vein
SUCV = subcardinal vein
VD = venous duct
VS = venous sinus
VV = vitelline veins
a Early embryonic stage.
b Late embryonic stage.

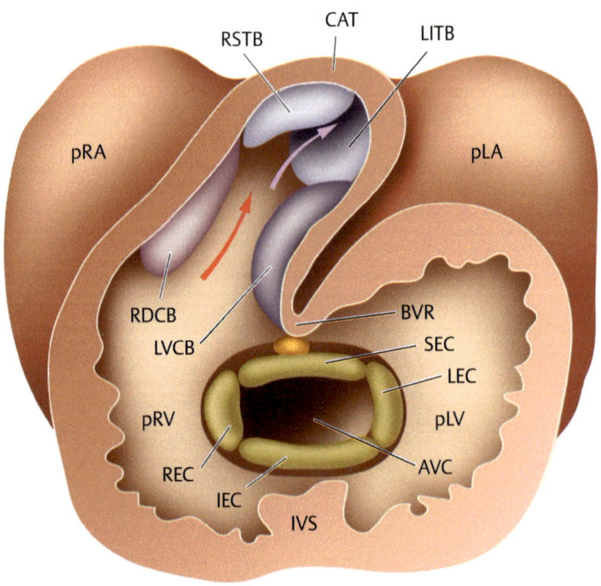

Fig. 1.9 Morphogenesis of the atrioventricular valves. Schematic depiction. Separation of the atrioventricular canal and the outflow tract via the coordinated fusion of endocardial cushions, conus bulges, and truncus bulges, taking into account the muscular ventricular septum and the bulboventricular fold. Ventricle, conus, and truncus, coronary opening, ventral view.

AVC = atrioventricular channel
BVR = bulboventricular ridge
CAT = common arterial trunk (truncus arteriosus)
IEC = inferior endocardial cushion
IVS = interventricular septum
LEC = left endocardial cushion
LITB = left inferior truncus bulge
LVCB = left ventral conus bulge
pLA = primitive left atrium
pLV = primitive left ventricle
pRA = primitive right atrium
pRV = primitive right ventricle
RDCB = right dorsal conus bulge
REC = right endocardial cushion
RSTB = right superior truncus bulge
SEC = superior endocardial cushion

muscles. In contrast, the mesenchymal material in the trabecular meshwork near and between the base transforms into fibrous cuspids or fibrous tendinous threads.

Since only two presumptive atrioventricular valves form in the human cardiac apparatus within the mitral and tricuspid ostium, the septal cusp of the tricuspid valve takes on a unique role in its solitary development. The merging of the superior and inferior endocardial cushions is important not just with regard to separating the common atrioventricular canal; rather, it also contributes significantly to the adequate closure of the interatrial crux via regional fusion with the septum primum.

Clinical Relevance

Ebstein's anomaly, characterized by the congenital right ventricular-apical displacement of individual or multiple (dysplastic) cusps of the tricuspid valve, leads to partial "atrialization" of the morphologic right ventricle. Its embryogenetic foundations are apparently caused by a disorder within the cavity in the right ventricular wall, which exposes the inner layer of the ventricular myocardium during normogenesis.

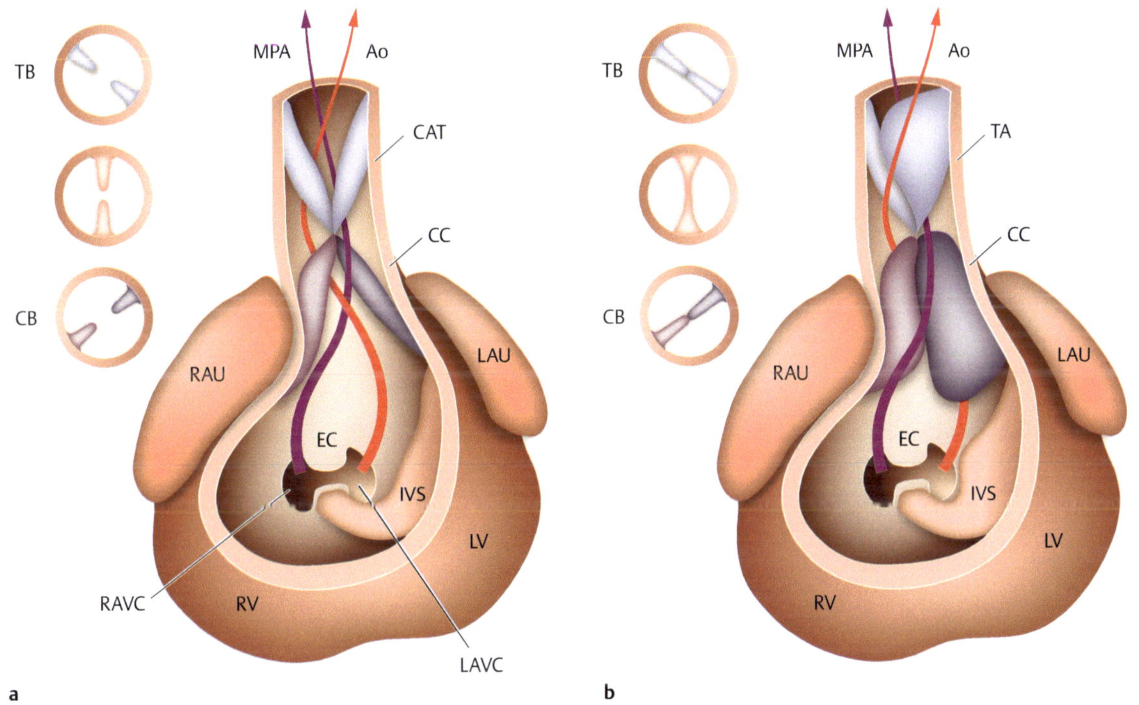

Fig. 1.10 Separation of the atrioventricular canal and outflow tract. Schematic depiction of helical morphogenesis. The coordinated merging of the conus and truncus septa, endocardial cushions, and muscular ventricular septum is the foundation of atrioventricular and ventriculoarterial concordance. Size-appropriate cross-section mapping, outflow tract open, ventral view.

Ao = aorta
CAT = common arterial trunk (truncus arteriosus)
CB = conus bulge
CC = conus cordis
EC = endocardial cushion
IVS = interventricular septum (muscular septum interventriculare)
LAU = left auricle
LAVC = left atrioventricular channel
LV = left ventricle
MPA = main pulmonary artery (truncus pulmonalis)
RAU = right auricle
RAVC = right atrioventricular channel
RV = right ventricle
TB = truncus bulge
a Early stage.
b Late stage.

Morphogenesis of the Ventricular Region

Between days 26 and 30 p.o. the ventricular and atrial regions separate via the development of atrioventricular septa and the atrioventricular sulcus within the scope of cardiac looping (▶ Fig. 1.2). As a result, the morphologic left ventricle develops disproportionately from the ventricular tube, whereas the true morphologic right ventricle is formed solely from a subordinate portion of the right-lateral circumference of the developing crus.

The primitive right ventricle septates via the complex interaction of the interventricular septum, the conus septa, and the atrioventricular septa (▶ Fig. 1.10). The pars muscularis of the true interventricular septum develops around day 30 p.o., as a medial muscular fold in the ventricular tube fundus. The anterior, left-oriented crus passes between the ventricular portion and the outflow tract of the cardiac loop to the transition area. The posterior crus, in contrast, is right-oriented and extends to the right-lateral circumference of the inferior atrioventricular septum, so that the tricuspid ostium will later theoretically be assigned to the final right ventricle. As of day 28 p.o., a cylindrical outflow tract is distinguishable, the proximal and distal segments of which are known as the "conus cordis" (conus segment) and "truncus arteriosus," respectively.

The conus septa—from which aortic and pulmonary outflow tracts later form, and which, like the conus as a whole, are incorporated into the final ventricle during the ongoing transformation of the cardiac loop—form on the respective sidewalls at the level of the conoventricular transition. Unlike the outflow tract, muscular trabeculae in the inflow area of the ventricular portion connect to the inlet septum, which extends into the cavum in a slightly different direction compared to the interventricular septum. Thus, a bulge that can be recognized as a septomarginal trabecula or moderator band on the final heart, and which characterizes the morphologic right ventricle, must form at the contact point with the interventricular septum (▶ Fig. 1.11).

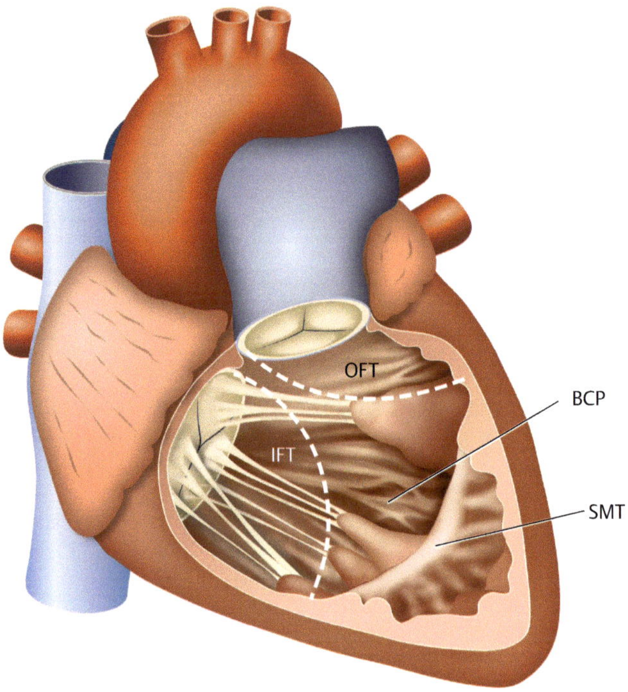

Fig. 1.11 Characterization of the morphologic right ventricle. Schematic depiction.
BCP = broad component (broad trabecular components)
IFT = inflow tract (inflow tract with tricuspid valve)
OFT = outflow tract (outflow tract with infundibulum)
SMT = septomarginal trabeculae (aka moderator band)

Clinical Relevance

- Fully arresting endocardial cushion fusion leads to a *common (persistent) atrioventricular ostium,* which enables pathological communication among all four chambers of the heart due to an extensive central septal defect.
- Merging of the endocardial cushions only in the center may lead to development of a right or left atrioventricular ostium; however, *fissure formation* may occur on the anterior cusp of the mitral valve (known as mitral cleft) or on the septal cusp of the tricuspid valve.
- *(Left) ventricular noncompaction cardiomyopathy* (spongy myocardium) is caused by an arrest of physiological myocardial compaction (see Chapter 4.6.1).

The distal truncal outflow tract septates approximately between days 28 and 35 p.o. The paired truncal septa fuse to the anterior and posterior circumference of the conotruncal transition, respectively. The aorticopulmonary septum contributes to complete subdivision of the initial common truncus arteriosus into separate arterial and pulmonary outflow tracts.

Clinical Relevance

A double outlet complex can be attributed to the lack of regression of the bulboventricular folds, followed by a lack of fusion of the conus and outlet septum. In cases of *Taussig–Bing anomaly*—the combination of DORV II with side-to-side orientation of the great arteries—the aorta develops fully from the morphologic right ventricle via a hypertrophied subaortic conus, whereby the pulmonary valve ostium overrides a malalignment VSD.

Final closure of the interventricular foramen also occurs during the septation process. As a result, the pars membranacea septi develops from the proximal portions of the conus septa. The characteristic topology of the ventricular outflow tracts and the typical left-helical rotation of the great arteries result from the fusion of primary paired septal primordia. They assume left-anterior and right-posterior configurations in the proximal conus, anterior-posterior configurations in the conotruncal transition, and, finally, left-cranial and right-caudal configurations in the distal segment of the truncus.

Clinical Relevance

- *TGA* is caused by a disorder of complex, helically occurring truncus septation.
- It is believed that cases of *anatomically corrected MGA*, in which the spatial relationship of the arteries to one another is disturbed despite retained ventriculoarterial concordance, are caused by persistent, isolated inversion of the conus for both a subaortic and subpulmonary conus.
- *Tetralogy of Fallot* is caused by asymmetrical septation of the conus cordis, whereby the ventral displacement of the conus septum leads to infundibulum stenosis and the lack of contact to the crista supraventricularis impedes closure of the interventricular septum.
- *APSD* and *perimembranous VSD* can be explained by the incomplete fusion of the outflow tract's respective septa.

Morphogenesis of the Major Vessels near the Heart

Morphogenesis of the aortic arch, the pulmonary arteries, and the ductus arteriosus are closely coordinated with one another and are coordinated based on the development and differentiation of the primitive cardiac tube. The first intraembryonic vessels are defined between days 17 and 19 p.o. in the form of paired, paramedian symmetrical dorsal aorta situated alongside the chorda dorsalis. Between days 19 and 21 p.o., they establish close contact with the caudally positioned umbilical arteries and are connected cranially to the outflow tract of the embryonic heart—the truncus arteriosus—via the first pair of pharyngeal arteries. A primary right-left symmetrical system then forms from six pharyngeal arch arteries (known as aortic arches; ▶ Fig. 1.12a) in a craniocaudal sequence from the subordinate saccus aorticus. On the dorsal truncus wall, they attach themselves to the two dorsal aorta, which initially fuse into an unpaired, left paramedian singular aorta, which later becomes the descending aorta. In addition, the intersegmental arteries that supply blood to the individual segments of the body begin to form from the dorsal aortic system. The vessels of the head and neck form from the first three arch arteries via segmental obliteration of the dorsal aorta (▶ Fig. 1.12b). The later subclavian artery is derived from the cranially positioned intersegmental artery VII.

Finally, on day 46 p.o., the distal segment of the right dorsal aorta obliterates up to the left dorsal aortic junction after the left subclavian artery develops. From now on, the left aortic arch remains as a persistent segment of the fourth left pharyngeal arch artery, and the rostral segment of the contralateral arch artery as the initial portion of the right subclavian artery, respectively.

Clinical Relevance

- *Double aortic arch* results from persistence of the right dorsal aorta; in this case, the right arch is predominant and the ductus arteriosus is localized on the left (see Chapter 4.5.3).
- Atresia of the fourth branchial arch artery causes an *IAA*; a *right descending aorta* results from persistence of the right dorsal aorta concurrent with full obliteration of the fourth left aortic arch.
- Lusoria artery is the result of obliteration of the right fourth aortic arch (subclavian segment) with persistence of the right dorsal aorta, which is obliterated in normal cases. In cases of right aortic arch, the left common carotid artery emerges as the initial branch of the aortic arch, followed by the right common carotid artery, the right subclavian artery, and a retroesophageal vessel segment. This segment, from which the left subclavian artery and the ductus arteriosus are formed, is also known as "Kommerell diverticulum" postnatally (Chapter 4.5.3).

The main pulmonary trunk is derived from the proximal half of the left sixth arch artery. The distal half—ductus arteriosus Botalli—is subject to regression postnatally. The peripheral pulmonary arteries emerge during differentiation of the pulmonary apparatus. They are first connected secondarily to the sixth pharyngeal arch; during this process, the pharyngeal plexuses which initially formed from the dorsal aorta recede.

Clinical Relevance

The intermittend aortopulmonary collaterals, which constitute the primitive, early embryonic vascular connections between the dorsal aortae and the pulmonary vessel plexus, may become of importance due to their persistence, e.g., within the scope of pulmonary atresia, as *MAPCA* (see Chapter 4.5.5).

Morphogenesis of the Semilunar Valves

Between days 35 and 38 p.o., two endocardial cushions not connected to the continual septum system form on the embryo (initially approximately 7 cm long) from the conotruncal transition, at the narrow ends of the oblique transverse section. Cushion-like valve protrusions known as intercalated valve swellings supply the material to the anterior and posterior semilunar valve of the aortic and pulmonary valves, respectively. In contrast, the right and left sinuses of the pulmonary and aortic valves, respectively, stem from the lateral sections of the truncus septum. Beginning on day 57 p.o., elastic fibers that later become collagenous—and in whose development neural crest cells are involved significantly—are visible within the extracellular matrix of the semilunar valves.

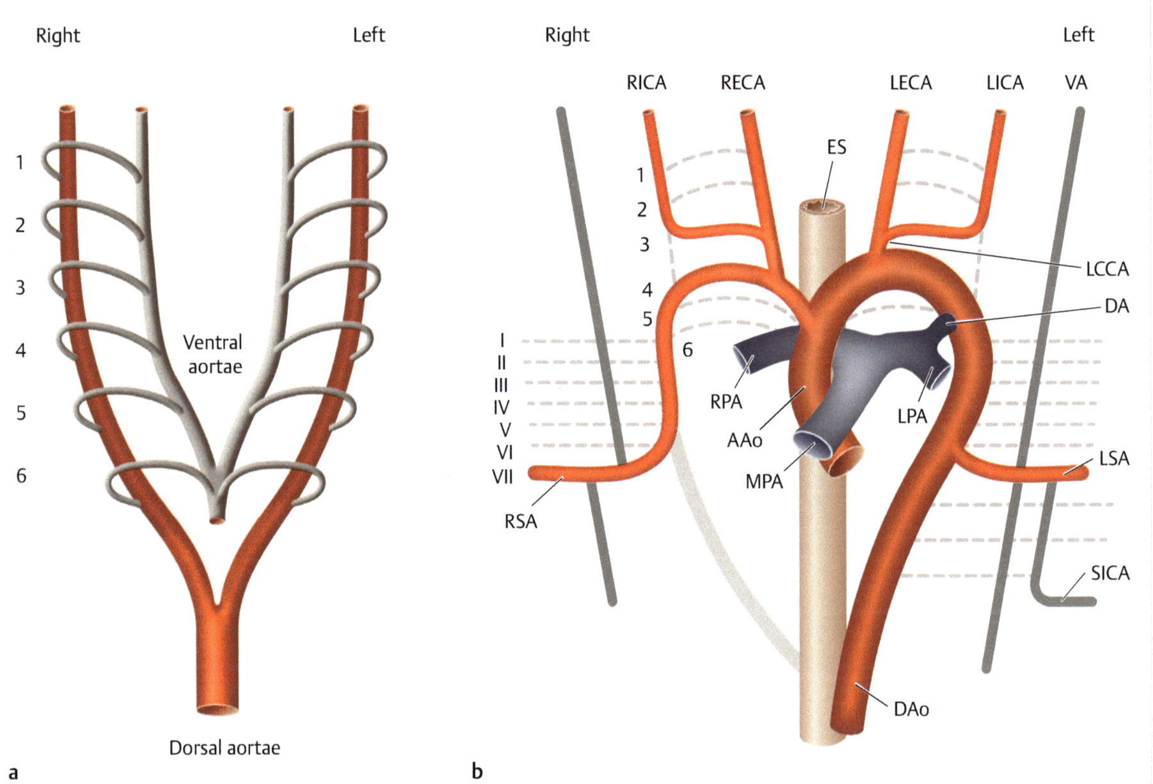

Fig. 1.12 Morphogenesis of the major vessels near the heart. Schematic depiction. Transformation of the primary symmetrical system of the pharyngeal arch arteries and formation of the final aorta, truncus pulmonalis, ductus arteriosus, and arteries near the heart. Arabic numerals 1–6 indicate the right-left symmetrical aortic arch system and derivates, while roman numerals I–VII indicate the intersegmental arteries. Regressive structures are shown in light gray.

AAo = ascending aorta
DA = ductus arteriosus
DAo = descending aorta
ES = esophagus
LECA = left external carotid artery
LICA = left internal carotid artery
LPA = left pulmonary artery
LSA = left subclavian artery
MPA = main pulmonary artery (truncus pulmonalis)
RECA = right external carotid artery
RICA = right internal carotid artery
RPA = right pulmonary artery
RSA = right subclavian artery
SICA = supreme intercostal artery
VA = vertebral artery
a Early stage.
b Final form (left-running, left-descending aortic arch).

Morphogenesis of the Coronary Vessels

The first signs of coronary vessels are visible on day 32 p.o. It is believed that, as of day 41 p.o., functionally adequate coronary circulation that replaces the previous circulatory system, which was intended only to diffuse the luminal blood pool-based supply of the myocardium, begins to develop. Development of a capillary plexus is induced within the subepicardial ventricular mesenchyme. The first thin subepicardial coronary truncal veins that drain into the venous sinus are visible as of day 35 p.o. As the sole vessel that drains blood from the heart, the coronary sinus develops from the left sinus horn after the primary merging cardinal, umbilical, and vitelline veins have been obliterated. The final outlet of the coronary sinus reaches its ultimate position to the right of the developing septum primum. Signs of coronary arteries communicating with the endothelium of the outflow tract are first visible as of day 40 p.o. The coronary ostia are only visible after the truncus has septated completely within the right and left sinuses of the aortic valves.

1.2 Classification and Nomenclature

1.2.1 Overview, Segmental Analysis, and Regulatory Algorithm

In addition to innovations in diagnostics and treatment, progress in the understanding of congenital defects is reflected, in particular, changes to nomenclature and classification. Since, from a historical standpoint, congenital defects could only be diagnosed post mortem and thus solely by pathologists, the primary significance of these defects' influence was explained via visual-morphological analysis performed on the autopsy table. Initial attempts at classification can be traced back to Lev, who attempted to establish universally applicable classifications for complex defects based on morphological analysis of the individual cardiac structures.[3] Essential amendments and modifications can be traced back to Van Praagh[4] and De la Cruz,[5] in particular. These authors performed a fundamental segmental analysis, which took into account intersegmental connections, in the mid-1970s. Additional progress was made primarily thanks to Anderson,[6] who established a universally recognized (albeit not universally implemented) nomenclature based on a strictly morphologyoriented analysis of segment-specific characteristics of complex cardiac malformations (known as segmental analysis). Certain reservations exist, not merely with respect to practicality in a clinical context, but also based on limitations in terminology and the limited "convertability" of historically established, primarily clinical entities such as *univentricular heart*.[7] The major group of septal defects (known as shunt defects) and obstructions or anomalous pulmonary venous connections are difficult to integrate into segmental analysis.

The original, oldest clinical classification of congenital defects was based on strictly hemodynamic, visible differences between cyanotic and acyanotic (non-cyanotic) defects. The increase in diagnostic options led to further differentiation between defects of the right and left heart. Certain descriptions and classifications have long since been established in everyday clinical practice for commonly concurrent defects, such as Tetralogy of Fallot, ASD, PFO, and PDA.

Formal diagnosis of malformations occurs within the scope of segmental analysis,[6] which uses a descriptive algorithm to analyze the three main cardiac segments (the atrial and ventricular segments and the outflow tract) independently of etiology and previously established complex entities. ▶ Table 1.3 provides an overview of the various malformations that may occur within the individual segments.

Since additional information aside from pathomorphological aspects is required in a clinical context and for interdisciplinary understanding, this information must take terminology and classification into account.

1.2.2 Primary Malpositions

The following differentiations can be made with regard to aberrant position of the heart and orientation of the apex cordis in the thoracic area: the usual position of the heart in the left hemithorax with left-anterior-inferior orientation of the apex *(levocardia)* contrasts with *dextrocardia* and *mesocardia*. In cases of the former, the apex has a right-anterior-inferior orientation; in cases of mesocardia, in contrast, the apex has a medial-anterior-inferior orientation and is generally located in the mid-sagittal plane.

Particular malpositions occur in cases of special clinical entities, such as ectopia cordis and congenital pericardial defects.

1.2.3 Secondary Malpositions

Secondary malpositions can result from unilateral pulmonary hypoplasia or thoracic or spinal column deformities, or from displacement of the heart in cases of intrathoracic masses, while largely maintaining normal organ axes and the spatial orientation of the heart's apex. In these cases, the usual *levoposition* contrasts with *dextroposition* or *mesoposition*.

Based on the common association between malpositions and cardiovascular malformations, it is necessary to analyze the topology, connections, and relations of cardiac segments, as occurs within the scope of the pathomorphological method,[6] with great precision for diagnostic purposes.

Site

The *visceral site* is determined by the lateralization of the unpaired parenchymatic abdominal organs (liver, spleen, stomach, and pancreas) as well as by the course and branching method of the main bronchi. Generally, the liver and its suprahepatic segments of inferior vena cava and the morphologic right atrium are located on the same side of the body (visceroatrial concordance). This same concordance is true of the morphologic left atrium and the spleen, stomach, and pancreas. A morphologic right main bronchus (eparterial bronchus) is more rigid and tends to branch; in doing so, the right superior lobar bronchus runs dorsally to the left pulmonary artery. In contrast, the course of a morphologic left bronchus (hyparterial bronchus) is more level; it is generally longer, and the left superior lobar bronchus extends cranially in front of the left pulmonary artery. In normal cases (situs solitus), these anatomical structures are assigned ultimately to their respective sides of the body. In cases of situs inversus, however, the configuration is mirrored, and the situs ambiguus (heterotaxia) is characterized by isomerism. Spleen anomalies are often encountered in cases of visceral heterotaxia; in these cases, right isomerism is often accompanied by asplenia with sagittal-symmetric liver and concordant right position of the great abdominal arteries. In contrast, left isomerism is often accompanied by polysplenia and azygos continuation in cases where the hepatic segment of the inferior vena cava does not develop.

Table 1.3 Overview of the various cardiac malformations.[8]

Malformation	Acronym	Term	Synonyms
Venous segment			
Partial anomalous pulmonary venous connection/return	PAPVR/PAPVC	Partial Anomalous Pulmonary Venous Return/Connection	Partial pulmonary vein transposition
Total anomalous pulmonary venous connection/return	TAPVC/TAPVR	Total Anomalous Pulmonary Venous Connection/Return	Total pulmonary vein transposition
Atrial segment			
Atrial septal defect	ASD	Atrial Septal Defect	
• **Ostium primum type**	ASD I	ASD primum type	Ostium primum defect
• **Ostium secundum type**	ASD II	ASD secundum type	Ostium secundum defect
Cor triatriatum sinistrum	CTS		Supravalvular mitral stenosis
Persistent foramen ovale	PFO	Persistent Foramen Ovale	Open foramen ovale
Atrioventricular septal defect			
Atrioventricular septal defect	AVSD	Atrioventricular Septal Defect	Endocardial cushion defect
• **Partial atrioventricular septal defect**	PAVSD	Partial Atrioventricular Septal Defect	Partial atrioventricular canal defect, endocardial cushion defect
• **Complete atrioventricular septal defect**	CAVSD	Complete Atrioventricular Septal Defect	Complete atrioventricular canal defect
Double inlet left/right ventricle	DILV/DIRV	Double Inlet Left/Right Ventricle	Single left/right ventricle
Mitral atresia	MA	Mitral Atresia	HLHS
Mitral stenosis	MS	Mitral Stenosis	
Mitral insufficiency	MI	Mitral Insufficiency/Incompetence	
Tricuspid atresia	TA	Tricuspid Atresia	
Ventricular segment			
Univentricular heart	CU	Cor Univentriculare	Single ventricle (cor triloculare biatriatum)
Ventricular septal defect	VSD	Ventricular Septal Defect	
Left ventricular non-compaction cardiomyopathy	LVNC	Spongy myocardium	Arrest of physiological compaction of the left ventricular myocardium
Ventriculoarterial segment			
Aortic valve atresia	AoVA	Aortic Valve Atresia	Aortic atresia - HLHS
Aortic insufficiency	AI	Aortic Insufficiency/Incompetence	Aortic valve insufficiency
Aortic stenosis	AS	Aortic stenosis (subvalvular, valvular, supravalvular)	
Double outlet left/right ventricle	DOLV/DORV	Double Outlet Left/Right Ventricle	
Pulmonary atresia	PA	Pulmonary Atresia	
Pulmonary stenosis	PS	Pulmonary Stenosis	
Subvalvular aortic stenosis	SAS	Subaortic Stenosis	Subaortic or conus stenosis of the aorta
Infundibular pulmonary stenosis	inf.PS	Infundibular Pulmonary Stenosis	Subpulmonary or infundibular stenosis
Aortic atresia	AoA	Aortic Atresia	HLHS

Table 1.3 *(Continued)* Overview of the various cardiac malformations.[8]

Malformation	Acronym	Term	Synonyms
Arterial segment			
Truncus arteriosus communis	TAC	Truncus Arteriosus Communis	
Aortopulmonary septal defect	APSD	Aortopulmonary Septal Defect	Aortopulmonary window
Congenitally corrected transposition of the great arteries	CC-TGA	Congenitally Corrected Transposition of the Great Arteries	
Complete transposition of the great arteries	TGA IVS	Transposition of the Great Arteries	
Aortic coarctation (preductal, juxtaductal, postductal)	CoA	Coarctation of the Aorta	Infantile/adult aortic coarctation
Interrupted aortic arch	IAA	Interrupted Aortic Arch	(Aortic arch atresia)
Supravalvular aortic stenosis	SVAS	Supravalvular Aortic Stenosis	(Williams–Beuren syndrome if concurrent with other arterial stenoses)
Patent ductus arteriosus	PDA	Patent Ductus Arteriosus	Open ductus arteriosus

HLHS, Hypoplastic left heart syndrome.

The *ventricular site* is defined based on the side of the body in which it is located (right-hand and left-hand rule; ▶ Fig. 1.13); the morphologic right ventricle possesses a right-handed orientation due to the D-loop configuration in cases of situs solitus with levocardia. These positioning issues result from topographical variation, particularly the positions of the great arteries to one another—which, in principle, can run along different courses independently of site and ventriculoarterial connection. In this context, eight principal positions of the aorta (similar to a clock face) are possible with respect to the centrally located pulmonary trunk.

Clinical Relevance

Physiological organ lateralization disorders are expressed as *heterotaxy syndrome* ("disorder") and as physiologically asymmetrical preformed organ structures with isomeric symmetry (*lateralization disorders*). Heterotaxy syndromes are associated almost exclusively with complex cardiac defects in cases of asplenia or polysplenia, and are further aggravated by additional morphogenetic disorders (midline defects). Not uncommonly, juxtaposition of the auricles in the sense of lateral displacement is associated with complex defects and displacement disorders of the heart.

Atrial Morphology

Unambiguous identification based on basal, segment-intrinsic criteria must occur during segmental analysis before defining the connections and relationships between the atria, ventricles, and great arteries.

The obligatory definition of the atrial segment occurs primarily based in auricular form, independently of the merging vessels. A *morphologic right atrium* is characterized by a triangular auricle with a large lumen attaching it to the remaining atrium, and is separated by a typical muscular border structure (crista terminalis; ▶ Fig. 1.14). The pectinate muscles are additional characteristics of the morphologic right auricle. In contrast, elements of the smooth-walled atrial segment, such as the limbus fossae ovalis or the remnants of embryonic venous valves (Thebesian and Eustachian valves), are considered secondary and variable.

Consistent characteristics of *morphologic left auricle* are its fingerlike or cylindrical shape, the close connection to the rest of the atrium with a lack of muscular separation, and limited development of the pectinate muscles.

Ventricular Morphology

The definition of the ventricular segment occurs primarily by means of the typical apical trabecularization pattern and the associated atrioventricular valves. A *morphologic right ventricle* possesses a rough trabecularization pattern with the subapically defined septomarginal trabecula, also known as the moderator band (▶ Fig. 1.11, ▶ Fig. 4.76, ▶ Fig. 4.77, and ▶ Fig. 4.78). Furthermore, there is a discontinuity between the tricuspid and semilunar valves via the interposed muscular conus. Superimposing the surface of the hand with an extended thumb upon the interventricular septum is helpful in determining the position of the morphologic right ventricle. In doing so, the thumb indicates the direction of the inflow tract (atrioventricular valve) and the other

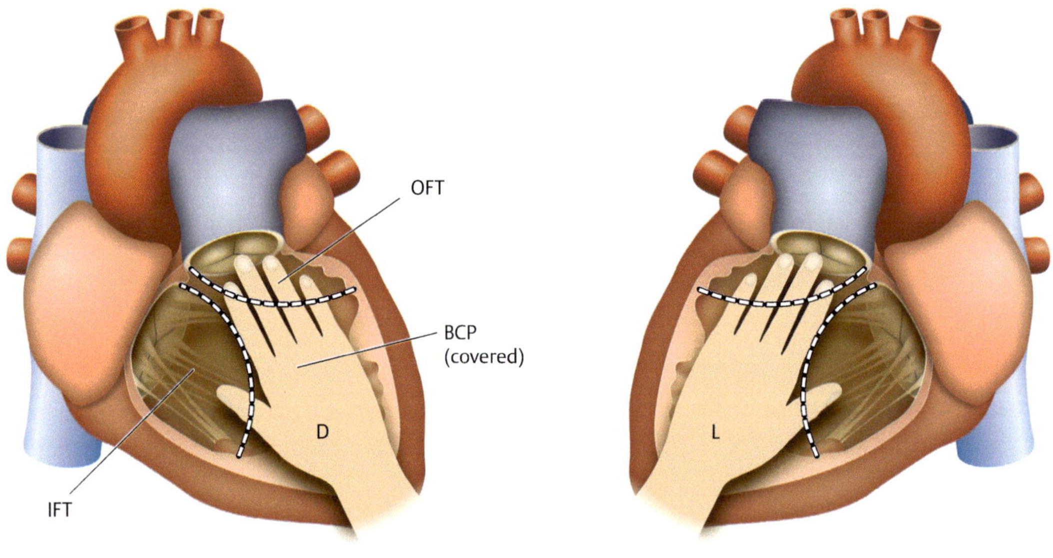

Fig. 1.13 Right-hand and left-hand rule. Schematic depiction. Definition of the topology of the morphologic right ventricle by superimposing the hand's surface on the interventricular septum. In this case, the thumb indicates the atrioventricular ostium (inflow tract), and the extended fingers indicate the outflow tract. Differences between the isomers.
BCP = broad component (broad trabecular components)
IFT = inflow tract
OFT = outflow tract
a Right-hand topology (ventricular D-loop).
b Left-hand topology (ventricular L-loop).

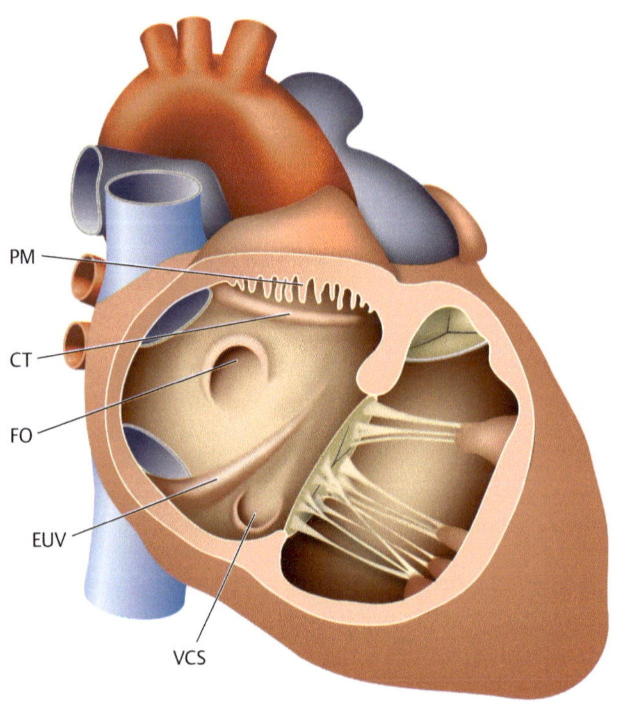

Fig. 1.14 Characterization of the morphologic right atrium. Schematic depiction. Blunt triangular auricle with pectinate muscles, broad connection to the atrial segment, delimited by the crista terminalis. Facultative fossa ovalis, coronary sinus valve, and inferior vena cava valve. Remnants of embryonic sinus valves can persist as a Chiari meshwork.
CT = crista terminalis
EUV = Eustachian valve (valve of the inferior vena cava)
FO = fossa ovalis
PM = pectinate muscles
VCS = valve of the coronary sinus (Thebesian valve)

fingers indicate the outflow tract (semilunar valve). In this manner, a right-hand architecture in cases of situs solitus (▶ Fig. 1.13a) can be differentiated from a left-hand architecture in cases of situs inversus (▶ Fig. 1.13b). In cases of full aplasia of the interventricular septum, a distinction must be made between solitary morphologic right or left ventricle and an indeterminate ventricle with extremely rough trabecularization. A *morphologic left ventricle*, in contrast, is characterized by a fine apical trabecularization pattern. Furthermore, a fibrous continuity develops between the mitral and semilunar valves.

In addition to apical morphology (trabeculated body), a ventricle can also be defined based on the presence of two additional components: the *inflow tract* (inlet) and *outflow tract* (outlet). A ventricle lacking an inlet tract is considered a "rudimentary ventricle." In these cases, the existence of an outflow tract is less decisive. A ventricular body that lacks an inflow tract but does possess an outflow tract is considered an "outlet ventricle" (outlet chamber). If only a trabeculated body is present, the term "trabecular valve" is used. In contrast, a ventricle with more than 50% of the opening surface of the semilunar valve is considered an outlet ventricle (outlet chamber).

Morphology of the Great Arteries

The great arteries are identified primarily based on the vascular branches and branching pattern. The *aorta*, characterized by its archlike course and the origin of the carotid arteries, supplies blood for coronary and systemic circulation. In contrast, branching into pulmonary arteries and supplying blood for pulmonary circulation are crucial for the *pulmonary trunk*.

Morphology of the Atrioventricular Connection

During sequential segmental analysis (segmental approach), the atrioventricular and ventriculoarterial connections are defined and placement positions (relations) are analyzed in accordance with unambiguous segment assignment (segmental approach).

The atrioventricular connection depends primarily upon the location and manner of connection (type), and only secondarily upon the morphology of the atrioventricular valve (mode). In cases of *atrioventricular concordance*, a morphologic right atrium is attached to a morphologic right ventricle, or a morphologic left atrium to a morphologic left ventricle, respectively. In cases of *atrioventricular discordance*, however, a morphologic right atrium is attached to a morphologic left ventricle, or vice versa.

Clinical Relevance

Special atrioventricular forms exist in cases of *atrial isomerism* or the lack of an atrioventricular connection in cases of an overriding contralateral connection:

- In cases of biatrial univentricular atrioventricular connections, a distinction is made between a *DIRV*, a *DILV*, and a *double inlet single ventricle*.
- In terms of the mode of atrioventricular connection, the morphology of the atrioventricular valve is decisive —pathological forms are differentiated into the following categories: stenotic, overriding (or straddling), non-perforated (atretic), or non-developed (aplastic).
- The existence of a single atrioventricular valve overriding a VSD in cases of *common atrioventricular ostium* constitutes another variant.
- *Criss-cross atrioventricular connections*[9] in cases of potential superior-inferior ventricular connections are an extremely rare form of atrioventricular connection. The criss-cross arrangement of atrioventricular inflow tracts deviating from the otherwise normal, parallel arrangement characterizes this disorder (▶ Fig. 1.15). A rotational anomaly of the ventricle causes a significantly foreshortened inlet zone of the morphologic right ventricle accompanied by a well-developed infundibulum. Concordant and discordant atrioventricular connections and additional superior-inferior ventricular relations with horizontally arranged interventricular septa are possible. In these cases, an additional VSD often occurs via a septal defect concurrent with criss-crossing of the tendinous cords (known as straddling).

Morphology of Ventriculoarterial Connection

Ventriculoarterial connection concurrent with the existence of two ventricles and outflow tracts each are analyzed similarly to atrioventricular connections: if an exclusive connection exists between the morphologic right ventricle and the pulmonary artery, or between the morphologic left ventricle and the aorta, *ventriculoarterial concordance* is the result. Conversely, if the morphologic right ventricle connects to the aorta and the morphologic left ventricle connects to the pulmonary artery, *ventriculoarterial discordance* is the result.

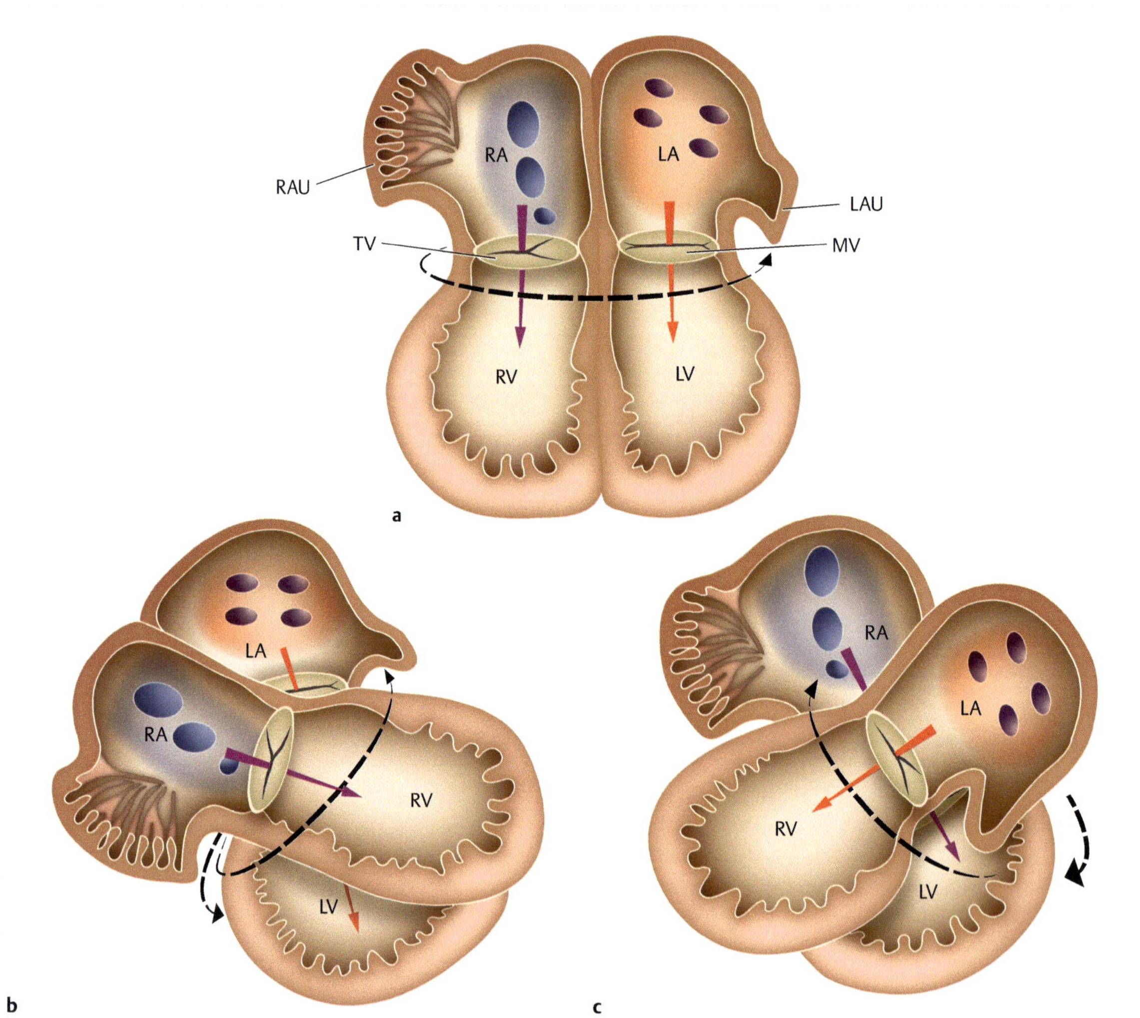

Fig. 1.15 Formal genesis of criss-cross heart (also known as twisted chambers). Schematic depiction. Ventral view. The arrows indicate the direction of blood flow.

LA = left atrium
LAU = left auricle
LV = left ventricle
MV = mitral valve
RA = right atrium
RAU = right auricle
RV = right ventricle
TV = tricuspid valve
a Counterclockwise torque in a case of atrioventricular concordance.
b Counterclockwise torque in a case of atrioventricular concordance.
c Clockwise torque in a case of atrioventricular discordance.

Clinical Relevance

Special forms occur in cases of single ventricle, truncus arteriosus, and atresia of an outflow tract (▶ Fig. 1.16):

- In cases of univentricular atrioventricular connections, a distinction is drawn between a *DORV*, *DOLV*, and a *double outlet single ventricle*. Concordance or discordance of a single ventricle in cases of atresia of an outflow tract or truncus arteriosus constitute additional possible connections.
- Special forms of ventriculoarterial connection with aberrant origin of a pulmonary artery are sometimes known as a "*hemitruncus*." In these cases, a pulmonary artery stems from the aorta. This primarily affects the right pulmonary artery, which originates in the ascending aorta, often immediately superior to the aortic valve. In contrast, the contralateral pulmonary artery, as a direct continuation of a pulmonary trunk correctly originating from the right ventricle, passes through a normal pulmonary valve.
- In cases of *double outlet ventricle*, both great arteries —each with more than 50% of the ostial cross-sectional area—originate in the same ventricle, so that the second ventricle is only connected to the great arteries via a VSD. If a bilateral conus exists, both great arteries are connected exclusively or primarily to the morphologic right ventricle (DORV). In contrast, if no subaortic and subpulmonary conus or rudimentary stenosing subpulmonary conus is present, the great arteries are displaced dorsally with respect to the base of the heart, meaning that they originate primarily from the morphologic left ventricle (DOLV).
- In cases of *single outlet ventricle*, only one of the great arteries is connected to the ventricular mass (two divided or one singular ventricle); in addition, either there is no direct connection to the second vessel, or this connection is only secondary, via a VSD. In these cases, the solitary artery can be the aorta, pulmonary artery (in cases of atresia of the respective pendant), or a common arterial trunk.

Note

Within the scope of interdisciplinary communication, a strict distinction between the terms "ventriculoarterial discordance" and "TGA" is important in order to avoid misinterpretations due to changing foci with respect to changes in position *(relation)* and anomalies in origination points *(connection)* of the great arteries.

Relation of Ventriculoarterial Connection and Great Vessels

A distinction is made between *D-loop* (dextrobulboventricular orientation of the bulboventricular loop) or *L-loop* (levobulboventricular) with regard to the spatial relation of the ventricles. In normal cases, the morphologic right ventricle has a right-anterior position with respect to the morphologic left ventricle (D-loop). The relation of the great arteries to one another is defined by their position with respect to the base of the heart. In cases of normogenesis and situs solitus, the pulmonary ostium has a left-anterior position and the aortic ostium has a right-posterior position, with a concurrent, helical course. Therefore, the pulmonary artery is positioned to the left, and the aorta, to the right (▶ Fig. 1.16).

Clinical Relevance

D-MGA is defined as the right-anterior position of the aortic ostium (▶ Fig. 1.16c) and the left-posterior position of the pulmonary ostium. Consequently, *L-MGA* is the left-anterior position with respect to the pulmonary arterial ostium (▶ Fig. 1.16f); in these cases, the aorta is also positioned dextrally with respect to the pulmonary artery (see also Chapter 4.4.1).

In contrast to the original understanding of transposition as a relative positioning or location anomaly of the great arteries, a more stringent nomenclature of TGA—in the sense of swapping the position of the great arteries with respect to the ventricular septum and thus with respect to the ventricular origin—has been established based on the work of Van Praagh et al.[4] Within this duct, *D-TGA* corresponds to the term "ventriculoarterial discordance." In contrast, *L-TGA* is characterized by atrioventricular and ventriculoarterial discordance (isolated ventricular inversion). This means that if concordant atrioarterial connections remain, the malformation complex can be interpreted as congenitally or functionally "corrected," since the disastrous parallel positioning of the systemic arterial and pulmonary venous circulatory systems, does not occur, as in cases of *D-TGA*. However, according to the "International Society for Nomenclature of Paediatric and Congenital Heart Disease," the common, colloquial designations for the types of transposition of the great arteries (*D-TGA* and *L-TGA*) do not adequately describe these heart defects in unambiguous terms. These defects must therefore be more accurately termed *complete transposition of the great arteries with intact ventricular septum* (TGA IVS) or *congenitally corrected transposition of the great arteries* (ccTGA), which henceforth will be utilized consistently throughout the following chapters of this book.

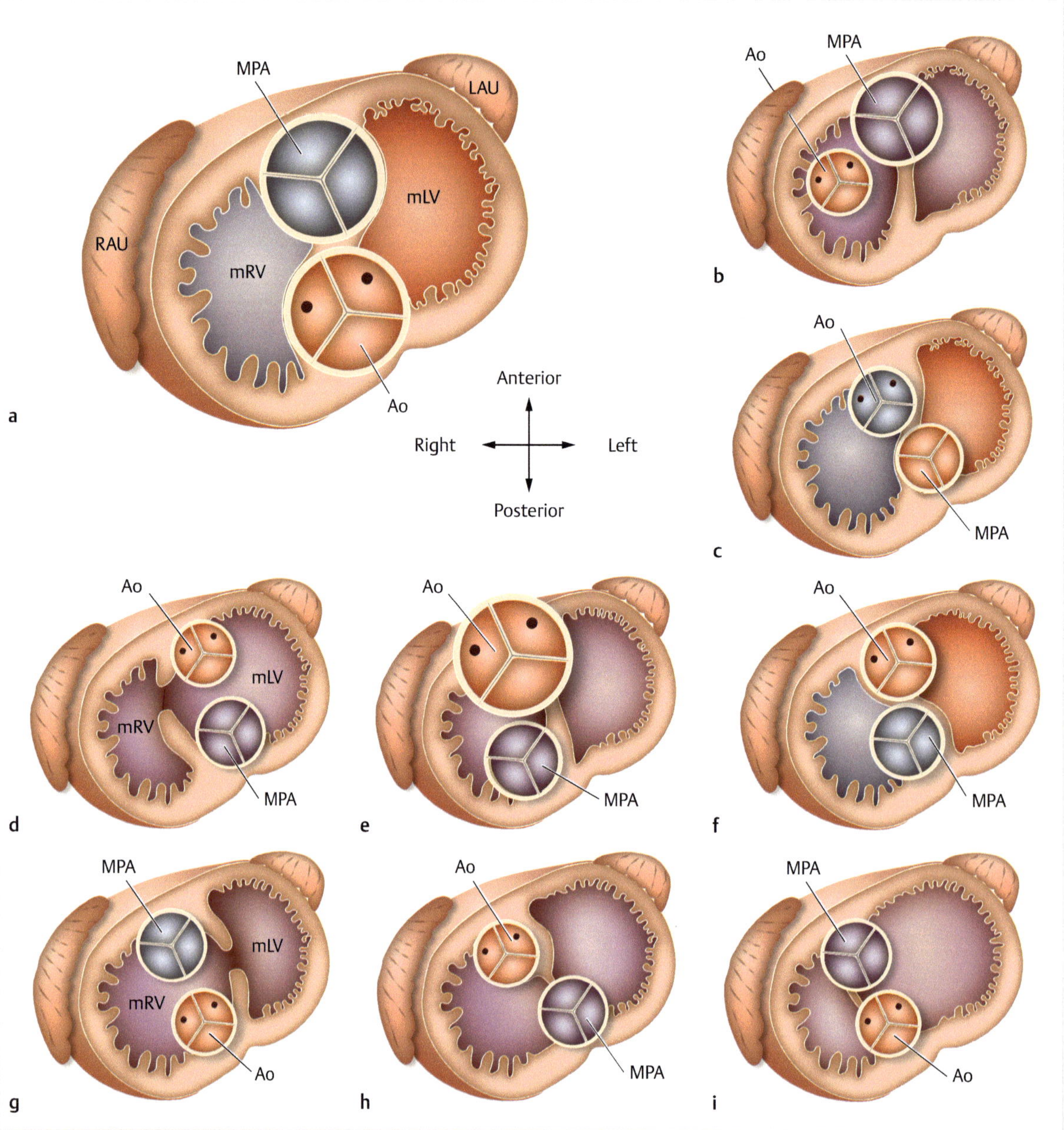

Fig. 1.16 "Transpositions" with and without septal defects in cases of situs solitus. Schematic depiction. Open ventricle, caudal view.
Ao = aorta
LAU = left auricle
mLV = morphologic left ventricle
MPA = main pulmonary artery (truncus pulmonalis)
mRV = morphologic right ventricle
RAU = right auricle
a Normal heart
b Taussig–Bing heart
c Dextro TGA
d DOLV
e Overriding aorta
f L-MGA of the great arteries
g DORV
h Overriding pulmonary trunk
i Overriding aorta and pulmonary trunk

References

[1] O'Rahilly R. Developmental stages in human embryos. Carnegie Inst Washington Pub. 1973; 631:1–167

[2] Chuaqui B, Farru O. Die Missbildungen des Herzens und der grossen Gefässe. In: Doerr W, Seifert G, Uehlinger E, ed. Pathologische Anatomie des Herzens und seiner Hüllen. Spezielle pathologische Anatomie; 22.1. Berlin: Springer; 1993; 237–461

[3] Lev M. Pathologic diagnosis of positional variations in cardiac chambers in congenital heart disease. Lab Invest. 1954; 3(1):71–82

[4] Van Praagh R. Terminology of congenital heart disease. Glossary and commentary. Circulation. 1977; 56(2):139–143

[5] De la Cruz MV, Berrazueta JR, Arteaga M, et al. Rules for diagnosis of arterioventricular discordances and septal identification of ventricles. Br Heart J. 1976; 38:341–354

[6] Anderson RH, Becker AE, Freedom RM, et al. Sequential segmental analysis of congenital heart disease. Pediatr Cardiol. 1984; 5(4):281–287

[7] Macartney FJ, Partridge JB, Scott O, Deverall PB. Common or single ventricle. An angiocardiographic and hemodynamic study of 42 patients. Circulation. 1976; 53(3):543–554

[8] Schumacher G, Hess J, Bühlmeyer K, Eds. Klinische Kinderkardiologie. Berlin: Springer; 2001: 105–106

[9] Anderson RH, Shinebourne EA, Gerlis LM. Criss-cross atrioventricular relationships producing paradoxical atrioventricular concordance or discordance. Their significance to nomenclature of congenital heart disease. Circulation. 1974; 50(1):176–180

Suggested Reading

DeHaan RL. Development of pacemaker tissue in the embryonic heart. Ann N Y Acad Sci. 1965; 127(1):7–18

2 Surgical Treatment for Congenital Heart Defects

2.1 Fundamentals of Surgical Treatment

Martin Kostelka, Farhad Bakhtiary, Friedrich Wilhelm Mohr

2.1.1 Evolution of Congenital Heart Surgery

The first successful surgical interventions for treating congenital heart defects were the correction of a PDA by Dr. Robert E. Gross at Children's Hospital of Boston in 1938[1] and correction of an aortic coarctation in 1945.[2] The decisive breakthrough in congenital cardiac surgery was first achieved with the development of the heart–lung machine, which made it possible to perform open-heart surgery. Generally speaking, these surgeries were first performed after infancy. Anesthesia, intensive care, and surgical instruments for newborns were still in early stages of development, and before echocardiography was introduced, diagnosing congenital heart defects was dependent upon invasive techniques and their corresponding rates of complication. For this reason, gradual therapies with non-corrective palliative interventions were generally used instead of the early correction that is common nowadays. For simplicity's sake, the pathophysiology of congenital heart defects can be reduced to the following main issues:

- *Volume overload:* Right-side load in cases of septal defects (ASD, VSD) is one example of volume overload.
- *Pressure overload:* This affects one or both ventricles and develops secondarily due to a stenosis in the outflow tract of the right or left ventricle.
- *Cyanosis:* Cyanosis can develop secondarily as a result of reduced pulmonary artery flow or in cases of ineffective mixing between parallel operating circulatory systems, as in cases of TGA.

2.1.2 Cardiac Surgery for Congenital Heart Defects within the Scope of Gradual Therapy or Palliative Treatment

The following depiction of a surgical procedure serves as an example of the treatment process.

> **Note**
>
> The goal of *gradual therapy* for congenital heart defects is to minimize the aforementioned pathophysiological issues. No complete correction of the congenital heart-defect occurs at a young age. This allows patients to grow and their size and weight to increase, thereby establishing the opportunity to operate upon these patients at an age where the risk of final surgical treatment is significantly lower.

Aortopulmonary Shunts

A systemic aortopulmonary shunt reduces cyanosis by increasing pulmonary arterial blood flow. Selecting an appropriate shunt size is a critical point during this usually technically simple procedure. A shunt that is too small can cause residual cyanosis, and a shunt that is too large can cause volume load or even the development of congestive heart failure. Shunt types include:

- *Blalock-Taussig shunt* (▶ Fig. 2.1): The Blalock–Taussig shunt was introduced by surgeon Alfred Blalock and cardiologist Helen Taussig at John Hopkins Hospital in Baltimore in 1947.[3] In this surgery, the subclavian artery is anastomosed directly to the pulmonary artery in order to increase pulmonary blood flow. This method also allows the shunt to grow along with the child, but is very technically demanding (especially for small children), and is associated with the risk of early thrombosis. This was also one reason why other shunts that are technically easier to insert became more common.
- *Waterston shunt* (▶ Fig. 2.2): The Waterston shunt is an artificial connection between the ascending aorta and the right pulmonary artery. It is inserted into both vessels via partial unclamping within the scope of a right thoracotomy. The shunt's size is crucial. Pulmonary volume overload occurs frequently. As the child grows, torsion or narrowing, primarily of the right pulmonaryartery, can also occur. Imaging can be helpful not merely for visualizing morphology, but also for determining shunt volume noninvasively.
- *Pott shunt* (▶ Fig. 2.3): The Pott shunt is an artificial connection between the descending aorta and the left pulmonary artery. It is inserted into both vessels via partial unclamping within the scope of a left thoracotomy. The Pott shunt has the same drawbacks as the Waterston shunt. In addition, it is often extremely difficult to remove it at a later date during final corrective procedures.

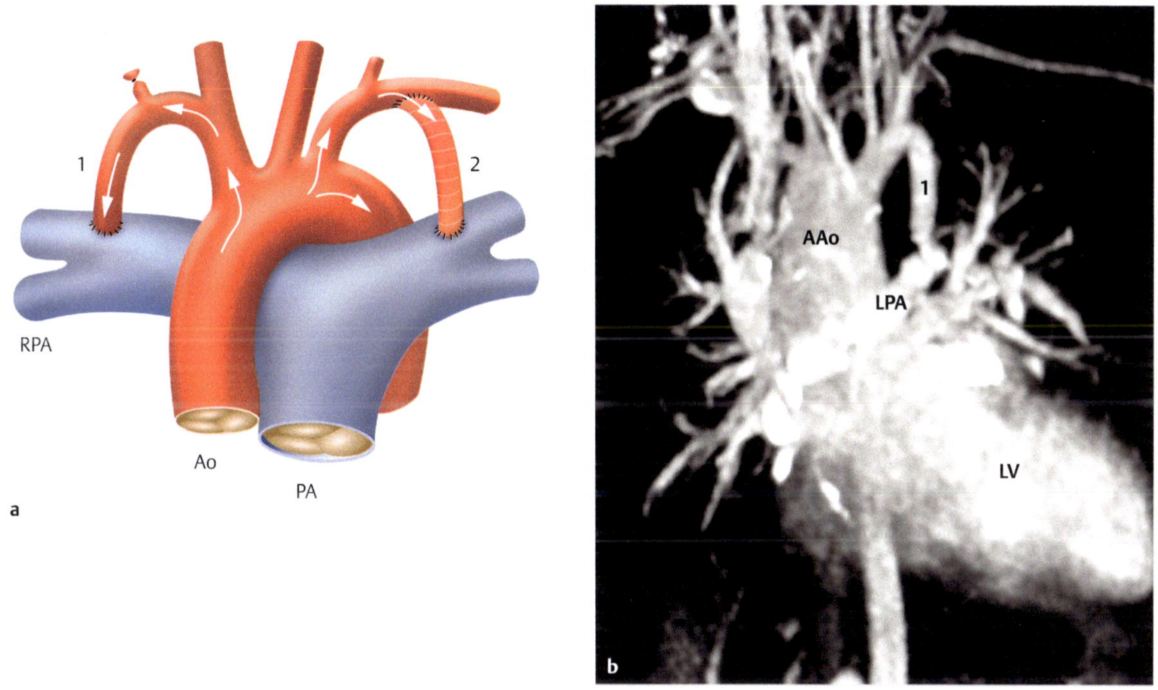

Fig. 2.1 Blalock–Taussig shunt.
AAo = ascending aorta
LPA = left pulmonary artery
LV = left ventricle
PA = pulmonary artery
RPA = right pulmonary artery

a Schematic depiction of a Blalock–Taussig shunt, a connection between the subclavian artery and pulmonary artery branches, right (1) using the native subclavian artery, left (2) via a GORE-TEX prosthesis.
b MIP reconstruction of an MRA with contrast after placing a Blalock–Taussig shunt (1) in the left pulmonary artery (LPA).

Pulmonary Artery Banding

VSD is, by far, the most common congenital heart defect. This defect leads to volume overload in both ventricles. If the defect is large and pulmonary resistance is also low, the patient will develop symptoms of congestive heart failure. Increased flow and pressure in the pulmonary arteries can lead to irreversible damage to pulmonary microcirculation, namely the development of pulmonary vascular disease. Muller and Darmann[4] first described pulmonary artery banding to reduce flow and pressure (▶ Fig. 2.4) in the 1950s. Similar to pulmonary artery shunts, pulmonary artery bands do not grow as the patient does. After a pulmonary artery band is placed, children can become cyanotic again as they grow. If scarring occurs, this can lead to distortion of both pulmonary arterial outflow tracts and pulmonary valves.

Atrial Septostomy

Cyanosis generally occurs due to reduced pulmonary blood flow. It can, however, also occur in cases of TGA. If neither PDA nor a septal defect is present, the newborn will die as a result of cyanosis. Blalock and Hanlon described a refined method in 1950: they surgically removed a large portion of the atrial septum in order to create an iatrogenic ASD in newborns with TGA. After the introduction of the Rashkind balloon septostomy, also known as the Rashkind maneuver (▶ Fig. 2.5) in 1966,[5] the Blalock and Hanlon surgical method is seldom used.

Surgical Treatment of Functional Univentricular Heart

A general goal in pediatric cardiac surgery is to correct the congenital heart defect as soon as possible. Biventricular correction, however, is often not possible. If only one functional ventricle is capable of independently sustaining one of the two circulatory systems—either systemic or pulmonary—independently, this is known as "univentricular heart." The most common forms of a functional univentricular heart occur due to the following defects:

- Tricuspid atresia
- DIV
- HLHS
- Pulmonary atresia with intact septum
- Heart with a univentricular atrioventricular connection
- Straddling atrioventricular valves
- Unbalanced hearts (AVSD)

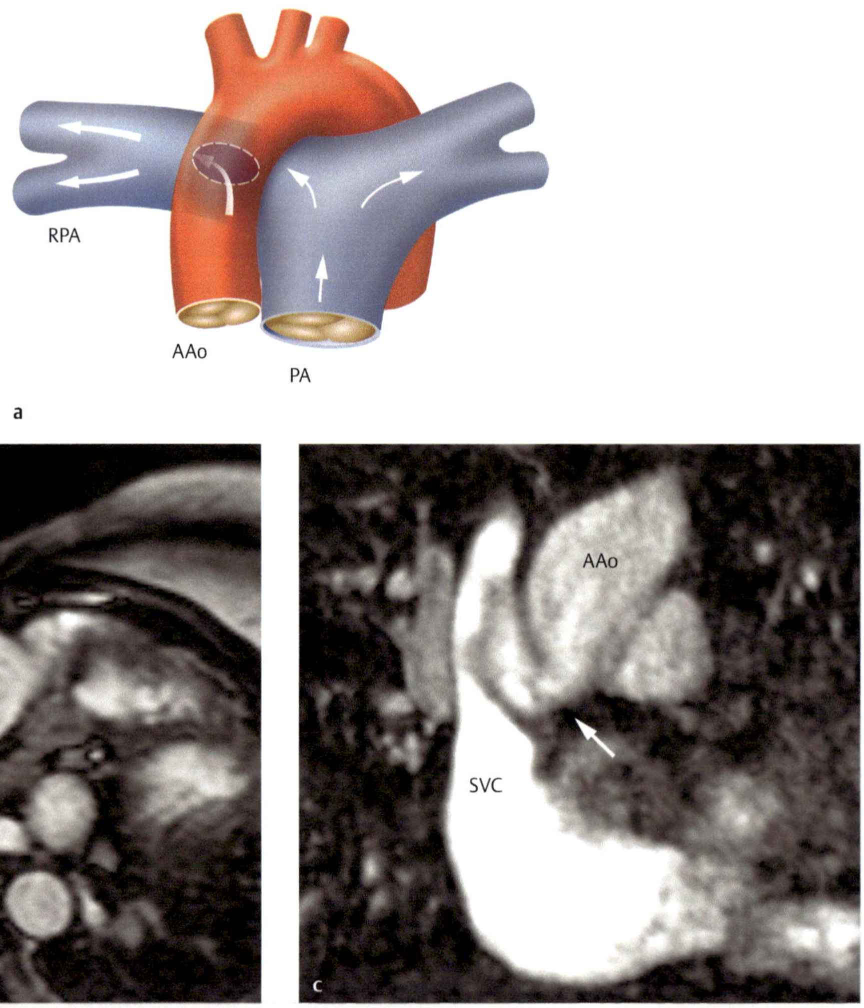

Fig. 2.2 Waterston shunt.
AAo = ascending aorta
PA = pulmonary artery
RPA = right pulmonary artery
SVC = superior vena cava

a Schematic depiction of a Waterston shunt between the dorsal wall of the ascending aorta and the right pulmonary artery.

b Transverse cine MRI of a patient with a Waterston shunt. Note the connection between the dorsal wall of the ascending aorta and the right pulmonary artery. There are visible differences in signal intensity between the ascending aorta and the right pulmonary artery (arrow) caused by stronger flow in the ascending aorta and by the shunt. The increased signal indicates stronger flow.

c Raw data for an MRA with contrast in coronal orientation also depicts the Waterston anastomosis (arrow).

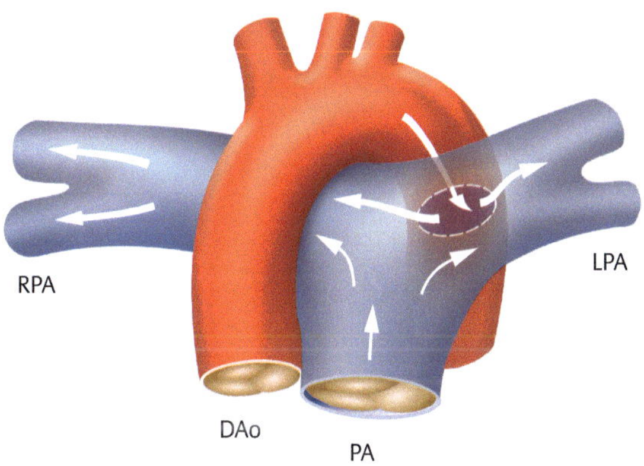

Fig. 2.3 **Pott shunt.** Schematic depiction of a Pott shunt between the descending aorta and the left pulmonary artery.
DAo = descending aorta
LPA = left pulmonary artery
PA = pulmonary artery
RPA = right pulmonary artery

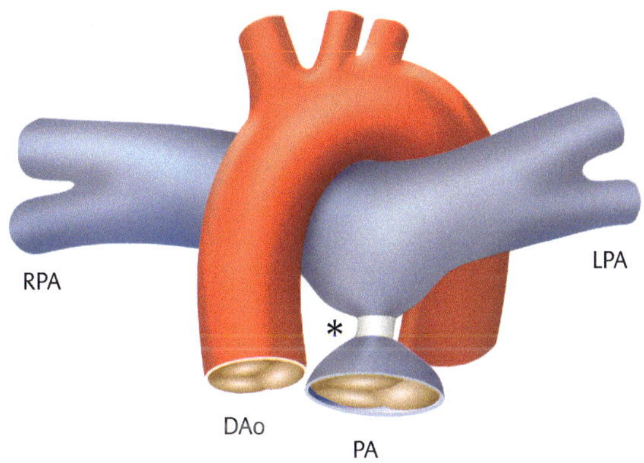

Fig. 2.4 **Pulmonary artery banding.** Schematic depiction. Pulmonary artery banding (asterisk) serves to reduce pulmonary volume load, e.g., in the case of a large VSD.
Ao = aorta
LPA = left pulmonary artery
PA = pulmonary artery
RPA = right pulmonary artery

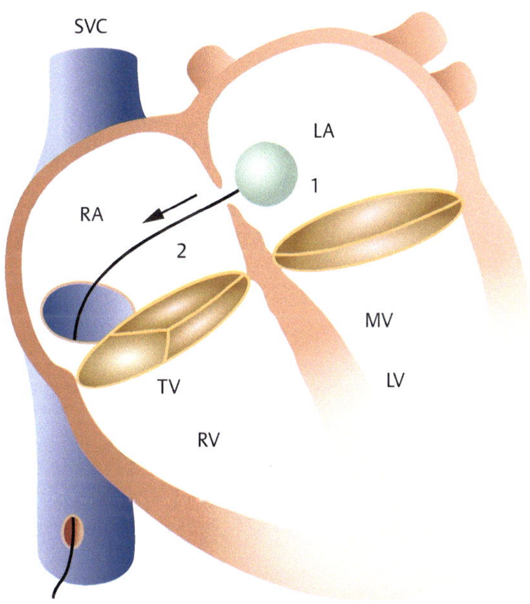

Fig. 2.5 **The Rashkind maneuver.** Schematic depiction. In this maneuver, a balloon catheter (1) that is introduced through the foramen ovale, opened, and then retracted (2) is used to establish a shunt connection between the right and left atrium for acute treatment of complete TGA.
LA = left atrium
MV = mitral valve
RA = right atrium
SVC = superior vena cava
TV = tricuspid valve
LV = left ventricle
RV = right ventricle

The umbrella term "hypoplastic left heart syndrome" encompasses a broad spectrum of heart defects with varying degrees of expression of the underdevelopment of the left ventricular structures:

- Aortic valve atresia
- Aortic stenosis
- Mitral stenosis
- Mitral valve atresia
- Hypoplasia of the left ventricle
- Lack of left ventricle
- Pronounced hypoplasia of the ascending aorta (a diameter smaller than 3 mm in 55% of cases)
- Aortic coarctation (in 80% of cases)

The most commonly associated defects are IAA, TAPVR, or an abnormal atrioventricular valve.

In cases of univentricular heart, the main treatment goals are to separate systemic and pulmonary circulation, ensure normal volume load for the functional singular ventricle, and reach normal arterial saturation. Surgical management generally occurs in three steps:

1. Up to the age of 7 days, only a palliative surgery is performed, regardless of functional status. In cases of pulmonary overflow, pulmonary artery banding is performed (▸ Fig. 2.4), while a Blalock–Taussig shunt is placed in cases of deficient pulmonary perfusion (▸ Fig. 2.1). HLHS presents as a very specific anatomical and functional entity that can generally be treated neonatally using the complex Norwood I operation (▸ Fig. 2.6). During this surgery, a neoaorta and an aortopulmonary shunt are placed, and an atrial septostomy is performed.

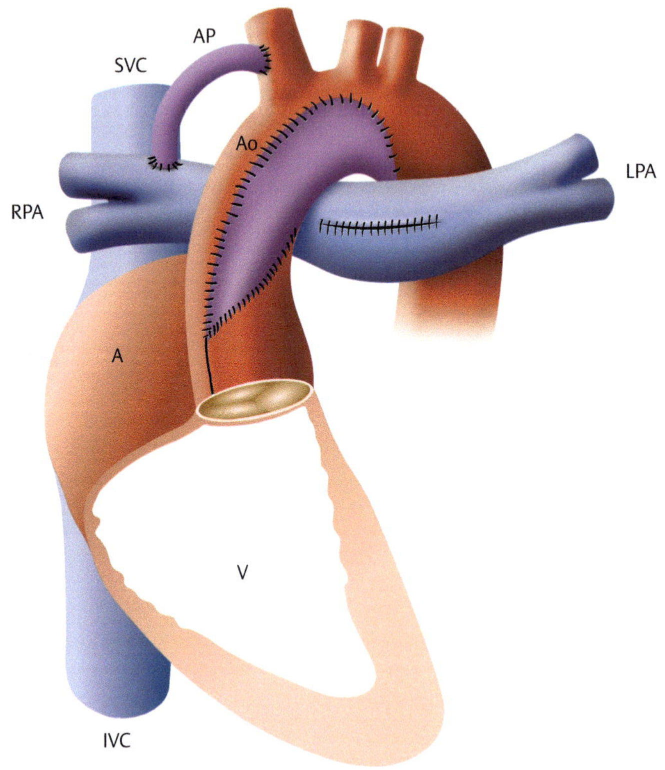

Fig. 2.6 Norwood I operation. Schematic depiction of the Norwood I operation for treating HLHS by forming a neoaorta and aortopulmonary shunt and performing an atrial septostomy.
A = atrium
Ao = aorta
AP = aortopulmonary shunt
IVC = inferior vena cava
LPA = left pulmonary artery
RPA = right pulmonary artery
SVC = superior vena cava
V = ventricle

2. The second step, generally occurring at the age of 4–6 months, is the Glenn procedure, meaning placement of a bidirectional cavopulmonary connection (▶ Fig. 2.7).
3. The last step, generally occurring at the age of 3–4 years (at a body weight of 12 kg), is placement of a TCPC. This step completes Fontan circulation. The TCPC can be placed intracardially, with a GORE-TEX tunnel, through the right atrium. Alternatively, it can be placed extracardially, which has become the preferred surgical technique for avoiding intraatrial manipulation. The extracardiac tunnel is placed outside of the right atrium, between the inferior vena cava and the right pulmonary artery, and connected to the superior vena cava (▶ Fig. 2.8).

2.1.3 Early Correction vs. Gradual Treatment

Drawbacks of Gradual Therapy for Congenital Heart Defects

All aforementioned palliative interventions render a thoracotomy necessary. The latter can lead to scarring in the mediastinum and vessels, distortion, or even dissection. Furthermore, gradual therapy always means a minimum of two interventions, and thus an additional burden.

Benefits of Early Correction of Congenital Heart Defects

Early correction of congenital heart defects has only become possible with the introduction of open-heart surgery. Temporary interruption of circulation, supported by hypothermia, allows early correction of less complex congenital heart defects. The first complex cardiac surgical interventions—TOF or AVSD—were performed either via cross-circulation (in which one parent was utilized as oxygenator[6]) or cardiopulmonary bypass. In the 1950s and 1960s, however, the two-step treatment with initial palliative and subsequent corrective intervention remained standard for older patients.

Brian Barrat-Boyes and his successor Castañeda completed numerous procedures at Children's Hospital of Boston using a heart–lung machine in 1972. The introduction of Prostaglandin E1 in the late 1970s made it possible to hold the ductus arteriosus or ductus Botalli open in newborns purely via medication, and thus achieve preoperative stabilization for the early correction of certain congenital heart defects. Optimizing invasive and noninvasive diagnostics also improved the conditions for early surgical correction.

The differences between the right and left ventricle do not develop until shortly after birth. Compared to the left ventricle, the right ventricle is significantly thinner. The left

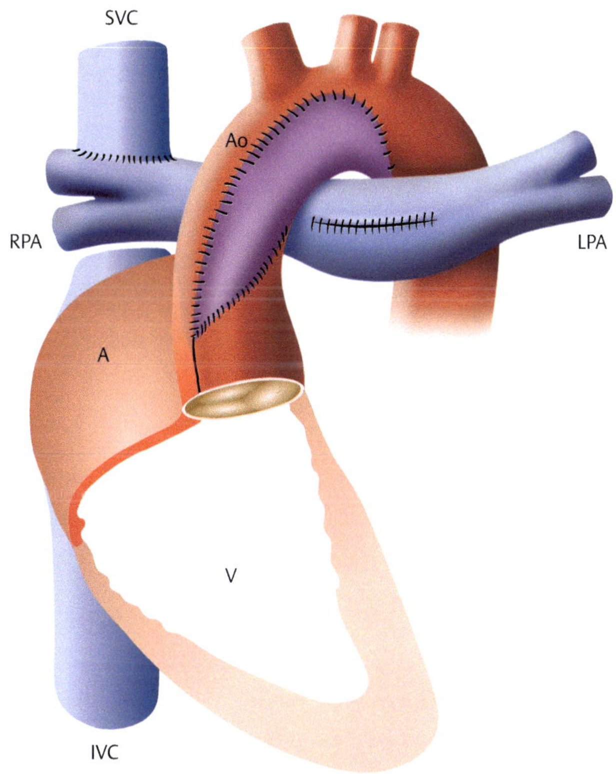

Fig. 2.7 Norwood II or Glenn operation. Schematic depiction of the Norwood II operation with placement of a bidirectional cavopulmonary anastomosis instead of an aortopulmonary shunt (▸ Fig. 2.6).
A = atrium
Ao = aorta
IVC = inferior vena cava
LPA = left pulmonary artery
RPA = right pulmonary artery
SVC = superior vena cava
V = ventricle

ventricle rapidly increases in thickness and mass. This is achieved by hyperplasia and hypertrophy of the left ventricular myocytes. The myocytes' ability to divide is believed to persist only until the third month of life. Developing new myocytes within a growing individual requires the concurrent formation of new coronary arteries by means of angiogenesis. Muscular hypertrophy, e.g., sustained high blood pressure, reduces the ability to form collateral arteries. Cardiac development can be disrupted by the palliative intervention, itself. The best-known examples are a large VSD accompanied by tetralogy of Fallot, which must then be treated using a shunt, and complete atrioventricular canal that must then be treated via pulmonary artery banding. In these cases, the right ventricle is exposed to pressure overload—with the corresponding hypertrophy—and thus assumes a round form rather than a semicircular one.

Note M!

This altered geometry has considerable consequences for the tricuspid valve, whose tendinous cords (unlike those of the mitral valve) insert primarily into the ventricular septum. These cases often result in tricuspid valve insufficiency, meaning that volume overload of the right ventricle occurs in addition to pressure overload.

Early correction, on the other hand, allows the pulmonary vessels to develop normally during the first year of life. Pulmonary resistance is reduced with the involution of the smooth musculature in the arterioles. If pulmonary arterial pressure and flow are not reduced within the first 1–2 years of life, this can begin to contribute to the development of pulmonary hypertonia. Generally speaking, a child is considered inoperable if pulmonary vessel resistance has exceeded three-fourths of systemic resistance and remains fixed. From that point onward, the child becomes increasingly cyanotic due to reduced pulmonary blood flow. The initial left–right shunt can convert to a right–left shunt. This phenomenon is known as the Eisenmenger reaction or Eisenmenger syndrome. Palliative interventions are meant to prevent this conversion. Pulmonary bands are placed to maintain pressure well below that of half of systemic pressure.

2.1.4 Cardiac Surgical Treatment for Common Congenital Heart Defects

Certain surgical procedures are described below as examples of treatment processes.

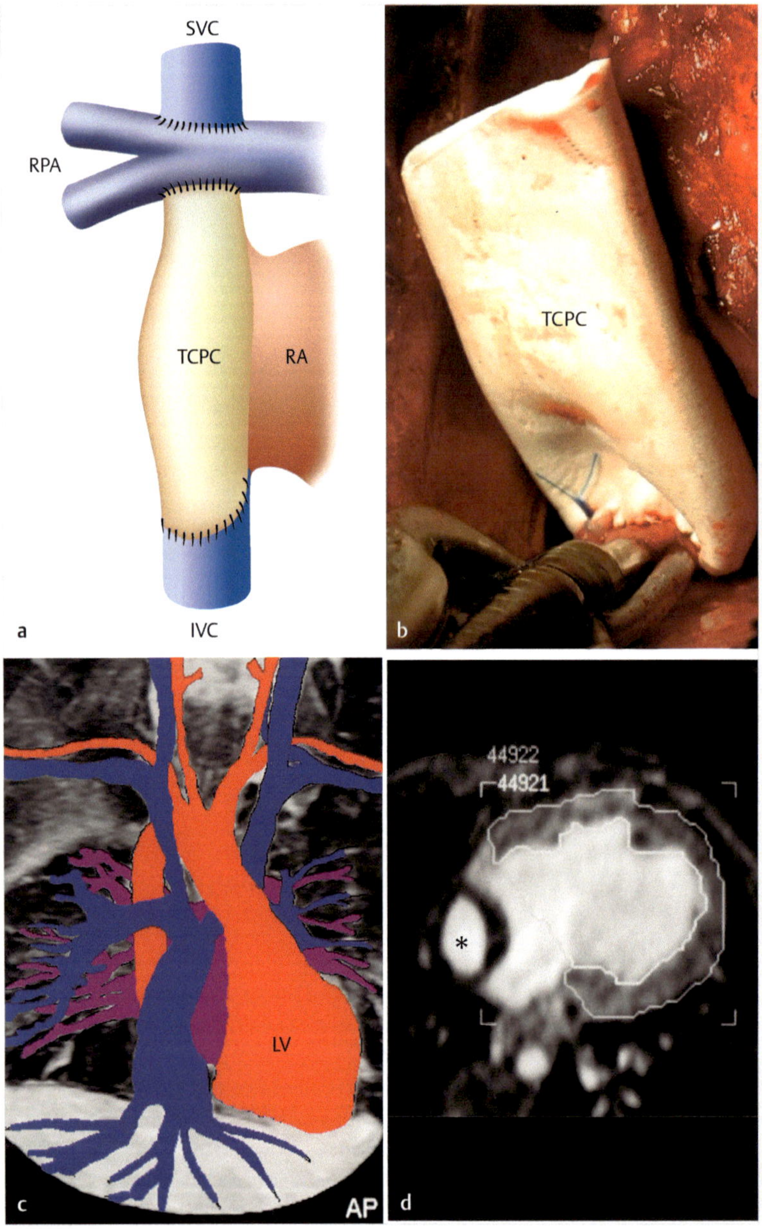

Fig. 2.8 Completing cavopulmonary anastomosis (TCPC).
IVC = inferior vena cava
LV = left ventricle
RA = right atrium
RPA = right pulmonary artery
SVC = superior vena cava
a Schematic depiction of TCPC.
b Extracardiac GORE-TEX tunnel.
c The colored MIP depiction of an MRA with contrast represents an overview of the connection between the superior vena cava, inferior vena cava, and the right pulmonary artery (blue).
d The end diastolic image of the cine MRI depicts a transverse view of the TCPC tunnel (asterisk).

Surgical Treatment of a Ventricular Septal Defect

Indication for surgery—in the sense of large left–right shunts and pulmonary overflow—occurs in infancy for all cases of hemodynamically relevant ventricular septal defects.

The usual route to VSD correction consists of a median sternotomy with subtotal, bilateral thymectomy, longitudinal perdicardiotomy, and removal of the pericardial portion for later use as a VSD patch. VSDs are treated primarily with the assistance of a heart–lung machine and under conditions of mild-to-moderate hypothermia. In addition, the ascending aorta and the superior and inferior hollow veins are cannulated. After stabilizing the flow of the heart–lung machine, the ascending aorta is clamped off. A cardioplegic solution is used to induce cardiac arrest, which is then concluded with the closure of both hollow veins.

For children with pulmonary hypertonia, the PDA is inspected and may be clamped off. During cardiac arrest, a longitudinal incision is made in the right atrium. The fossa ovalis, tricuspid valve, and coronary sinus are then inspected. The type (membranous or muscular) and position of the VSD with respect to the aforementioned structures determine how surgery proceeds:

- In cases of *perimembranous VSD*, both intraoperative representation and patch closure are possible via the tricuspid valve; a portion of the anchoring stitches can

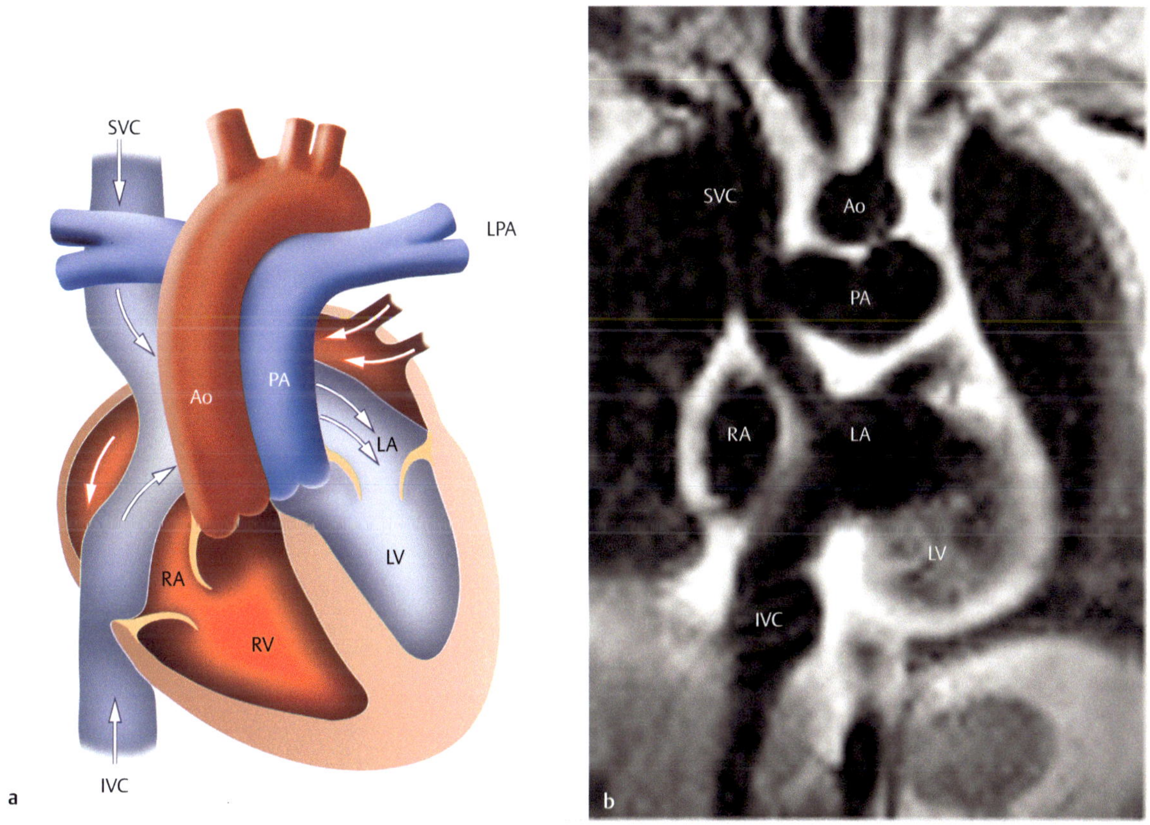

Fig. 2.9 Mustard or Senning atrial switch (atrial switch operation) to correct complete transposition of the great arteries with intact ventricular septum (TGA IVS). Both partial depictions show the venous baffle that diverts blood flow at the atrial level from the superior and inferior vena cavae toward the left atrium.
Ao = aorta
IVC = inferior vena cava
LA = left atrium
LPA = left pulmonary artery
LPV = left pulmonary vein
LV = left ventricle
PA = pulmonary artery
RA = right atrium
RV = right ventricle
SVC = superior vena cava
a Schematic depiction.
b Corresponding coronal T1w MR SE image (MR spin echo image).

be placed through the tricuspid valve ring. At the end of the procedure, the valve must be tested and the surgery may need to be supplemented by a commissuroplasty of the tricuspid valve.

- A high *membranous* or *subarterial VSD* may be reachable via the pulmonary valve and closed with a pericardial patch.
- In cases of *infundibular muscular VSD*, a right ventriculectomy with RVOT reconstruction and an additional pericardial patch (▶ Fig. 2.11d) is needed.
- *Muscular apical VSDs* cannot be reached via the tricuspid valve. They must be accessed via a right or left apical ventriculectomy in order to achieve adequate view of the VSD margins during the operation, so that a safe patch closure can be performed.

Surgical Treatment of Transposition of the Great Arteries

The arterial switch operation, also known simply as "arterial switch," is definitively one of the greatest success stories in pediatric cardiac surgery. Before the arterial switch operation was established by Jatene et al. in 1975,[7] surgical treatment consisted of the choice to perform physiological correction via either a Mustard[8] or Senning atrial switch operation. The blood from the superior and inferior hollow veins was diverted into the anatomic left ventricle via the mitral valve using a venous baffle (▶ Fig. 2.9). This blood was then transported into the lungs so that the blood from the pulmonary veins was pumped into the aorta via the right atrium and right ventricle.

Clinical Relevance

The weaknesses in non-anatomical surgical atrial switch surgical procedure have been proven over the long term; among other factors, patients suffer from rhythm disorders due to surgical manipulation of the atria in order to construct the venous baffle (bradyarrhythmia, sinus node dysfunctions, tachyarrhythmia, especially atrial reentry tachycardia [occurring in 50% of cases after approximately 20 years]) and subsequently die of sudden cardiac arrest. "Right heart failure" is typical, as the morphologic right ventricle now functions as a systemic ventricle. Additional common complications, which must be taken into consideration with the help of imaging procedures, include tricuspid valve insufficiency, baffle stenoses, and baffle leaks.[9]

Despite the intermittently increased rate of early mortality for the arterial switch operation, which is generally performed in infancy during the first (5–10) days of life and is thus extremely technically demanding, anatomical correction has established itself due to its significant benefits over the long term.

The arterial switch operation is performed as follows: after a median sternotomy and subtotal bilateral thymectomy (▶ Fig. 2.10a) have been performed, a piece of the pericardium is removed (▶ Fig. 2.10b) to be used for reconstructing the neopulmonary artery (▶ Fig. 2.10e) after the coronary button has been removed (▶ Fig. 2.10c and d). It may also be used to close the concurrent ASD. The pulmonary arteries are exposed up to the bifurcation, and the ductus arteriosus is dissected. After being attached to the heart–lung machine via bicaval cannulation, the left atrium is drained via the right superior pulmonary veins using a vent catheter, supported by the superior position of the aortic cannula (nearly in the aortic arch). During a total bypass, the patient is cooled to a state of moderate hypothermia. The blood flow within the pulmonary arteries has to be controlled and the ductus arteriosus doubly suppressed, divided, and overstitched. After cardioplegic cardiac arrest, the aorta is transected approximately 2 cm above the valve, and the commissures are marked with three retaining stitches. At the same time, the aorta is stretched. The area between the aorta and the pulmonary artery is dissected completely. Both coronary buttons are excised, taking care to protect the semilunar valves, and retaining stitches are placed. The defect in the aortic wall is covered using a pericardial patch of the appropriate size (▶ Fig. 2.10f). After transection of the pulmonary artery, the pulmonary valve is stretched using three retaining stitches. Then, based on the position of the commissures and the size, position, and anatomy of the coronary button, the pulmonary arterial root is reconstructed and the coronary buttons are sewn into the neoaorta, so that they are neither exposed to tension nor possess too much clearance. The aorta is closed using the Lecompte maneuver,[10] namely displacement of the pulmonary arterial bifurcation ventral to the aorta (▶ Fig. 2.10g). If the ASD is closed either directly or with a pericardial patch, the aortic clamp is removed, enabling coronary perfusion. The pulmonary artery is stitched on the beating heart (▶ Fig. 2.10h), and the atrium is then closed. The chest cavity is either closed or left open depending on the patient's hemodynamic and respiratory condition.

Note

All patients require the support of adequate catecholamine treatment during an arterial switch operation.

Surgical Treatment for Tetralogy of Fallot

Indication for correction occurs during infancy for patients with adequate oxygen saturation (between 80% and 90%). Early correction prevents the negative effects of chronic hypoxia. After the patient has been connected to the heart–lung machine and has entered a state of cardiac arrest (as occurs during surgical procedures for correcting other heart defects), and after retaining stitches have been placed, the pulmonary valve is exposed and an open commissurotomy is performed (▶ Fig. 2.11a). The size of the valve ring is tested using a Hegar dilator. If the ring is adequately sized, the valve is retained. In cases of valve ring hypoplasia, however, the ring must be incised and the entire right outlet tract must be expanded using a transannular pericardial patch. A ventriculectomy of the right ventricle is then performed (▶ Fig. 2.11b), and the obstructing musculature is transected or removed (▶ Fig. 2.11c). After determining VSD, which typically arises due to the anterior-cranial deviation of the ventricular septum in cases of tetralogy of Fallot, Teflon felt–supported sutures are placed on the margins of the VSD. A pericardial patch of the appropriate size is cut and attached appropriately. The tricuspid valve is inspected and its function reviewed via atriotomy. The atrial septum is also inspected. Any necessary additional shunt connections are closed. In cases of valve-preserving correction, both the RVOT (▶ Fig. 2.11d) and the pulmonary artery stem are expanded upon using two separate patches. The transannular patch is placed by means of an infundibulectomy for cases of valve ring hypoplasia (▶ Fig. 2.11c). The nature of the selected surgical technique influences the likelihood and extent of pulmonary valve insufficiency after the surgical correction of tetralogy of Fallot.[11]

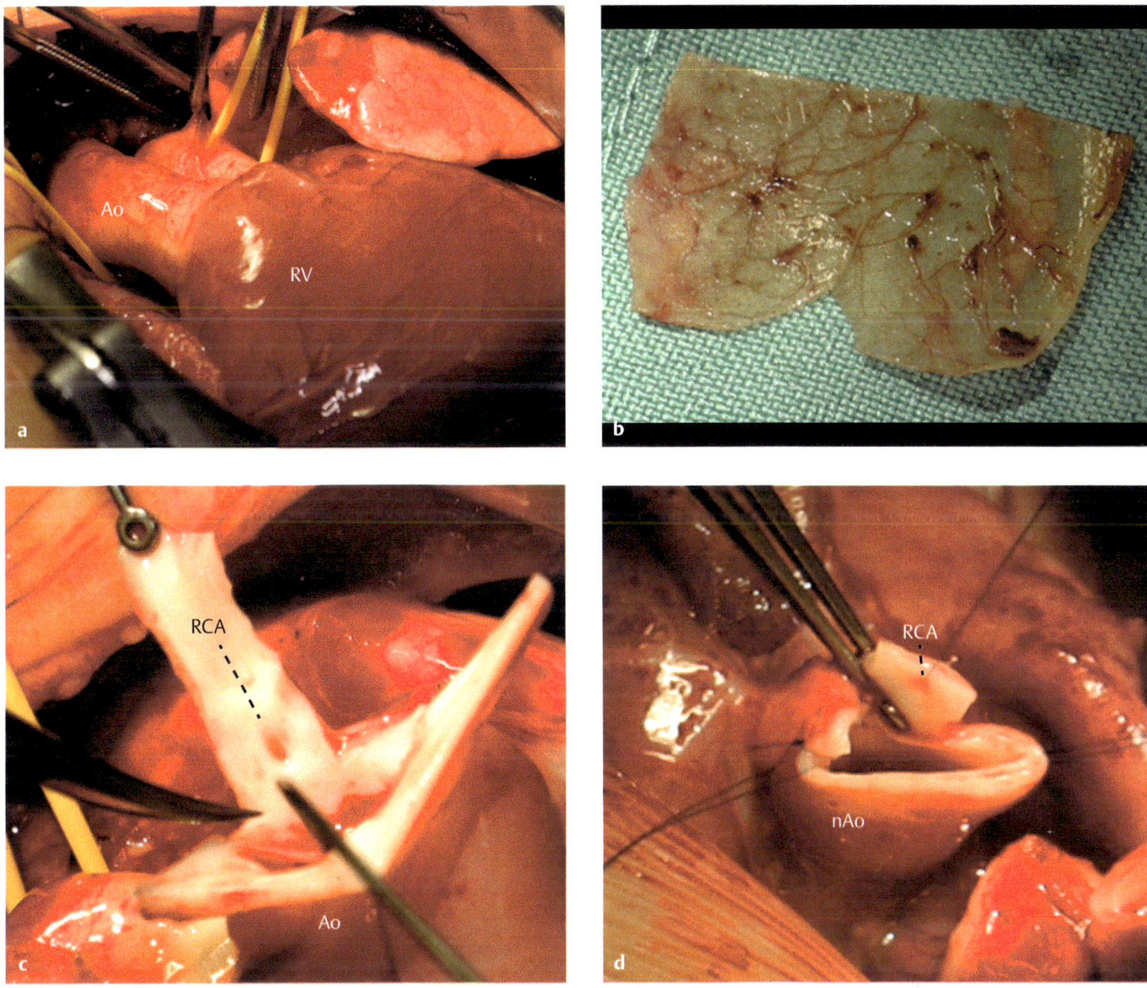

Fig. 2.10 Performing the arterial switch operation.
Ao = aorta
LPA = left pulmonary artery
nAo = new aorta (neoaorta)
nPA = new pulmonary artery (neopulmonary artery)
PA = pulmonary artery
PC = pericardium
RCA = right coronary artery
RPA = right pulmonary artery
RV = right ventricle

a Surgery site in a case of complete TGA with origin of the aorta from the right ventricle.
b Prepared pericardial patch for creating the neopulmonary artery.
c Surgery site with preparation of the aortic button from the right coronary artery.
d Introducing the button into the neoaorta.

(Continued)

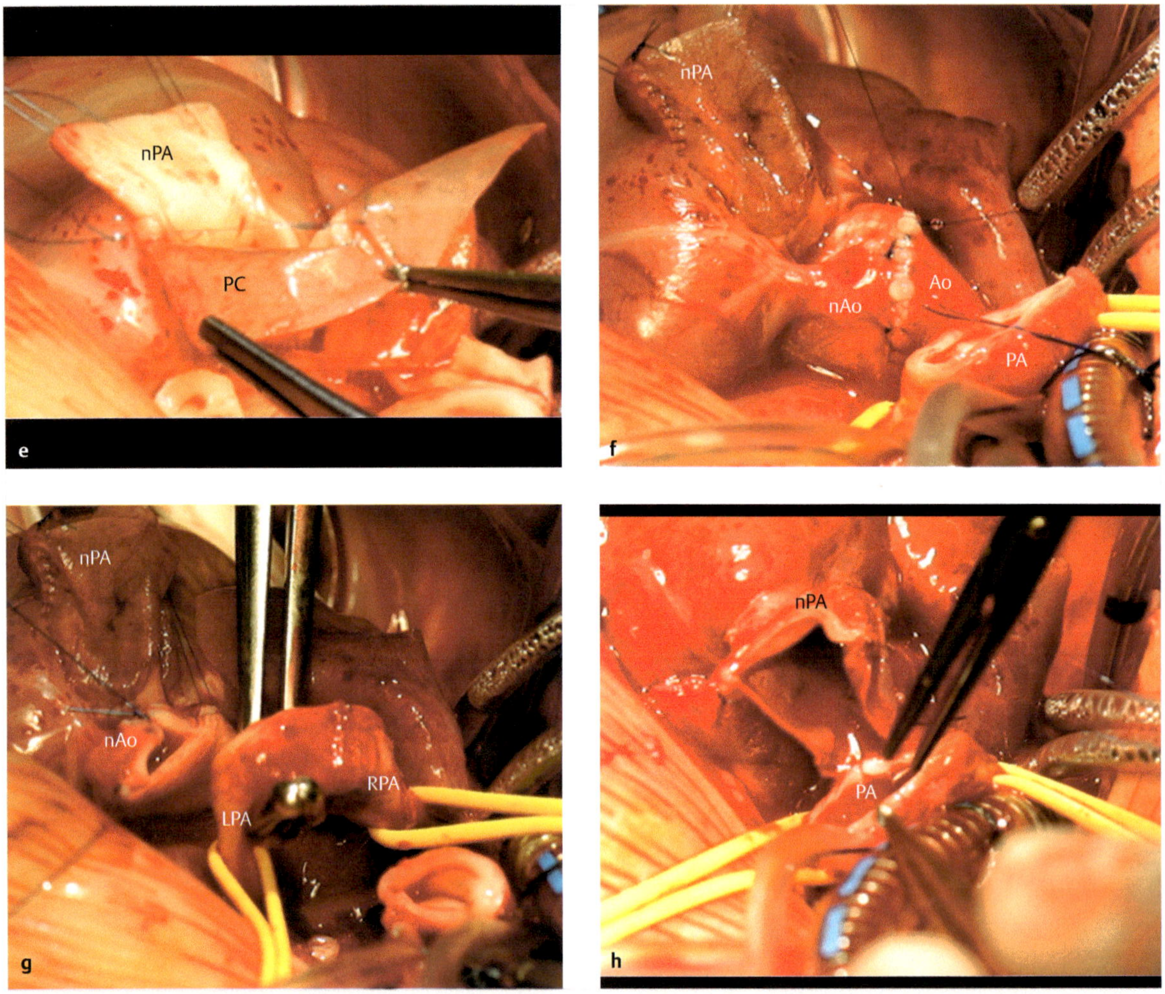

Fig. 2.10 (*Continued*) **Performing the arterial switch operation.**
Ao = aorta
LPA = left pulmonary artery
nAo = new aorta (neoaorta)
nPA = new pulmonary artery (neopulmonary artery)
PA = pulmonary artery
PC = pericardium
RCA = right coronary artery
RPA = right pulmonary artery
RV = right ventricle

- **e** Reconstruction of the neopulmonary artery using a pericardial patch (PC) (▶ Fig. 2.10b).
- **f** Surgery site for anastomosis of the neoaorta with the aorta.
- **g** Looping of the right and left pulmonary artery to prepare for the Lecompte maneuver, with ventral displacement of the pulmonary artery. As a result, the neoaorta is positioned dorsally to the neopulmonary artery.
- **h** Surgery site before preparing the end-to-end anastomosis of the neopulmonary artery with pulmonary arterial bifurcation.

2.2 Patient Preparation and Sedation

Axel Rentzsch, Hashim Abdul-Khaliq

Imaging diagnostics using echocardiography, CT, and MRI require cooperative patients who move as little as possible. Diagnostic conditions such as space, unusual noises, and especially placement of an esophageal tube for TEE can provoke fear even in growing and cooperative children, and thus can render it impossible to examine conscious patients. For this reason, examinations using these techniques can only be performed on younger children once they have been sedated.

> **Note**
>
> On principle, children should only be sedated by trained medical personnel, and their cardiorespiratory condition should be under continuous monitoring. Due to the increase in required sedation procedures, anesthetists should be limited to performing sedations where intubation is required.

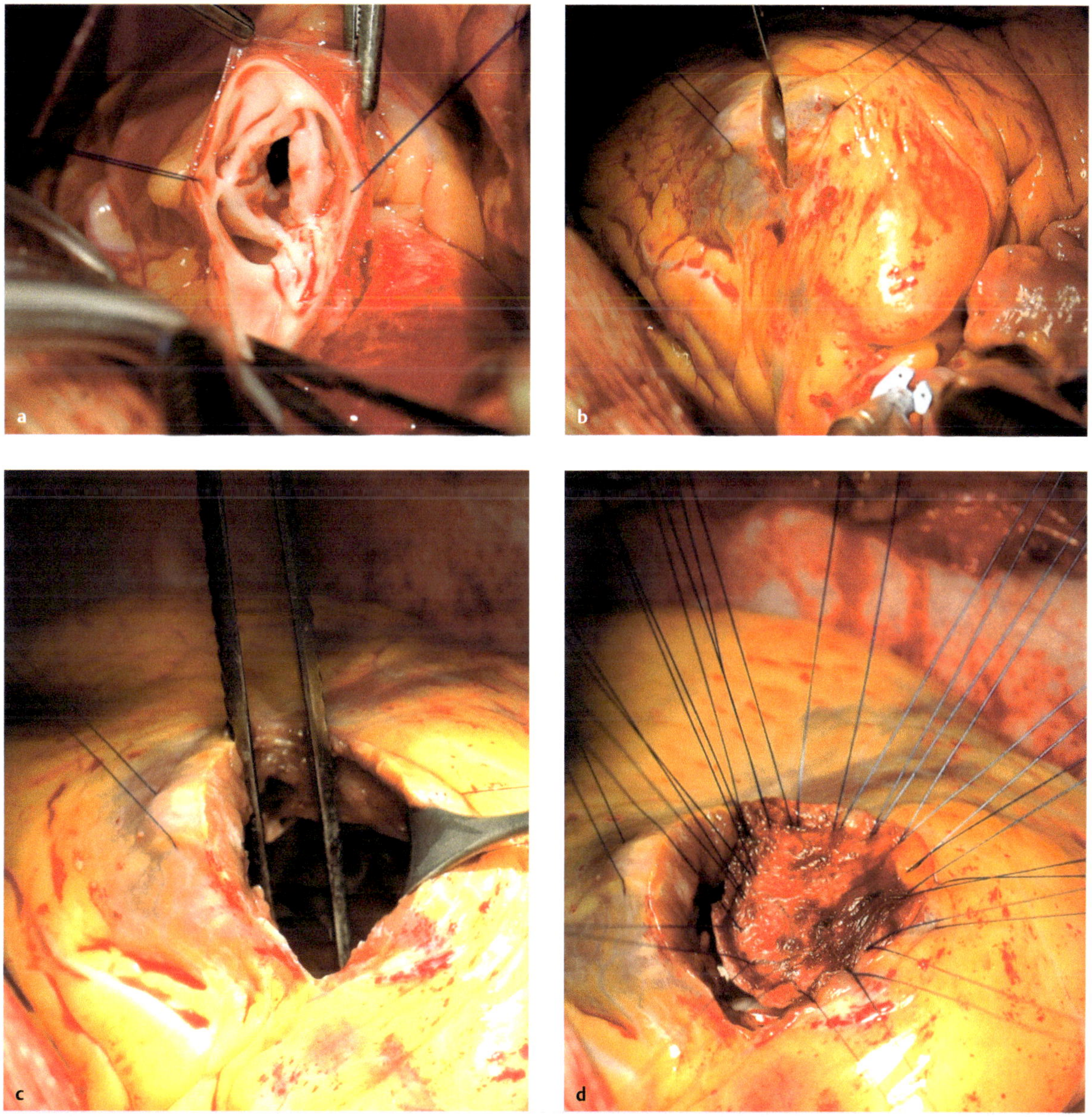

Fig. 2.11 Therapeutic correction of tetralogy of Fallot.
a Dysplastic and stenosed pulmonary valve of a patient with tetralogy of Fallot.
b Ventriculectomy of the right ventricle.
c Infundibulectomy.
d Placement of an RVOT patch.

Consequently, sedation and analgesia are being performed more frequently by non-anesthesiologists. Multiple studies have shown that sedation can be performed safely and effectively, provided that it is done in accordance with standards.[12,13,14,15,16]

2.2.1 Preprocedural Visits

Parents often find the sedation of their children to be a worrisome event, both because they are concerned about the exam results and because they have to see their child in a drastically altered state while in unusual surroundings. Sedation for purely diagnostic reasons in order to treat congenital heart defects poses an additional risk to the child, albeit a minor one. Consequently, the indication for treatment, the treatment's duration, and the method of sedation must be *explained* to the parents thoroughly, and while demonstrating sensitivity. For legal reasons, the preliminary exam and explanation should occur at least 24 hours before sedation.

During the *preliminary exam*, the presence of an obstruction in the upper respiratory tract, pathological or inflammatory changes in the lower respiratory tract, and signs of muscular weakness must be taken into consideration. Respiration, cardiac circulation, metabolism, the neuromuscular system, and psychomotor development are examined.

> **Note**
>
> Sedation should be postponed in cases of acute febrile, purulent respiratory infections, or obstructive bronchitis. If there is suspected exposure to childhood diseases, incubation time should be taken into account when scheduling appointments for unvaccinated children.

Children with chronic respiratory diseases are examined while in their best possible state. For children taking anti-seizure medications or children with psychomotor impairment or ADHD, it may be advisable to plan to use general anesthesia from the outset. Newborns up to a maturity age of approximately 43 weeks have an increased risk of apnea.[17]

Vaccinations with inactive vaccines can be administered no later than 3 days before the exam, and those with attenuated live vaccines, no later than 2 weeks before the exam. In theory, any systemic response to the vaccine can temporarily modulate or reduce immune response, since anesthesia, stress, and especially trauma reduce cell-mediated immune function. At any rate, there is no clinical evidence that a previous vaccination leads to increased risk associated with anesthesia or with the perioperative complication rate.[18] In order to avoid misinterpreting the side effects of vaccines as post-procedural complications and vice versa, it is advisable to comply with the aforementioned administration intervals.[19] A recently administered vaccine does not constitute a contraindication for urgent exams.

> **Note**
>
> Set times or exam days for imaging procedures can be helpful for planning, since entire families often must be mobilized for an exam appointment. A child-appropriate environment and the parents' presence should be encouraged.

2.2.2 Sedation

Level of Sedation

Sedation is the use of medication to achieve a neurophysiological state characterized by anxiolysis, hypnosis, and amnesia. This condition is desirable in smaller children for imaging procedures such as TEE, CT, and MRI. The European Guidelines for Sedation and/or Analgesia by Non-Anesthesiologists[20] describe levels of sedation using the sedation scale developed by Ramsay et al.:[21]

- *Stage 1:* awake
- *Stage 2:* drowsy
- *Stage 3:* asleep, responsive to speech
- *Stage 4:* asleep, responsive to physical stimuli
- *Stage 5:* asleep, unresponsive to physical stimuli (comatose)

According to the European guidelines, level 2 or 3 (light sedation) is adequate for performing uncomfortable diagnostic procedures on patients. Brief periods of stage 4 or 5 of sedation (deep sedation)—sometimes lasting mere seconds —cannot, however, be avoided completely. For this reason, the sedating physician must be capable of handling complications that may occur at deeper levels of sedation.

Safety

Goals of pediatric sedation:
- maximize patient safety;
- minimize discomfort, psychological trauma, fear, and pain;
- reach an adequate state of amnesia;
- avoid restless movements; and
- place the patient in a condition in which he or she can be released from medical supervision.

In order to achieve this, the lowest possible dose of the applied medication with the highest possible success rate should be selected.

Fasting

In order to avoid the risk of pulmonary aspiration, multi-hour fasting is recommended during preoperative management and while preparing for sedation. This constitutes abstaining from solid food and moderately solid food (such as baby food) for 6 hours, breastmilk for 6 hours, and clear fluids for 2 hours, respectively.[22,23] Multiple prospective examinations have shown, however, that failure to fast is not associated with an increased rate of aspiration or other adverse anesthesia events.[24,25] Ghaffar et al. have even demonstrated that for children under 6 months of age, fasting for more than 2 hours can lead to less effective sedation during echocardiograms.[26]

Discharge

It is most hospitals' standard to monitor and observe patients after sedation until they awake fully. After sedation for diagnostic purposes, children and adolescents should only be released once they have reached their previous mental clinical condition, their peripheral oxygen saturation is more than 95% below that of the ambient air, they are adequately hydrated, are showing no symptoms of stridor or vomiting, and are able to eat or drink without issue. The sedating physician decides when the patient may be released.

Sedation Procedure

Procedures for sedating children vary greatly among institutions. The success rate for elective radiological procedures for children is approximately 94–98%.[27,28] In general, smaller children require sedation. It is certainly possible, however, to convince children aged seven and older to cooperate if an explanation suitable to the child is provided and if the parents are allowed to be present. Since most imaging procedures are performed under IV sedation, it can be helpful to place the necessary indwelling venous catheters while the patient is in the pediatric unit in order to avoid delays.

Note

Children up to an age of 6 weeks can be examined in an MRI *during natural sleep after a meal*. Good time coordination between feeding time and the scan appointment is a prerequisite for this method. If the child is not asleep, he or she can be sedated using chloral hydrate or midazolam.

Chloral hydrate has the highest success rate for children with a body weight under 15 kg.[29] A dosage of 50–100 mg/kg body weight (maximum: 1.5 g), administered orally, achieves a sedation duration of 60–120 minutes.[30] This sedation goes into effect after 30–60 minutes. Good cooperation with the pediatric unit ensures that chloral hydrate is administered orally (via stomach tube) or rectally 30 minutes before the scan appointment. Liver or cardiac conduction disorders are contraindications, since higher dosages can sensitize the cardiac muscles to noradrenaline, leading to rhythm disorders. Chloral hydrate and benzodiazepines are considered the least acutely dangerous hypnotics. Adverse cardiorespiratory events occurred in 3% of cases with a sedation protocol for MRI exams, and were addressed rapidly by means of stimulation or improved positioning.[29] In a retrospective study of 1,095 patients—the majority with congenital heart defects—who were sedated prior to an echocardiographic exam via chloral hydrate, hypercapnia (defined as a 20% increase in carbon dioxide concentration above the end-tidal initial value) occurred in 6.6% of cases. Hypoxia and hypotension occurred in 5.9% of cases, and vomiting in 0.4% of cases, respectively. Children under the age of 6 months were at an increased risk of experiencing an adverse event.[31] Coté et al. analyzed the adverse sedation events occurring with the use of various pharmaceuticals,[32] and described 13 cases resulting in lasting neurological damage or death after administration of chloral hydrate. Of these cases, chloral hydrate was used in isolation in seven instances; in the other six instances, it was used in combination with other medications. These incidents were caused by dosage errors, a lack of monitoring, or monitoring by non-medical personnel. Two of these children had congenital heart defects, and thus cardiac arrhythmia was assumed to be the cause of the negative outcomes.

Alternatively, it can be helpful—especially for children with a body weight of over 10 kg—to administer *midazolam* at a dosage of 0.05–0.10 mg/kg body weight via slow titration until the desired effect is reached, since the required amount of chloral hydrate can lead to stomach irritation and vomiting. Midazolam goes into effect quickly due to its high lipophilia. It is anxiolytic, sedative, and a muscle relaxant, and causes antegrade amnesia. A waiting period of 2–5 minutes should be observed before administering another dose in order to be able to adequately assess the sedative effects. The elimination half-life is 2 hours. Respiratory depression or apnea may occur based on the dosage and rate of injection. For imaging procedures longer than 20–30 minutes, additional doses are necessary. Restlessness, aggression, ataxia, withdrawal-like phenomena, or general disinhibition and euphoria may still occur 3–4 hours after administration. Seizures are observed more commonly in premature babies and newborns, and the risk of apnea also increases within this age group.

Note

Since midazolam can lead to dangerous respiratory depression, the benzodiazepine antagonist *flumazenil* must be on hand. Flumazenil's short half-life of 30–60 minutes must be taken into account. Midazolam is not recommended for children under 6 months due to a lack of clinical experience for this age group.

It is not always necessary to place uncooperative children under deep sedation. For older children with misgivings, administering a single dose of an anxiolytic *benzodiazepine* can help examiners complete imaging procedures successfully.

Numerous studies describe *propofol* as the ideal short-term narcotic.[33] The patient loses consciousness 10–20 seconds after IV administration. The wake-up period is also very short (just 5–15 minutes), which is why propofol is well-suited to outpatient sedation. In order to reduce painful venous irritation during administration, propofol can be diluted with an equal measure of 0.9% sodium chloride solution. It is non-analgesic and is not a muscle relaxant. First, an initial bolus injection of 3–5 mg/kg body weight is administered, beginning with one-fourth of the bolus, and then more is administered based on effect. Then, a continuous infusion at a dosage of 2–7 mg/(kg body weight x h) is administered. For infants, an initial dosage of up to 15 mg/(kg body weight x h) may be needed, which can then be reduced to 5–8 mg/(kg body weight x h) during the exam. If the bolus is administered too quickly, this can lead to attenuated respiratory function and a drop in oxygen saturation. This issue can be addressed quickly by minor extension of the neck, the jaw-thrust maneuver, administering oxygen, and in some cases, applying an oxygen mask.[34] In addition, propofol has negative inotropic properties and is a peripheral vasodilator, which decreases blood pressure. Slow infusion can be used to manage these effects in children with cardiac disorders or hypovolemia. Because of this negative inotropic effect and a broad reduction in systemic resistance, particular caution should be exercised when administering boluses to newborns and patients with limited ventricular function, as well as to patients with pulmonary arterial hypertonia. In rare cases, the negative chronotropic effect may require treatment with atropines or sympathomimetics. Administration of midazolam before propofol, significantly reduces the required propofol dosage.[35]

A combination of *S ketamine* and *midazolam* is an alternative to sedating both newborns and patients with pulmonary hypertonia and poor cardiac function for imaging diagnostic purposes. Anesthesia accompanied by analgesia and amnesia occurs approximately 30 seconds after IV administration of S ketamine (0.5–1 mg/kg body weight). These effects last 5–10 minutes. S ketamine causes increased saliva production, which is why concurrent administration of anticholinergics is recommended. Advantages include minimized respiratory depression, the opportunity to complete even painful interventional procedures during the same session, and the amnestic and strong immobilization effects. It has a sympathomimetic effect; in cases of high sympathicotonia (e.g., in cases of hypovolemia), however, hypotension can occur. Thus, ketamine can be beneficial to patients with heart conditions. One disadvantage is hyperacusis, which limits use in MRI. Nightmares and hallucinations during the wake-up phase may also occur, and can be reduced by concurrent administration of benzodiazepines.

Monitoring and Equipment

> **Note**
>
> Children should always be sedated by adequately trained personnel who are not involved in performing the imaging procedure.[36] The presence of parents during the child's sedation has a calming effect and should be encouraged.

Monitoring during sedation comprises pulse oximetry, noninvasive blood pressure measurement, ECG readings, capnometry, and body temperature monitoring, particularly for lengthy procedures. In addition, video monitoring can increase safety if no direct contact with the child is possible. Monitoring should be begun before administering any type of IV sedation. The monitor must be visible to the person administering the sedation at all times, and must also display high-quality images. Equipment must be available in sizes appropriate for children and must be approved for use in MRI examinations performed using MRI devices. Any apparatus that is not suitable for MRI can influence image quality and often does not work optimally.

Continuous *ECG registration* using 3–5 leads allows the heart rate to be monitored and rhythm disorders to be detected. A high-quality ECG lead is crucial, particularly for stress MRI exams or when administering medication. Respiratory rate can be monitored via the ECG electrodes or a respiratory belt.

A nasal cannula for administering oxygen should be placed for each patient. Continuous *pulse oximetry* with acute variability in pitch corresponding to current oxygen saturation is an absolute minimum standard, regardless of the means of sedative administration. Since there is always a delay between the start of hypoventilation and the fall in oxygen saturation measured via pulse oximetry, particularly during continuous administration of oxygen,[37] pulse oximetry alone is not reliable for respiratory monitoring.

Capnometry measures the carbon dioxide content in the exhaled air and provides prompt notice of bradypnea and pauses in breathing, and thus indirect information regarding depth of sedation. During adverse sedation events, apnea and airway obstructions can be identified much more quickly using capnometry than via clinical observation or pulse oximetry.[38–40] The current guidelines of the American Academy of Pediatrics expressly recommend capnometry, especially for sedation cases where access to the patient is limited, such as in an MRI machine.[22]

If a longer exam (e.g., within the scope of a clinical trial) is anticipated, continuous *body temperature monitoring* via rectal probe should be performed, especially in infants. Shivering leads to restlessness in patients and a significant increase in oxygen requirements. A blanket or appropriate warming system (Bair Hugger™) can prevent hypothermia. The ambient temperature should be at least 22 °C.

Oxygen connectors and masks, respiration and intubation devices (laryngoscopes, endotracheal tubes, larynx masks) for all ages, suction devices and the corresponding catheters in various sizes, and emergency medication and antagonists (flumazenil, naloxone) must be available and functional during sedation and transport. A defibrillator should be easily accessible, and it should be possible to transfer the patient quickly to the intensive care unit.

Complications

Sedating children is associated with serious risks, such as hypoventilation, hypoxemia, apnea, airway obstruction, aspiration, laryngospasm, and adverse cardiopulmonary events. These risks can be minimized but not eliminated completely. An examination of the most common causes of adverse sedation events indicated that inadequate monitoring, incorrect dosages, overdoses, inadequate equipment in the working area, inadequately qualified personnel, and excessively early patient discharge contributed significantly to the adverse events.[32] An ASA status of III or IV (patients with severe general illnesses with functional limitations or with ongoing threats to survival) and an age of less than 1 year are predictors for increased risk.[41] In contrast, no connection was drawn between the occurrence of adverse events and the exam type or the patient's weight or sex. The odds ratios for an adverse event were approximately five times higher when using a combination of medication for sedation.[42] Hypoxia is three time as likely to occur during sedation in children with developmental retardation.[43]

Thus, it is recommended that anesthesia be administered to children and adolescents by specialized pediatricians or anesthetists, ideally with at least one of their assigned nurses. In order to be able to act appropriately in case of complications, personnel must receive periodic training for resuscitation including securing the airway, intubation, and respiration. Since resuscitation (e.g., with a defibrillator) cannot be performed within the MRI machine, itself, personnel should also practice transporting the patient from the MRI room, ideally using a detachable table. Very few, yet highly precise sedation plans should be used within an institution, and the following contraindications should be taken into consideration:

- Airway issues
- Risk of apnea (newborns, premature babies)
- Risk of aspiration
- Increased intracranial pressure
- Epilepsy (generalized occurrences in the last 24 hours)
- Complications with prior sedation (e.g., occurrence of adverse events)
- Resuscitation due to seizure within the last month
- Decompensating cardiocirculatory function.

Since problems often occur during the recovery phase for exams performed under sedation and/or analgesia, appropriate spaces with an adequate number of resting areas, qualified personnel, monitoring and devices, materials, and medications for treating any complications are indispensable.

Note

The patient should be monitored continuously, including via pulse oximeter, by qualified personnel until the patient has recovered fully.

2.2.3 Special Exam Methods

Transthoracic Echocardiography

Generally speaking, very few preparations are needed for TTE exams for children and adolescents, since these exams can usually be performed on patients who are awake. In some cases, resistant infants and young children may require mild sedation with chloral hydrate or midazolam. Simultaneous ECG monitoring should also be ensured for every exam. Particularly for babies and small children, the exam should be performed in a quiet room in order to provide a calming effect in the absence of parents or other trusted people. It can be helpful to distract restless children by feeding them or administering 20/24% glucose. Based on clinical experience, increasing the acoustic signals of rhythmic heart sounds while recording Doppler signals is calming to many young children.

Transesophageal Echocardiography

The exam is always performed with a second physician and potentially with an appropriately trained technical assistant. In rare cases with toddlers and young children, intubation narcosis may be necessary. Local anesthesia with lidocaine spray and additional sedation with midazolam, propofol, or ketamine are sufficient for most patients (▶ Fig. 2.12). Anticholinergic medications are

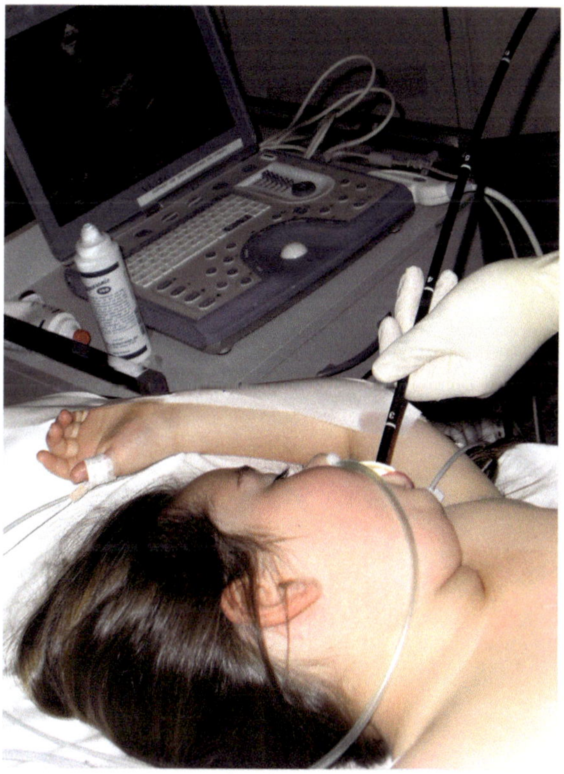

Fig. 2.12 Transesophageal echocardiography.

generally not recommended during exams. Administering atropine, however, can be helpful for younger patients who tend to salivate more profusely.[44] Venous access must always be available in order to quickly administer contrast agent or necessary medications, e.g., in cases of vasovagal response due to esophageal intubation. Local oral anesthesia often leads to unpleasant reactions and throat irritation shortly before placing the tube. Patients may not drink anything for 2 hours after receiving oral anesthesia. Outpatient monitoring with ECG and pulse oximetry should occur for 2–5 hours after the exam, depending on the patient's condition. The sonic probe should be attached and a functional test should be performed before the exam.

Computed Tomography

Computed tomography exams are painless and can be performed faster than echocardiographic and MRI exams, though these advantages come at the cost of radiation exposure. Under certain circumstances, this exposure is below that of a diagnostic cardiac catheter when using the newest generations of CT devices. Thus, CT is a reasonable, noninvasive alternative, particularly for depicting coronary arteries for patients with congenital heart defects. For children under the age of about 7, or for older, uncooperative, or developmentally delayed children, it can be difficult or impossible to hold the children still even for the few seconds needed for a scan. Furthermore, CT exams triggered by cardiac ECGs benefit from lower heart rates. For this reason, mild sedation is often helpful in these cases. Since administering contrast agent during the apnea phase is generally necessary depending on the device's age and generation, general anesthesia with tracheal intubation or larynx mask and mechanical ventilation should be taken into consideration. As with any CT exam with contrast, kidney functional limitations and thyroid function must be taken into account.

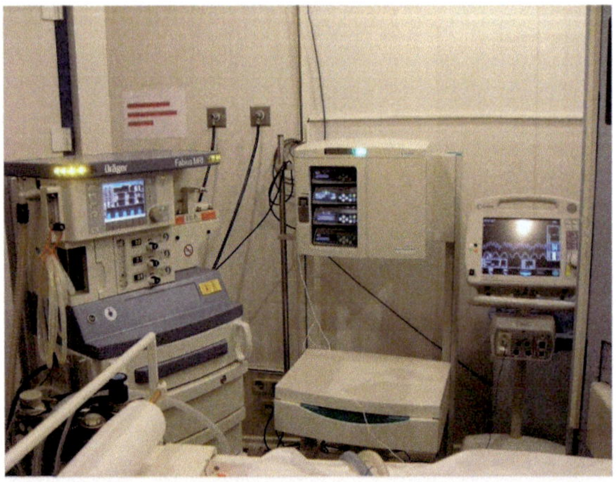

Fig. 2.13 Anesthesia unit in MRI.

Magnetic Resonance Imaging

MRI exams can also be performed painlessly, but they are usually lengthier than TTE or CT exams. As with CT exams, it is difficult to keep children under seven motionless for 30–60 minutes. Consequently, deep sedation (or general anesthesia with tracheal intubation or a larynx mask, if contrast must be administered during the apnea phase while the examination is being conducted) is necessary (▶ Fig. 2.13). The patient must not have any severe renal functional limitations if the examiner plans to use gadolinium contrast agent.

From an organizational perspective, it is simpler to plan a child's day in the MR than to try to examine children during a hectic working day. Furthermore, attempts should be made to coordinate the exam date with rest periods. Earrings, barrettes, and similar accessories must be removed before MRI scans, and it must be ensured that any clothing remaining on the body does not contain metal.

Cardiac Catheter Exam

For older, cooperative patients, light sedation with midazolam with good local anesthesia is often adequate. Most children over age 2, however, require deep sedation (▶ Fig. 2.14 and ▶ Fig. 2.15). Propofol infusions have been tried and tested in this context. Ketamine can also be administered to ensure that the patient remains motionless while the vessel is punctured. Endotracheal intubation with inhaled or propofol anesthesia may be necessary for infants and children under age 2, or for difficult, lengthy interventional procedures. A nasal cannula for administering oxygen should be placed for each patient. Regular suctioning is required to prevent a buildup of secretions. The arms are placed beside the head. Adequate elevation must be ensured to prevent plexus paresis caused by the patient's position.

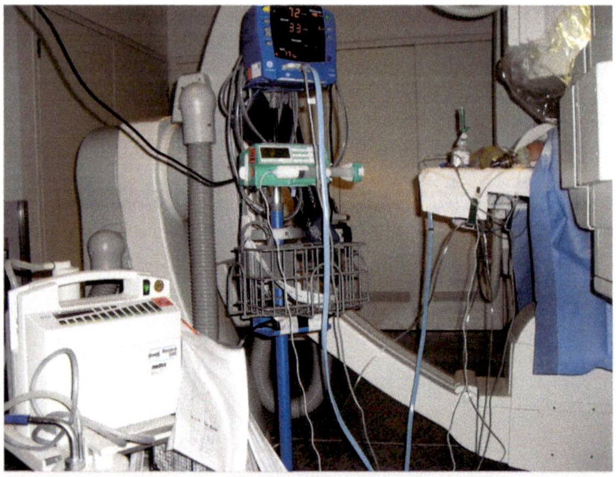

Fig. 2.14 Sedation in the cardiac catheter laboratory. The monitor, perfusor, and suction device should not limit access to the child.

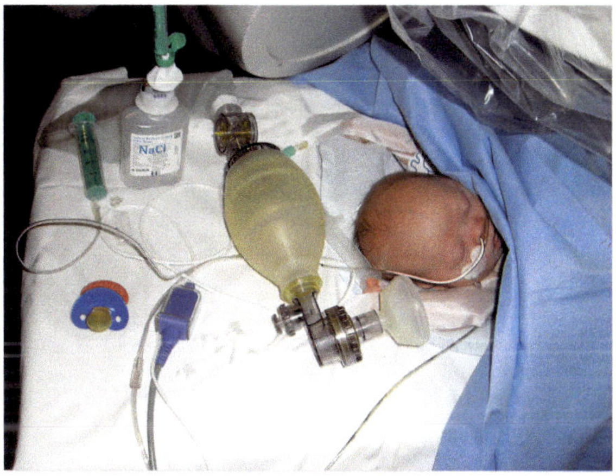

Fig. 2.15 Patient positioning and preparation for cardiac catheter exam. The arms are positioned upward and fixed on either side of the head during a cardiac catheter exam. A resuscitation bag should be within reach.

References

[1] Gross RE. Surgical management of the patent ductus arteriosus: with summary of four surgically treated cases. Ann Surg. 1939; 110 (3):321–356

[2] Gross RE. Surgical correction for coarctation of the aorta. Surgery. 1945; 18:673–678

[3] Taussig HB, Blalock A. The tetralogy of Fallot; diagnosis and indications for operation; the surgical treatment of the tetralogy of Fallot. Surgery. 1947; 21(1):145

[4] Smith GW, Thompson WM, Jr, Dammann JF, Jr, Muller WH, Jr. Use of the pulmonary artery banding procedure in treating type II truncus arteriosus. Circulation. 1964; 29 Suppl.:108–113

[5] Rashkind WJ, Miller WW. Creation of an atrial septal defect without thoracotomy. A palliative approach to complete transposition of the great arteries. JAMA. 1966; 196(11):991–992

[6] Warden HE, Cohen M, De Wall RA, et al. Experimental closure of interventricular septal defects and further physiologic studies on controlled cross circulation. Surg Forum. 1955; 5:22–28

[7] Jatene AD, Fontes VF, Paulista PP, et al. Successful anatomic correction of transposition of the great vessels. A preliminary report. Arq Bras Cardiol. 1975; 28(4):461–464

[8] Mustard WT. Successful two-stage correction of transposition of the great vessels. Surgery. 1964; 55:469–472

[9] Gutberlet M, Hoffmann J, Künzel E, et al. [Preoperative and postoperative imaging in patients with transposition of the great arteries]. Radiologe. 2011; 51(1):15–22

[10] Lecompte Y, Zannini L, Hazan E, et al. Anatomic correction of transposition of the great arteries. J Thorac Cardiovasc Surg. 1981; 82 (4):629–631

[11] Grothoff M, Hoffmann J, Lehmkuhl L, et al. Time course of right ventricular functional parameters after surgical correction of tetralogy of Fallot determined by cardiac magnetic resonance. Clin Res Cardiol. 2011; 100(4):343–350

[12] Hertzog JH, Havidich JE. Non-anesthesiologist-provided pediatric procedural sedation: an update. Curr Opin Anaesthesiol. 2007; 20 (4):365–372

[13] Pitetti R, Davis PJ, Redlinger R, White J, Wiener E, Calhoun KH. Effect on hospital-wide sedation practices after implementation of the 2001 JCAHO procedural sedation and analgesia guidelines. Arch Pediatr Adolesc Med. 2006; 160(2):211–216

[14] Pitetti RD, Singh S, Pierce MC. Safe and efficacious use of procedural sedation and analgesia by nonanesthesiologists in a pediatric emergency department. Arch Pediatr Adolesc Med. 2003; 157 (11):1090–1096

[15] Sauer H, Grünzinger L, Pfeifer J, Lieser U, Abdul-Khaliq H. Sedation and analgosedation performed by pediatricians—experience made with the implementation of an in-house sedation standard: sedation and analgosedation-implementation of an in-house standard. Wien Med Wochenschr. 2016; 166(1–2):54–61

[16] Smallman B. Pediatric sedation: can it be safely performed by non-anesthesiologists? Curr Opin Anaesthesiol. 2002; 15(4):455–459

[17] Ramanathan R, Corwin MJ, Hunt CE, et al. Collaborative Home Infant Monitoring Evaluation (CHIME) Study Group. Cardiorespiratory events recorded on home monitors: comparison of healthy infants with those at increased risk for SIDS. JAMA. 2001; 285 (17):2199–2207

[18] Short JA, van der Walt JH, Zoanetti DC. Immunization and anesthesia —an international survey. Paediatr Anaesth. 2006; 16(5):514–522

[19] Siebert JN, Posfay-Barbe KM, Habre W, Siegrist CA. Influence of anesthesia on immune responses and its effect on vaccination in children: review of evidence. Paediatr Anaesth. 2007; 17(5):410–420

[20] Knape JT, Adriaensen H, van Aken H, et al. Board of Anaesthesiology of the European Union of Medical Specialists. Guidelines for sedation and/or analgesia by non-anaesthesiology doctors. Eur J Anaesthesiol. 2007; 24(7):563–567

[21] Ramsay MAE, Savege TM, Simpson BRJ, Goodwin R. Controlled sedation with alphaxalone-alphadolone. BMJ. 1974; 2(5920):656–659

[22] Coté CJ, Wilson S, American Academy of Pediatrics, American Academy of Pediatric Dentistry, Work Group on Sedation. Guidelines for monitoring and management of pediatric patients during and after sedation for diagnostic and therapeutic procedures: an update. Pediatrics. 2006; 118(6):2587–2602

[23] American Society of Anesthesiologist Task Force on Preoperative Fasting. Practice guidelines for preoperative fasting and the use of pharmacologic agents to reduce the risk of pulmonary aspiration: application to healthy patients undergoing elective procedures: a report by the American Society of Anesthesiologist Task Force on Preoperative Fasting. Anesthesiology. 1999; 90(3):896–905

[24] Agrawal D, Manzi SF, Gupta R, Krauss B. Preprocedural fasting state and adverse events in children undergoing procedural sedation and analgesia in a pediatric emergency department. Ann Emerg Med. 2003; 42(5):636–646

[25] Roback MG, Bajaj L, Wathen JE, Bothner J. Preprocedural fasting and adverse events in procedural sedation and analgesia in a pediatric emergency department: are they related? Ann Emerg Med. 2004; 44 (5):454–459

[26] Ghaffar S, Haverland C, Ramaciotti C, Scott WA, Lemler MS. Sedation for pediatric echocardiography: evaluation of preprocedure fasting guidelines. J Am Soc Echocardiogr. 2002; 15(9):980–983

[27] Frush DP, Bisset GS, III. Sedation of children for emergency imaging. Radiol Clin North Am. 1997; 35(4):789–797

[28] Sury MR, Hatch DJ, Deeley T, Dicks-Mireaux C, Chong WK. Development of a nurse-led sedation service for paediatric magnetic resonance imaging. Lancet. 1999; 353(9165):1667–1671

[29] Dalal PG, Murray D, Cox T, McAllister J, Snider R. Sedation and anesthesia protocols used for magnetic resonance imaging studies in infants: provider and pharmacologic considerations. Anesth Analg. 2006; 103(4):863–868

[30] Low E, O'Driscoll M, MacEneaney P, O'Mahony O. Sedation with oral chloral hydrate in children undergoing MRI scanning. Ir Med J. 2008; 101(3):80–82

[31] Heistein LC, Ramaciotti C, Scott WA, Coursey M, Sheeran PW, Lemler MS. Chloral hydrate sedation for pediatric echocardiography: physiologic responses, adverse events, and risk factors. Pediatrics. 2006; 117(3):e434–e441

[32] Coté CJ, Karl HW, Notterman DA, Weinberg JA, McCloskey C. Adverse sedation events in pediatrics: analysis of medications used for sedation. Pediatrics. 2000; 106(4):633–644

[33] Sury MR, Smith JH. Deep sedation and minimal anesthesia. Paediatr Anaesth. 2008; 18(1):18–24

[34] Machata AM, Willschke H, Kabon B, Kettner SC, Marhofer P. Propofol-based sedation regimen for infants and children undergoing ambulatory magnetic resonance imaging. Br J Anaesth. 2008; 101 (2):239–243

[35] Paspatis GA, Charoniti I, Manolaraki M, et al. Synergistic sedation with oral midazolam as a premedication and intravenous propofol versus intravenous propofol alone in upper gastrointestinal endoscopies in children: a prospective, randomized study. J Pediatr Gastroenterol Nutr. 2006; 43(2):195–199

[36] Coté CJ. Round and round we go: sedation—what is it, who does it, and have we made things safer for children? Paediatr Anaesth. 2008; 18(1):3–8

[37] Shankar V, Deshpande JK. Procedural sedation in the pediatric patient. Anesthesiol Clin North America. 2005; 23(4):635–654, viii

[38] Anderson JL, Junkins E, Pribble C, Guenther E. Capnography and depth of sedation during propofol sedation in children. Ann Emerg Med. 2007; 49(1):9–13

[39] Lightdale JR, Goldmann DA, Feldman HA, Newburg AR, DiNardo JA, Fox VL. Microstream capnography improves patient monitoring during moderate sedation: a randomized, controlled trial. Pediatrics. 2006; 117(6):e1170–e1178

[40] Mason KP, Burrows PE, Dorsey MM, Zurakowski D, Krauss B. Accuracy of capnography with a 30 foot nasal cannula for monitoring respiratory rate and end-tidal CO2 in children. J Clin Monit Comput. 2000; 16(4):259–262

[41] Malviya S, Voepel-Lewis T, Tait AR. Adverse events and risk factors associated with the sedation of children by nonanesthesiologists. Anesth Analg. 1997; 85(6):1207–1213

[42] Sanborn PA, Michna E, Zurakowski D, et al. Adverse cardiovascular and respiratory events during sedation of pediatric patients for imaging examinations. Radiology. 2005; 237(1):288–294

[43] Kannikeswaran N, Mahajan PV, Sethuraman U, Groebe A, Chen X. Sedation medication received and adverse events related to sedation for brain MRI in children with and without developmental disabilities. Paediatr Anaesth. 2009; 19(3):250–256

[44] Lutterotti N, Clinical Committee of the German Society of Cardiology. Quality guidelines in echocardiography. Z Kardiol. 1997; 86 (5):387–401

3 Technical Basics of Diagnostic and Interventional Imaging

3.1 Echocardiography

Hashim Abdul-Khaliq, Matthias Gutberlet

3.1.1 Introduction

Echocardiography, which was introduced in the 1950s, leverages the physical characteristics of ultrasound. Echocardiography[1] uses special transducers whose design allows intercostal views by using frequencies between 2 and 7 MHz to achieve the necessary penetration depth (▶ Fig. 3.1). Due to the prevalence of these devices and the universal applicability of the method (including in intensive care units), echocardiography is the method of choice for noninvasive imaging diagnostics, in that it depicts cardiac morphology and function, even in children and infants with congenital or acquired heart diseases.[2,3] In most cases, the entire cardiac structure and possible malformations in the heart and adjacent vessels can be depicted even prenatally by using specifically adjusted probes. Echocardiography has established itself as the method of choice for diagnosing functional and structural heart diseases in both children and adults. In addition to universal applicability and real-time image acquisition, the large variety of functional parameters that can be measured via echocardiography constitute a decisive benefit to this method as compared to other imaging modalities. Over the past 10 years, traditional 2-D echocardiography has been supplemented by 3-D and even 4-D echocardiography and tissue Doppler, which have been introduced as new procedures in all modern echo devices.

Fig. 3.1 Echocardiography transducer. Schematic depiction. The transducer permits intercostal views.

3.1.2 Standard Techniques

The following techniques are considered standard:

- 1-D (M-mode) echocardiography,
- 2-D echocardiography,
- 3-D echocardiography, and
- Doppler echocardiography.

The exam is usually performed in a left lateral position with a slightly elevated upper body.[4] The examiner faces the patient and performs the exam from the left or right side.

One-Dimensional (M-mode) Echocardiography

The sonic waves emitted by the transducer at a certain frequency are reflected by interfaces and converted into electronic signals based on the interfaces' depths. For A-mode echocardiography, echogenicity corresponds to the height of the amplitude, and for B-mode, the brightness (also known as intensity; ▶ Fig. 3.2). If the B-mode image is recorded over time, it is considered to be "M-mode" (motion). 1-D echocardiography only retains practical importance in the form of M-mode (▶ Fig. 3.3), which can be used to determine ventricular diameter and valve level in a standardized manner.[1]

Two-Dimensional Echocardiography

The echocardiographic window to the heart and major vessels is better in children than in adults. Both in terms of transthoracic imaging (by means of standard sectional planes) and subcostal/subxiphoidal or suprasternal imaging (▶ Fig. 3.4), additional views of the heart and the major vessels are easier to achieve in pediatric patients. A 2-D image is achieved by taking scans of the organ in multiple layers and depicting the images in B-mode. In general, two standard views—left parasternal and left apical (▶ Fig. 3.4)—are used. These views are oriented to the anatomical long axes of the heart with its three distinct angulations. These standard sectional planes, well-known in echocardiography, can also be used for other imaging modalities (for MRI, by means of the corresponding angulation during data acquisition, and for MDCT, by means of corresponding multiplanar reconstructions of the 3-D data sets).[5]

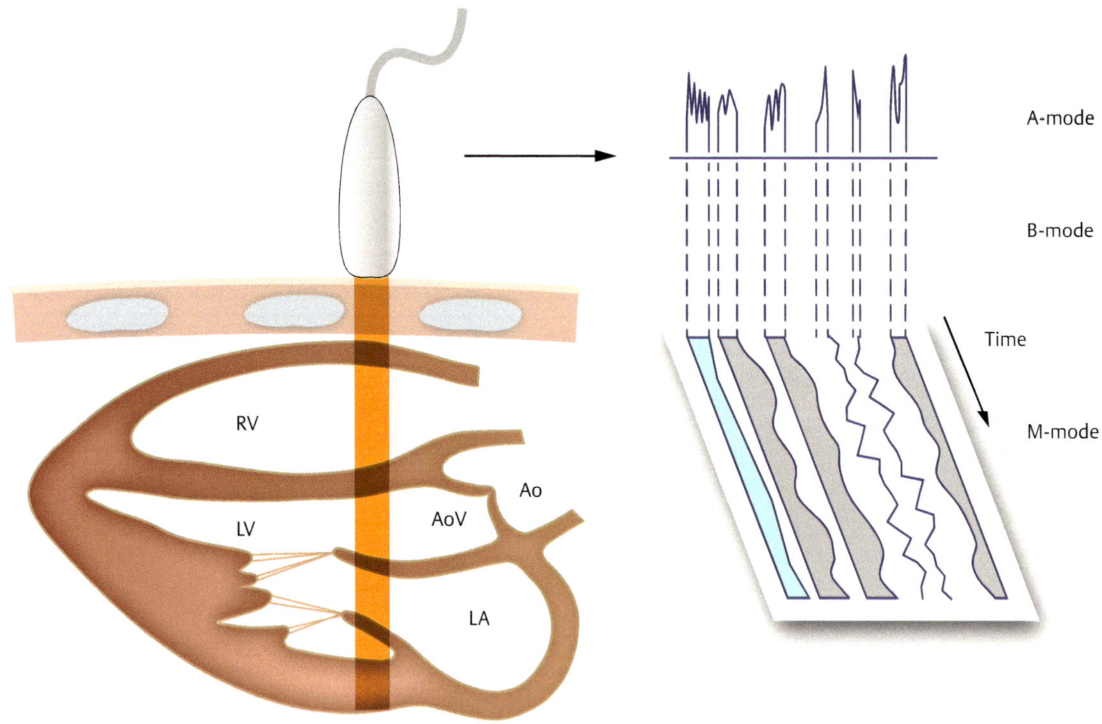

Fig. 3.2 Principles of 1-D echocardiography. Schematic depiction. Parasternal view with recordings in A-mode, B-mode, and M-mode.
Ao = aorta
AoV = aortic valve
LA = left atrium
LV = left ventricle
RV = right ventricle

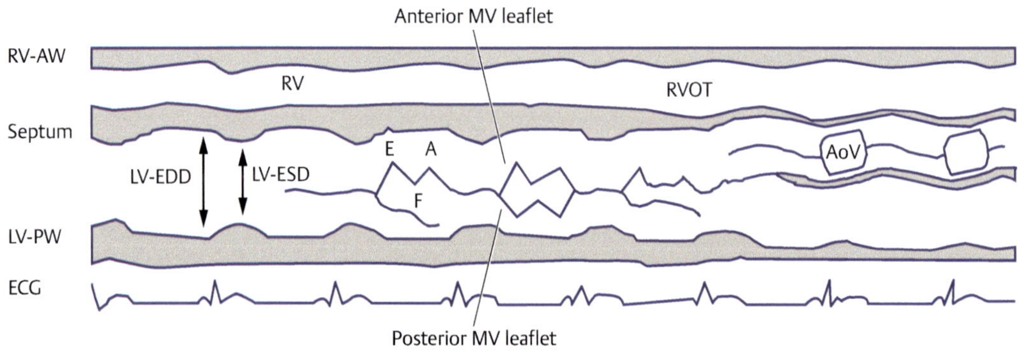

Fig. 3.3 1-D echocardiography in M-mode. Schematic depiction. M-mode sweep along the parasternal long axis with a recording of typical movement patterns of the left and right ventricles and the mitral and aortic valves during the cardiac cycle. Fractional shortening can be determined as a measure of left ventricular global function based on the LV-EDD and LV-ESD parameters.
A = A-wave (mitral valve movement during atrial contraction)
AoV = aortic valve
E = E-wave (mitral valve movement during diastole, known as early filling)
ECG = electrocardiogram
LV = left ventricle
LV-EDD = left ventricular end diastolic diameter
LV-ESD = left ventricular end systolic diameter
LV-PW = left ventricular posterior wall
MV = mitral valve
RV = right ventricle
RV-AW = right ventricular anterior wall
RVOT = right ventricular outflow tract

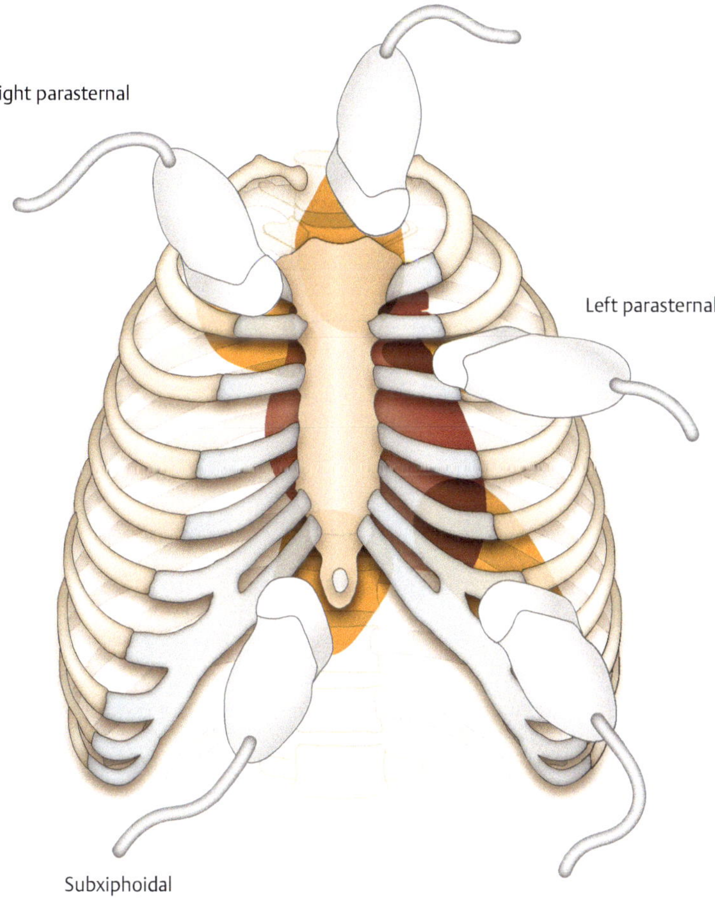

Fig. 3.4 Typical transducer positions during TTE. Schematic depiction. By using the depicted views, the heart and adjacent vessels can generally be depicted well in pediatric patients during a TTE. For children, even the suprasternal view often allows an aortic isthmus to be visualized.

The left-parasternal view allows the following sectional planes to be examined, based on transducer rotation and angulation[4]:

- *Parasternal long axis of the left ventricle* (▶ Fig. 3.5): This view primarily allows left ventricular size and function to be evaluated. In addition, this view allows 2-D and color Doppler visualization of the presence of a VSD in the perimembranous and muscular portion of the septum.
- *Parasternal short axis of the left ventricle* (after rotating the transducer 90° and shifting it accordingly)
  - with a depiction of the aortic and pulmonary valves (▶ Fig. 3.6), the pulmonary arterial stem, possible abnormal vascular connections such as a coronary fistula, abnormal connection of the coronaries to the pulmonary arterial stem (Bland–White–Garland syndrome), and, above all, PDA.
  - with a depiction of the mitral valve, the papillary muscles, or the apex (▶ Fig. 3.7). This sectional plane allows the size and function of the left ventricle and the mitral valve opening to be assessed.

Note

Under favorable conditions, a parasternal long axis of the right ventricle can also be acquired from a parasternal position (▶ Fig. 3.4).

The following standard planes can be acquired from an apical view:

- *Apical 4-chamber and 5-chamber views:* These views can depict the LVOT and aortic valve (▶ Fig. 3.8). Abnormal structures and functional abnormalities, such as turbulences or regurgitation via the aortic valve, can be visualized using color Doppler.
- *Apical left 2-chamber view and apical long axis* (by rotating the transducer 90° and angulating it appropriately): These views can depict the LVOT (▶ Fig. 3.9).

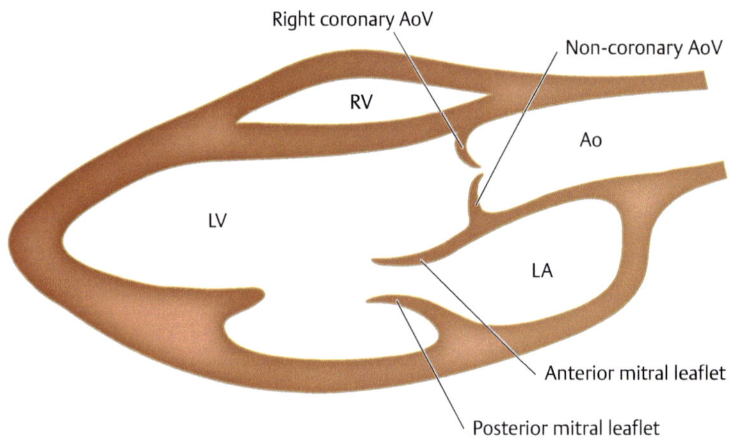

Fig. 3.5 2-D echocardiography—parasternal long axis of the heart. Schematic depiction.
Ao = aorta
AoV = aortic valve
LA = left atrium
LV = left ventricle
RV = right ventricle

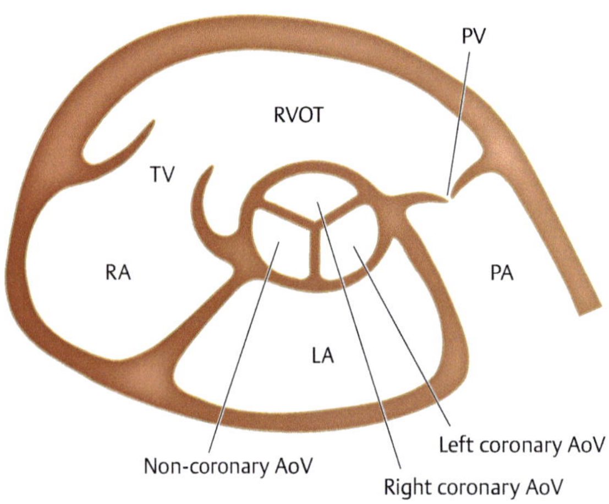

Fig. 3.6 2-D echocardiography—parasternal short axis of the heart. Schematic depiction. This sectional plane allows the aortic and pulmonary valve views to be depicted.
AoV = aortic valve
LA = left atrium
PA = pulmonary artery
PV = pulmonary valve
RA = right atrium
RVOT = right ventricular outflow tract
TV = tricuspid valve

a

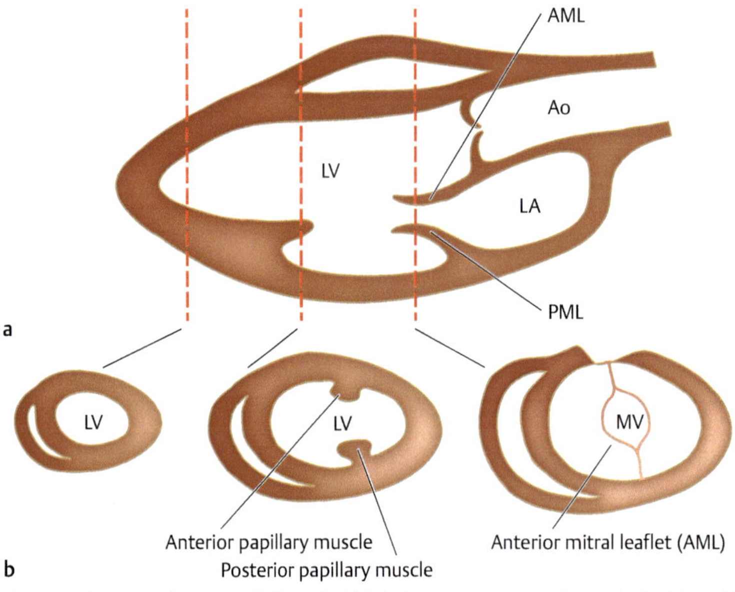

b

Fig. 3.7 2-D echocardiography—parasternal short axis of the heart. Schematic depiction. The parasternal long axis (**a**) is depicted with the corresponding short-axis slices (**b**) that occur when the transducer is rotated 90°. The red lines indicate the corresponding transducer position.
Ao = aorta
AML = anterior mitral leaflet
LA = left atrium
LV = left ventricle
MV = mitral valve
PML = posterior mitral leaflet
a Parasternal long axis.
b Short axis slices.

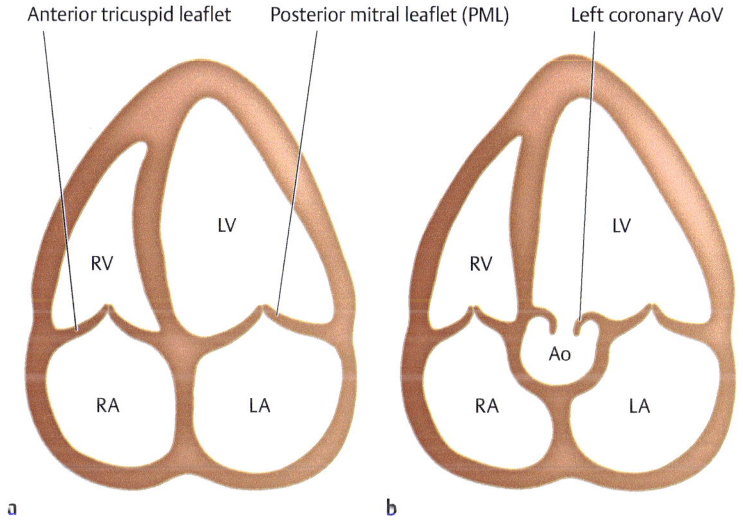

Fig. 3.8 Apical 4-chamber and 5-chamber view. Schematic depiction.
Ao = aorta
AoV = aortic valve
LA = left atrium
LV = left ventricle
MV = mitral valve
RA = right atrium
RV = right ventricle
TV = tricuspid valve.
a Four-chamber view.
b Five-chamber view.

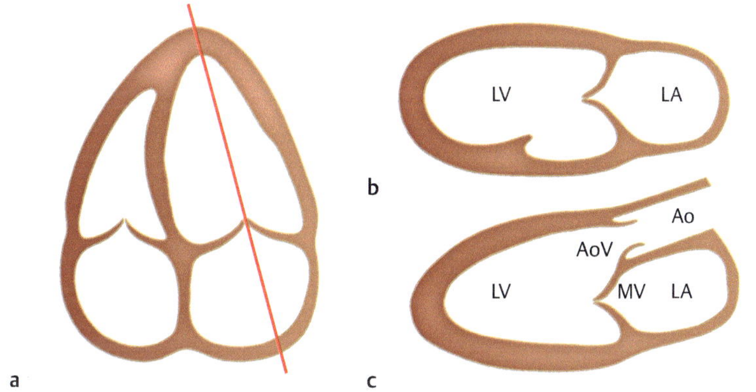

Fig. 3.9 Apical 2-chamber view and LVOT cross-section. Schematic depiction. From an apical view, by rotating the transducer 90° in the 4-chamber view (**a**, red line), the apical 2-chamber view (**b**) and the apical long axis or LVOT cross-section (**c**) can be acquired by rotating the transducer appropriately.
Ao = aorta
AoV = aortic valve
LA = left atrium
LV = left ventricle
MV = mitral valve
a Four-chamber view.
b Apical 2-chamber view.
c Apical long axis or LVOT cross-section.

A suprasternal view (▶ Fig. 3.4) is used to depict the aortic arch and the vessels branching off from it, whereas subcostal or subxiphoidal access is often also selected to depict a 4-chamber view.

Using the named sectional planes, the morphology and function of various different regions of the heart, including the valves, can be evaluated visually and quantitatively in real time. This is of great significance for heart defects that correlate to abnormal positioning of the atrioventricular valve.

M-mode is generally used to determine cardiac diameter (e.g., left-ventricular end diastolic diameter) in the parasternal long and short axes in a standardized manner (▶ Fig. 3.2 and ▶ Fig. 3.3). Segmental fiber shortening can be determined using these diameters from M-mode. This shortening represents the shortening fraction percentage of the left ventricle and is determined using the following formula[1]:

$$\text{FS}\ (\%) = \left(\frac{\text{LV} - \text{EDD} - \text{LV} - \text{ESD}}{\text{LV} - \text{EDD}}\right) \times 100$$

where

FS = segmental fiber shortening in %
LV–EDD = left ventricular end diastolic diameter
LV–ESD = left ventricular end systolic diameter.

Three-Dimensional Echocardiography

This newer development is based either on data sets acquired using multiplanar reconstruction with 2-D echocardiography in regular intervals of the transducer held in a parallel, rotated, or fanlike fashion[4,6,7] or using data acquired via real-time 3-D echocardiography.[8] The latter requires recording only a single cardiac cycle. Modern echo devices make it easier and faster to acquire 3-D volumes. Most high-performing echo devices possess digital 3-D volume transducers. In particular, acquiring 3-D volume data from a single cardiac cycle appears to be of particular importance (▶ Fig. 3.10 and ▶ Fig. 3.11).

For younger children who cannot hold their breath or patients with frequent extrasystole, this new technique has made it possible to collect 3-D data sets for reconstructing intracardiac structures or measuring *ventricular volume.* Most importantly, however, the new software can help record and calculate the volumes of the left and, increasingly, the right ventricle in real time, and thus very rapidly (▶ Fig. 3.12). The end systolic volume (ESV), end diastolic volume (EDV), and ejection fraction of the left ventricle can be calculated easily using this data.

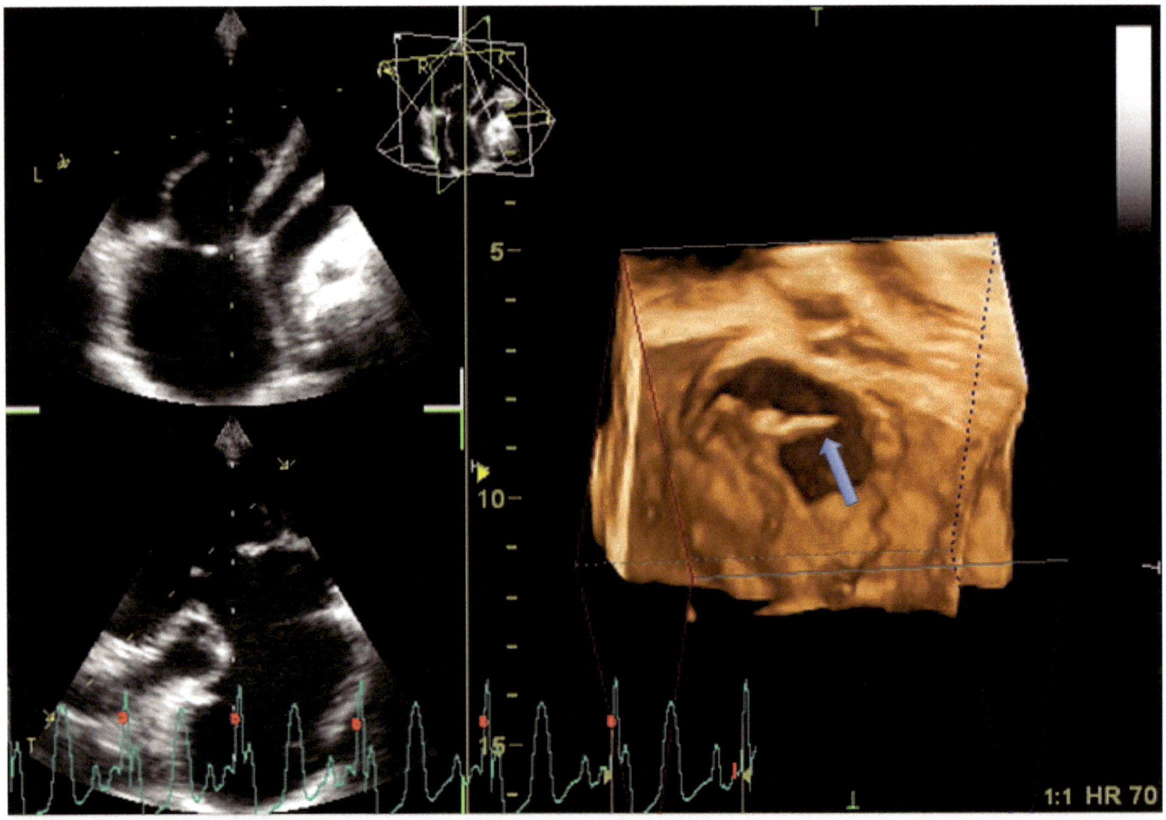

Fig. 3.10 3-D echocardiography. 3-D reconstruction of the tricuspid valve (before surgical reconstruction) for an 11-year-old girl with Ebstein's anomaly, a free-floating leaflet (blue arrow), and chordal rupture.

By dividing left ventricular volume into 17 segments, changes can be calculated in the respective segments of the left ventricle during a single cardiac cycle. Heterogeneous changes can be identified in cases of dyssynchrony. An index known as the *SDI* (Systolic Dyssynchrony Index) can be determined using the changes calculated in the left ventricle's individual volume segments (▸ Fig. 3.13).[9]

Note

Modern 3-D echo devices only need relatively short processing times after data acquisition, thanks to modern, fast, high-performance transducers, and are no longer subject to movement, arrhythmia, or respiratory artifacts due to the introduction of single cardiac cycle acquisition. Under favorable imaging conditions, there is a very strong correlation of the recorded volumes with MRI results for the left ventricle, as well as for the right ventricle (though in a more limited scope).[6,7]

Doppler Echocardiography

Doppler Principle

Compared to purely imaging 2-D echocardiography, Doppler echocardiography technology also provides the opportunity to acquire information about flow direction, velocity, and flow quality (laminar or turbulent flow). Noninvasive determination of blood flow velocity[3,10] is based on the application of the Doppler effect. This means that sonic waves reflected by moving objects perceive a change in frequency directly proportional to the object's velocity. Velocity v is calculated using the Doppler equation:

$$\mathrm{Fd} = \left(\frac{2 \times \mathrm{v} \times \cos\alpha}{\mathrm{c}}\right) \times \mathrm{f}_0$$

where

fd = change in frequency (Doppler frequency or shift)
f_0 = emitted frequency (e.g., 3.5 MHz)
v = blood flow velocity
α = angle between ultrasound waves and blood flow
c = sonic velocity in human tissue (approx. 1,530 m/s).

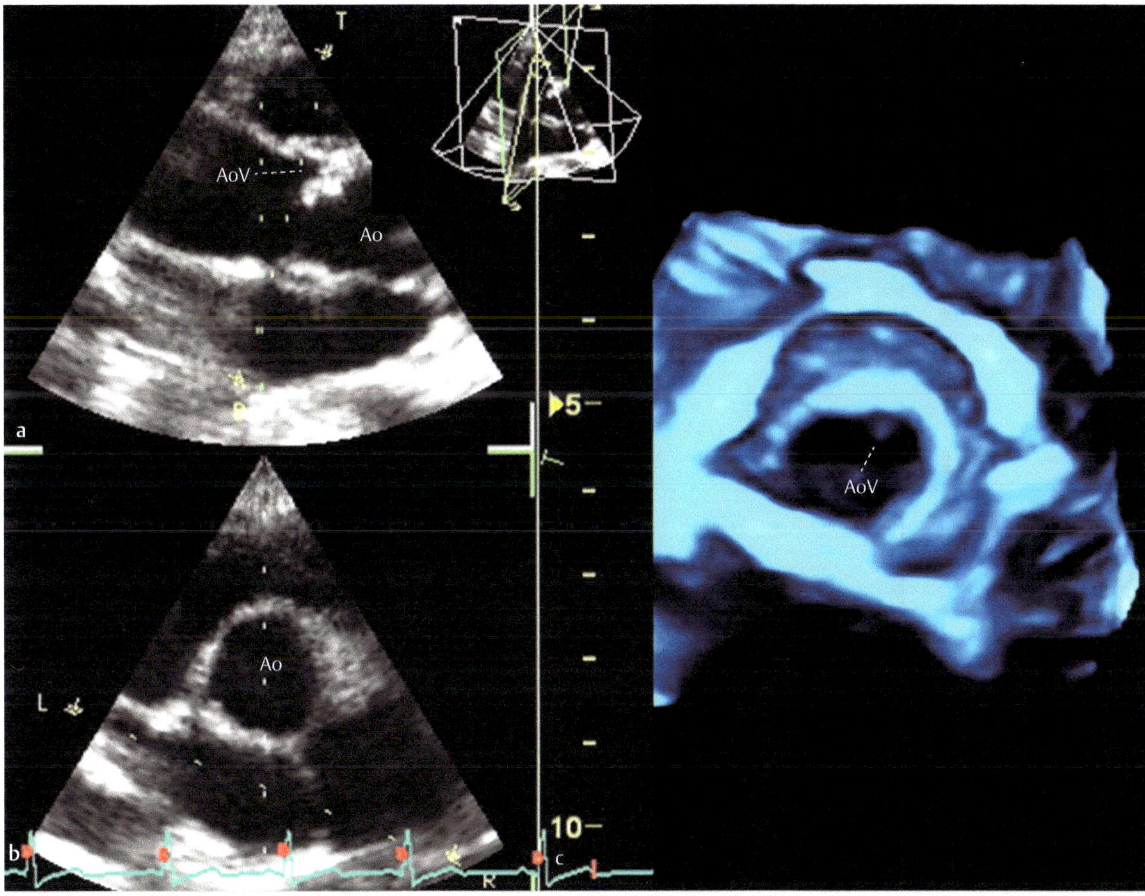

Fig. 3.11 3-D echocardiography.
Ao = aorta
AoV = aortic valve

a LVOT reconstructed from a 3-D data set with a thickened aortic valve.
b 5-chamber view with a central ascending aorta.
c 3-D reconstruction of a unicuspid aortic valve (before surgical valve reconstruction) in a 15-year-old girl with a combined aortic vitium.

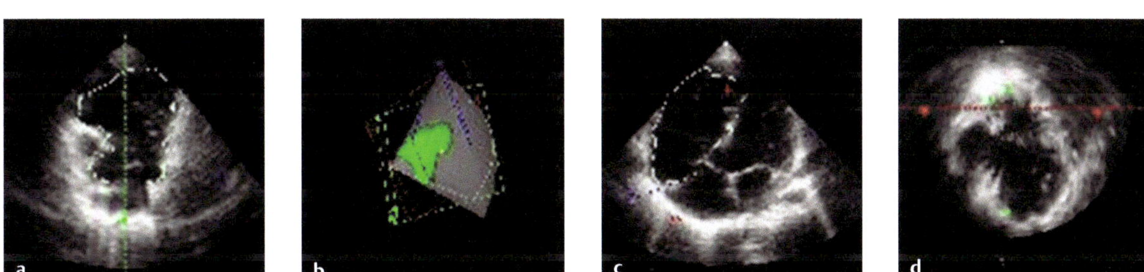

Fig. 3.12 3-D echocardiography. 3-D volume reconstruction of the right ventricle in a patient with surgically treated tetralogy of Fallot and a significantly enlarged right ventricle.

a Long-axis planimetry of the right ventricle (2-chamber view).
b Total volume of the enlarged right ventricle determined using planimetry.
c Long-axis planimetry of the right ventricle (4-chamber view).
d Short-axis planimetry of the right ventricle.

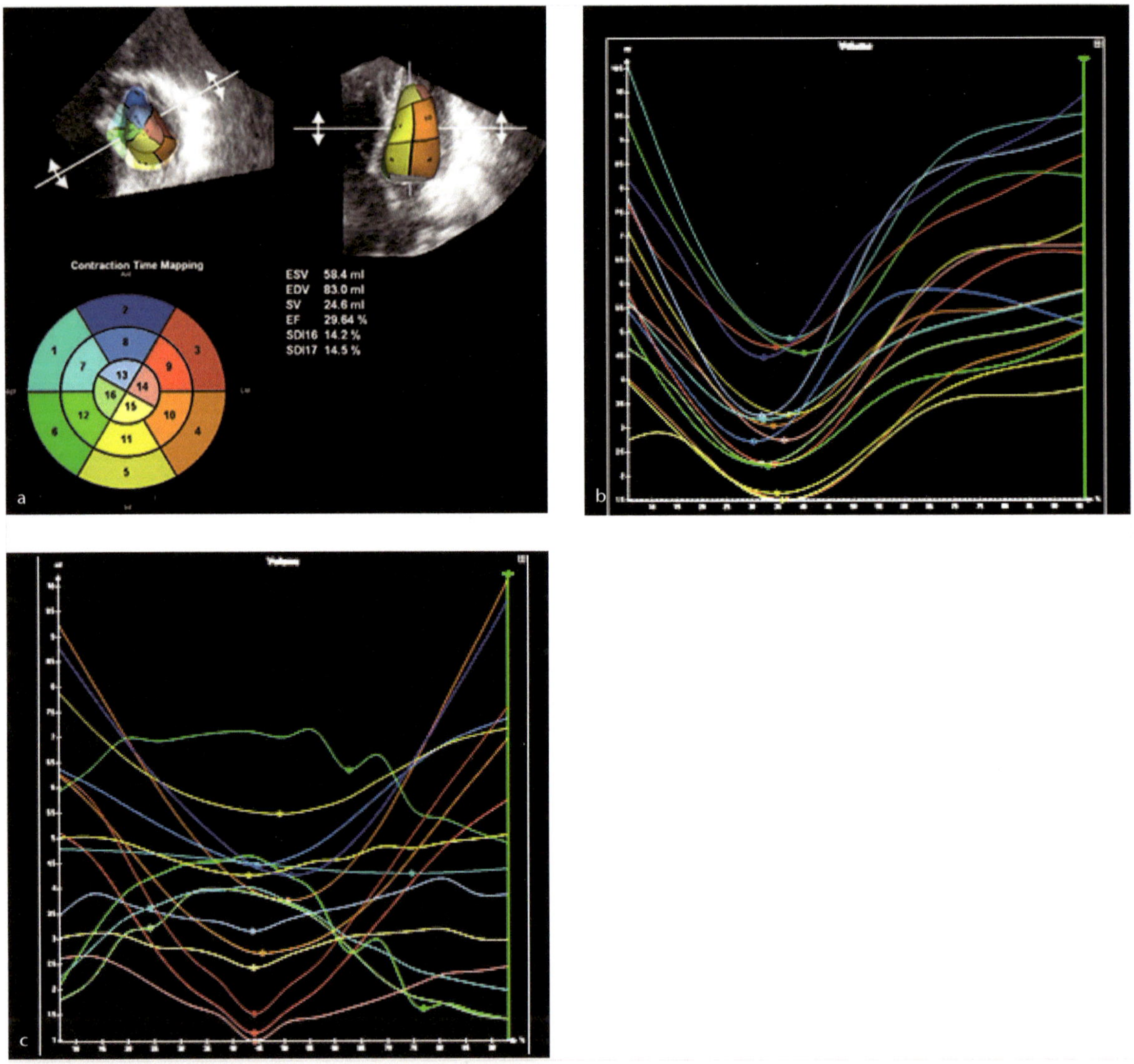

Fig. 3.13 3-D echocardiography.
EDV = end diastolic volume
EF = ejection fraction
ESV = end systolic volume
SDI = systolic dyssynchrony index
SV = stroke volume

a Real-time 3-D reconstruction of a male patient's left ventricle after correcting his pulmonary atresia correction. The left ventricular volume is subdivided into 17 segments according to the AHA, and the decrease in volume is measured and recorded in the individual segments during systole within a single cardiac cycle. At 29.64%, the patient's left ventricular ejection fraction is reduced significantly.
b Segmental curves of a test subject's homogeneous volume change. All of the curves demonstrate a largely synchronous course.
c Dyssynchronous volume changes in a male patient a from which an SDI can be calculated, which appears to be closely associated with left ventricular function. In particular, septal segments 1, 6, 7, and 12 demonstrate significant asynchrony after correcting the patient's pulmonary atresia.

The three systems of Doppler echocardiography[10] are as follows:

- *Continuous-wave Doppler (CW Doppler):* CW Doppler records all flow velocities along the sonic ray. It possesses a large penetration depth and allows high flow velocities to be recorded and quantified. Unlike a PW Doppler, however, it cannot precisely localize the site with the highest flow velocity.
- *Pulsed-wave (PW) Doppler:* PW Doppler allows flow velocities to be recorded only within a "measuring range," in a sample volume (measured volume). It possesses less penetration depth than a CW Doppler. Unlike the CW Doppler, however, PW Doppler allows precise localization of the recorded flow velocity.
- *Color Doppler:* This type of Doppler is represented primarily by color Doppler, and constitutes the most

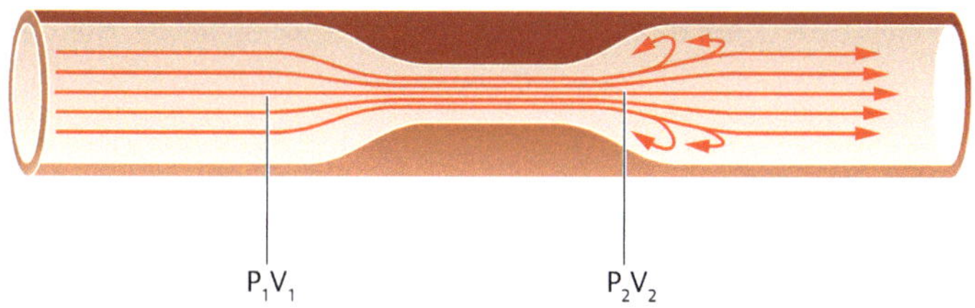

Fig. 3.14 Flow ratios in vascular or valvular stenoses. Schematic depiction. Application of the Bernoulli equation to assess pressure gradients based on maximum flow velocity using Doppler sonography.

Table 3.1 Graduation of the aortic valve stenosis in Doppler ultrasound.[4]

Parameter	Degree of severity of aortic valve stenosis			
	Low	Moderate	Significant	Severe
Δp_{max} (mmHg)	<30	30–60	61–90	>90
Δp_{mean} (mmHg)	<20	20–30	31–50	>50
AVOA (cm^2)	>1.00	1.00–0.75	0.74–0.50	<0.5

AVOA, aortic valve orifice area; Δp_{max}, maximum pressure gradient over the aortic valve, determined using CW Doppler; Δp_{mean}, mean pressure gradient over the aortic valve, determined using PW Doppler.

common type of Doppler echocardiography. The median flow velocities determined using many measurement volumes (sample volumes) are depicted in a color-coded 2-D image. Color Doppler echocardiography delivers not just information about blood flow velocity, flow turbulence, and flow volume, but also information about the direction and quality of blood flow in real time. Thus, it can be used for orientation, qualitative assessment of the extent of valve insufficiency or stenosis, or assessment of shunt size in cases of ASD or VSD.

Stenosis Quantification

If an obstruction (stenosis) is present in a vessel or valve, this leads to increased blood flow velocity in this area. When blood flow velocity is measured immediately before and immediately after the stenosis (▶ Fig. 3.14), the Bernoulli equation is applicable. This means that maximum velocity (velocity behind the stenosis) and the pressure gradients measured at the site of the stenosis are directly proportional to one another. Since velocity before the stenosis is generally relatively low (less than 1 m/s), it can often be disregarded.[11] This results in a simplified formula for calculation, which can also be used to evaluate gradients in MRI flow measurements[5,12]:

$$p_1 - p_2 = 4 \times v_2^2$$

where

p_1 = pressure before the stenosis
p_2 = pressure after the stenosis
v_2 = maximum flow velocity immediately after the stenosis.

In addition to assessing pressure gradients for valvular and vascular stenoses, Doppler echocardiography also collects data for a number of additional parameters to assess valve function.[1,3,4,10] Calculating aortic valve orifice area via the continuity equation from aortic diameter caudal to the aortic valve and maximum flow velocity in LVOT and distal to the aortic valve is of particular practical significance.

$$\text{AVOA} = \pi \times \left(\frac{d}{2}\right)^2 \times \left(\frac{v_{LVOT}}{v_{max}}\right)$$

where

AVOA = aortic valve orifice area
d = diameter of LVOT caudal to the aortic valve
v_{LVOT} = maximum flow velocity in the LVOT
v_{max} = maximum flow velocity distal to the aortic valve.

The *graduation of the aortic valve stenosis* should be recorded via Doppler as an example (Table 3.1). The mean gradient above the aortic valve correlates best to aortic valve gradients measured invasively.

Note

Care should be taken that the maximum and mean pressure gradient of the aortic valve are taken subaortically in the 5-chamber view, suprasternally from the jugulum, or right-parasternally. Additional criteria, such as hypertrophy of the left ventricle and ECG changes, must be taken into account when assessing the degree of severity.

Unlike in MRI, *valve incompetence grading* in Doppler echocardiography (in contrast to stenoses grading) can usually be only assessed only semiquantitatively due to the jet length and width in color Doppler or by using signal intensity or signal gradient in CW Doppler (Table 3.2).[3,4] In addition, the influence of the insufficiency on peripheral flow in the ascending aorta can also be assessed using Doppler. The volume and duration of diastolic regurgitation in the aorta provide additional qualitative information regarding the degree of aortic valve insufficiency.

3.1.3 Special and Newer Techniques

Transesophageal Echocardiography

For respirated patients or for patients who cannot be imaged easily from a transthoracic view, the heart can be assessed using echocardiography and Doppler echocardiography via a transesophageal probe with an integrated transducer. This improves the depiction of cardiac structures and vessels adjacent to the esophagus, since it leads to less sonic absorption compared to TTE.[4] For these reasons, high-frequency transducers (5–9 MHz) can also be used, which improves spatial resolution significantly. A distinction is made between monoplanar (only allows transverse imaging), biplanar, and multiplanar probes.

Main areas of application for transesophageal echocardiography (TEE) include the following:

- Assessing atrial structures (e.g., clots, tumors, intraatrial septal defects, valve morphology and function, changes in valves in the sense of endocarditis vegetation)
- Assessing LVOT morphology
- Assessing the aortic valves (unicuspid, bicuspid, or tricuspid aortic valves) and their function
- Assessing the morphology and size of the ascending aorta (e.g., aortic dissection)

Note

The size and morphology of interatrial septal defects, in particular, can be examined better from different angles using TEE (▶ Fig. 3.15 and ▶ Fig. 3.16).

Table 3.2 Graduation of aortic valve insufficiency measured via Doppler.[4]

Parameter	Aortic valve insufficiency		
	Low	Moderate	Severe
Jet width in color Doppler/LVOT width	< ⅓	< ⅔	> ⅔
Signal gradient in CW Doppler (m/s²)	< 2.5	> 2.5–4.0	> 4.0

CW, continuous wave; LVOT, left ventricular outflow tract.

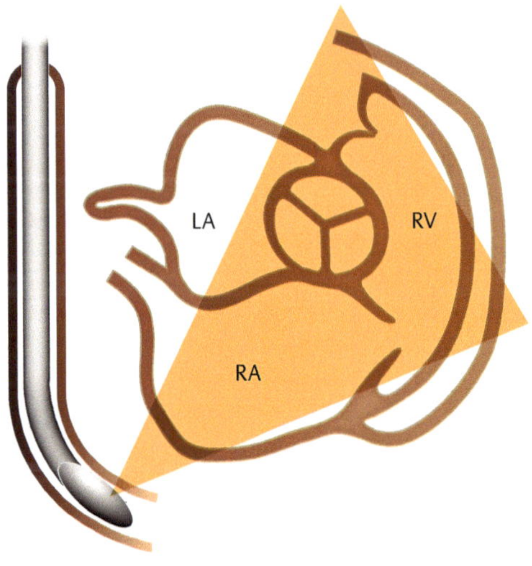

a

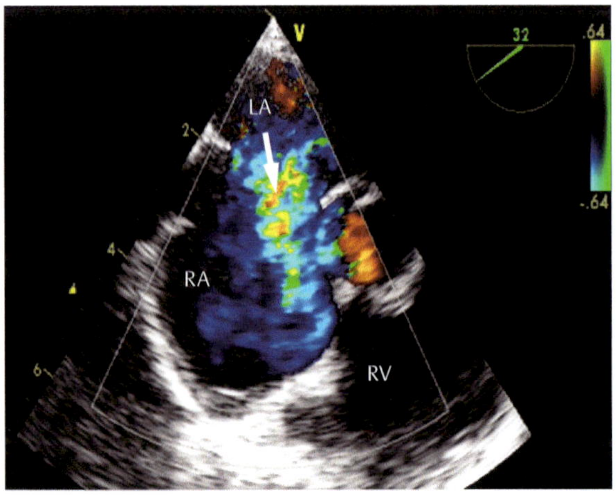

b

Fig. 3.15 TEE. Depiction of an ASD.
LA = left atrium
RA = right atrium
RV = right ventricle

a Schematic depiction of a TEE being performed and the most clearly visualized cardiac structures.
b Large ASD depicted using TEE, with a significant left-right shunt (arrow) in a male patient with a limited transthoracic acoustic window.

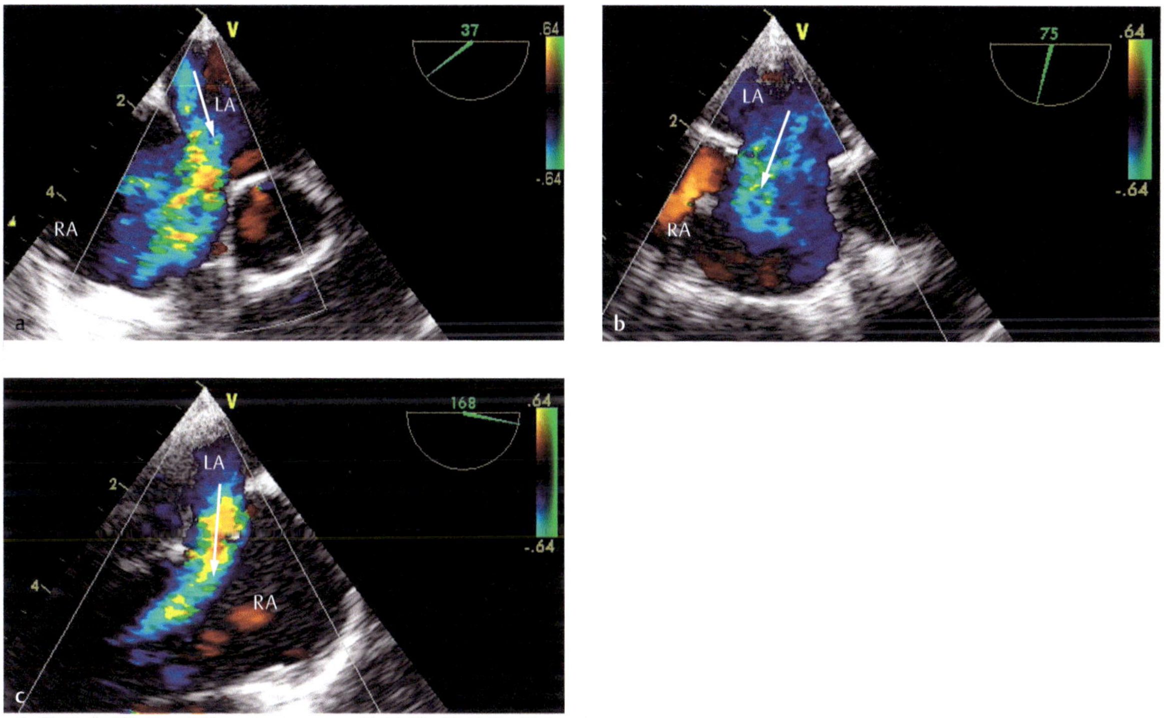

Fig. 3.16 TEE. Depiction of an ASD. The interatrial septum can be clearly depicted via TEE. Multiplanar depiction of the septal defect (**a–c**, arrows) from various angles (0–180°; three angles are shown as an example [angular display listed top right in green]) allowing the size, extent, and shape of a defect to be visualized with precision before an interventional closure.

LA = left atrium
RA = right atrium

a 37° angle.
b 75° angle.
c 168° angle.

In principle, interventional treatments (such as closure of intraatrial communication) can also be performed during TEE exams. Since atrial structures can be depicted so well via TEE, any atrial maneuvers—from probing the defect and pulmonary veins up to placement of an Amplatzer™ septal occluder—can be performed without X-ray exposure (▶ Fig. 3.17).

Stress Echocardiography

Stress echocardiography became widely used in clinical routines for detecting coronary heart disease, particularly as a noninvasive imaging procedure,[13] in the 1990s. Since then, it is used only rarely to diagnose disorders during preinterventional and postinterventional diagnostic procedures for patients with congenital heart defects—and even then, mostly to diagnose ischemia. This is particularly true for patients with limitations in performing, assessing, or interpreting stress ECG tests, or with positive clinical pictures but negative stress ECG results.[4] Stress can be induced via bicycle ergometry or, more commonly, using pharmacological means. The latter has been tried and tested particularly in patients with limited exercise capacity or physical compliance due to age or illness. The main principle of stress echocardiography is based on proving the presence of wall motion abnormalities in the left ventricle after stress-induced ischemia (▶ Fig. 3.18). For this reason, the stressor dobutamine[13,14] is often preferred over vasodilators (dipyridamole, adenosine)[15] in stress echocardiography. Recently, there have been promising trials using echo contrast agents[16] to examine myocardial perfusion under stress conditions. Thus, vasodilators are becoming more prominent.

The known methods of wall motion analysis in stress echocardiography have also been applied to MRI in recent years. This has led to significant improvement in image quality, particularly for patients with limited feasibility for echocardiography due to a poor acoustic window. Overall, these improvements have expressed themselves via higher sensitivity and specificity in detecting coronary heart disease.[17]

Stress echocardiography is used not just for diagnosing ischemia, but also for myocardial viability diagnostic purposes in the form of low-dose dobutamine stress (5–20 µg/[kg x min]). The examiner takes advantage of the positive inotropic effects of the sympathomimetic, in that improved contractility in areas previously afflicted with disrupted contractions under low-dose dobutamine stress[13,14] is seen as an indication of a viable myocardium.

Exam Procedure

The following views are generally recorded for all types of stress tests—both at rest and under stress conditions—in order to be able to draw conclusions about wall motion in the various segments of the left ventricle:

- *Parasternal* (▸ Fig. 3.4): long and short axis
- *Apical:* 2-chamber and 4-chamber view, long axis

The American Society of Echocardiography's 18-segment model is a common segment model for the left ventricle (▸ Fig. 3.19)[18]: The acquired sectional planes are saved on video or in digital form and then assessed visually or quantitatively at various stress levels. Continuous monitoring of ECG and blood pressure at regular intervals during the stress test is mandatory.

Atropine Administration

In cases of inadequate increase in frequency (target frequency = 220 - age in years × 0.85) under pharmacological stress, a fractional dose of a total of 1 mg of atropine can be administered intravenously (▸ Fig. 3.20).[4]

Termination of Stress ECG Exams

The same termination criteria apply as with stress ECG exams. In addition, a stress ECG exam is terminated if new wall motion abnormalities or side effects to medications occur.

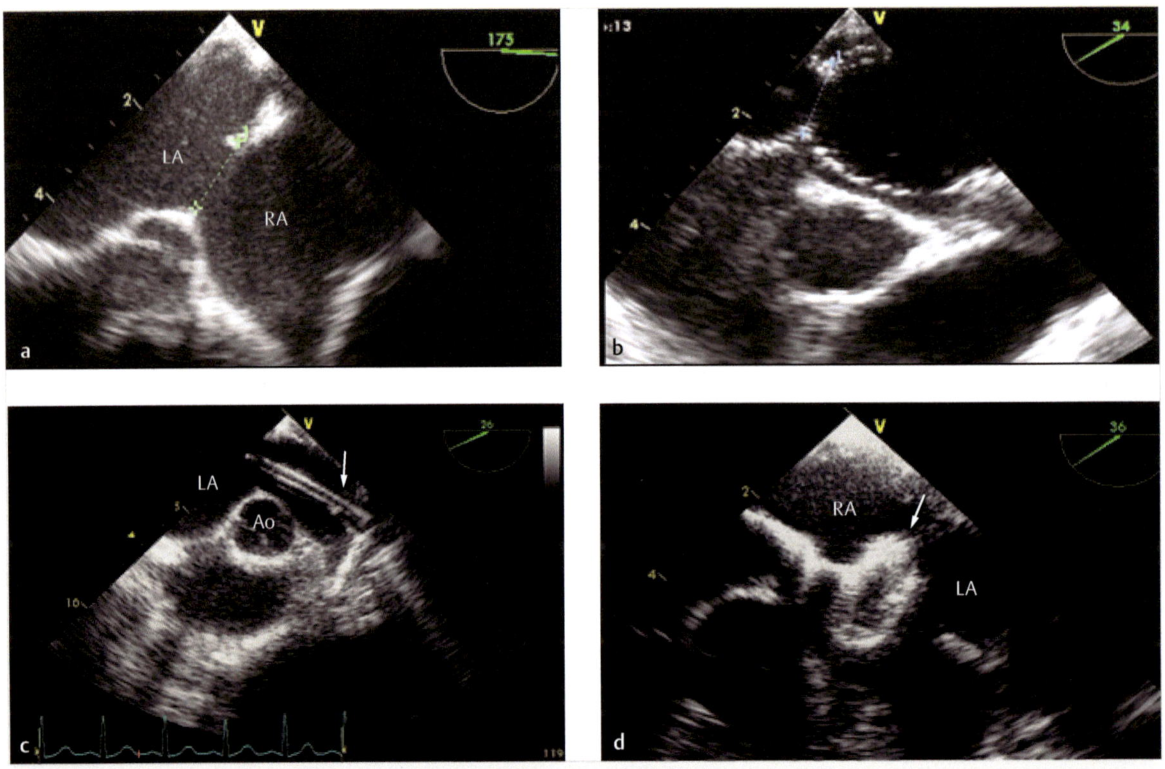

Fig. 3.17 Therapeutic closure of intraatrial communication during a TEE exam.
Ao = aorta
LA = left atrium
RA = right atrium

a Thorough measurement of the defect's native size.
b A guide wire is subsequently placed in the left pulmonary vein via a catheter.
c The sizing balloon is then introduced into the defect via the wire and inflated carefully. This allows precise assessment of the defect's size. An appropriate catheter (arrow) is then introduced into the left atrium using the same guide wire.
d The appropriate Amplatzer™ septal occluder is placed using the catheter during TEE monitoring, and only the left atrial disc is deployed (arrow). *(Continued)*

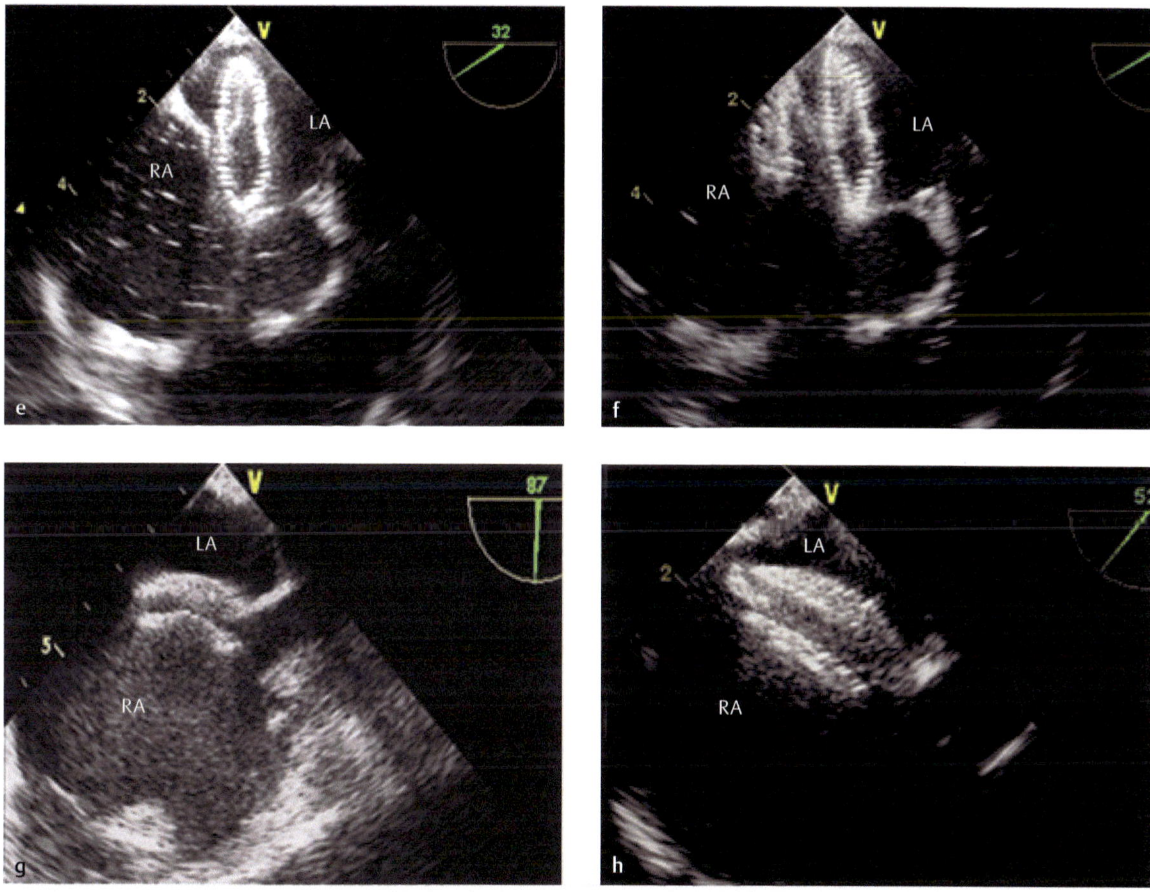

Fig 3.17 (*Continued*) **Therapeutic closure of intraatrial communication during a TEE exam.**
Ao = aorta
LA = left atrium
RA = right atrium

- **e** The left atrial disk is then adapted carefully to the intraatrial septum or defect.
- **f** The right atrial disc is carefully released by slowly withdrawing the wire, thereby closing the defect.
- **g** During TEE monitoring, a stress test is performed by pulling and pushing on the probe before the occluder is detached from the wire.
- **h** The placement and position of the occluder are examined and monitored from different angles while the occluder is still attached to the wire.

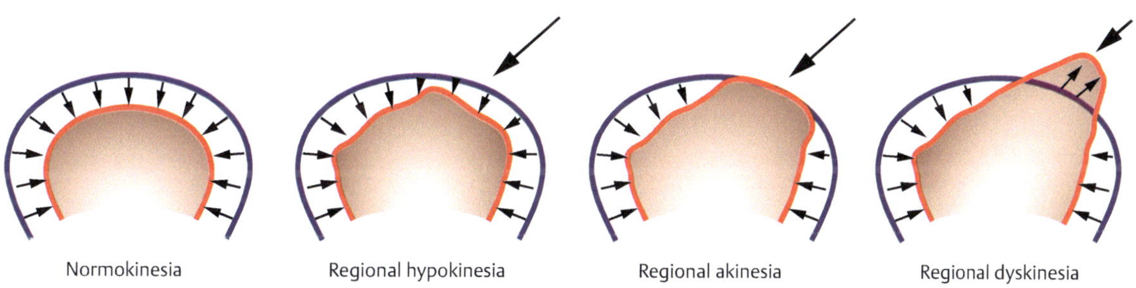

Fig. 3.18 Echocardiographic wall motion analysis. Schematic depiction. The blue contour indicates the end diastolic and the red contour, the end systolic border of the left ventricle in a 4-chamber view in a healthy patient and in the presence of various pathologies.

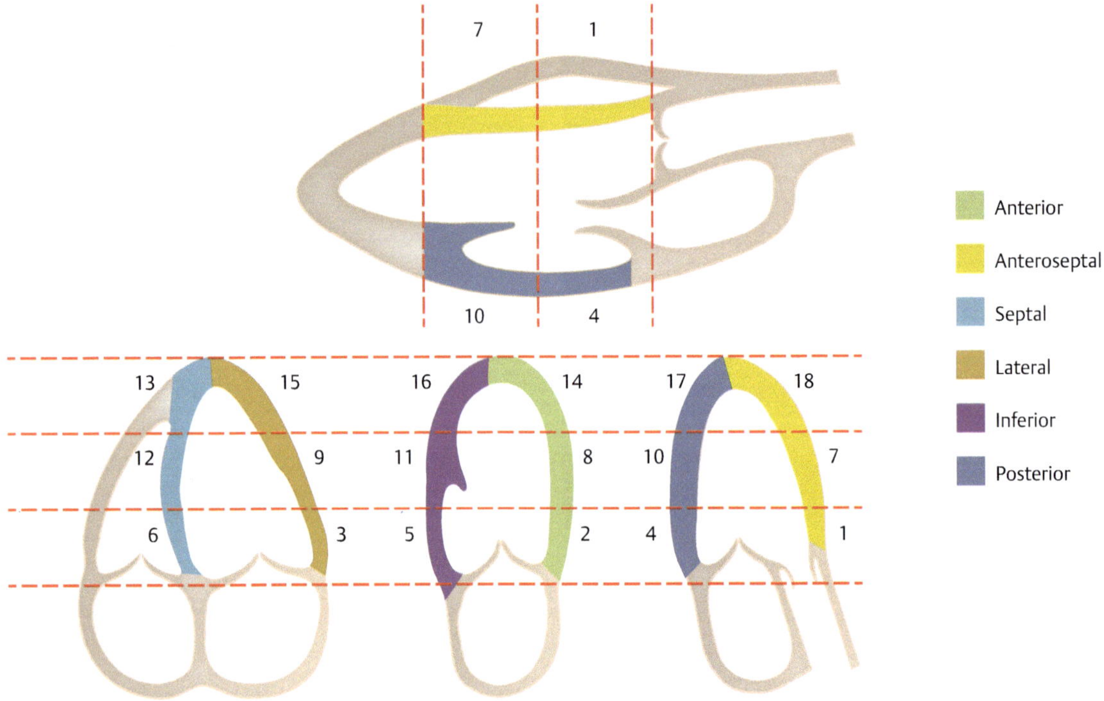

Fig. 3.19 American Society of Echocardiography's modified 18-segment model. Schematic depiction. The numbers indicate the 18 segments.

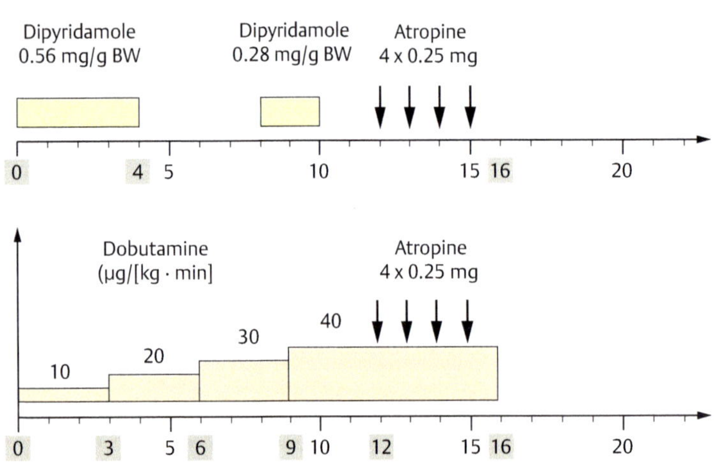

Fig. 3.20 Atropine administration. Schematic depiction. Stress protocols with dipyridamole and dobutamine. The highlighted minute labels indicate the point of recording.
BW = body weight

Stress ECG in Cases of Congenital Heart Defects

To date, only limited experience exists for stress ECG in the field of congenital heart defects. In addition to malformed semilunar valves or seemingly insignificant morphological narrowing near the isthmus, latent structures can be identified and visualized under pharmacological stress conditions. Increases in heart frequency can likewise be identified by administering Alupent. This could become more important in the future; to date, it has only been possible to perform many invasive and noninvasive exams on children with congenital heart defects while the patients were sleeping or sedated. The German Competence Network for Congenital Heart Defects, among others, has performed the first patient trials under low-dose dobutamine stress conditions after surgical correction of tetralogy of Fallot. The initial results indicate that it may be possible, in the future, to diagnose right ventricular failure at an earlier stage, and thus to provide better treatment management options.[19]

Furthermore, it is to be expected that quantitative analyses of regional myocardial velocities and deformations under stress conditions will also permit important and interesting conclusions to be drawn regarding abnormal

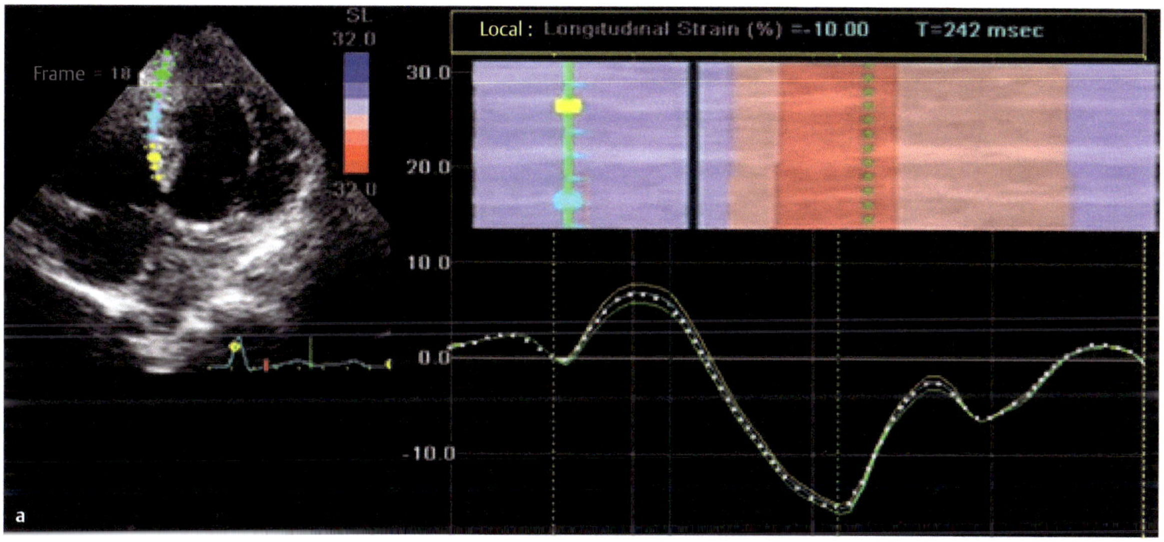

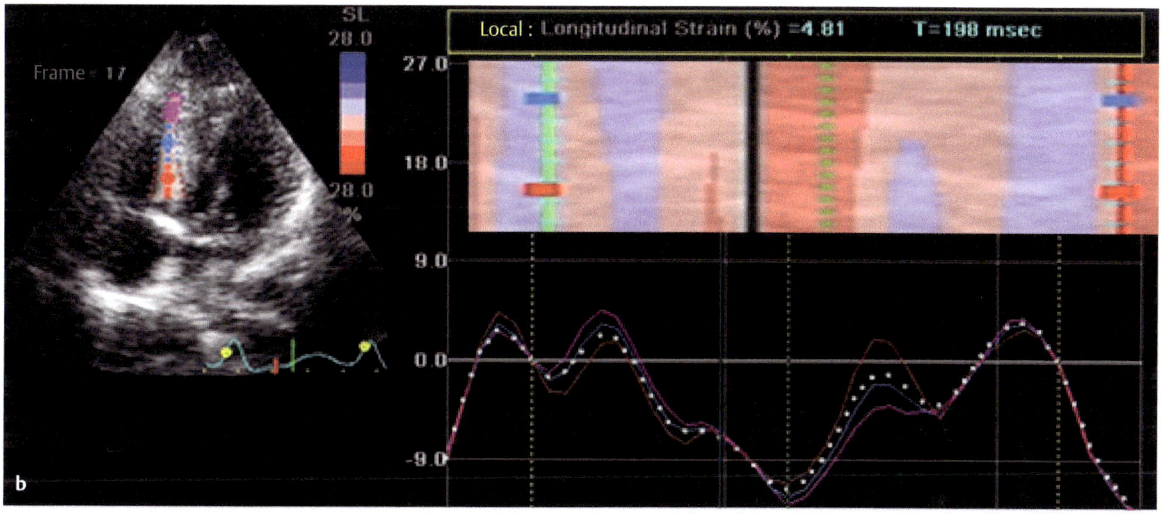

Fig. 3.21 Quantitative analyses of regional myocardial velocity and deformation under stress conditions.
a Deformation (strain) in the interventricular septum of a boy with pressure overload in the left ventricle due to an aortic valve stenosis.
b Clear visibility of post-systolic contraction as an expression of possible myocardial fibrosis after a pharmacological stress test using Alupent.

regional myocardial function or dyssynchronous contractile behavior in the left and right ventricles. In the example case of a boy with aortic valve stenosis and myocardial hypertrophy of the interventricular septum, a significant change in the deformation was visible before and after being subjected to pharmacological stress conditions (▶ Fig. 3.21). The new methods of 2-D strain or speckle tracking should also be considered when assessing myocardial function under stress conditions.

Second-Harmonic Imaging

The image quality in native 2-D echocardiography was improved significantly by implementing tissue-harmonic imaging. Nowadays, this technology is a standard option. When using echo contrast agents (known as micro bubbles),[20] the use of second-harmonic oscillation allows the contours of the endocardium to be depicted more clearly and artifacts to be suppressed more consistently.[21,22] Special transducers that emit with a single ultrasound frequency and receive with a double ultrasound frequency are used. This approach is recommended for patients who are difficult to image.[23] Image quality is not, however, improved immediately adjacent to the transducer (within 3 cm).[4] This echo contrast agent also makes it possible to visualize myocardial perfusion.[16]

Tissue Doppler Echocardiography and Strain Analysis

The Doppler principle is used by these relatively new examination methods in order to quantify myocardial motion (myocardial velocity) by applying special velocity and amplitude filters. Low-velocity (under 20 cm/s),[24,25] high-amplitude myocardial signals are recorded, while high-velocity, low-amplitude blood flow signals are filtered out. Both PW and color Doppler are used. Myocardial tissue Doppler has not yet established itself in routine diagnostics. A combined approach using color Doppler to assess myocardial wall motion during stress, however, appears useful. Earlier approaches hope for improved characterization of diastolic wall motion abnormalities,[26] meaning also in cases of complex congenital heart defects.[27]

Tissue Velocity

Tissue velocity is the velocity with which the myocardium moves during the cardiac cycle. Velocity is defined as displacement over time:

$$v = \frac{\Delta x}{\Delta t}$$

where
v = velocity
x = distance
t = time.

Tissue velocity is listed in cm/s. Movement toward the ultrasound probe is considered positive velocity, while movement in the opposite direction is considered negative velocity. The velocity curve is a direct result of the Doppler data (▶ Fig. 3.22 and ▶ Fig. 3.23).[28]

Deformation (Strain)

An object's deformation with respect to its original size is called "strain." The myocardium is a 3-D body that can deform in any direction during contraction. If we simplify matters and only consider deformation in a single spatial dimension, then average deformation can be expressed mathematically as follows (▶ Fig. 3.24)[28,29]:

$$\text{deformation} = \frac{(L - L_0)}{L_0}$$

where
deformation = strain
L = length at the end of deformation
L_0 = length at time t_0

The deformation is a non-dimensional size indicated in percent (%). Increased object length compared to the initial length is indicated as a positive value, and a decreased length, as a negative value. Linear dimensions are necessary for calculating deformation (strain). Since no changes in length can be recorded during echocardiographical measurements, the size of the strain must be calculated using velocity gradients. These gradients can be recorded via tissue Doppler—or, more recently, via B-mode images—by dividing the distance in myocardial velocity between two points

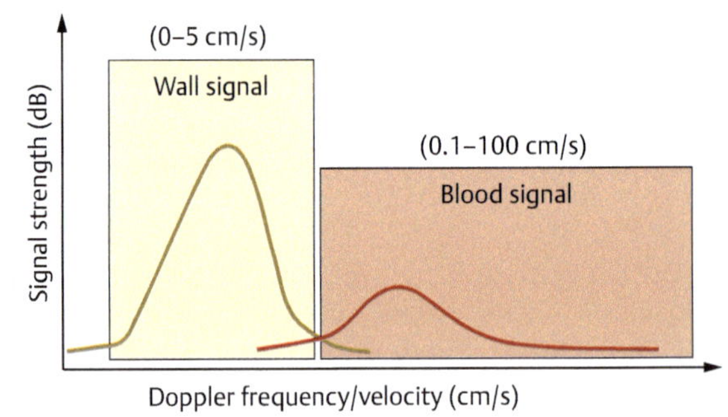

Fig. 3.22 Tissue Doppler ECG. Schematic depiction. Recording of wall velocities and deformations at defined points. Special filters are applied in order to suppress signals from the blood and record only signals from the myocardial wall.

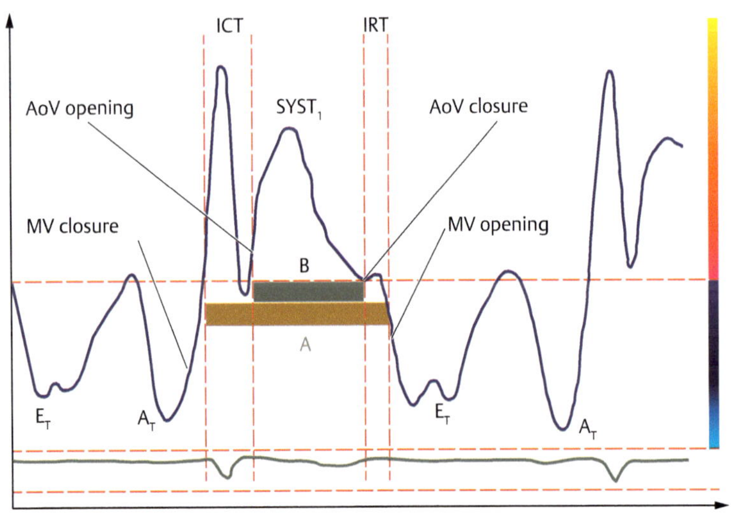

Fig. 3.23 Tissue Doppler ECG. Example schematic depiction of wall velocities and time intervals derived from a tissue Doppler during a cardiac cycle. In addition to determining systolic, early diastolic, and late diastolic velocity, it is also possible to calculate important time intervals, such as isovolumetric contraction and relaxation time. This allows the Tei index to be calculated as a parameter of the global function using the following formula: Tei index = (A – B)/B.
AoV = aortic valve
A_T = late diastolic velocity
E_T = early diastolic velocity
ICT = isovolumetric contraction time
IRT = isovolumetric relaxation time
$Syst_T$ = systolic velocity

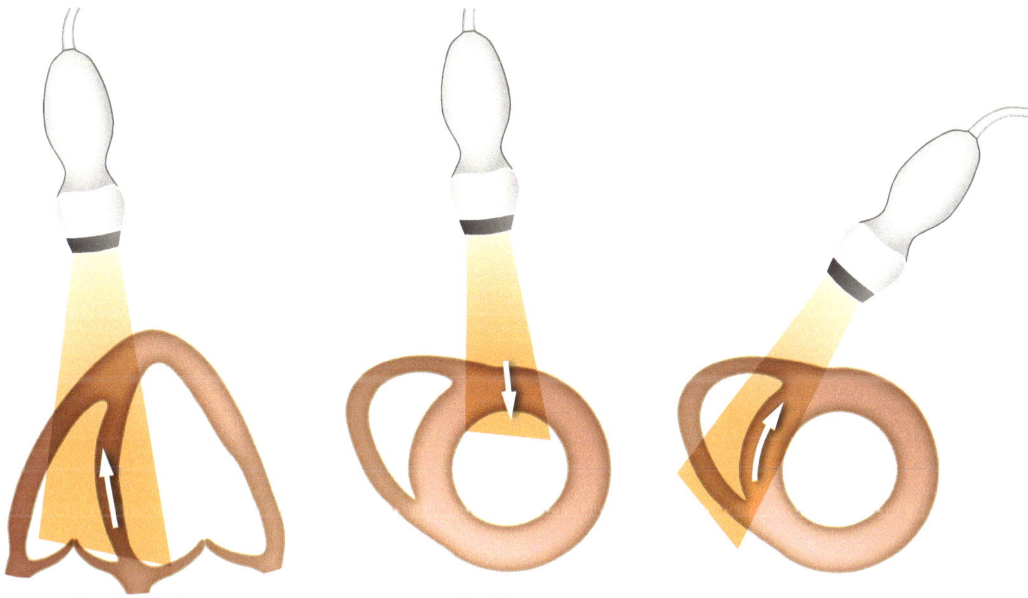

Fig. 3.24 Myocardial strain or deformation. Schematic depiction. The longitudinal, radial, and circumferential myocardial wall deformations can be determined using special software and a more precise configuration for data acquisition.

(along the ultrasonic beam) at a defined distance from one another by the original distance between those two points. This allows us to calculate the deformation rate (strain rate):

$$SR = \frac{(v_2 - v_1)}{L}$$

where
SR = strain rate = deformation rate
v_1, v_2 = velocities between two different points separated by distance L.

If an integral forms over any time interval of the strain-rate curve, the change in length during this interval is calculated as follows:

$$\frac{L(t)}{L_0} = \int SR \times dt$$

where
L(t) = length of object at time t
L_0 = length of object at time t_0
SR = strain rate = deformation rate
t = time

The equation can be further adapted to reflect the relationship between strain and strain rate, as follows[30]:

$$\text{deformation} = \exp\left(\int SR \times dt\right) - 1$$

where
deformation = strain
SR = strain rate
t = time

Deformation Rate (Strain Rate)

The strain rate is the deformation rate of the myocardial tissue. It is considered to be the deformation of the myocardium within a specific time interval, and uses the unit s^{-1}. Average strain rate can be calculated mathematically as a quotient of deformation and time:

$$SR = \frac{\Delta strain}{\Delta t}$$

where
SR = strain rate
t = time

Strain represents the degree of myocardial deformation between end diastole and end systole, whereas strain rate represents the velocity of the deformation. Thus, a strain rate of 0.2 describes a 20% reduction in length per second. The maximum systolic strain rate represents maximum deformation during systole.

Speckle Tracking (2-D Strain)

This method of measuring wall velocity is based on a different physical principle than the common Doppler method. Estimated velocity can be determined for any point on the myocardial wall, regardless of angle. In doing so, a search pattern is selected around this point in the first image (frame 1). In the following image (frame 2), the analysis program searches for the new position of the previously recorded point (▶ Fig. 3.25). Then the program determines the route over which the point travelled during this time. Thus, velocity can be calculated using displacement within the sequence of images relative to time. Strain and strain rate can both be determined based on velocity (▶ Fig. 3.26).

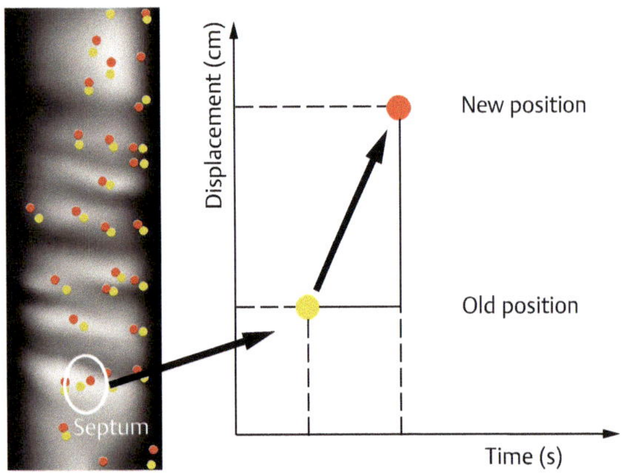

Fig. 3.25 Speckle tracking or 2-D strain. Schematic depiction. Speckle tracking does not use the Doppler principle to calculate myocardial velocity.

3.2 Computed Tomography and Radiation Protection

Willi A. Kalender

3.2.1 Introduction

X-ray CT has been in clinical use since 1972, though it made only minor contributions to cardiac imaging during its first two decades of existence. The scan times were too long to deliver reliable results that could be incorporated into clinical routines. The same was true of MRI, the other tomographic imaging procedure available at that time.

The 1990s, however, brought rapid technological development that continues to this day. The fact that the newest modern technologies can depict the entire heart in less than 1 second with an effective slice scan time of under 100 ms can be attributed to the early development of electron beam CT. This technique of electron beam CT allowed cardiac imaging with a temporal resolution of 50 ms, albeit with limited spatial resolution. In particular, the development of helical CT with the subsequent significant increase in rotational velocity, the development of

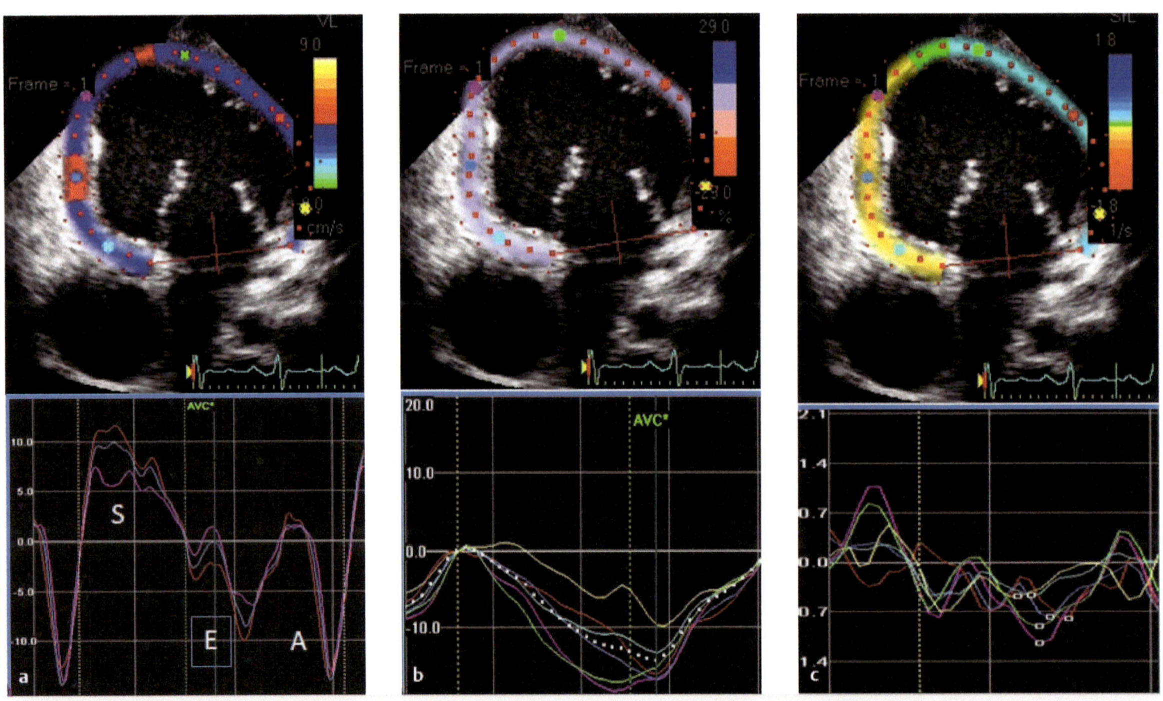

Fig. 3.26 Speckle tracking. The myocardial walls can be recorded semi-automatically using this new method. Wall velocities, deformations, and deformation rates can be calculated in the recorded region using special software.

A = atrial peak
AVC = aortic valve closure
E = early filling peak
S = systolic peak

a Determining wall velocity.
b Determining deformations.
c Determining deformation rates.

multiple-row detector systems, and DSCT (dual source CT) were the primary contributors to cardiac CT as it is performed today.

Accordingly, cardiac CT possesses great potential, especially for the noninvasive visualization of the coronary arteries. To date, it has rarely been used on children with congenital heart defects due to high radiation exposure. The different sections in this chapter will depict and discuss the following subjects: modern CT technology, special technological solutions for CT images of the heart and the resultant image quality, aspects of patient dose and radiation protection, and, finally, recommendations for scan techniques and dose optimization during pediatric cardiac exams.

3.2.2 Modern Computed Tomography Technology

The development of the CT technique and the underlying principles has already been discussed in many publications, including those by Kalender.[31] Therefore, this section will provide only a brief discussion of the newest developments relevant to cardiac CT in cases of congenital heart defects. Since 1989, the basis of modern CT has been the *spiral scan procedure*.[32] It is based on modern slip ring technology—whereby the detector and tubes continually rotate around the patient—and has been implemented in all modern CT scanners for more than a decade. Helical CT allows very rapid, continual scanning of the patient with no gaps along the body's longitudinal axis and, depending on patient compliance, virtually no respiratory artifacts.

The development of *multiple-row detectors* was another extremely significant step in the development of helical CT: this technology, which allowed four slices to be acquired at once, was made available simultaneously by virtually all manufacturers in 1998. Rapid further development has been noted since then, such as the 16-slice scanner in 2001, the 64-slice scanner in 2004, and numerous other detectors that have been placed on the market since then. At times, this was referred to as the "slice race," since development seemed to continue more or less independently of clinical requirements.

Note

Today, there is a broad consensus that the 64-slice scanner is optimal for standard clinical applications. Newer scanners that can record up to 320 slices at once benefit the detector as a whole only for special applications, such as cardiac imaging. They typically use only 64 slices in the inner detector range during the aforementioned standard tasks due to image quality.

A further technological development meant specifically to support cardiac imaging was *DSCT*, namely scanners that use two complete measurement systems, meaning two X-ray tubes and two detectors (▶ Fig. 3.27).[31,33] Both measurement systems are placed at the same level and attached rigidly to one another so that the data from both systems can be combined and contribute jointly to image generation. Devices designed in this fashion offer decisive advantages: the combination of data measured by both

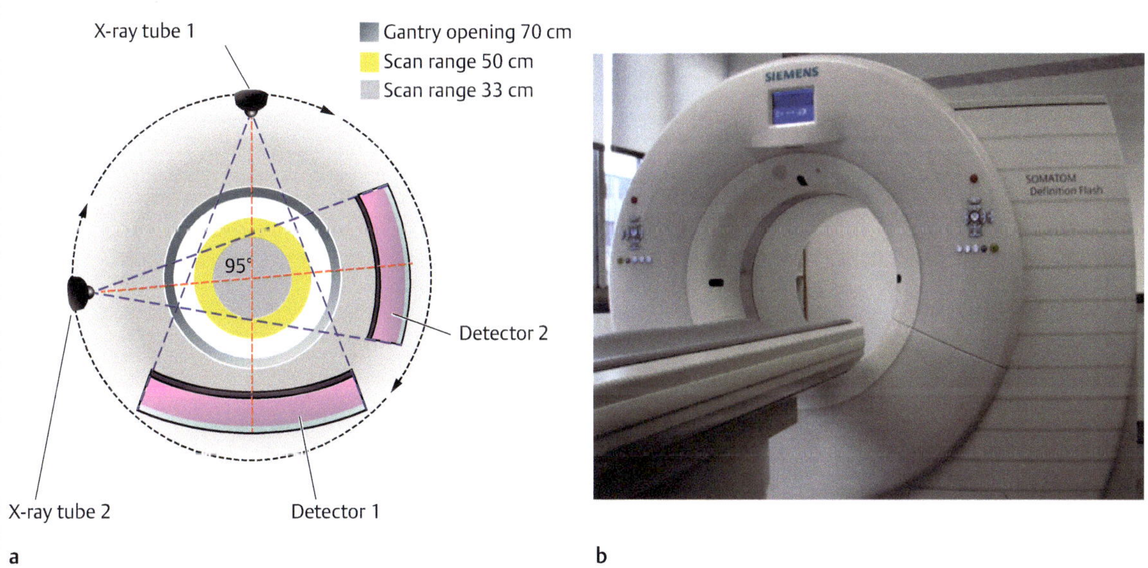

Fig. 3.27 DSCT. CT with two complete measurement systems.[31]
a Schematic depiction of the principle of the scanner.
b Photo of a clinical installation.

systems allows the effective scan time to be cut in half. At minimum, a scan range of 180° plus fan angle is needed for image reconstruction. DSCT scans can provide this information after only a 90° rotation. Furthermore, double X-ray power is available. This is of great importance particularly to images with short effective scan times, since this exposes the patient to the required radiation dosage for the shortest possible period of time.

The most important *scanner and image quality parameters* are summarized in ▶ Table 3.3. Nowadays, modern scanners offer rotation times of 0.27–0.35 seconds for a full 360° rotation. This means that for partial scans, the minimum acquisition time per image is 140–200 ms for simple scanners, but only 75–85 ms for DSCT. The minimum slice thickness is 0.500–0.625 mm, which also yields high 3-D resolution (meaning along the body's longitudinal axis) in all multiplanar and 3-D views. This ensures high, isotropic local resolution; in this context, *isotropic* means that local resolution is approximately the same in all three spatial dimensions, and thus that the examined volume can be viewed and evaluated 3-dimensionally from any orientation. This is of particular importance when examining the coronary arteries, for example. Resolution may be less than 1 mm, but isotropic resolutions of 0.5 mm can be achieved routinely.

Note

The combination of spiral scan, multirow detectors, and high-pitch DSCT (i.e., rapid table shift) permits astonishingly fast acquisition times: it has become possible to routinely perform exams with a table shift of up to 40 cm/s without compromising image quality. This means that images of a complete adult thorax can be acquired in less than 1 second, and less than 0.5 seconds for a child's thorax, respectively. Acquisition times for the heart are circa 0.25 seconds for both cases, and thus are well-suited both for pediatric cardiac imaging without ECG triggering and for less cooperative patients.

Image quality is generally good (▶ Fig. 3.28), and increased acquisition speed does not generally correlate with reduced image quality.[34] Another positive effect of increased acquisition speed is that the patient dosage is reduced significantly due to increased table shift. This will be discussed in greater detail later in this chapter.

Table 3.3 Features of modern high-performance CT scanners.

Parameter	Value
360° rotation time	0.27–0.35 s
Minimum effective scan time	0.75 s
Slice thickness	0.5–0.6 mm
Slices acquired simultaneously	64 (–320)
Z coverage per rotation	40–160 mm
Scan time for full body exams	2–20 s
Scan range	> 1000 mm
Isotropic local resolution	0.4–0.6 mm
Effective dose E	1–10 mSv

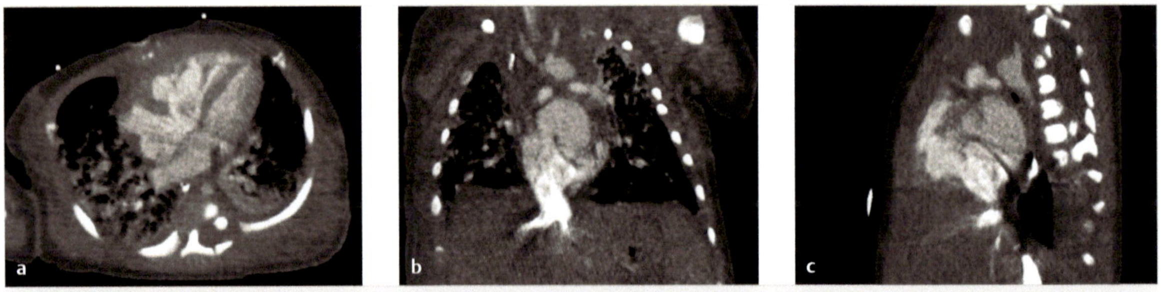

Fig. 3.28 DSCT image of a heart. One-year-old child. Measurement parameter: 75 ms effective slice scan time, 0.26 s overall scan time, 1.1 mSv effective dose.
a Axial reconstruction.
b Coronal reconstruction.
c Sagittal reconstruction.
(Courtesy of Prof. Dr. M. Lell, Erlangen.)

3.2.3 Technical Approaches to Cardiac Imaging

The main goal of cardiac imaging is to depict the anatomy without blurring or imaging artifacts caused by movement. Thus, the effective scan time must be significantly shorter than the length of a cardiac cycle. Furthermore, it is desirable that the scan time, typically indicated in % of the contraction cycle, can be predetermined and selected freely based on cardiac phase. Precise assignment to a cardiac phase is important for diagnostic purposes, e.g., if it is necessary to depict the heart over the entire cardiac cycle as a 4-D data set for functional analysis, or if the data needs to be collected for the phase of the cardiac cycle involving the least movement—namely end diastole. For this reason, it is generally necessary to record an ECG simultaneously with all image acquisitions of the heart in order to achieve a depiction with few movement artifacts. Two different procedures—prospective ECG triggering and retrospective ECG gating—are implemented in order to ensure assignment to a cardiac phase. In the former, measurements generally begin during diastole, based on the desired ECG time. In the latter, continually acquired CT data is assigned retrospectively to the ECG data collected in parallel in order to reconstruct images.

In principle, *prospective ECG triggering* is easier to perform and also generally means a lower dose for the patient, since the patient is only exposed to radiation during the desired cardiac phase. Prospective triggering, however, can fundamentally only be performed in cases of low heart rate, and thus frequently cannot be used in children with high heart rates. When taking contraindications into account, it is occasionally possible to administer a beta blocker to reduce heart rate. The movement of the heart or valves cannot, however, be evaluated via prospective triggering.

Retrospective ECG gating procedures, on the other hand, still allow imaging data to be acquired after reconstruction, and thus at the optimal time, thereby increasing the likelihood of good image quality. Furthermore, retrospective procedures allow the reconstruction of temporally resolved 4-D exams—such as exams of the heart's valves or the ventricles over the entire cardiac cycle—which can then be observed in motion. Dynamic exams of this type have been performed successfully for years via spiral CT with retrospective gating, though this is associated with a higher radiation exposure than prospective triggering. Only a very low table shift or pitch is possible for retrospective gating, since data must be collected for every cardiac phase.[31]

M!

Note

Pitch p is defined as the ratio of table shift per rotation to detector width.

For retrospective gating, scans are performed with a pitch of 0.2–0.4, which means overlapping data acquisition and thus generally a higher patient dose. In order to reduce dose, prospectively triggered single scans have been performed sequentially ("step and shoot") over the past few years, corresponding to a pitch of 1 and thus a lower dose. These scans cannot, however, depict any motion over time, which is necessary for functional analysis.

Broad detector scanners can depict a child's entire heart in a single rotation and are thus especially attractive, particularly for dynamic exams. For example, a device that offers 320 slices at 0.5 mm each can image approximately 12 cm during a single rotation. While this is not always adequate to depict a full adult heart, it generally suffices for small children. One current drawback of these scanners is their somewhat lower temporal resolution.

DSCT can be implemented with a pitch greater than 3 and/or in conjunction with prospective triggering (▶ Fig. 3.28). If high-pitch mode can be implemented, this results in a very high temporal resolution of circa 75 ms, a very short overall scan time of approximately 0.25 seconds (meaning acquisition during a single heartbeat), and a low dose of circa 1 mSv (▶ Fig. 3.29). Though high-pitch mode can only be used with a low heart rate, image quality corresponds to that during normal operation.[34]

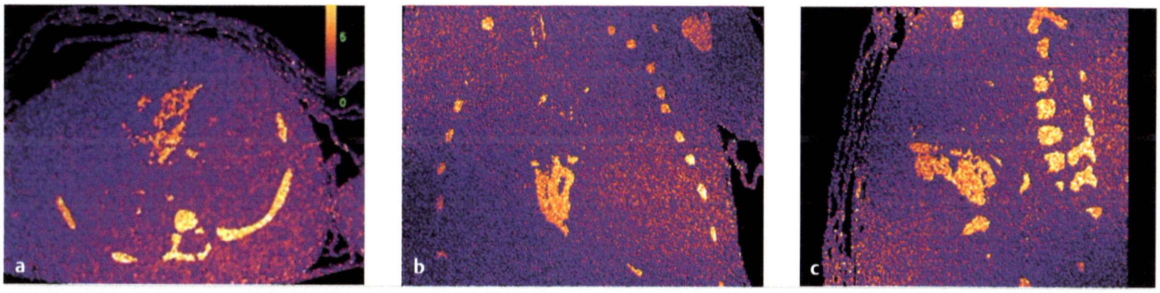

Fig. 3.29 DSCT image of a heart. 3-D dose distributions calculated using the Monte Carlo approach for the CT exam shown in ▶ Fig. 3.28.
a Axial.
b Coronal.
c Sagittal.

3.2.4 Patient Dose and Radiation Protection

We cannot and should not go into great detail in this book regarding the technical and physical aspects of dosimetry in CT. This information is discussed in depth in the literature in this field.[31,35,36]

The most significant variables are the CT dose index and the dose–length product, which nowadays are displayed on the operation console of every modern CT scanner and, according to the German X-Ray ordinance, must also be documented. The *CT dose index* is a value specific to each device and scan mode (independent of tube voltage and slice thickness) that is specified by the manufacturer and must be recorded during quality inspection. Constancy tests for the CT dose index performed regularly by technical personnel and/or a medical physicist (generally at least twice per year) ensure that the patient dose does not change. The CT dose index is determined using 10-cm-long ionization chambers in Acrylic Glass phantoms (cylinders made of polymethyl methacrylate with diameters of 16 and 32 cm for skull or thoracic exams, respectively). The CT dose index measured on the phantoms without table shift must then be corrected by the pitch value p for the respective patient exam. The volume CT dose index is calculated by division:

$$\mathrm{CTDI_{vol}} = \frac{\mathrm{CTDI}}{\mathrm{p}}$$

whereby

$\mathrm{CTDI_{vol}}$ = volume CT dose index
CTDI = CT dose index
p = pitch.

> **Note**
>
> Using this formula, it becomes apparent that dose decreases when table shift (pitch) increases, even without changing the other scan parameters.

The volume CT dose index, which is indicated using a dose unit of Gy or mGy, is not used to estimate the patient's radiation exposure. Rather, this index is only used to document that the device is functioning properly and that the correct exam parameters were chosen for the respective patient exam. The volume CT dose index does, however, allow an initial estimate of local dose (e.g., organ doses in the examined area), provided that the patient data is interpreted correctly (patient thickness compared to the Acrylic Glass phantom).

The *dose–length product*, on the other hand, provides values that allow an initial, preliminary estimate of the patient's radiation exposure (effective dose). An automatic recording is created for each CT exam specifically for the implemented CT protocol and the selected scan parameters. This recording is then displayed on the CT scanner's operating panel. The following formula is used:

$$\mathrm{DLP} = \sum_{i}^{n} \mathrm{CTDI_{100,w,i}} \times \mathrm{C_i} \times \mathrm{N_i} \times \mathrm{M_i} \times \mathrm{S_i}$$

where

DLP = dose–length product
CTDI = CT dose index
C = tube current–time product
N = number of rotations
M = number of slices
S = slice thickness.
100 = measured over a 100 mm long ionization chamber
w = weighted
i = tissue weighting factor

In essence, this formula means that to calculate the dose–length product, the standardized CTDI value must be multiplied by the mAs value for the tube current–time product of the respective exam scan and the length of the examined area (slice thickness multiplied by the number of slices and rotations). For repeated exams, the product must be added up for all exam indices (index *i*). This results in values using the unit mGy × cm, which, like the values for the dose–area product in projection radiography, are a measure of radiation exposure, and can be referenced to compare exams in the same section of the body.

Thus, the dose–length product, in addition to the volume CT dose index, is also a basis for defining *diagnostic reference dose values*. These diagnostic reference dose values have been legally binding in the European Union since 2000 and in Germany since 2002, with the amended X-Ray Ordinance. The diagnostic reference dose values are stipulated by law in Germany by the Federal Agency for Radiation Protection[37] and are adapted to the most up-to-date technological methods every few years. Specifying diagnostic reference dose values provides the examiner with comparative values for optimizing his scan parameters for patient dose via benchmarking. The diagnostic reference dose values are determined by the Federal Agency for Radiation Protection, based on national surveys. Thus, a diagnostic reference dose value for a dose size for a specific exam type is compared to the value for the third quartile (75th percentile) while distributing mean value for the individually recorded institutions. This means that, based on specifications, circa 25% of German institutions that perform this exam need to lower their values (for CT, the volume CT dose index, and the dose–length product). Long-established medical authorities regularly check the dose value to be set by the examiner compared to diagnostic reference dose values on a regular basis, in addition to justified indication, adequate image quality, and correct findings. If the statistical mean dose value exceeds the diagnostic reference dose value by more than 30%, supervisory authorities may be informed due to unjustifiably high exam doses. The medical authority will, however, first attempt to consult with examiners to reduce median dose values.

The actual dose unit relevant to patient risk is the *effective dose*. This dose can generally be estimated using the Monte Carlo method for average people (average man: 70 kg, 170 cm tall) based on information from the dose–length product.[35,38] This procedure is established, and the corresponding 3-D distribution of patient dose can be seen in ▶ Fig. 3.29. These distributions determine the dose for individual organs in the direct path of radiation as well as all other organs exposed to radiation. The effective dose is calculated as a weighted median of the relative sensitivity of the individual organs from the whole of organ dose values.[31,36] This procedure, which estimates effective dose in this manner using the dose–length product, is established[35] and is an approach for estimating doses in a manner appropriate for daily practice.

Note

It must also be noted, however, that in 2008, the ICRP published new tissue weighting factors that in some cases differ significantly from the values listed in literature and in the X-Ray Ordinance of 2002. This difference is especially notable for thoracic exams and in its dependency upon the patient's sex.[38]

Procedures for evaluating *CT doses in children* are not defined and standardized to the same extent as those for CT in adults. The information for volume CT dose indices and dose–length products cannot be easily applied to pediatric exams. The skull and thoracic thicknesses of 16 and 32 cm phantom diameters, respectively (which are used for estimating doses in adults) do not adequately represent the anatomical proportions in children. The common conversion values from the dose–length product for effective dose calculations as listed in the literature should be evaluated critically. To date, the Federal Agency for Radiation Protection has made no statements on this matter. The American Association of Physicists in Medicine provides recommendations for using conversion factors,[39] which were also taken into account in ▶ Table 3.4. A direct dose calculation based on concrete patient profiles and organ dose values (thus providing an estimate of effective dose) would be more precise (▶ Fig. 3.29), though this is not always feasible in everyday practice. Since 2010, it has been recommended that, at minimum, CT manufacturers refer to the smaller Acrylic glass phantom diameter of 16 cm value for the volume CT dose index and the dose–length product shown on the CT during pediatric exams. Special phantom diameters for pediatric CT protocols, a topic of discussion in recent years, have not yet been introduced. It is expected, however, that the Federal Agency for Radiation Protection will soon publish graded reference dose values for pediatric CT exams for children in various age groups. An approach based on size with standard phantoms for all age groups, similar to the procedure for adults (▶ Fig. 3.30), might offer additional benefits.[38]

For these reasons, any patient dose values for pediatric cardiac CT scans published in the literature thus far should

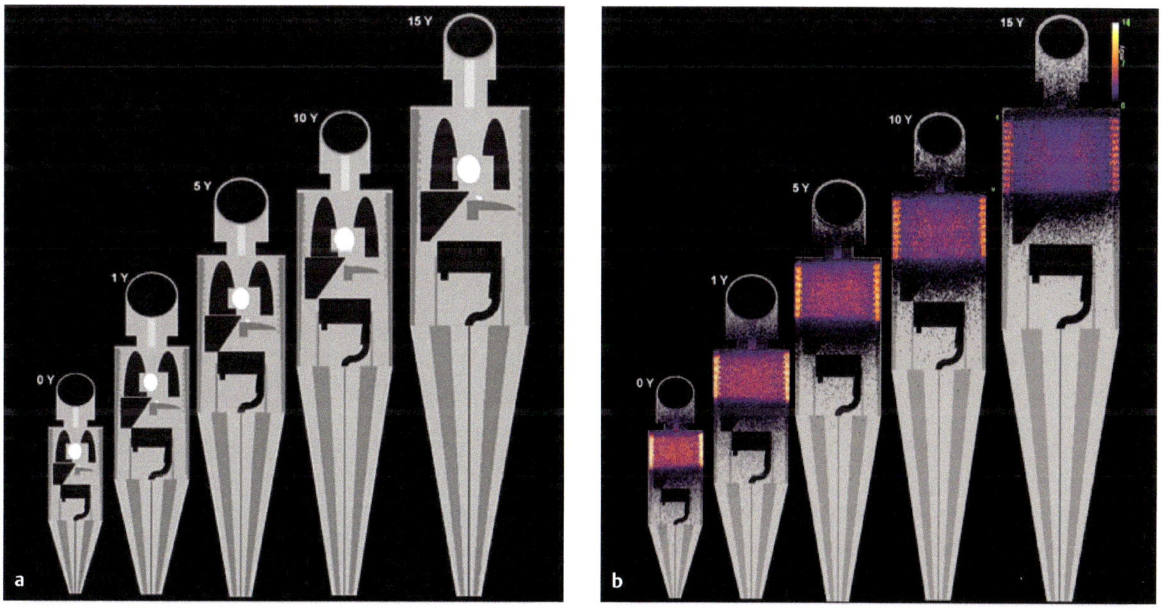

Fig. 3.30 Dose calculation for various age groups.
a ORNL phantoms corresponding to male children ages 0, 1, 5, 10, and 15 years (Y).
b 3-D dose distribution for a cardiac CT scan.

Table 3.4 Typical dose value for CT thoracic exams in children of various ages with the associated conversion factor for estimating effective dose based on the dose-length product; in accordance with higher sensitivity to radiation, the conversion factors are more than twice as large as for adults.

Age (years)	Dose-length product DLP (mGy x cm)	Conversion factor (DLP to E)	Effective dose E (mSv)
0	100–200	0.039	3.9–7.8
1	150–300	0.026	3.9–7.8
5	150–400	0.018	2.7–7.2
10	200–500	0.013	2.6–6.5
15	200–500	0.014	2.8–7.0

be viewed with criticism, particularly with regards to statements concerning effective dose. Table 3.4 provides an overview of typical values. Smal et al. have published a current work with listed references.[40] For questions of dose, the established Monte Carlo dose calculation procedure that can record every parameter is recommended. This dose calculation should be favored over elaborate and in some cases, more error-prone measurements. One example of this is the examination of the influence of *pitch factor* on dose based on a simulation with measured CT data where pitch = 1 (▶ Fig. 3.31). As pitch increases, dose decreases correspondingly while other scan parameters remain unaltered. Increasing the pitch value by 0.3 (retrospective gating) to more than 3 means a reduction in dose by a factor of 10 for the same tube current.

In a similar fashion, other procedures for reducing and optimizing dose have also been developed and assessed. Important opportunities and recommendations, many of which are based on dose calculation, are summarized in the next section.

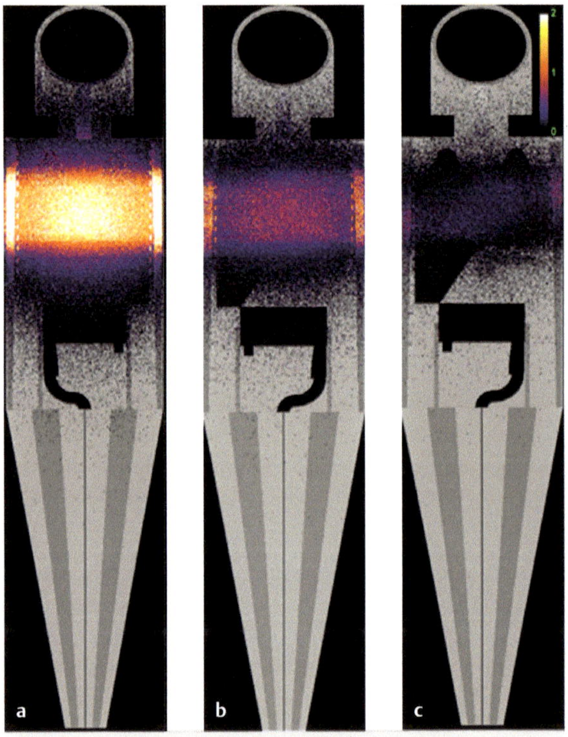

Fig. 3.31 Dose calculation for various pitch values (p). As expected, increased pitch leads to a significant reduction in dose while the other scan parameters remain unchanged (see the colored scaling standards for dose values in **c**, upper right).
a p = 0.3 for retrospective gating and 4-D imaging.
b p = 1.0 for sequential imaging.
c p = 3.4 with prospective triggering.

3.2.5 Recommendations for Scan Techniques and Dose Optimization

In principle, a reliable, meaningful diagnostic result is the goal of all radiological examinations. Measures for reducing dose during CT cannot result in any non-permissible compromises in image quality. Modern CT technology makes promising measures available, yet the technological options have not yet been optimized and tested for all pediatric protocols. When these options for optimizing dose are not yet available for a particular scanner, a retrofit should be created to also enable children with congenital heart defects to be examined with appropriate radiation exposure via cardio CT. The options for dose optimization on the devices should be reviewed at length before making a purchase decision.

General recommendations for reducing dose without limiting image quality include the following:

- *Apply strict standards for determining indication for pediatric CT exams:* Possible alternative procedures such as MRI should be taken into consideration.[41]
- *Limit the examined area strictly to the area required:* This common-sense measure minimizes the dose-length product and thus the effective dose.
- *Implement specially adapted pediatric protocols* (by using tube current modulation and dose automation, if available): Modern scanners offer dose automation, allowing examiners to achieve the desired noise level with minimum dose by adapting the tube current automatically.

- *Reduce the tube current:* For small children, lower kV values (e.g., 80 kV) are preferable to more commonly used values such as 120 kV, since this allows dose to be reduced significantly without reducing image quality.[42]
- *Perform cardiac exams during a single phase:* Generally speaking, in order to clarify anatomical relationships and coronary morphology in cases of congenital heart defects, the heart only needs to be visualized during a single phase (generally during diastole) rather than during the entire cardiac cycle. Limiting exposure to a single phase with the use of prospective triggering allows significantly lower dose values.
- *High-pitch spiral scan:* The highest possible pitch should be selected in order to reduce overall scan time and slice overlap, and thus dose.
- *Comply with diagnostic reference values:* It is useful to compare the achieved values of the dose–length product displayed on the scanner with the recommended reference values. When using modern CT technology, it is often possible to fall well below the diagnostic reference values. A median should be used for orientation purposes (second quartile rather than third).
- *Provide consultation when choosing exam protocols:* In cases of uncertainty, a consultation should be requested from the manufacturer, medical physics experts, or other qualified consultants.

If the indicated measures are implemented appropriately, this can lead to a significant reduction in radiation exposure, particularly for children, whose risk for radiation exposure is much higher than for older patients. Regardless, this can constitute a good reference point for hospitals and medical practices, and is considered the "as low as reasonably achievable" patient dose for general optimization requirements.

► **Acknowledgment.** The author thanks Ms. Yulia Smal, Mr. Paul Deak, Mr. Lukas Lehmkuhl, and Mr. Michael Wucherer for their assistance in creating this chapter.

3.3 Cardiac Magnetic Resonance Imaging

Matthias Gutberlet

3.3.1 Introduction

The technological basics of cardiac MRI can be described only briefly within the scope of this book, and are explained primarily with regard to special requirements for imaging in cases of congenital heart defects. Otherwise, we refer you to the extensive works regarding magnetic resonance physics.[43,44] Despite the special requirements of imaging for congenital heart defects due to patient age and the defects' complexities, it was one of the first ever indications for cardiac MRI.[45] Due to the lack of radiation exposure, the freely selectable slice orientation, and a versatility comparable to or, in some cases, superior to echocardiography (e.g., for 4-D flow measurements) without the drawbacks of a limited acoustic window, it remains the one of the first indications for cardiac MRI, even today.[45–47]

Based on the often very long exam times and the patients' ages, preparation via coil selection, potential sedation, and placement, as already discussed in Chapter 2.2, is of particular importance. A dedicated MRI-compatible incubator and coils for newborns and children now exist for premature babies (► Fig. 3.32). Otherwise, universally usable surface coils can be used for smaller children, and head (► Fig. 3.33) or knee coils can be used for newborns.

Since the examined patients are often incapable of providing statements and the treating physician is thus

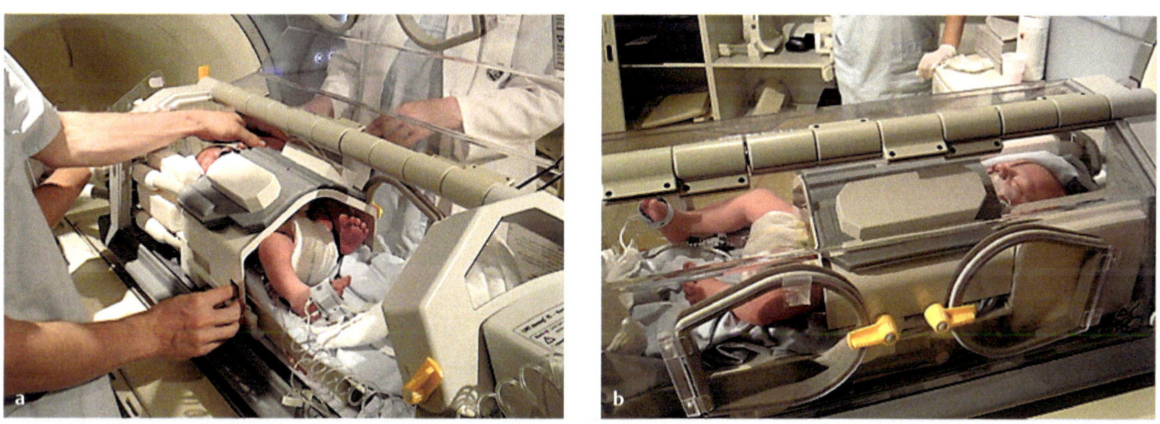

Fig. 3.32 MRI-compatible incubators used with multi-channel body coils. Nomag incubator (manufactured by LMT Medical Systems). 20-day-old, mature male newborn.
a View from the foot end of the incubator.
b Side view.
(Courtesy of Prof. Dr. med. Hans Mentzel, IDIR, University Hospital Jena.)

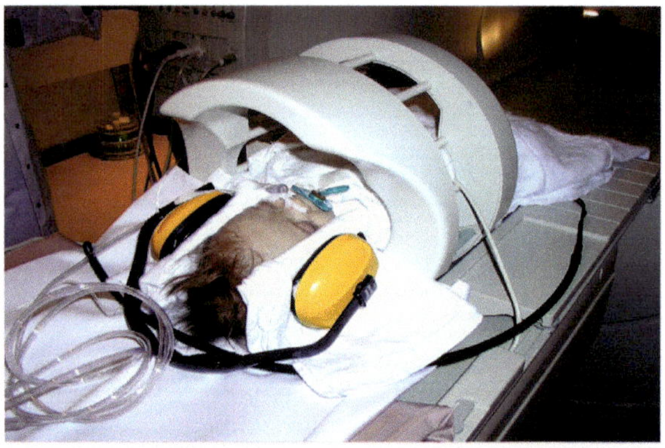

Fig. 3.33 Examination of a newborn using a head coil.

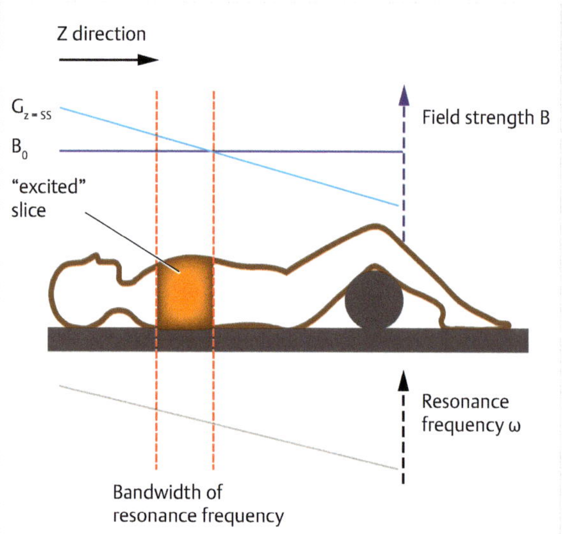

Fig. 3.34 Location dependency of resonance frequency ω on gradient G_z in the Z direction. The gradient is superimposed on static magnetic field B_0. This gradient is also called "slice-selective" (index "ss"). Slice thickness can be determined by limiting the bandwidth of the resonance frequency pulse's frequencies, since only spins with frequencies falling within this bandwidth can be excited.

reliant upon the third-party anamnesis of parents and their assistants in the exam room, special attention should be paid to the safety aspects of MRI before the exam, even though MRI exams are now able to be performed on patients with pacemakers and implantable cardioverter defibrillator (ICD) under certain circumstances. It should be noted that though most manufacturers now have "conditional" MRI-appropriate pacemakers (known as MRI-conditional pacemakers) on the market, no fully MRI-compatible pacemakers yet exist.[48]

Note

In particular, accompanying personnel and accompanying relatives must be informed of the following: the magnet is always on, even if no gradient noises are audible!

3.3.2 Slice Selection and Spatial Encoding

A few brief comments on image formation (spatial encoding, k-space) should render the following sections easier to understand.

Radio frequency stimulation and the corresponding MRI signals (echoes) only occur if the radio frequency of the excitation pulse coincides with the resonance frequency of the excited spin. In order to enable spatial encoding of the excited spin, a dynamic magnetic field (known as a gradient G) must be switched on—in addition to the static magnetic field B_0—so that the resonance frequencies of the stimulated spin differ along the gradient (▶ Fig. 3.34). The resonance frequency is then considered location-dependent, and thus allows precise spatial encoding. To this end, gradients are selected along all three spatial axes (x, y, and z). The gradient on the z axis, meaning perpendicular to the slice, is known as a slice-selective gradient.

In order to allow spatial encoding within the excited slice (2-D) or the excited volume (3-D), gradients must also be switched on in the perpendicular x and y axes, in addition to the slice-selective gradients on the z axis. The x axis is then known as a "frequency-encoding direction" or "readout direction," while the y axis is known as the "phase-encoding direction." The G_x gradients on this axis are known as "frequency-encoding" or "readout" gradients, and G_y is known as a "phase-encoding gradient," respectively.

A second gradient perpendicular to the first is switched on shortly after excitation, and causes controlled dephasing of the spin, such that the spin has a different phase during each image row of the spin's precession (phase-encoding gradient). The third gradient is switched on during measurement, at a right angle to the other two gradients. It ensures that the spins of each image column have a different precession velocity, meaning that they send a different Larmor frequency (selective and frequency-encoding gradients). In order to be able to generate an image from the complex recorded frequency spectrum, the signals must be parsed into their frequency components using the Fourier transformation, and the data must be deposited in a virtual space, known as the k-space.

All three gradients together thus encode the signal on three spatial planes. The received signal corresponds to a specific slice of the body and includes a combination of frequency and phase encoding, which the computer can translate into a 2-D image using the Fourier transformation.

Note

The k-space is a type of mathematical storage, a virtual space with particular qualities important to image generation:

- The k-space is constructed symmetrically.
- Complete image information is included within every point in the k-space.
- Contrast (low spatial frequency) is determined by the center of the k-space.
- Resolution (high spatial frequency) is determined by the periphery of the k-space.

All frequency components can be measured in one direction (frequency-encoding direction) with a single echo signal. For the second direction (phase encoding), only one of the respective strengths of the frequency components corresponding to the gradient can be measured. In order to receive all frequency components, the measurement must be repeated with various values of the phase-encoding gradient.

The number of phase-encoding steps in this slice has the largest influence on the overall measurement time for a 2-D MRI slice. This can be calculated using the following formula:

Note

T = TR x PES

PES = phase-encoding steps
T = overall time in s
TR = repetition time in s

The symmetrical characteristics of the virtual k-space can be used in various ways in order to reduce measurement time, by taking advantage of symmetry to calculate data rather than measuring all data. This does, however, negatively affect the signal to noise ratio.

3.3.3 Avoiding Motion Artifacts

In addition to patient movement, cardiac and phrenic movement, specifically, constitute a particular challenge to imaging. The latter can be addressed via appropriate placement, patient preparation, and sedation, particularly for babies and small children.

In order to "freeze" cardiac movement, it is simplest to limit data acquisition to the phase in the cardiac cycle in which cardiac movement is least pronounced, namely diastole. In addition to data acquisition, a surface ECG must generally also be recorded in these cases.

Gating and Triggering with Electrocardiography

A distinction is made between two types of ECG triggering, true triggering and gating:

- *ECG triggering:* During triggering, data is acquired with a certain temporal delay, known as the trigger delay, with respect to the R peak; this means the repetition time of the individual echo sequence is oriented to this trigger delay and the length of the RR interval. This type of triggering allows individual slices of the previously defined phases of the cardiac cycle (meaning end diastole or end systole) to be triggered. The duration of systole during the cardiac cycle indicates a relatively constant length throughout the cardiac cycle. The duration of diastole, however, is highly dependent on frequency. The orientation values for the corresponding selection of trigger delay can be seen in the tables; in order to determine the exact moment during the cardiac cycle on an individual basis, a test cine MRI, e.g., in a 4-chamber view, can be acquired.
- *ECG gating:* If images are acquired at various phases of the cardiac cycle using different repetition time intervals, this is considering gating. Retrospective gating is a specific type of gating. The ECG is recorded and saved continually during acquisition, and the acquired images are subsequently first assigned during the reconstruction phase of the individual phases of the cardiac cycle. Using this type of sequence control, recordings of the heart can be gleaned throughout the entire cardiac cycle with various temporal resolutions. This is particularly advantageous for functional exams (wall motion analysis, flow measurement, etc.).

Note

If ECG triggering is not possible due to inadequate recording, triggering can also be performed using the pulse curve of a pulse oximeter. The temporal delay of the pulse waves with respect to the R peak must, however, be taken into account.

Generally speaking, prospective triggering is used for pure imaging by means of SE (spin-echo) sequences using a fixed trigger delay with respect to the R peak of the superficial ECG. In doing so, it should be noted that the surface electrodes also register other electrical signals, including those induced by the magnetic field of blood flow within the aorta and ventricles. This field can be so pronounced that it is misinterpreted by the system as a T wave or even as an R peak.[45] In general, these effects can be recognized and addressed when positioning the electrodes by placing them elsewhere—for example, further from the aorta.

Respiratory Compensation

Significant respiratory excursion during imaging can lead to ghosting artifacts (▶ Fig. 3.35). The easiest way to avoid this is to use very rapid *real-time sequences*. These sequences are, however, limited by a significantly worse signal-to-noise ratio and worse spatial resolution. This means that, for the most part, they can only be implemented as localization sequences. For this reason, sequences in breath-holding techniques are generally used.

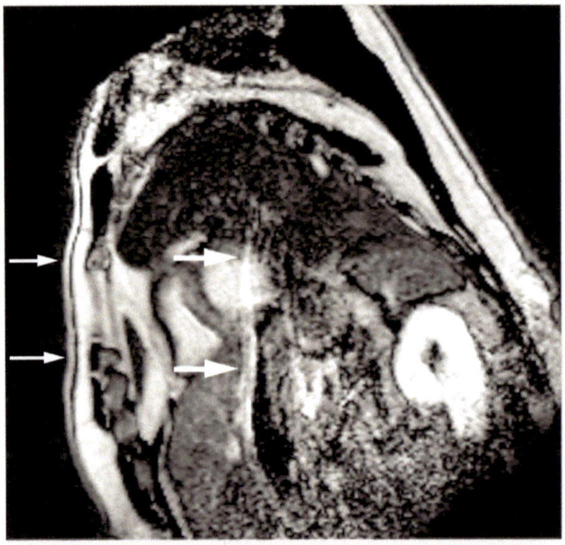

Fig. 3.35 Ghosting artifacts. Short-axis slice with ghosting artifacts (thick arrow) in phase-encoding direction parallel to the thoracic wall (thin arrow) caused by respiratory excursion during image acquisition.

Naturally, it is usually impossible to use breath-holding techniques for babies and small children. Consequently, acquisition occurs either via an external sensor such as a *respiratory belt* that registers "abdominal breathing" or via the navigator technique.

The position of the diaphragm is depicted in temporal resolution using the *navigator technique* (▶ Fig. 3.36). Data acquisition then occurs only during a particular portion of the respiratory cycle, namely the gating window, without the patient needing to follow any commands. For this reason, these sequences are especially well-suited for children with congenital heart defects. With the navigator technique, a trigger signal is recorded in sagittal orientation through the diaphragm, right lateral to the heart, before the actual measurement. Because of the large difference in contrast between the liver, diaphragm, and lungs, a single line in the k-space suffices to visualize the movement of the diaphragmatic dome.[45] Continuous measurements depict the diaphragm's motion in temporal resolution, similar to M-mode in echocardiography. A particular portion of the respiratory cycle can be measured based on the desired imaging technique. If the corresponding height of the diaphragm is reached, a trigger impulse is generated at the start of the actual measurement sequence. Overall, this type of data acquisition requires

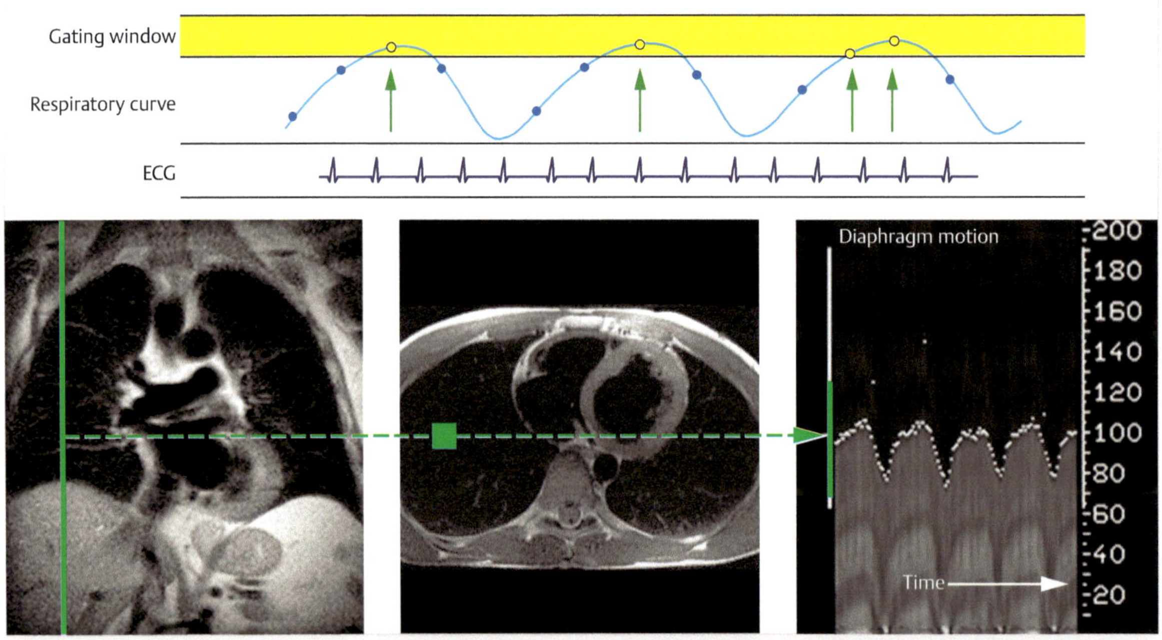

Fig. 3.36 2-D excitation via navigator (left) and positioning on the patient near the dome of the diaphragm. One navigator measurement is performed for each heartbeat; this allows the diaphragm's motion to be depicted in temporal resolution (right). Actual image acquisition occurs only during a predetermined gating window (green arrow, yellow surface)—in this case, during end expiration.

significantly more time than the use of breath-holding techniques, but leads to very high image quality. To date, this technique has been used primarily to depict the coronary arteries within a whole-heart sequence. It can, however, also be combined with other sequences (such as black blood sequences or certain edema-sensitive T2-weighted (T2w) sequences with otherwise relatively long acquisition times) for breath-holding techniques.

For smaller children with often very flat respiration but high respiratory frequency, who are also unable to follow breath-holding commands, *acquisition during free breathing and multiple repetitions* (3–4 times) with a subsequent averaging may be attempted, in addition to acquisition using the navigator technique. The corresponding sequence parameters include:

- *NSA:* Number of signals averaged
- *NEX:* Number of excitations

3.3.4 Rapid Imaging

In order to be able to acquire dynamic images (such as in a cine MRI) to assess cardiac function as quickly as possible, faster and faster gradient systems and GE (gradient-echo) sequences are being used. These signals are, among other factors, limited by potential peripheral neural stimulation or tissue warming caused by the high-frequency excitation pulse—known as specific absorption rate (SAR)—with their corresponding thresholds, especially in children.

Parallel Imaging

Parallel imaging offers a solution to this issue and is one of the most widely used acquisition and reconstruction techniques for fast imaging, meant to avoid these limitations. Fundamentally, nearly all sequence types can be combined with parallel imaging.

> **Note**
>
> During parallel imaging, MRI signals are recorded simultaneously, meaning parallel to multiple (at least two) surface coils. The phase-encoding steps are not accelerated; rather, the number of phase-encoding steps is reduced. The corresponding acceleration factor corresponds exactly to the factor of phase-encoding step reduction. In everyday clinical practice, acceleration factors of 2–4 are used.

Increasing intervals in the k-space (▶Figs. 3.37a,b) reduces the number of phase-encoding steps. The field of view with its corresponding foldover and overlapping images—which can be separated from one another using various "view axes" for the depicted object—is reduced when distributing image acquisition among multiple coil elements. SENSE (Philips), iPAT (Siemens), ASSET (GE), RAPID (Hitachi), and SPEEDER (Toshiba) are examples of this type of processing algorithm. This results in a reconstructed image without foldover. The signal-to-noise ratio is reduced

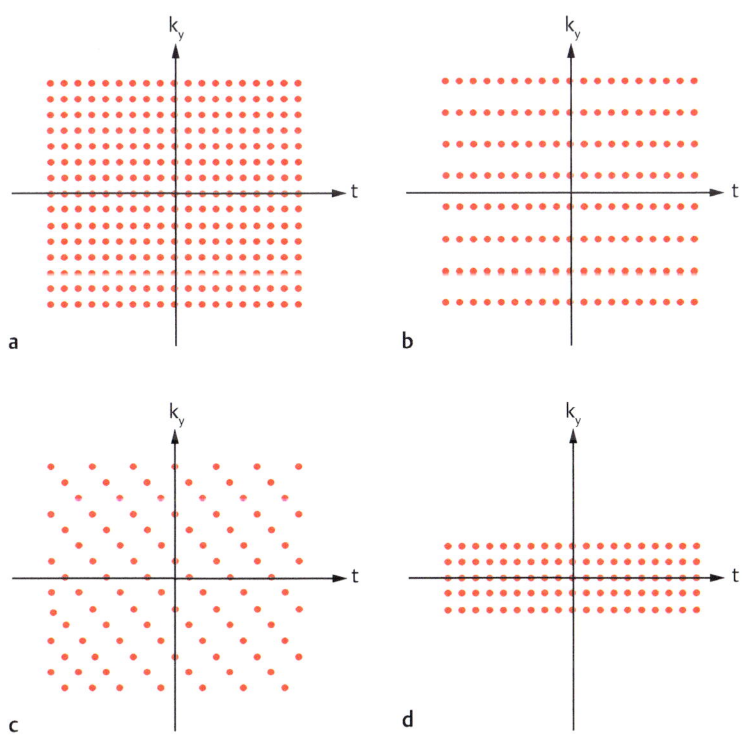

Fig. 3.37 Overview of various algorithms for filling k-space. Schematic depiction.
a Traditional complete performance of all phase-encoding steps of a dynamic sequence along the y axis.
b Leaving out every second phase-encoding step during parallel imaging, e.g., SENSE.
c Data set with "temporal" gaps during a k-t BLAST.
d k-t BLAST training data set with a central data set without any temporal gaps, and corresponding low spatial resolution.

based on the acceleration factor and the coil used, meaning that the procedure is especially suited to sequences with an already high intrinsic signal-to-noise ratio (such as SSFP sequences) and at higher field strengths (such as 3T[49]):

> **Note**
>
> $$SNR_{\text{with parallel imaging}} = \frac{SNR_{\text{without parallel imaging}}}{(g \times \sqrt{R})}$$
>
> where
>
> SNR = signal-to-noise ratio
>
> g = geometric factor based on coils
>
> R = acceleration factor.

3-D procedures, such as 3-D cardiac MRA, are also well-suited for use in parallel imaging due to the two phase-encoding directions.

k-t BLAST

Even higher acceleration values are possible when using additional data reduction techniques (such as UNFOLD, k-t BLAST) when imaging during dynamic processes, as they occur in great numbers during cardiovascular imaging. Acceleration factors of up to 10x are possible, primarily with k-t BLAST (where "k" stands for k-space and "t" for time).[43,50] These techniques take advantage of the redundancy of imaging data for movable objects in order to accelerate data acquisition. Unlike with parallel imaging, phase-encoding components are measured in full, though not for the entire period of time *t* (▶ Fig. 3.37c). This results in a "temporal" data set with gaps. Similar to parallel imaging, this leads to overlap distortion which must be filled in using data sets with no temporal gaps and with only limited spatial resolution, known as training scans (▶ Fig. 3.37d). This scan can be measured separately or in conjunction with the actual sequence. Parallel imaging and k-t BLAST techniques can also be implemented in conjunction with this scan. Fundamentally, this also allows 3-D cine images of the entire heart to be performed within a breath command.

Black Blood Sequences

Particularly for congenital heart defects with complex anatomy, it is necessary to achieve a rapid overview of thoracic and cardiac anatomy at the beginning of the exam. This often occurs using rapid black blood sequences triggered for end diastole, in which two (180°) initial inversion pulses "nullify" the blood signal in the vessels and cardiac cavities. The two 180° pulses include a non-slice-selective initial pulse that ensures that the blood flowing into the slice is "saturated" and no more signals occur, and a slice-selective 180° pulse that re-inverts magnetization in the imaging layer with the exception of the influent blood. One of the sequences most commonly used to this end is the HASTE sequence, a single-shot turbo SE sequence that takes advantage of the symmetry of the k-space by means of half-Fourier acquisition. This sequence can be implemented using multiple breath-holding commands or during normal breathing using the navigator technique. The initial pulse interval with respect to image data acquisition is selected independently of heart rate, so that the influent blood is "nullified." Using contrast agents postpones the black blood delay accordingly due to a shortening in T1 relaxation time, and must be adapted on a case-by-case basis.

Whole Heart Sequences

Because of the good contrast, the high signal-to-noise ratio, and the opportunity to accelerate these sequences significantly using parallel imaging—meaning that they no longer have to be used exclusively with the navigator technique, but can now also be used during a single breath command to depict the entire thoracic area—static SSFP sequences (known as 3-D whole heart sequences) triggered by diastole are being used more and more frequently to depict patients' anatomy. Originally, these whole heart sequences were used primarily for MRI depictions of coronary arteries, and generally suffice at least for detecting coronary outlet abnormalities. The decisive advantage of this type of 3-D acquisition is the ability to generate isotropic voxels 1.5–2.0 mm in size. This means that in-plane resolution is identical to slice thickness. Thus, reformatting is possible in any spatial dimension using the 3-D data set, including in angled perspectives. If the goal is to depict cardiovascular structures within the entire thoracic cavity, it has proven effective to use angled sagittal slices with subsequent preparation of multiplanar reformatting in all other spatial dimensions rather than transverse acquisition. This means that significantly fewer slices are needed for this task.

> **Note**
>
> The longest trigger delay possible during diastole (based on heart rate) should be selected when acquiring 3-D whole heart sequences. This allows an acquisition window of 45–100 ms.

These 3-D SSFP sequences have been improved by integrating a fat saturation and a T2 preparation pulse (two 90° pulses) and the intensive use of parallel imaging, so much so that 3-D bright blood SSFP sequences have replaced black blood sequences in many medical centers.

3.3.5 Cine Magnetic Resonance Imaging

Originally, simple, rapid GE sequences were used for functional assessments of the heart. In recent years, however, a special variant known as the "steady state free precession" or SSFP sequence has become predominant. This SSFP sequence is characterized primarily by a high contrast between the myocardium, blood, and fatty tissue based on T2/T1 mixed weighting (▶ Table 3.5). Thus, the signal depends primarily on the T2/T1 ratio. The same sequence is given different names by various manufacturers, e.g., bFFE (Philips), TrueFISP (Siemens), and FIESTA (GE).

Because of SSFP sequences' greater susceptibility to magnetic field inhomogeneity,[49] there has been more reliance on the original standard GE sequences for higher field strengths ≥ 3 T in recent years. For all cine sequences, data is acquired over multiple heartbeats and then distributed among the individual cardiac phases within a single heartbeat (▶ Fig. 3.38). This means that cine MRIs do not represent a single heartbeat, but rather data averaged from multiple heartbeats. Averaging this data leads to errors in cases of large differences between the length of RR intervals (deviations of more than 25%). For this reason, this data is not reconstructed, and is instead discarded. If still no adequate image can be generated, it may be necessary to rely on fast real-time sequences without ECG triggering, albeit with worse spatial resolution.

Volumetric Analysis

The volumes and function of the atria and ventricles can be determined reliably by using cine MRI and SSFP sequences, via manual, semi-automatic, or automatic contour findings of the endocardial and epicardial contours. For the left ventricle, these measurements can be approximated using the area-length method from a single (monoplanar) axis or two long (biplanar) axes, if we assume roughly ellipsoid geometry. In cases of pathological geometry, including that of the right ventricle, the strengths of MRI as a 3-D imaging modality must be used (particularly in cases of congenital heart defects) and the entire ventricle must be imaged using continuous slice coverage. This can be performed along the short axis or along the long axis, especially for the right ventricle and the atria. Under this condition, MRI constitutes the current gold standard for cardiac volumetric analysis.[45–47]

Tagging and Feature Tracking

Analogous to echocardiography, there exist various methods for determining myocardial strain (also known as tissue strain). This allows not only for visual or quantitative analysis of endocardial wall motion, but also for analysis of diastolic and intramyocardial dysfunction.

The newest method, known as *feature* tracking,[51] uses standard SSFP sequences to this end. Thus, unlike older tagging procedures, feature tracking can also be used in cases of non-hypertrophied right ventricle, with a good correlation to strain analysis using the tagging procedure.

The various tagging sequences are specialized cine GE sequences. Unlike with feature tracking, the myocardium is "tagged" (or marked) by saturation grids or lines during the tagging procedure. This tagging occurs via initial saturation pulses immediately after the R peak and, depending on contractility during the cardiac cycle, encounters a deformity (▶ Fig. 3.39) that can be assessed visually or quantitatively by determining myocardial strain.

3.3.6 Quantitative Flow Measurements

Using rapid GE sequences, flow within vessels can be quantified with great precision, e.g., in order to determine the regurgitation fraction in cases of valve insufficiency or shunt volumes. MR flow quantification is based on the phase shift of the moving spin, which is dependent upon velocity. Assuming a laminar flow, this phase shift is proportional to velocity. Bipolar gradients —which, in the case of static tissues, lead to phase shift 0—are used to best take advantage of these characteristics, since dephasing and rephasing are the same for stationary spins when using bipolar gradients, and magnetization is in phase again after using bipolar gradients. Since magnetic field inhomogeneity is among the additional factors besides flow leading to phase changes, two measurements should be taken right after one another with two different bipolar gradient polarities

Table 3.5 T1 and T2 relaxation times for various tissues. The highest T2/T1 ratio and thus a good contrast in the SSFP sequence is shown between the myocardium, fatty tissue, and blood.

Tissue	T1 (ms)	T2 (ms)	T2/T1
Blood	1200	250	0.21
Myocardium	870	55	0.06
Liver	500	45	0.09
Spleen	775	60	0.08
Fat	250	80	0.32

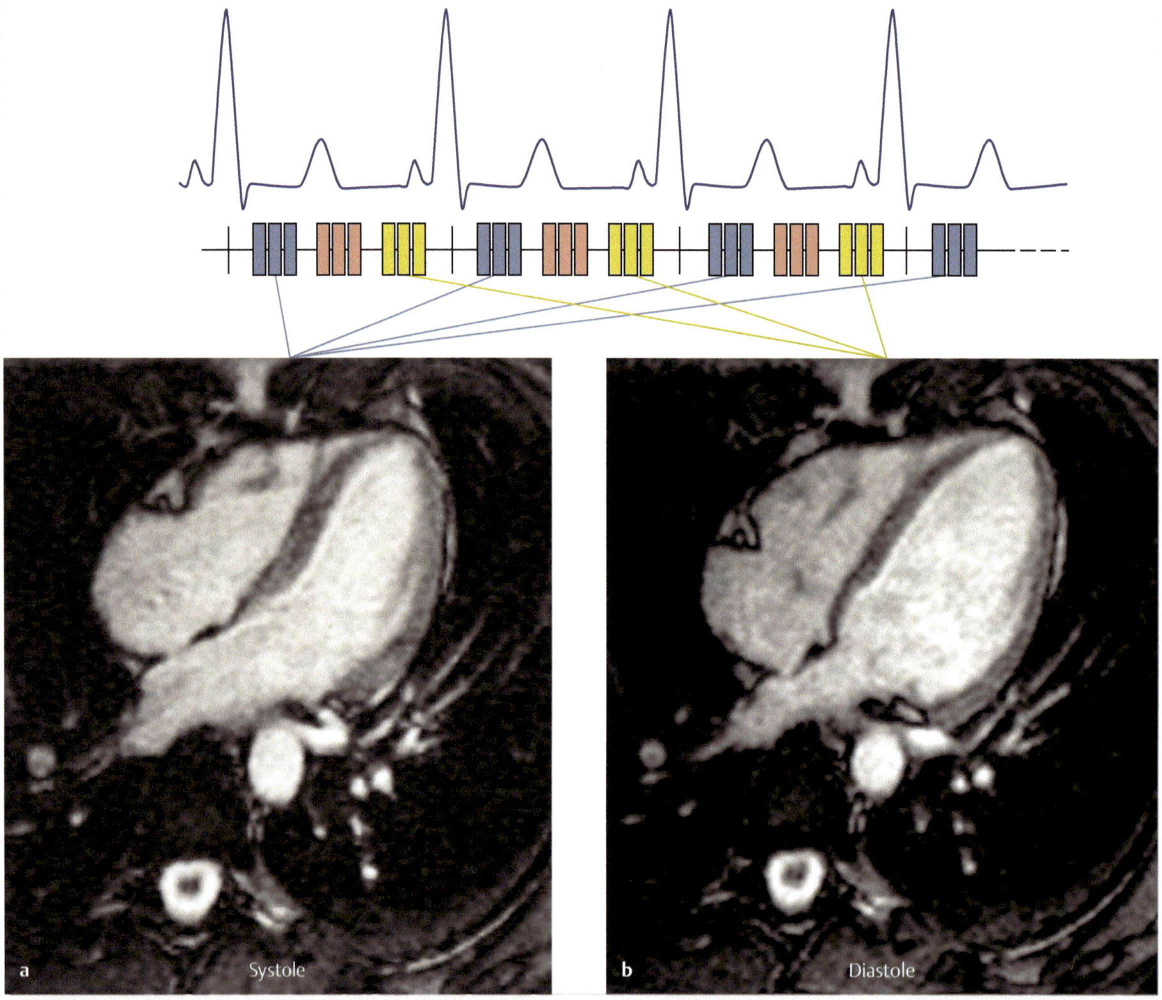

Fig. 3.38 Retrospective assignment of imaging data during different cardiac phases gathered over multiple heartbeats. Schematic depiction.

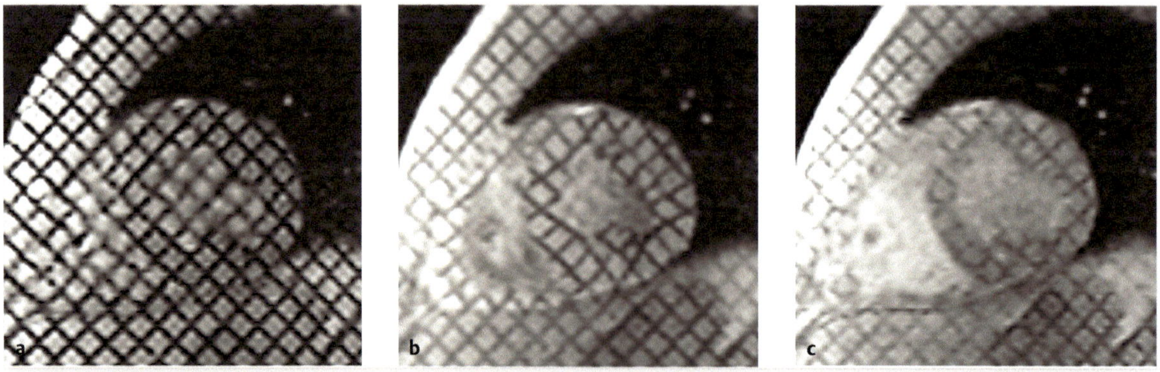

Fig. 3.39 Tagging procedure.

a Regular tagging grid of a volunteer using a 1.5 T MRI immediately after generation, meaning shortly after detecting the R peak at the beginning of the cardiac cycle. Note that even the blood in the ventricular cavum is tagged.

b During systole, the grid deforms due to the contracting myocardium. The static tissues of the thoracic wall and the liver, on the other hand, do not deform.

c Minor "fading" of the tagging grid occurs during late diastole. To achieve a longer tagging grid persistence until the end of the cardiac cycle, tagging sequences benefit from a higher field strength.[49]

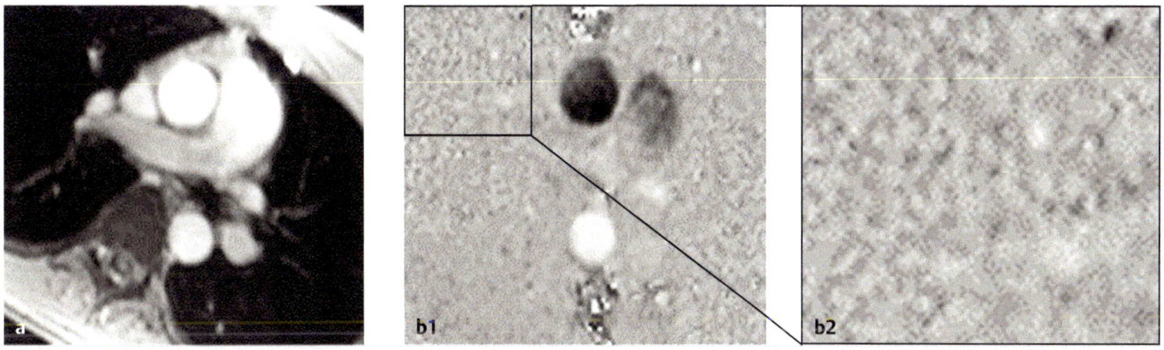

Fig. 3.40 Flow-sensitive GE sequences.

a The magnitude image of the flow-sensitive GE sequence corresponds to an anatomical GE image.

b Flow direction and velocity are encoded in the phase image: cranial flow in the ascending aorta is black, and the light color is the caudal flow in the descending aorta. Background noise in the lungs during the phase image are visible as a typical "salt-and-pepper" pattern (enlarged).

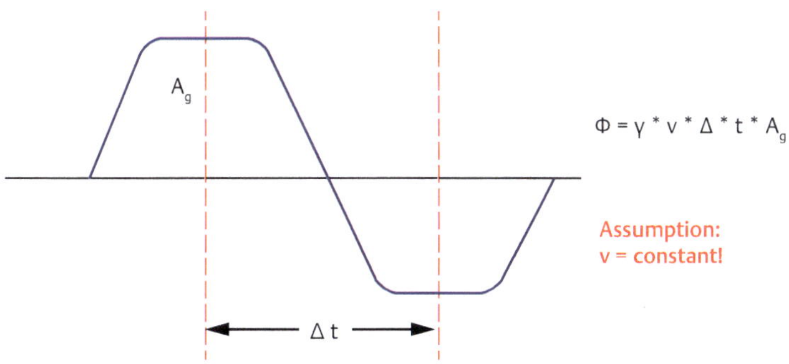

Fig. 3.41 Effect of a bipolar gradient with surface area A_g on phase ϕ of a moving spin with velocity v. Schematic depiction. While phase ϕ, according to the gradient, is unchanged for static spins (v = 0), a phase angle ϕ proportional to velocity occurs for moved spins. See text for additional information.
A_g = area under the curve of the gradient pulse
Δt = time between the midpoints of the bipolar gradient pulse

(negative-positive and positive-negative). This allows elimination of temporally constant phase changes by simply subtracting the two data sets from one another.

Flow velocity, gray tone intensity, and flow direction are depicted as positive or negative values on a voxel in cm/s when using flow-sensitive GE sequences (black versus white intensity scales: positive signals scale from white to medium gray, and negative signals scale from medium gray to black; ▶ Fig. 3.40). Similar to Doppler sonography, a 360° radian with ranges of + 180° to − 180° is used.

Retrograde flow leads to a negative phase difference, and antegrade flow to a positive one; in MRI, this is generally depicted as a gray value on the phase image. The image data can also be color-coded, similar to color Doppler sonography. The measured mean flow velocities of each voxel can be used to convert this value into volume flow in ml/s using the product of pixel area and pixel velocity.

This method of flow quantification is fundamentally similar to data acquisition for *phase contrast angiography*. One difference lies in the fact that, generally speaking, for 2-D flow measurements used in clinical routines, flow is only measured in one direction (ideally perpendicular to the main flow vector), and the encoded velocity (maximum anticipated flow velocity in the vessel) must be set higher (circa 10%) in order to avoid signal loss due to aliasing. Since phase changes of more than 360° or more than ±180° indicated on the radian are no longer clearly defined and thus lead to phase wrapping and aliasing, this definition must instead be determined by the user.

The following linear correlation between the resultant phase shift and flow velocity exists when using a bipolar gradient (▶ Fig. 3.41):

> **Note** (M!)
>
> $$\phi = v \times (\gamma \times \Delta t \times A_g)$$
>
> where
> ϕ = phase shift
> v = flow velocity in m/s
> γ = gyromagnetic constant
> Δt = time between the midpoints of the bipolar gradient pulse
> A_g = area under the curve of the gradient pulse.

Turbulences can lead to dephasing, which limits the precision of flow measurements. The signal intensity of each pixel stands for local flow velocity during quantitative flow measurements. This velocity value is an average that is proportional to the phase of the sum vector of the signals of all spins within the voxel. Therefore, errors in flow measurements can occur because of this partial volume effect. If the distribution of velocity values within a voxel is very broad, then the corresponding phase differences are also large, meaning that the net signal can even sink to zero. Even in static tissues, however, no null value is reached during the phase image, but rather a random value corresponding to background noise. Unlike anatomical magnitude images, *background noises* are clearly visible on phase images and influence the measured value. They can, however, be clearly distinguished from areas with normal flow due to their salt-and-pepper appearance (▶ Fig. 3.42b, enlargement). The salt-and-pepper appearance occurs primarily in areas with air, meaning in the lungs and outside the patient's body. Quantitative flow measurements are normally performed using thin (3–10 mm thick), single 2-D slices.

During MR flow measurements, *retrospective gating* should be used if possible in order to be able to fully capture all phases of the cardiac cycle in cases of pulsatile flow.

In order to minimize *partial volume effects*, acquisitions should always be taken perpendicular to the course of the vessel. Because of the relatively long measurement periods, measurements are generally taken during normal respiratory cycles with multiple acquisitions in order to reduce respiratory artifacts. Measurements last several minutes, and can also be taken when using breath-holding techniques or even as real-time sequences by using acceleration procedures, such as parallel imaging. In the former case, prospective gating must be used, which may not record everything during diastole.

In addition to partial volume effects, *angle errors* also constitute an issue, just like in Doppler echocardiography. Unlike Doppler, however, there are no fundamental limitations, since flow can be measured in any direction if the MRI is set up appropriately beforehand. In cases of 2-D flow measurements, only the main flow vector is measured in the vessel perpendicular to the slice level for through-plane measurements, and at the slice level for in-plane measurements. Deviations from the main flow vector lead to underestimating maximum flow velocity. Spatial resolution should be as high as possible (e.g., more than 10 pixels per vessel diameter) in order to minimize partial volume errors. For this reason, MR flow measurements can only be performed on a limited basis in the coronary arteries, but works quite well in the great vessels.

The newest developments allow simultaneous acquisition of flow measurements in all three spatial dimensions; in doing so, bipolar gradients are applied in all three dimensions. Thus, flow measurement is also known as *"4-D flow measurement"* (▶ Fig. 3.42). This does, however, significantly lengthen measurement times, meaning measurements can no longer be gathered within a single breath-holding command. 4-D flow measurement is thus generally combined with the navigator technique, which allows acquisition during normal respiration.

> **Note** M!
>
> Even though multiple factors fundamentally influence the reliability of MR flow measurements, numerous in vitro and in vivo studies indicate that it is a very reliable method of flow quantification whose informative value relies less on the examiner's experience than Doppler echocardiography.

3.3.7 Magnetic Resonance Angiography

Of the many options for performing an MRA, only three will be detailed here. Contrast enhancement is of the greatest clinical significance because of its numerous advantages, especially for patients with congenital heart defects.

Time-of-Flight Magnetic Resonance Angiography

Before the option to use contrast-enhanced MRA was available, MRA was performed by taking advantage of the inflow effect via unsaturated spins that reached the image plane inside the blood vessels and generated a signal using an appropriate pulse selection. For the larger vessels, this type of MRA allows adequately precise depictions, under the condition that ECG triggering is used and the patient is able to lie absolutely still for up to 10 minutes. Time-of-flight MRA is still widely used to depict intracerebral vessels. The basic concept of inflow MRA is based on the following principles:

- *Saturation of stationary tissue* (in the examined volume): In order to depict a vascular tree as optimally as possible, the surrounding tissue in the measurement volume should, ideally, emit no signal. This is achieved by applying multiple successive high-frequency pulses to the measured volume. In order to accomplish this, the shortest possible repetition time between the high-frequency pulses is necessary. This is most easily achieved by using GE sequences.
- *Contrast enhancement using influent blood:* If fully magnetized, fresh, unsaturated blood (i.e., blood that has not yet been excited by any high-frequency pulses) flows into the measurement volume, the blood generates a strong MR signal when excited by the first high-frequency pulse. This only enhances contrast during a time-of-flight MRA, since the surrounding tissues is already saturated by the initial pulse at this time. Maximum inflow effect is achieved if the fresh, influent blood only experiences a single high-frequency pulse

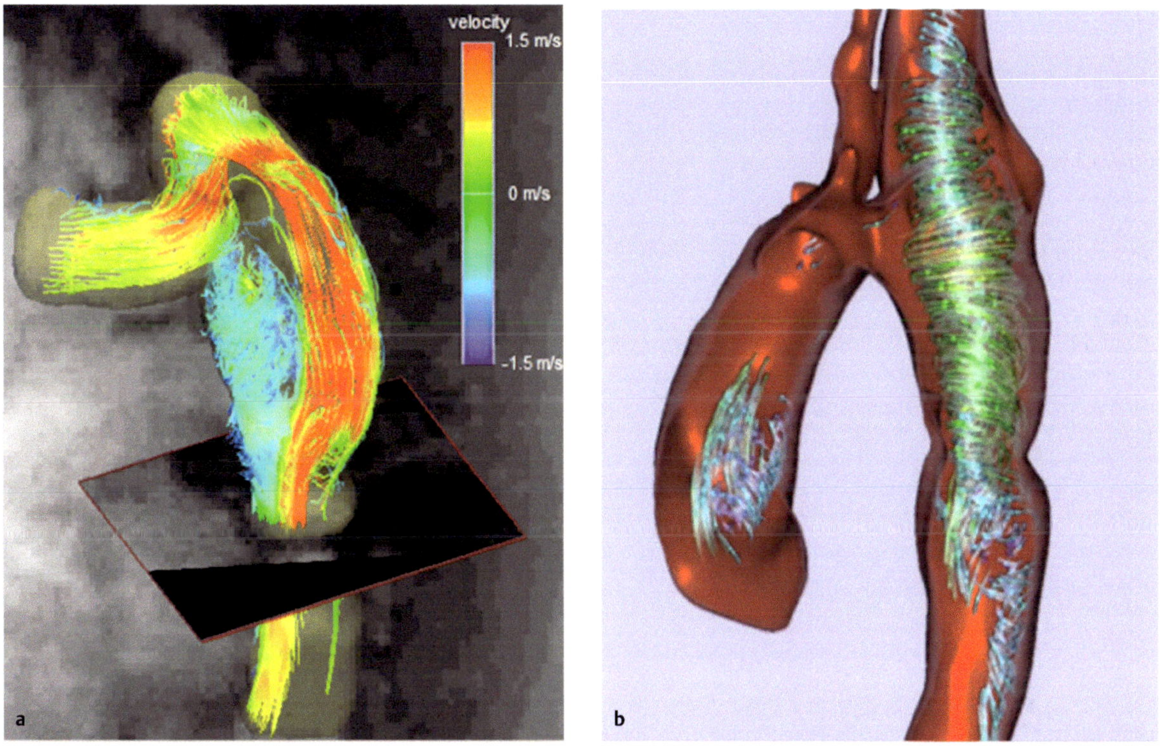

Fig. 3.42 4-D flow measurement.
a The depicted streamlines in 4-D flow analysis represent peak systolic flow (here, circa 1.5 m/s) in an extra-anatomical bypass from the left subclavian artery to the descending aorta, for treating a high-grade, unresected aortic coarctation.
b "Helical" flow in this same patient's bypass.

while images of the examined measurement volume are being acquired. Once the blood has been excited by more than one high-frequency pulse, a saturation effect similar to those used to suppress the signals in the tissue surrounding the vessels sets in.

The blood in the scan volume will only encounter a single high-frequency pulse under the following conditions:

> **Note**
>
> $$v \geq \frac{d}{TR}$$
>
> where
> v = blood velocity component perpendicular to the scan volume
> d = slice thickness based on the measurement technique used (**2-D:** d = slice thickness, **3-D [single slab]:** d = slab thickness; **3-D [multi-slab]:** d = thickness of each individual slab)
> TR = repetition time.

The conditions for the aforementioned equation are best fulfilled when flow runs perpendicular to the measurement volume. Since flow velocity within the vessel cannot be influenced, the other parameters must be selected carefully. The slice to be measured should, however, run perpendicular to the main direction of flow. The flip angle is another factor that influences the inflow effect. In general, the largest possible flip angle should be selected, since this leads to a stronger inflow signal and better suppression of background signals.

Phase Contrast Magnetic Resonance Angiography

For phase contrast angiography, the phase shift of the MR signal caused by the flowing blood is used to distinguish between vessels and the surrounding tissue. Nevertheless, phase contrast techniques are also based on renewing inflowing blood in the measurement volume, though less strongly than with inflow techniques. The pulse sequences used are arranged such that the measured phase shift is proportional to the flow velocity of the flowing blood.[45] Using the phase contrast technique, it is possible to fully suppress the stationary tissue by subtracting various acquisitions of flow-compensated and flow-sensitive images from one another (▶ Fig. 3.43). Furthermore, the phase contrast technique can also depict small vessels with very slow flow. Based on the flexible configurability

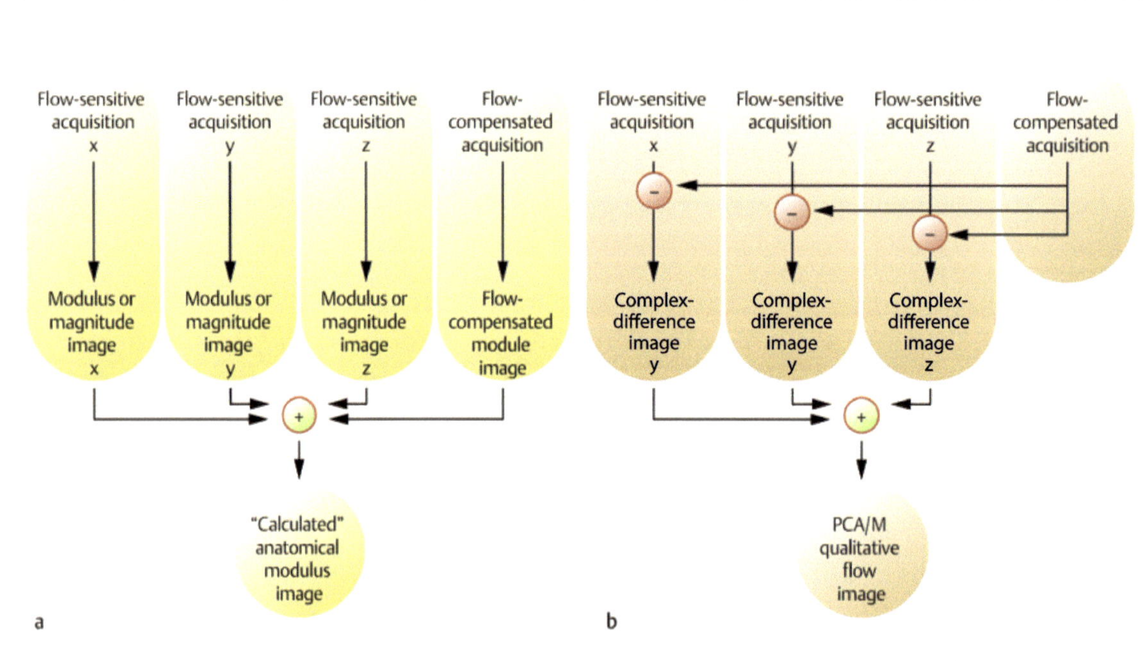

Fig. 3.43 Various forms of calculation for phase contrast angiography. Schematic depiction.
PCA/M = phase contrast angiography
a "Averaged" anatomical magnitude or modulus image.
b Qualitative flow image.

of sequence sensitivity to various flow velocities (encoded velocity) and flow directions, it is possible to adapt the sequence appropriately for the task at hand. Fundamentally, phase contrast angiography can be used for both purely morphological and functional assessments (flow velocity, flow volume). Both functional and morphological data can be gathered using a single-phase contrast angiography acquisition. The approaches for purely morphological and functional examinations differ only in the form of their data reconstruction. In principle, four different reconstruction algorithms are possible:

- Traditional "anatomical" magnitude or modulus image that only includes inflow (magnitude) information, but no phase information (▶ Fig. 3.43a)
- Magnitude image that only includes qualitative flow information
- Up to three phase images, whereby each contains one component (on the x, y, or z axis) of the total flow vector (▶ Fig. 3.43b)
- Speed image that includes the amplitude of the flow vector, but no information regarding direction.

Information is generally reconstructed using the difference in amplitudes for the purely morphological depiction of vessels. Using this method, a maximum intensity projection (MIP) can be used to reduce the volume of reconstructed data to a reconstructed volume in various projections. In addition, magnitude images that only include qualitative flow information are less susceptible to signal loss via aliasing. This phenomenon is analogous to the Doppler procedure if the physical flow velocity exceeds the set maximum flow velocity (encoded velocity). For purely imaging purposes, the encoded velocity can thus be slightly below the expected maximum flow velocity. The encoded velocity must, however, be set above the expected maximum flow velocity in the vessel (more than 10%) for quantification purposes.

Precipitation during a specific phase is a fundamental characteristic of all spins. Flow-sensitive sequences can thus be used, because moving spins experience a flow-induced phase shift in a magnetic field. This shift depends upon the strength of the magnetic field and the flow velocity of the spins. Because of inhomogeneities in magnetic fields, the phase for stationary tissue is never exactly zero—thus, various images must be subtracted. The simplest method of generating this type of reference image is to acquire a flow-compensated image in which all spins (either stationary or moving) indicate the same phase. An important aspect of phase contrast angiography is that measurement can only ever occur in one direction for a particular encoded velocity. Unlike with the inflow technique, simultaneous recording in multiple directions is not possible. As a result, at least three acquisitions taken orthogonally to one another are necessary to capture all three dimensions during phase contrast angiography (▶ Fig. 3.43). This means that a total of four

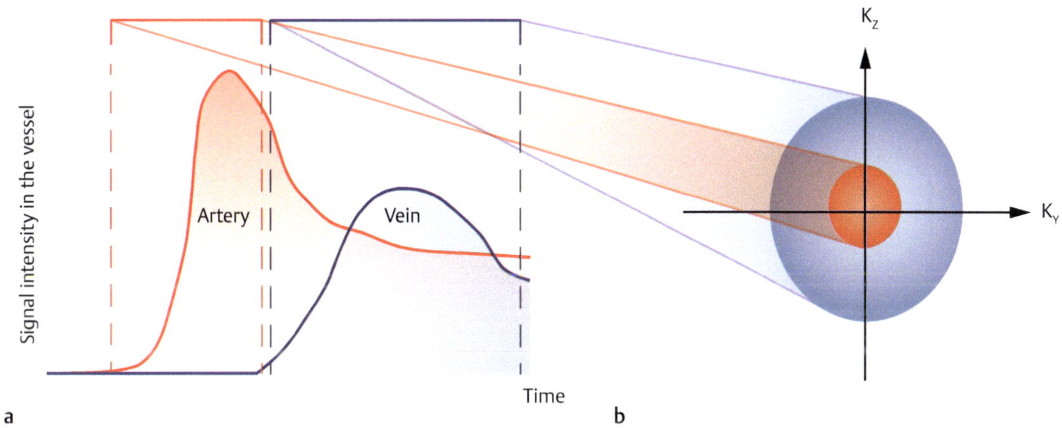

Fig. 3.44 Chronology of the phase-encoding steps (profile order) for a contrast-enhanced MRA. Schematic depiction.

a Temporally different signal-time curves of the contrast agent enhancement in the artery and vein.

b Corresponding chronology for filling the k-space, first internally (arterial phase) for the contrast, and then externally, the relevant portion of the k-space for the spatial resolution (venous phase).

acquisitions are needed to generate a phase contrast angiography image. Compared to time-of-flight angiography, this significantly increases measurement time. Despite this, the excellent background noise suppression means that phase contrast angiography is used for smaller scan volumes.

Contrast-Enhanced Magnetic Resonance Angiography

Most patients are not able to remain still long enough to complete a traditional inflow MRA. Contrast-enhanced MRA with or without breath-holding techniques is well-suited to these patients. The high signal, which is normally achieved by using contrast agent, is extremely well-suited for 3-D reconstructions. Correct timing for administering the contrast agent bolus plays a crucial role in the quality of the contrast-enhanced MRA images. Its use is especially helpful if abnormal vessels would otherwise be masked by slow or turbulent flow. The first pass of contrast agent is used to depict arterial vessels, as is also done in myocardial perfusion analyses (▶ Fig. 3.44). Rapid T1-weighted (T1w) 3-D GE sequences are used for this purpose.

In order to determine the correct measurement point for the first pass, a rapid, dynamic MRI sequence is used—a sort of MR fluoroscopy technique named differently by different manufacturers, including Bolus TRAK (Philips), Care Bolus (Siemens), and Fluoro Triggered MRA (GE). A single slice several cm thick is acquired at various points with a temporal resolution of at least 1 image/s. The sequence is started by applying a small test bolus of contrast agent (e.g., 1 ml). By playing the acquired images in cine mode (▶ Fig. 3.45), contrast agent flooding can reach the target area, which helps determine the optimal point for starting the sequence. The sequence can, however, also be used to start the high-resolution 3-D sequence directly, upon flooding the target vessel.

> **Note**
>
> In patients with congenital heart defects, especially ones already treated via surgery, pulmonary perfusion can be partially limited, or a difference in sides may occur. The point of bolus administration can be determined very well using this rapid, temporally high-resolution, yet spatially low-resolution sequence (▶ Fig. 3.45).

The measurement periods for a spatially high-resolution 3-D MRA would normally be too long to make a sharp distinction between arterial and venous signals, since the arterial window before the contrast agent also reaches the veins is only a few seconds long. If the special characteristics of the k-space are used, the phase-encoding steps responsible for the contrast are acquired during the first seconds (meaning during the arterial phase), and the later phase-encoding steps are then used to determine image sharpness; the veins will not be depicted despite containing contrast agent (▶ Fig. 3.44). This profile order can be configured for the sequence and is described differently by different manufacturers—it is known as CENTRA, Elliptic Centric, and Centric-elliptical, among other names. Another "venous" phase from which the arterial phase may be subtracted should be acquired after the arterial phase so that the contrast-enhanced MRA is most effective.

Particularly for congenital heart defects with numerous vessel variants and postoperative changes, time-resolved

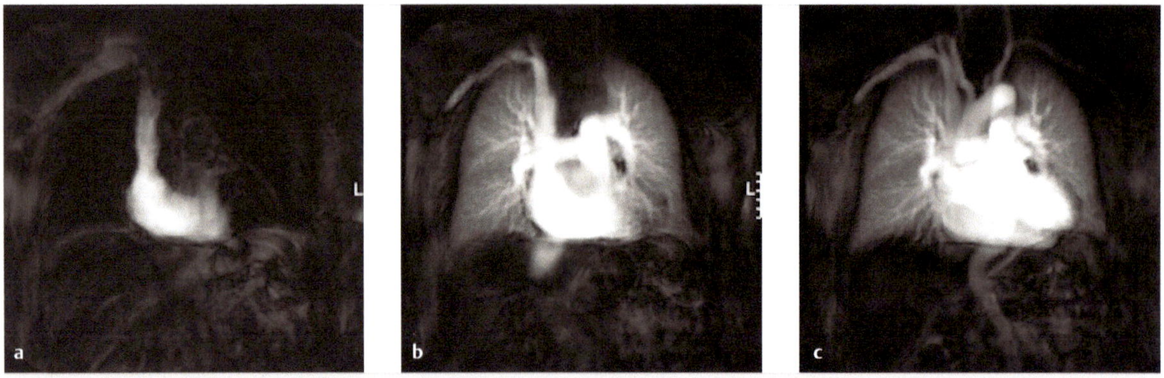

Fig. 3.45 Depiction of three example points of a bolus TRAK sequence in coronal orientation through the thorax.
a Contrast agent inflow in the right time-ventricle via the superior vena cava.
b Contrast agent inflow in the pulmonary arteries of the right and left lungs.
c Contrast agent inflow in the ascending aorta.

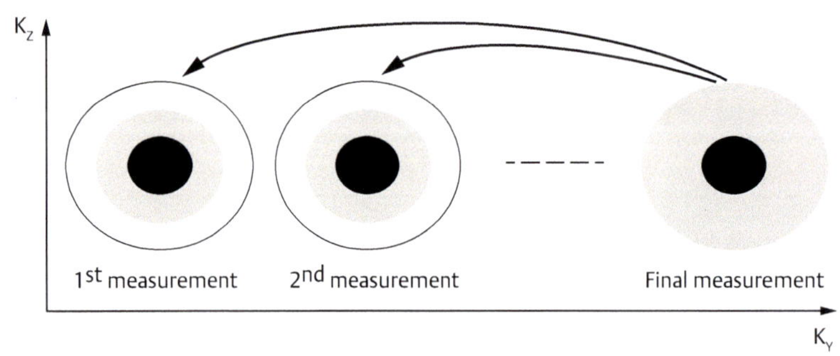

Fig. 3.46 3-D keyhole technique. Schematic depiction. For the keyhole technique, the internal area of the k-space (black and gray circle) is measured repeatedly at the start of the acquisition. All the data in the k-space is not collected until the last measurements are taken, and the previous measurements are copied over into all of the missing areas (arrows). This makes rapid 4-D MRAs with high temporal resolution possible.

contrast-enhanced MRA sequences that show dynamic depictions with contrast agent flooding and run-off (similar to those in digital subtraction angiography) are very useful and can help avoid more extensive invasive diagnostic procedures. To this end, numerous techniques for shortening acquisition time must be combined with one another. The characteristics of the k-space with measurement of partial data and the use of parallel imaging with higher acceleration factors are nearly always used. A temporal resolution of circa 1 second has been reached for the numerous time-resolved contrast-enhanced MRA sequences now available on the market, including 4-D Trak (Philips), Twist (Siemens), or TRICKS (GE). One particular technique for filling the k-space, known as the keyhole technique, is used for 4-D MRA. Only the internal area of the k-space, which is responsible for the image contrast, is measured repeatedly during contrast agent passage (▶ Fig. 3.46).

Only in the very last data set is all of the k-space data completely selected and copied over to all other data sets, which previously were only partially acquired. At the end of the acquisition period, both the arteries and veins are filled with contrast agent, meaning that information regarding image sharpness for both vessels is available in high spatial resolution during all phases, while the contrast-determined portions reflect the contrast agent flooding in the 4-D MRA with a high temporal resolution after the Fourier transformation.

3.3.8 Depiction of Scars and Fibroses

Based on the data from various cardiac MRI registries,[52,53] depicting MR scars, viability, and fibroses is one of the most common indications for cardio MRI, and is being used more and more frequently in patients with congenital heart defects, particularly for postoperative exams. Depicting scars and fibroses in the myocardium is of relevance to prognosis and also helps with the differential diagnosis of numerous acquired or congenital cardiomyopathies.

To date, the most widely spread method of depicting necrosis, scars, and fibroses is the delayed contrast agent enhancement technique, also known as late gadolinium enhancement (LGE) or delayed enhancement.

The principle of delayed contrast agent enhancement (circa 10–20 minutes after injection) in scar tissue is based on a combination of multiple, sometimes concurrent pathomechanisms, namely delayed contrast agent inflow and delayed contrast agent outflow. This leads to a larger contrast agent distribution volume caused by concurrent acute edema and an enlarged extracellular space due to destruction of the myocardium after an infarction or an inflammation. The contrast agent leads to a reduction in T1 relaxation time, which is expressed more visibly in the scar than in the viable myocardium. The principle of delayed contrast agent accumulation in the scarred tissue was already depicted in the 1980s during animal trials with CT, and was then later depicted via MRI. Nevertheless, the procedure only became widespread in cardiac MRI in the mid-1990s, with the introduction of contrast-rich inversion recovery GE sequences.[46]

Using this sequence (which is generally acquired during end diastole), it is possible to use a non-slice-selective 180° inversion pulse to "nullify" the healthy (meaning not delayed in absorbing contrast agent) myocardium so that it is depicted in black, while the scar appears bright. This effect can be further enhanced by using fat suppression. This technique takes advantage of the differing T1 relaxation times of the myocardium, blood, and scar tissue after a 180° prepulse ($T1_{myocardium} > T1_{blood} > T1_{scar}$). The prepulse delay must be selected so that the T1 relaxation time curve of the healthy myocardium passes through its "zero-crossing" point and appears black on the LGE images (▶ Fig. 3.47).

The ratio of relaxation times for the various relevant tissues and the optimal initial pulse changes mostly during the first 10 minutes after administering contrast agent, in addition to being reliant on the type of contrast agent used. Ten to thirty minutes after administering contrast agent, the ratio of relaxation times of the tissues to one another is relatively constant.

Choosing the correct inversion time is a critical point for MR depictions of scars using standard inversion recovery GE sequences. Thus, it is helpful to perform a test sequence with high temporal resolution and various inversion times prior to the actual measurement. The optimal inversion time at which the healthy myocardium

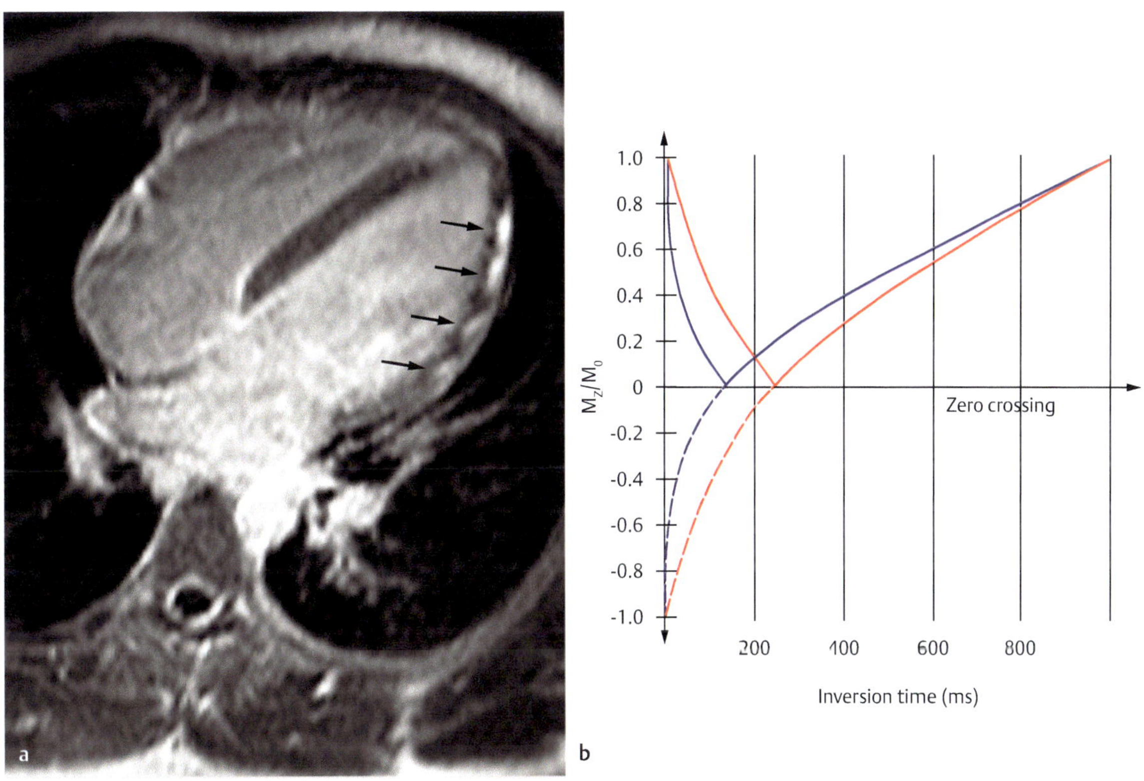

Fig. 3.47 Optimal scar depiction.
M_0 = initial magnetization
M_z = longitudinal magnetization

a Image of a subepicardial scar (arrow) in a patient with previous myocarditis, with optimal contrast (scar: white, myocardium: black, blood: medium gray). Measurement occurs during diastole with an inversion time of 220 ms.

b Signal intensity curves of the scar tissue (blue) and the healthy, viable myocardium (red) after the inversion pulse (180° pulse), at various inversion times. The inversion time must be selected such that the longitudinal magnetization of the myocardium (red line) passes through its "zero-crossing" point and is thus depicted as black. In this depicted example, zero crossing occurred at circa 220 ms. The scar (blue line) displays a zero crossing at circa 150 ms after administering contrast agent. If the selected inversion time is too short (in this case, 150 ms), the scar would appear black in the image (▶ Fig. 3.48b). Since the image does not depict any negative signal intensity values (dotted line), the values (solid lines) of the signal intensity curves (always positive) are actually depicted in the image.

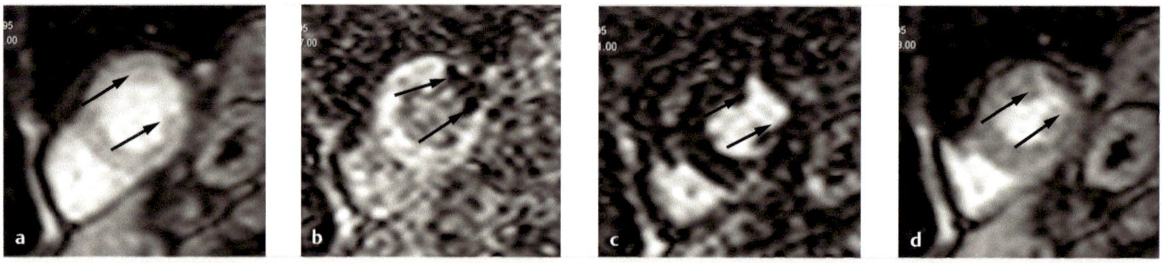

Fig. 3.48 Scar depiction with the Look-Locker sequence. Example selected images from a dynamic Look-Locker sequence series after administering contrast agent, in a patient with chronic infarction of the lateral wall of the left ventricle (**a–d**, arrows), using various inversion times.

a Approximately the same signal intensity values are displayed in the viable myocardium and in the scar at an inversion time of 14 ms.
b The scar's zero-crossing point occurs at an inversion time of 127 ms and is depicted in black (arrows).
c Optimal selection of an inversion time of 211 ms: the healthy myocardium passes through its zero-crossing point and is depicted in black, while the scar is depicted bright.
d If too long an inversion period is selected (in this case, 408 ms), the scar and viable myocardium can no longer be differentiated.

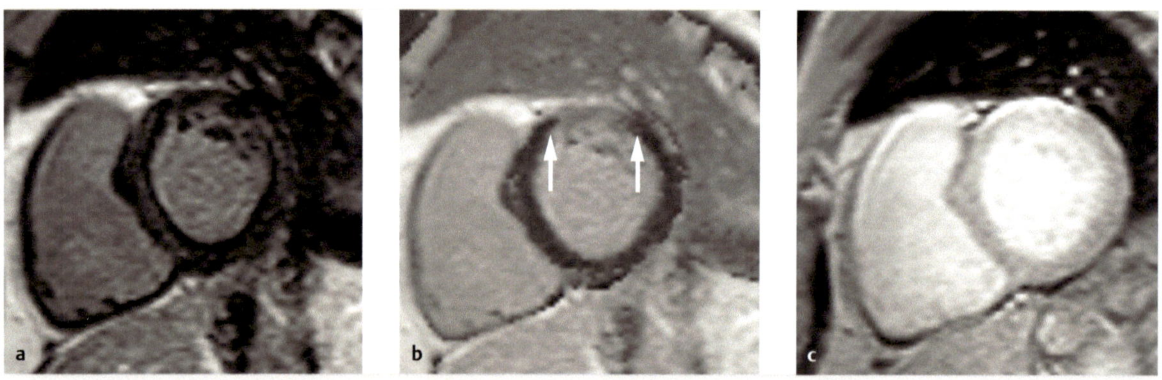

Fig. 3.49 Fibrosis and scar depiction using a PSIR sequence. 2-D PSIR sequence of a 67-year-old male patient with discrete fibrosis and scar formation near the anterior wall, which can only be identified clearly during the phase image (**b**, arrows).

a Short-axis slice of the modulus image.
b Short-axis slice of the phase image.
c Short-axis slice of the reference image.

appears black can be read directly from the images (▶ Fig. 3.48). The sequences are commercially available and are also known by other names, such as Look-Locker sequence (Philips) or TI Scout (GE).

When depicting signal intensities, the algebraic signs of signal intensity curves (▶ Fig. 3.47b) are commonly not taken into account. This means that the values are depicted as the mathematical modulus so that the viable myocardium shows the same signal, whether the selected inversion time is too short or too long. This can present difficulties, especially when interpreting smaller scars or fibroses. The phase-sensitive inversion recovery (PSIR) sequence constitutes an alternative that is relatively independent of inversion time. This is a depiction of a signal dependent upon algebraic signs, which enables real images to be calculated (▶ Fig. 3.49 and ▶ Fig. 3.50) with somewhat longer acquisition times.[54] Using traditional modulus imaging methods and an inversion recovery GE sequence, only one image is acquired during diastole. In contrast, two images from consecutive heartbeats are acquired during diastole with the PSIR sequence. The actual data is then measured with a fixed inversion time (generally 300 ms) and then measured at the same time during the cardiac cycle with a smaller flip angle (5°), so that all tissue already demonstrates a positive signal.

This second data set serves as a reference data set (▶ Fig. 3.49c) for correcting the first one (▶ Fig. 3.49a) and reconstructing a real image (▶ Fig. 3.49b), which generates an LGE image—largely independent from the inversion time selected (▶ Fig. 3.49a)—with high contrast between the myocardium and the scar (▶ Fig. 3.49b and ▶ Fig. 3.50b).

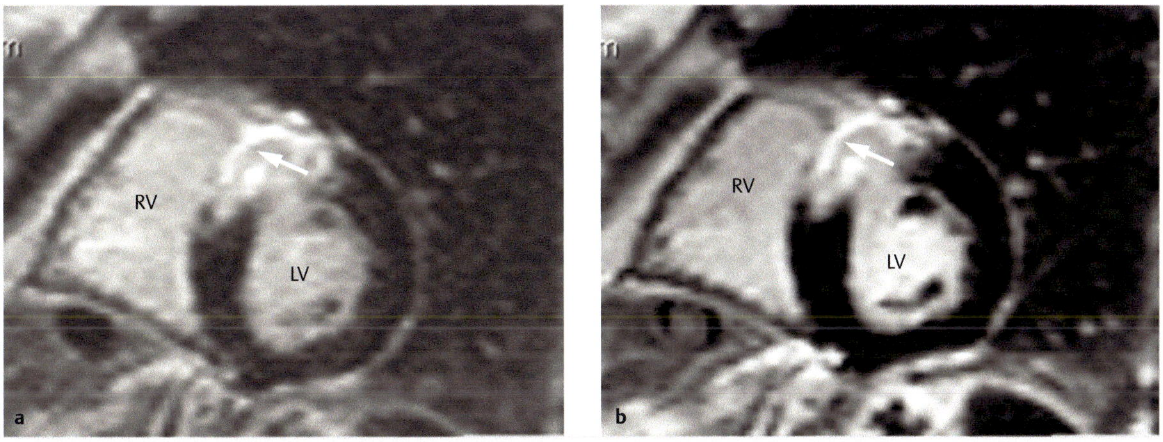

Fig. 3.50 Fibrosis and scar depiction using a PSIR sequence. Sixty-year-old male patient after an anterolateral infarction (**a**, **b**, arrows). During the inversion recovery GE sequence (**a**), the inversion time is set to 230 ms on an individual basis in order to nullify the myocardium. (**b**) The PSIR sequence demonstrates a much better "nulling" of the viable myocardium and also a better delineation of the scar tissue (arrow).
LV = left ventricle
RV = right ventricle.
a 2-D inversion recovery GE sequence.
b Phase image of the 2-D PSIR sequence.

Table 3.6 Imaging procedure for percutaneous transluminal interventions on the heart and great vessels.

Physical basis	Imaging procedure	Image dimensions
X-ray radiation	Monoplanar or biplanar fluoroscopy/angiography C-arm rotation tomography CT	2-D summation 3-D, 2-D cross-section 3-D, 2-D cross-section
Ultrasound	TTE TEE Intracardiac echocardiography	3-D, 2-D cross-section 3-D, 2-D cross-section 2-D cross-section
Magnetic field	MRI	3-D, 2-D cross-section
Electrical signals of the heart	Electroanatomical mapping	3-D

CT, computed tomography; MRI, magnetic resonance imaging; TEE, transesophageal echocardiography; TTE, transthoracic echocardiography.

3.4 Imaging-Guided Interventional Treatment

Ingo Dähnert

3.4.1 Introduction

Preparations for both interventional and surgical procedures are made using various imaging procedures for diagnostic purposes. During the procedure, however, the processes differ fundamentally. The surgeon gains significant information via direct visual observation and palpatory perception. The interventionalist, on the other hand, relies on additional imaging procedures that allow him or her to perform the procedure in a controlled manner and provide adequate anatomical and functional information before, during, and after the intervention, as well as information regarding any complications that may occur. In principle, various imaging procedures can be used to guide interventional procedures, many of which can be combined with one another (▶ Table 3.6). Catheter procedures without imaging guidance have become the exception. Catheter exams and interventions on the heart and adjacent vessels are traditionally performed under fluoroscopic monitoring. Angio(cardio)graphy provides anatomical information. For certain applications, it can be helpful to superimpose 3-D anatomical information gleaned from prior CT, MRI, or echocardiography over the fluoroscopic image. For electrophysiological interventions, these images, as well as the local electrical signals of the heart acquired during electroanatomical mapping, are also superimposed on the fluoroscopic image. C-arm rotation tomography is a new, rapidly developing field that allows 3-D angiograms to be performed

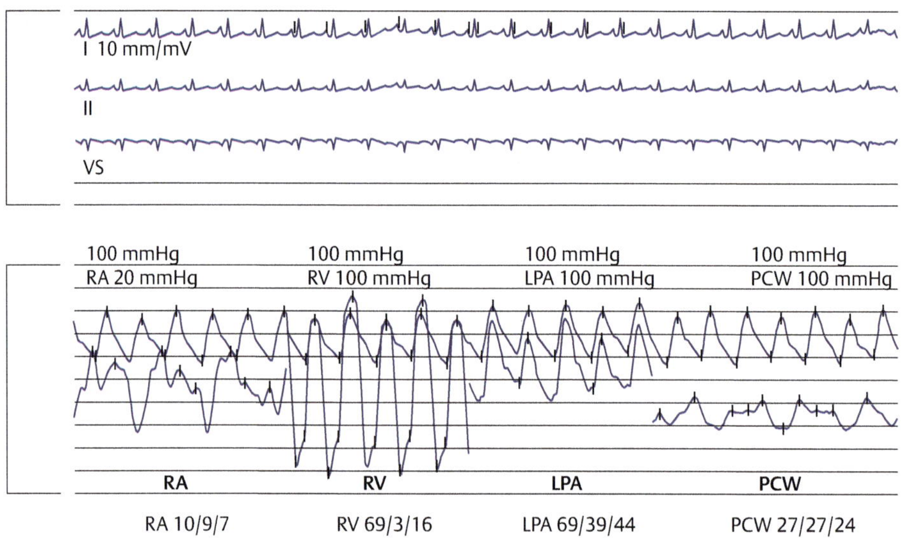

Fig. 3.51 Flow-directed catheter exams. Six-month-old infant with mitral stenosis. The pressure curve shows the location of the catheter tip: concurrent with the continuous arterial pressure curve (pressure: 69/50–59 mmHg), normal pressure is present in the right atrium (RA pressure: 7 mmHg, measurement range: 20 mmHg), elevated pressure in the right ventricle (RV pressure 69/0–16 mmHg, measurement range: 100 mmHg), elevated pressure in the pulmonary artery (LPA pressure: 60/39–44 mmHg, measurement range: 100 mmHg), and pulmonary arterial occlusion pressure is significantly elevated (PCW or wedge pressure: 24 mmHg, measurement range: 100 mmHg) as an indirect measure of left atrial pressure.
LPA = left pulmonary artery
PCW = pulmonary capillary wedge pressure (wedge pressure [left atrial pressure])
RA = right atrium
RV = right ventricle

during the intervention. Combined imaging using fluoroscopy and echocardiography has been tried and tested for certain interventions. Pure echocardiography imaging is also possible, but has not yet become standard for individual indications. The field of MRI-guided interventions is promising, but currently remains largely experimental.

3.4.2 Catheter Procedures without Imaging Guidance

Nearly all diagnostic and therapeutic cardiovascular catheter interventions are performed while under some sort of imaging monitoring. Exceptions include diagnostic right heart catheter exams (known as flow-directed catheters), placement of pulmonary catheters (Swan-Ganz catheters), and transfemoral implantation of intra-aortic balloon pumps in the ICU. In the former, monitoring via imaging is replaced by simultaneous ECG observation and observation of the peak of a pressure curve derived from a balloon catheter floating along with blood flow (▸ Fig. 3.51). For the latter two cases, correct catheter placement is subsequently monitored using a thoracic X-ray (▸ Fig. 3.52 and ▸ Fig. 3.53). The complication rates for these interventions are low, but not negligible in individual cases, allocating all of the introduced devices can constitute a challenge.[55,56]

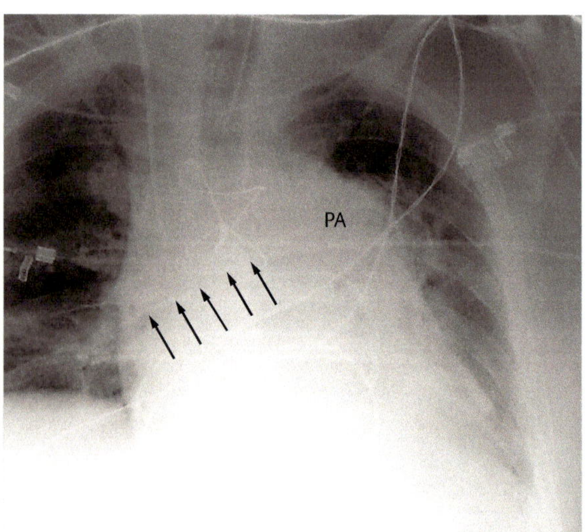

Fig. 3.52 Thoracic X-ray for monitoring catheter placement. Thoracic image in the supine position with documentation of a correctly placed pulmonary artery catheter (Swan-Ganz catheter) for intensive monitoring of pulmonary pressure and cardiac output in the right pulmonary artery (arrows).
PA = pulmonary artery

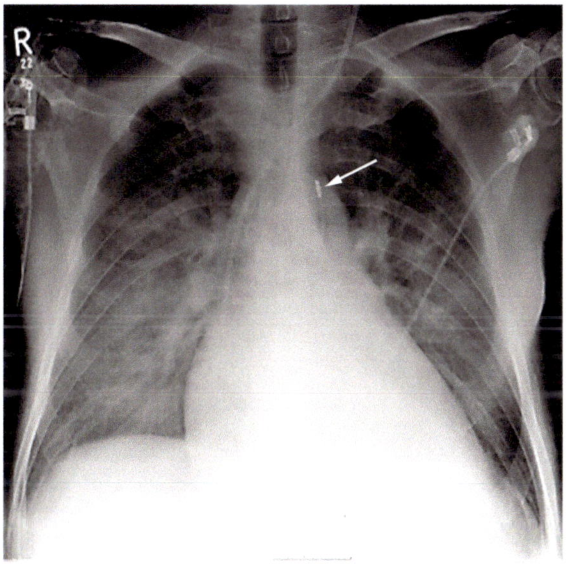

Fig. 3.53 Thoracic X-ray for monitoring catheter placement. Thoracic image in the supine position for a patient with left heart failure and pulmonary edema. The image shows a central venous access placed superior to the left jugular vein in the upper hollow vein, and an intra-aortic balloon pump in the descending aorta (arrow).

> **Note**
>
> It is inadvisable to use blind catheter positioning for patients with congenital heart defects. Instead, we recommend monitoring catheter movement.[57]

3.4.3 Methods of Imaging Guidance

Imaging via Conventional Fluoroscopy and Angiography

Diagnostic and imaging treatments for the heart and the great vessels are closely intertwined with X-ray diagnostics. For decades, angiographic images were the only method of depicting images of the anatomy and function of cardiovascular structures. Even today, they remain the gold standard, particularly for unusual findings (▶ Fig. 3.54). All interventional procedures were developed using this type of imaging, and continue to be performed under its use (▶ Fig. 3.55). Solutions for problematic situations and complications (▶ Fig. 3.56) are well-known and documented.

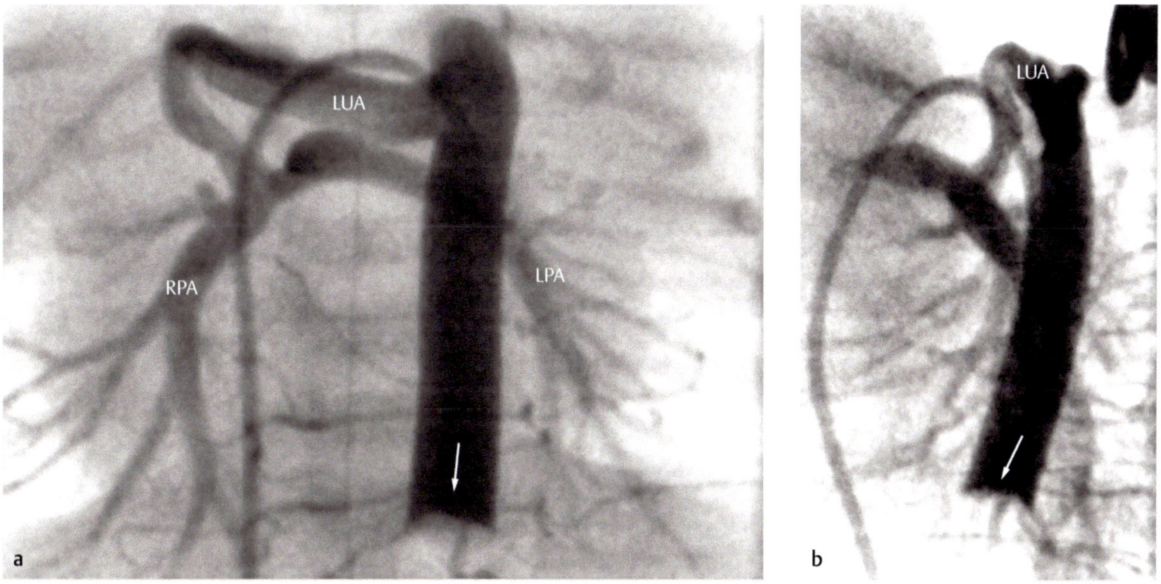

Fig. 3.54 Aortogram. Right PDA from the right lusoria artery near the left aortic arch in a cyanotic newborn with pulmonary atresia and a VSD. A Berman angiographic balloon catheter (**a**, **b**, arrows) is pushed from the right femoral vein deep into the descending aorta (via the right atrium, right ventricle, VSD, ascending aorta, and left aortic arch), blocking it on the lower margin of the image (**a**, **b**, arrows). Injection of the contrast agent identifies an aberrant right subclavian artery (lusoria artery) originating as a final branch of the aortic arch, from which a right PDA perfuses the pulmonary arterial branches.
LPA = left pulmonary artery
LUA = aberrant right subclavian artery
RPA = right pulmonary artery
a Aortogram, RAO 0°.
b Aortogram, LAO 90°.

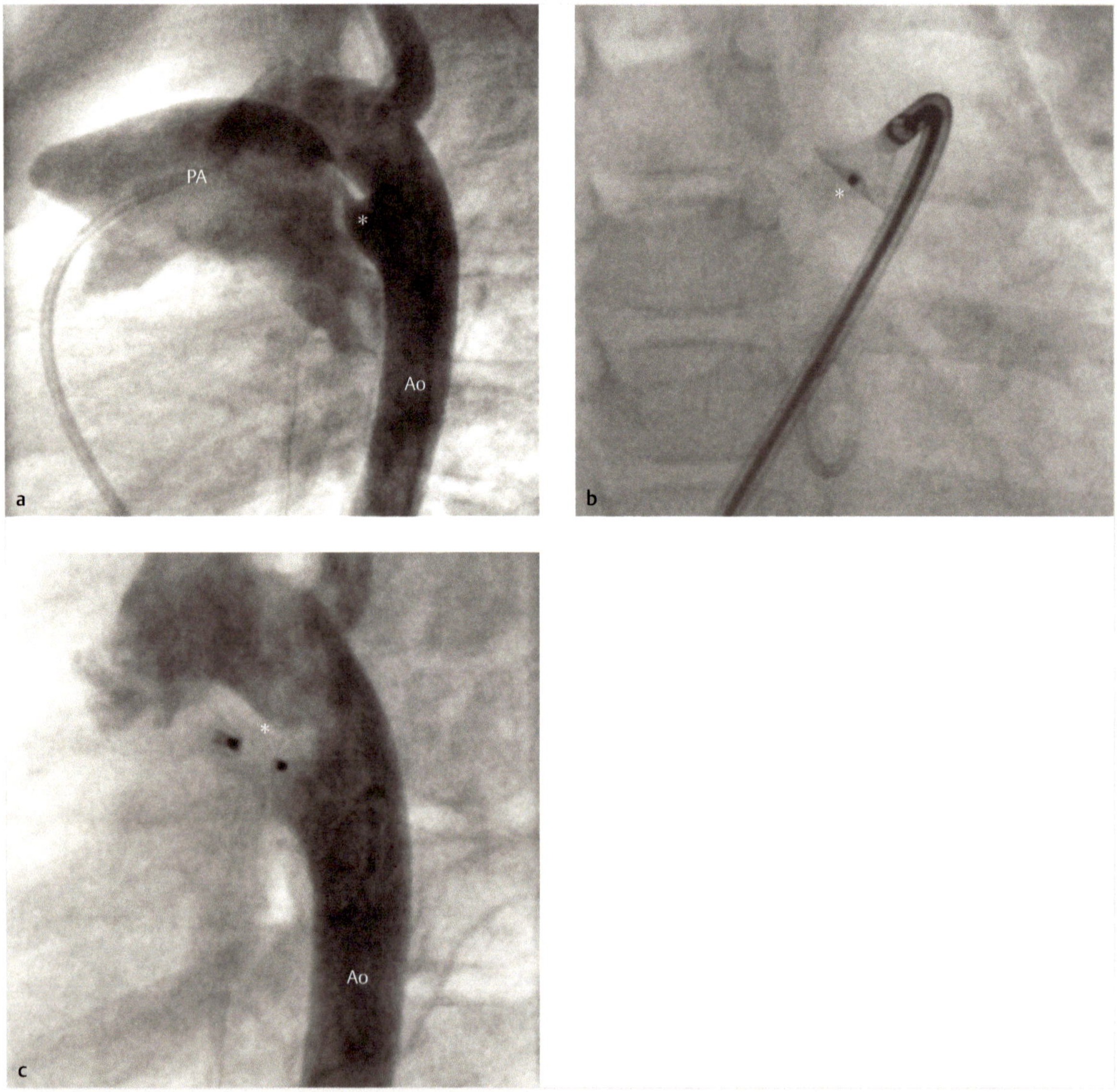

Fig. 3.55 Aortogram. Six-month-old infant with a PDA (**a–c**, asterisk).
Ao = aorta
PA = pulmonary artery
a Aortogram, LAO 90°: access to the descending aorta via the main pulmonary arterial trunk. Ampulla of the PDA (asterisk).
b Occlusion device (asterisk) in place (a.–p. projection).
c Aortogram, LAO 90°: Occlusion device (asterisk) after the intervention.

Modern catheter laboratories in Germany that are suitable for interventional procedures are generally known as "*left catheter measurement facilities*" even though they often also treat congenital heart defects via interventions on the right heart. They possess a (biplanar) system with two mobile fluoroscopy devices. Digital flat panel detectors generate images that allow both fluoroscopic imaging for catheter manipulation (while sparing the patient exposure to radiation) and simultaneous registration of up to 50 images/s in two levels for angiographic exams. The electronically saved images can be processed, measured, and depicted by the examiner on an additional monitor or "map" (also known as a road map), upon which the subsequent fluoroscopic image can be superimposed. Equipment also includes an injection pump for contrast agent, as well as a multi-channel

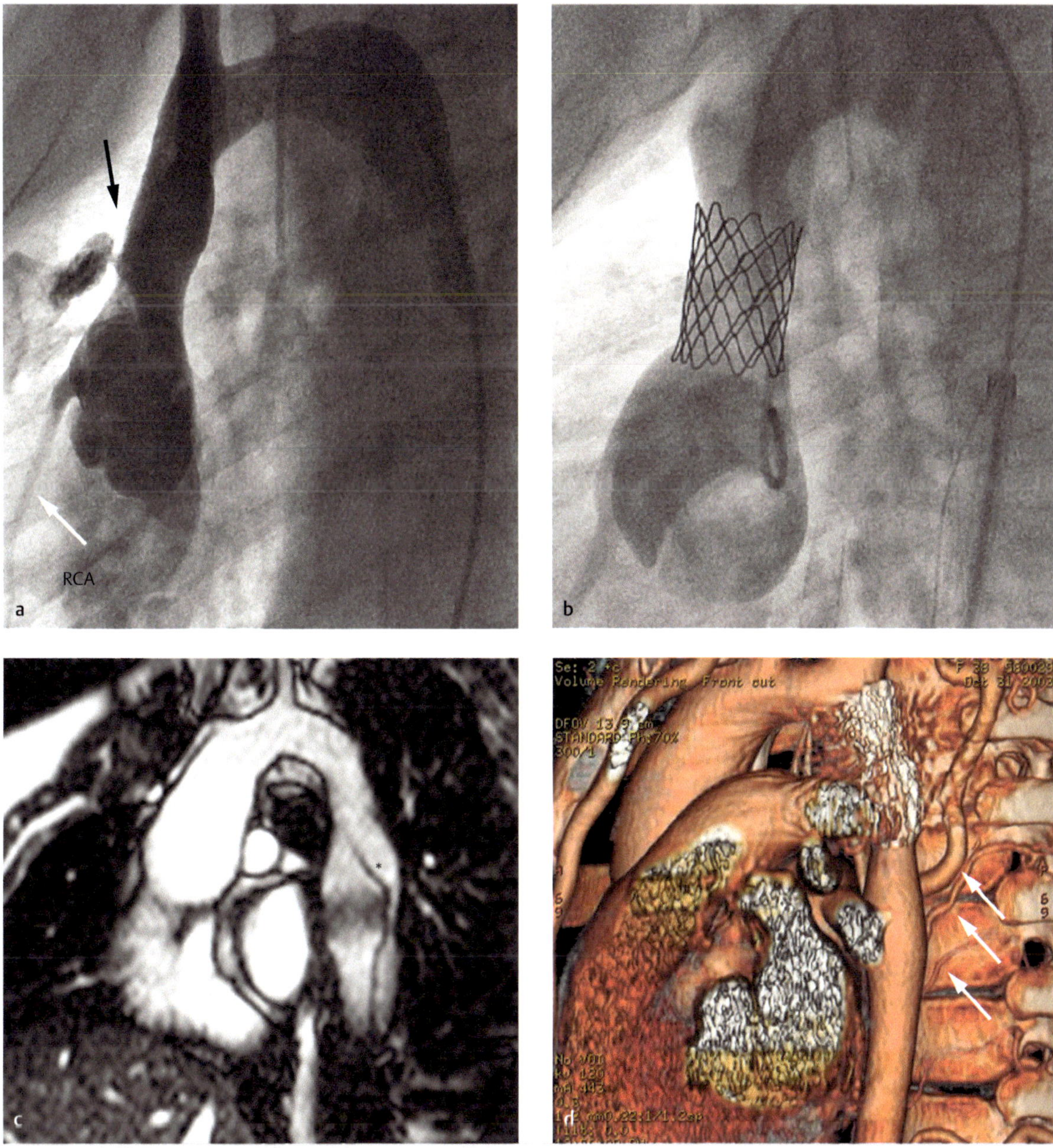

Fig. 3.56 Aortogram. Three different patients.
RCA = right coronary artery—white arrow

- **a** Rupture of the ascending aorta during balloon angioplasty of a postoperative supravalvular aortic stenosis in a 12-year-old boy. Aortogram, LAO 90°: anterior rupture site (black arrow). This rupture caused an acute, life-threatening situation.
- **b** Repeat aortogram, LAO 90°, after emergency placement of a covered stent; correct closure of the perforation. Rapid stabilization and restoration to previous condition after placement of the stent.
- **c** Parasagittal transverse cine MRI of another patient during systole: dissection membrane after implanting a covered nitinol stent with only minor obliteration after dilating an aortic coarctation. The stent is not completely flush with the wall (asterisk).
- **d** 3-D reconstruction of a control CT after stent placement to treat an aortic coarctation. Residual collaterals are still visible (arrows).

measurement and registration system for depicting ECG and blood pressure curves and hemodynamic calculations, and for documenting additional vital signs and exam parameters. It is crucial that facilities also be properly equipped with the following devices in case of complications or emergencies:

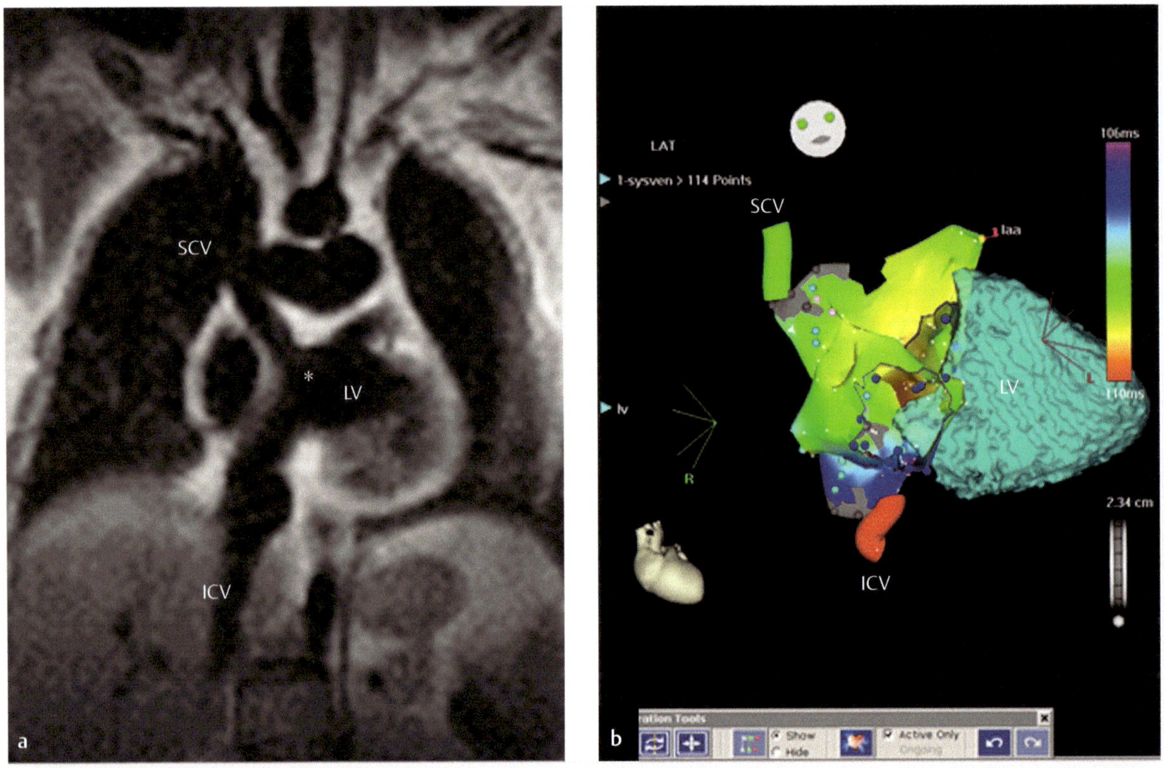

Fig. 3.57 Imaging integration of MRI/CT data.
IVC = inferior vena cava
LV = left ventricle
SVC = superior vena cava

a Coronal SE image of a male patient with complete transposition of the great arteries and an intact ventricular septum (TGA IVS) after an atrial switch operation (also known as Senning/Mustard procedure), during which atrial flow was diverted using a venous baffle (asterisk)—thus, the TGA underwent physiological correction.

b Imaging integration into the Carto electrophysiological ablation system of CT data and electroanatomical mapping for a patient after an atrial switch operation.

- Cardioverter defibrillators
- Intubation equipment
- Suction systems
- Respiration devices
- Pleural drainage sets
- Pericardial puncture sets
- Oxygen supply
- Emergency medications

No literary references are listed here, since comprehensive standard works (e.g., the work of Mullins[57]) already exist in this field.

Imaging via Fluoroscopy and Angiography by Superimposing or Integrating Images from Other Procedures

Previous integration of 3-D data sets acquired via CT, MRI, or echocardiography with the fluoroscopic images is a promising idea that has already gained some traction[58] in interventional electrophysiology (▶ Fig. 3.57). Its application for coronary interventions remains in the experimental stages.[59]

To date, it has only been possible to use this technique for interventions in patients with congenital heart defects in rare cases, because the change in bodily posture, respiration, and larger intraluminal devices (rigid guide wires, balloon catheters, large-lumen sheaths) during the intervention can change the position and course of anatomical structures significantly compared to preinterventional exams.

Imaging Using C-Arm Rotation Tomography

The prevalence of flat panel detectors has made it possible to also prepare images similar to CT images via a 3-D rotational angiogram with the C-arm that is generally available in most catheter laboratories (▶ Fig. 3.58), thus allowing 3-D imaging.[60] Its applications for interventions due to congenital heart defects have been documented.[61] In order to generate optimal images, it is necessary to induce temporary respiratory and cardiac arrest. This necessitates the use of intubation narcosis and adenosine injection, or rapid ventricular pacemaker stimulation.[62,63]

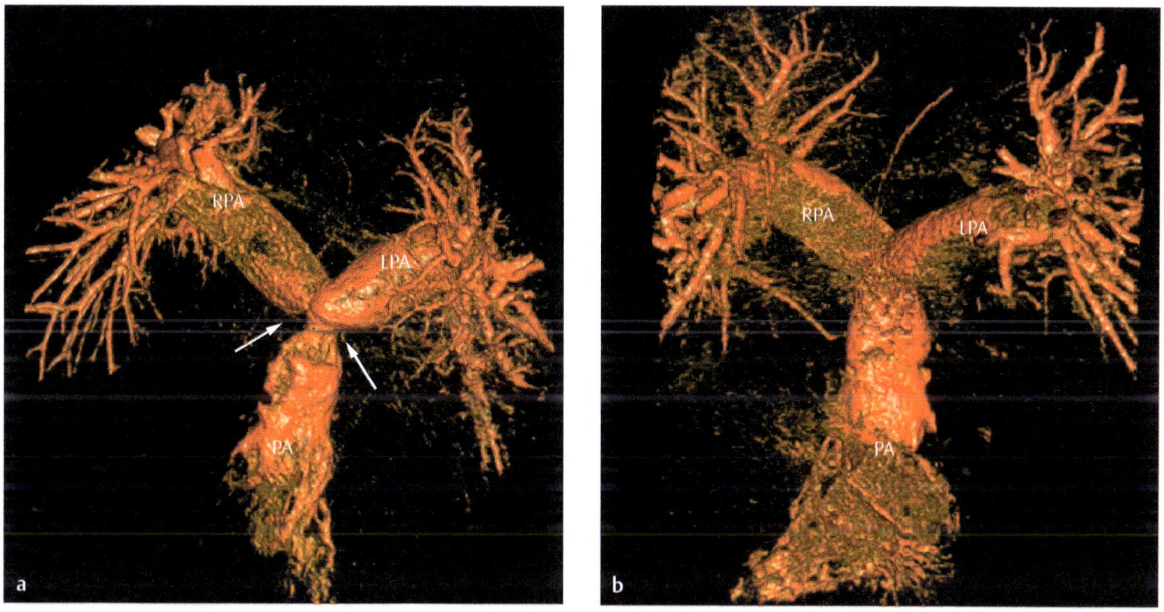

Fig. 3.58 C-arm rotation tomography. 3-D reconstruction of a rotational angiogram image dataset for a patient with supravalvular pulmonary stenosis (**a**, arrows).
LPA = left pulmonary artery
PA = pulmonary artery
RPA = right pulmonary artery

a Before stent implantation.
b After stent implantation.

Table 3.7 Interventions in which a combination of traditional fluoroscopy and echocardiography have been tried and tested.

Intervention	Role of echocardiography
Transseptal puncture (TSP)	Positioning the puncture needle
Myocardial biopsy	Checking bioptome position
Mitral valve balloon valvuloplasty	TSP, checking catheter position, assessing results of the intervention
Interventional mitral valvuloplasty	TSP, checking device position, assessing results of the intervention
Balloon atrial septostomy	Checking catheter position, assessing results of the intervention
Interventional ASD closure	Measuring size, checking occlusion device position
Interventional PFO closure	Measuring size, checking occlusion device position
Interventional VSD closure	Checking occlusion device position
Interventional closure of the left auricle	TSP, ruling out thrombi, measuring size, checking occlusion device position
Closure of paravalvular leaks	Determining location of the defect
Septal ablation in cases of HOCM	Marking the target area with contrast

ASD, atrial septal defect; HOCM, hypertrophic obstructive cardiomyopathy; PFO, patent foramen ovale; TSP, transseptal puncture; VSD, ventricular septal defect.

Imaging Using a Combination of Traditional Fluoroscopy and Angiography with Echocardiographical Methods

Radiation exposure and dependence on administering contrast agents are a few of the significant drawbacks of traditional, X-ray based imaging. In addition, thin (e.g., interatrial septum) and/or movable structures (e.g., mitral valve) cannot always be depicted with the necessary precision. Thus, a combination of traditional fluoroscopy and angiography with echocardiographic procedures (▶ Table 3.7) has been tried and tested for certain interventional procedures.[64] Transthoracic, transesophageal, and intracardiac probes are available for echocardiography, which allow 2-D slice depiction and color Doppler depictions of blood flow in accordance with standards. Systems that also provide real-time 3-D depictions are gaining popularity.[65] Echocardiographical imaging allows continual cross-sectional depiction of small and rapidly moving structures without contrast agent and radiation exposure. The position and movement of catheters, balloons, and other interventional devices can be observed and guided in direct relation to the intracardiac structures (▶ Fig. 3.59, ▶ Fig. 3.60, ▶ Fig. 3.61, ▶ Fig. 3.62). The result of the intervention can be assessed and, if needed, can be corrected immediately. However, a combination of fluoroscopy, echocardiography, and other cross-sectional procedures (MRI, CT) is often necessary, particularly for more complex interventions or complications (▶ Fig. 3.63).

Exclusive Echocardiographic Imaging

Individual interventions have been described exclusively as being carried out under echocardiographic monitoring (▶ Table 3.8). One reason for the development of this technique is that it allows bedside interventions to be performed in the ICU while avoiding potentially dangerous transport and repositioning of the patient.[66–68] To date, this type of approach has only established itself as a standard for balloon atrial septostomies in newborns with TGA (▶ Fig. 3.60); refer to the chapter on TGA.[69] Another reason is the ability to avoid burdening the patient with ionizing radiation and contrast agent. When closing an ASD, fluoroscopy and angiography serve solely to determine orientation and general position within the thorax. All significant information is gleaned by means of echocardiography.[70] Thus, it is suggested that the intervention be performed under exclusive echocardiographical monitoring (▶ Fig. 3.61 and ▶ Fig. 3.62), as is done in the authors' institutions and in other medical centers on a routine basis.[71,72] This allows a recoarctation to be treated under good echocardiographical imaging conditions.[73] Fetal interventions, which can also be performed under echocardiographical imaging monitoring, lie outside the focus of this chapter.[74]

Magnetic Resonance Imaging

MRI is especially well-suited to noninvasive multiplanar or 3-D depictions of the anatomy and function of cardiovascular structures. Thus, it will be discussed more thoroughly in Chapter 3.5, Interventional Magnetic Resonance Imaging. It does not use ionizing radiation. Small volumes of non-iodine contrast agent are administered, though only if absolutely necessary. In many respects, the development of MRI-based interventional techniques constitutes a significant challenge: many traditionally available interventional devices (wires, catheters, implants) are barely visible via MRI, cause artifacts, or are dangerous because of potential heating due to induction. Completely new materials and new techniques for signal transmission and processing must be developed, but are also expected to be used for new applications and interventional methods—this, in addition to current interventions, which remain under ongoing development.[77–79]

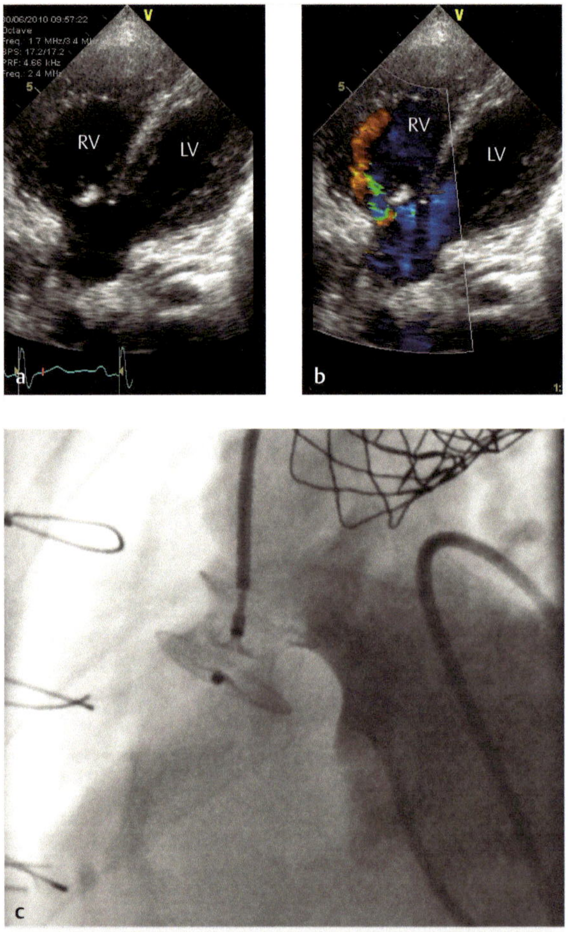

Fig. 3.59 Combination with ultrasound and angiography. Echocardiographic and angiographic depiction of a VSD closure.
LV = left ventricle
RV = right ventricle
a TTE of a membranous VSD without color Doppler.
b TTE of a membranous VSD with color Doppler.
c 90° LAO angiogram with implanted VSD occlusion device and no evidence of a residual shunt.

(Continued)

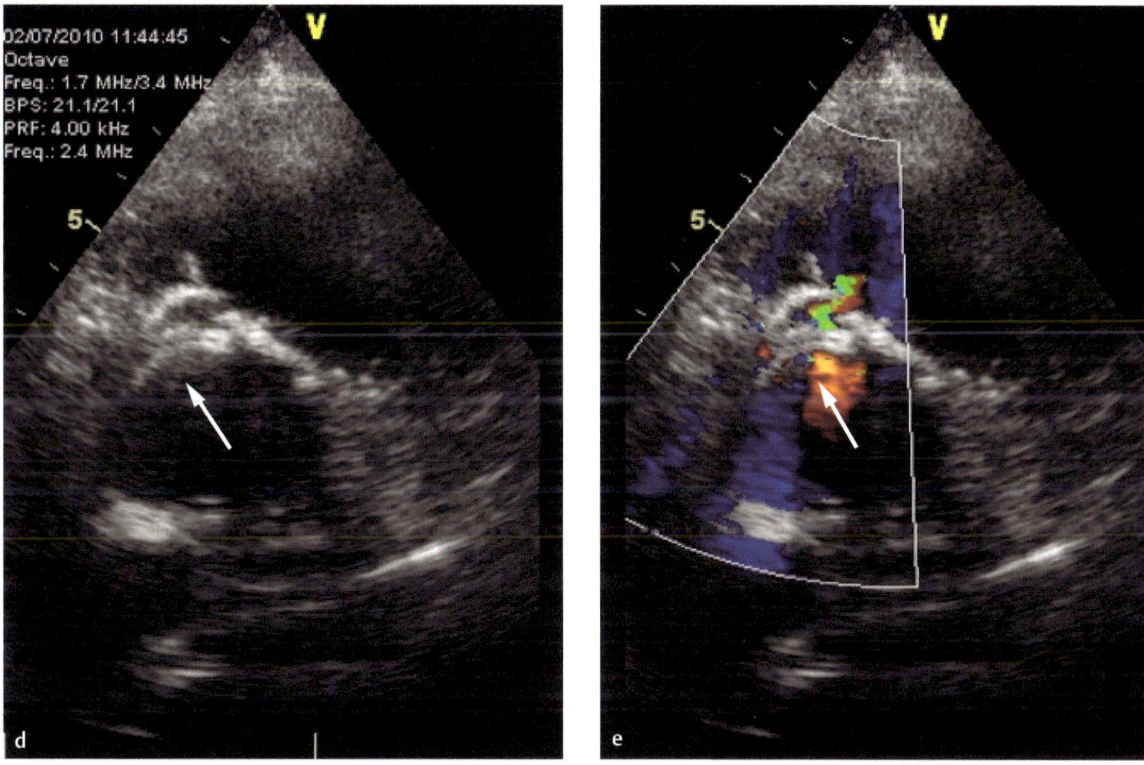

Fig 3.59 (*Continued*) **Combination with ultrasound and angiography.** Echocardiographic and angiographic depiction of a VSD closure.
LV = left ventricle
RV = right ventricle
d Echo follow-up after implantation of the VSD occlusion device (arrow), no color Doppler.
e Echo follow-up after implantation of the VSD occlusion device (arrow), color Doppler.

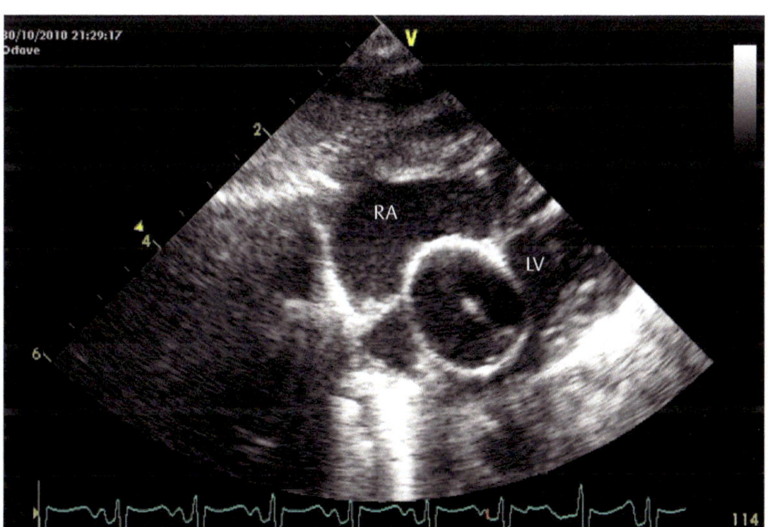

Fig. 3.60 Echocardiogram with balloon septostomy.
LV = left ventricle
RA = right atrium

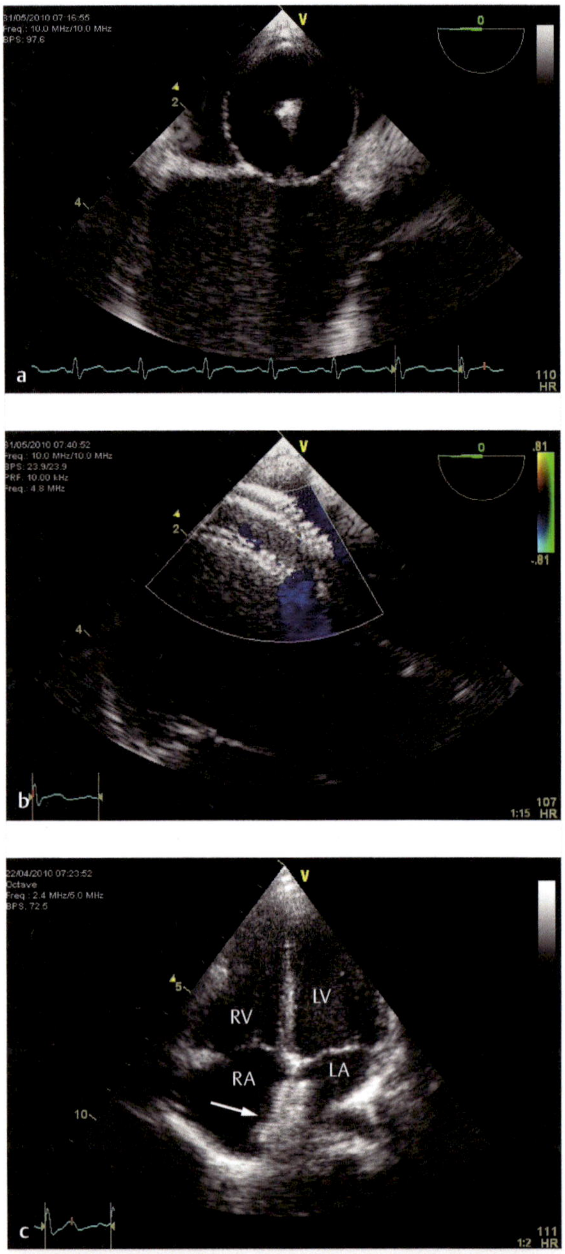

Fig. 3.61 Echocardiographic ASD closure.
LA = left atrium;
LV = left ventricle
RA = right atrium
RV = right ventricle

- **a** TEE measurement of defect size using a balloon (balloon sizing).
- **b** TEE after occlusion device implantation.
- **c** TTE in 4-chamber view after implantation of an atrial septal occlusion device (arrow).

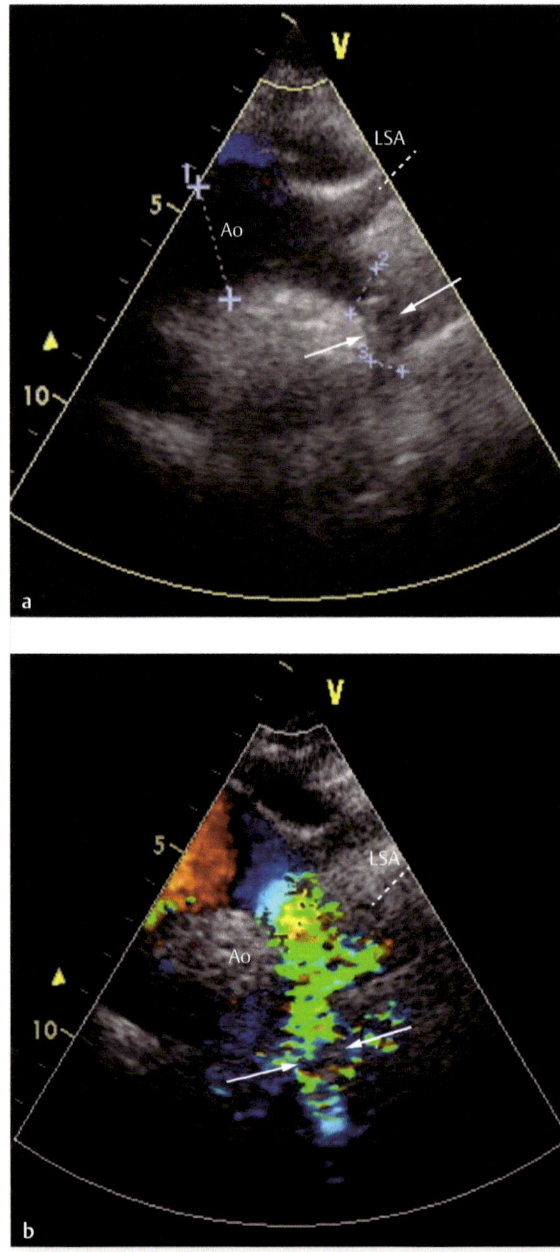

Fig. 3.62 Combination of ultrasound, X-ray, and angiography.
Diagnosing and treating recoarctation via stent implant.
Ao = aorta
LSA = left subclavian artery

- **a** Depiction of recoarctation (arrows) via a suprasternal echocardiographical view without color Doppler.
- **b** Depiction of a recoarctation (arrows) via a suprasternal echo view with color Doppler.

(Continued)

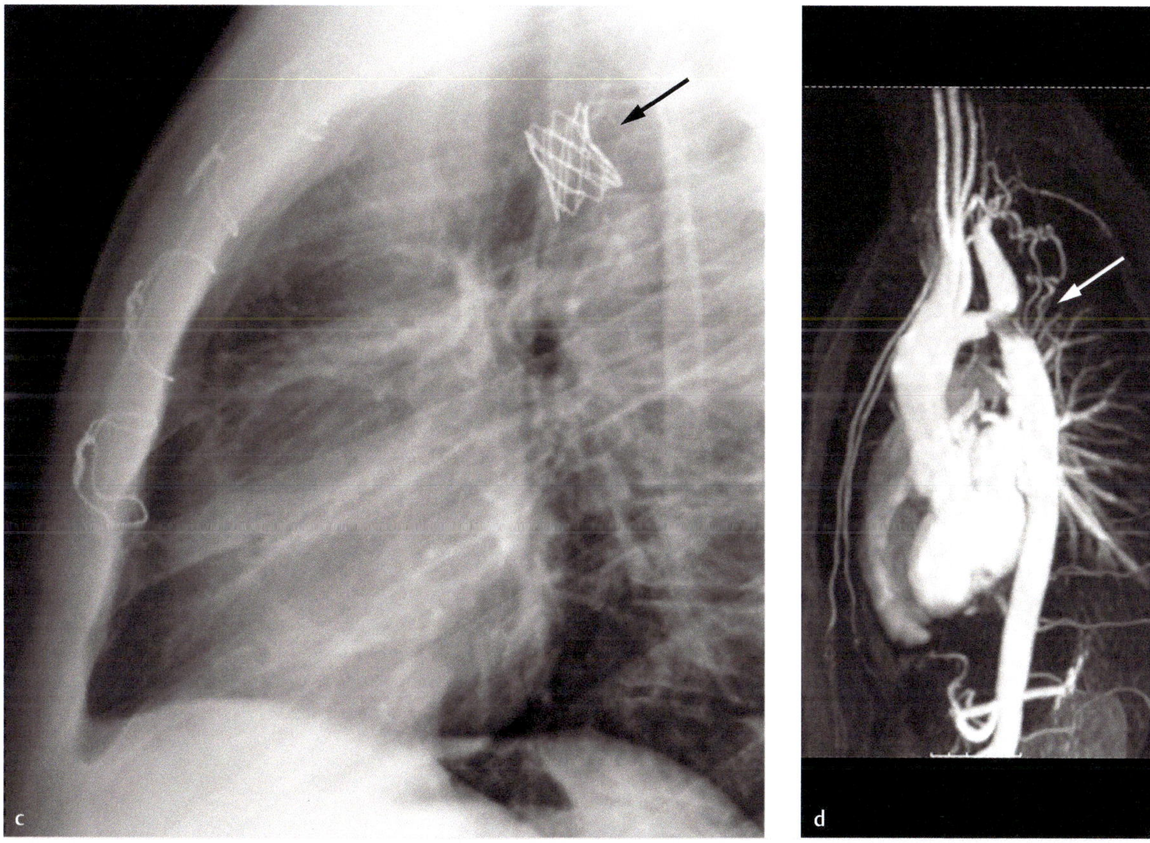

Fig. 3.62 (*Continued*) **Combination of ultrasound, X-ray, and angiography.** Diagnosing and treating recoarctation via stent implant.

Ao = aorta
LSA = left subclavian artery

c Lateral thoracic X-ray after stent implantation (arrow).
d MIP reconstruction of a contrast-enhanced MRA after stent implantation with obliteration (arrow).

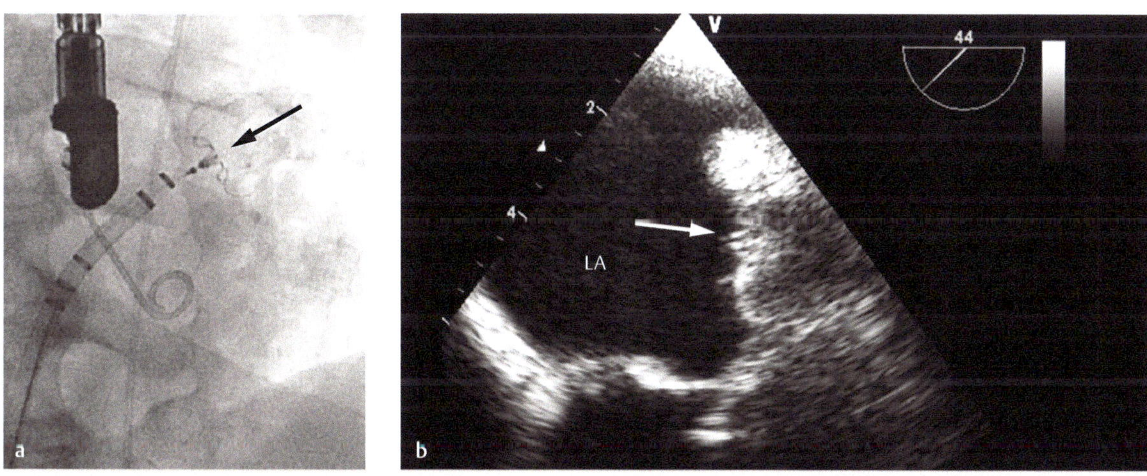

Fig. 3.63 Combination of angiography, X-ray, and CT with echocardiographical methods. Simultaneous angiographic and echo depictions of a Watchman closure device in the left auricle of a male patient with chronic atrial flutter and contraindication against oral anticoagulants.

LA = left atrium
LV = left ventricle
Rcx = ramus circumflexus

a Fluoroscopic image of the occlusion device positioned and opened in the left auricle (arrow). The exact position cannot be assessed accurately without administering contrast agent.
b TEE depiction allows exact localization of the occlusion device (arrow), which, in this instance, has properly closed the auricle.

(*Continued*)

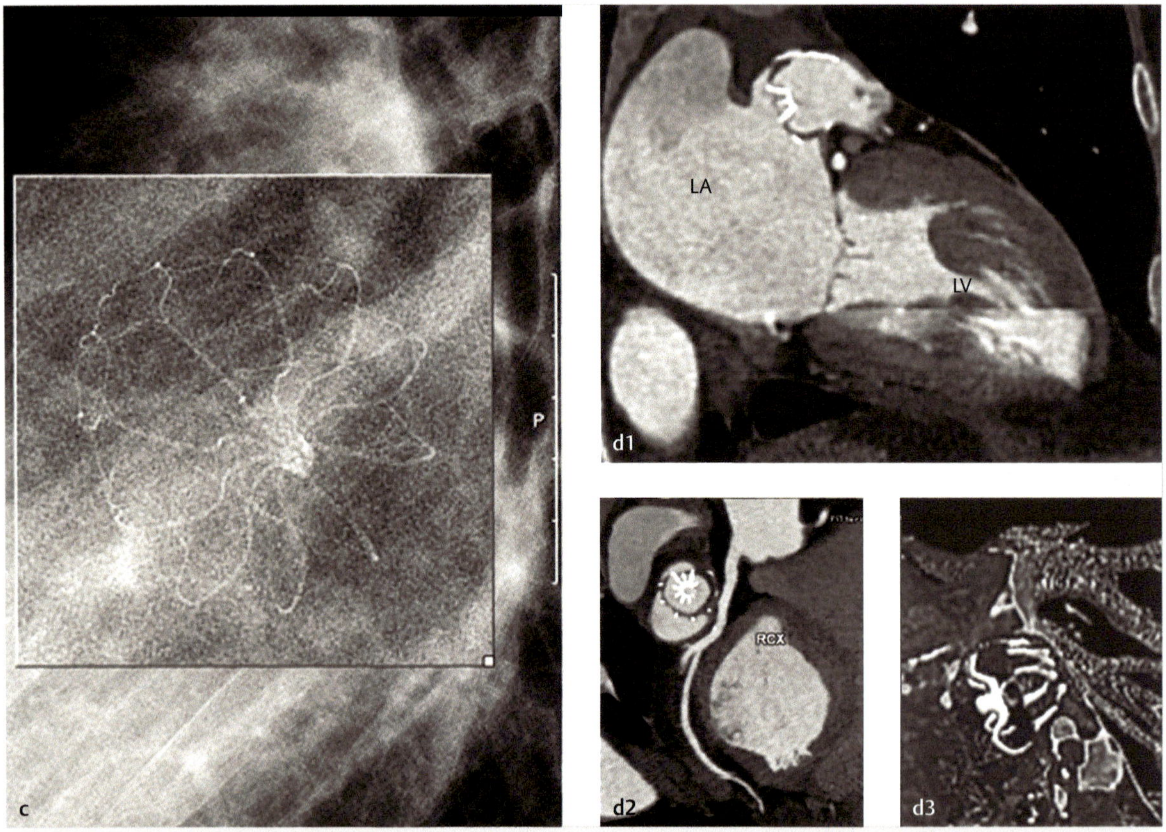

Fig. 3.63 (*Continued*) **Combination of angiography, X-ray, and CT with echocardiographical methods.** Simultaneous angiographic and echo depictions of a Watchman closure device in the left auricle of a male patient with chronic atrial flutter and contraindication against
oral anticoagulants.

LA = left atrium
LV = left ventricle
RCX = ramus circumflexus

c X-ray enhanced image of a Watchman closure device in the left auricle with insufficient closure.

d Depictions using multiplanar reformation of an ECG-triggered MDCT data set.

Table 3.8 Description of interventions using exclusively ECG imaging.

Interventional procedure	References
Balloon atrial septostomy	Steeg et al. (1985)[66]
ASD closure	Ewert et al. (2000)[70]
PFO closure	Daehnert et al. (2001)[75]
Balloon valvuloplasty of the aortic valve	Weber et al. (2000)[68]
Balloon valvuloplasty of the mitral valve	Trehan et al. (2006)[67]
Balloon valvuloplasty of the pulmonary valve	Bouzas-Mosquera et al. (2008)[76]
Balloon angioplasty of a recoarctation	Springer and Dähnert[73]

ASD, atrial septal defect; PFO, patent foramen ovale.

3.5 Interventional Magnetic Resonance Imaging

Arno Bücker, Titus Kühne

3.5.1 Introduction

In many respects, MRI has replaced diagnostic catheter angiography for imaging purposes within the scope of congenital heart defects. Improvements in hardware and progress in terms of sequence development are responsible for this change. Nowadays, the anatomical depiction of the heart's chambers also falls within the domain of MRI. The low invasiveness of MRI exams is appealing, particularly for purely diagnostic procedures. The lack of radiation exposure is also a compelling argument within pediatric cardiology. The UK National Radiological Protection board operates under the assumption that, for children under 5 years of age, a solid tumor is formed in 1 of every 1,000 cardiac catheter cases (vs. 1 of every 2,500 corresponding cases in adults).[80] It quickly becomes apparent that avoiding ionizing radiation during diagnostic procedures is particularly important for children with cardiac disorders, who generally require multiple cardiac catheter exams.

3.5.2 Technology

Hardware

If the examiner is primarily interested in speed, then *high-field scanners* (with a magnetic field strength of at least 1 T) is prefereable for MRI-guided interventions, since these scanners offer a better signal-to-noise ratio. Thus, they fundamentally offer images with better local resolution in a shorter timespan compared to low-field scanners. These systems, do, however, have the disadvantage of being composed largely of closed magnets, which severely limits access to the patient.[81] There are a few newer 1-T devices whose horseshoe-like shape offers better access to the patient. In addition to limited patient access for high-field scanners, it is also noteworthy that these scanners are also more prone to pronounced susceptibility artifacts compared to low-field scanners (▶ Fig. 3.64).

In addition to magnetic field strength, the development of functional gradients has contributed significantly to improved image quality. In particular, the short repetition and echo times available today have made "SSFP" sequence technologies (also known as TrueFISP for Siemens scanners, FIESTA for GE scanners, and balanced FFE for Philips scanners) the most widely used technologies for

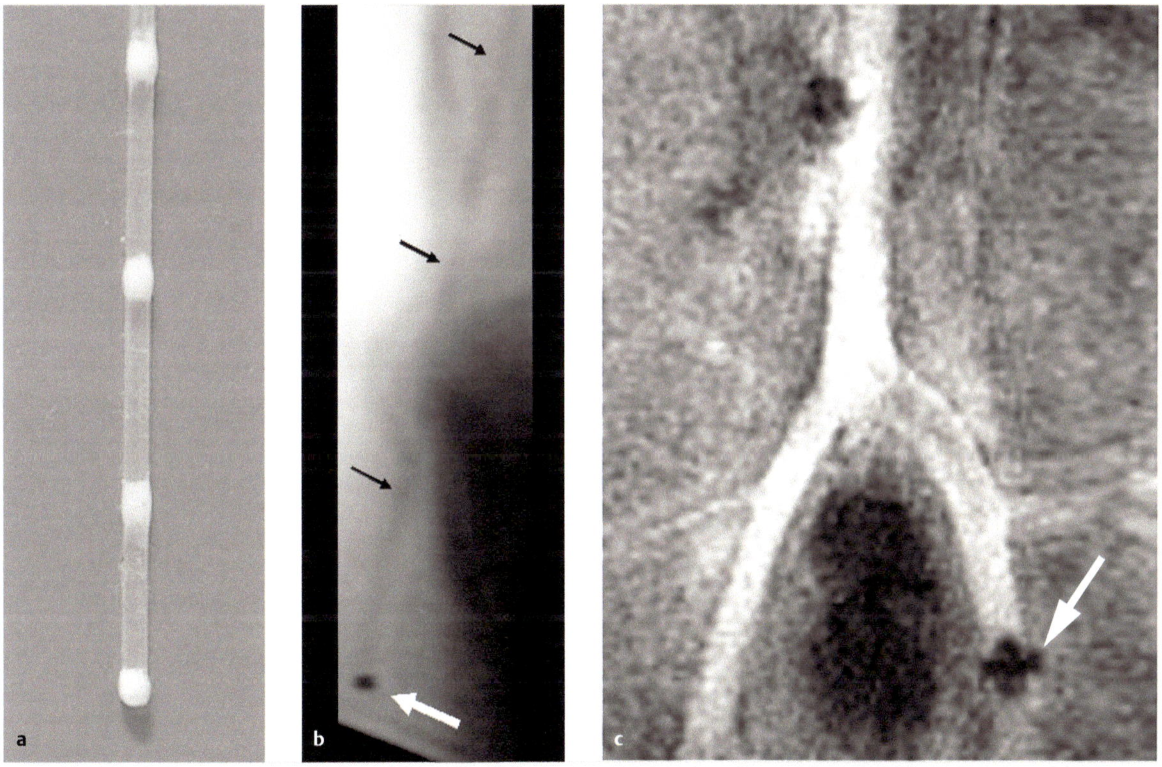

Fig. 3.64 MRI markers. MRI measurements (**a**, **b**) demonstrate that the markers (**b**, white arrow) can be distinguished easily. The instrument, itself, is much more difficult to see in a water bath (**b**, black arrows).

a A synthetic wire was equipped with dysprosium markers in order to generate easily localizable artifacts during an MRI exam.

b Positioning an instrument with an individual marker in the water bath.

c Positioning an instrument with an individual marker within the left iliac artery of a pig (black arrow).

anatomical cardiac imaging. Many vascular interventions have been performed using this technology.[82–84]

Performing MRI interventions requires additional modifications to the MRI room itself:

- The interventionalist requires a monitor that displays the MRIs in real time.
- Furthermore, it needs to be possible to issue at least simple commands, such as adapting the sectional plane in the MR room.
- Special communication equipment needs to be used to ensure communication with the operation console.
- It should also be possible to enter the high-frequency cage via a tube while a measurement is being performed.
- At this time, it is still necessary to have immediate access to an X-ray angiography unit in order to perform angiographic interventions, so that a fallback solution exists in the event of unforeseen complications during the MRI intervention.

Real-Time Magnetic Resonance Imaging

The physics of MRI causes an inverse relationship between the spatial and temporal resolution of MRIs. In addition to the commonly used Cartesian k-space sampling (another name for acquiring raw MR data), various other strategies are available—refer to the chapter on cardiac MRI. Explaining the technical details of radial or helical k-space sampling falls outside the scope of this book. Instead, we refer interested readers to supplemental literature.[85,86] Real-time imaging techniques with helical k-space sampling have already been described in detail.[87,88] Using helical k-space sampling for interventions has the significant drawback of generating relatively large and often unmanageable artifacts.[82] Using radial k-space sampling is less efficient. This technique is, however, less susceptible to movement artifacts[89] and can thus be used to suppress movement artifacts[87,88] and to guide interventions.[90]

X-rays provide a projection image that depicts a large volume. While it is possible to record 3-D volumes using MRI, there is currently no technology fast enough to acquire this type of 3-D data set in real time. This type of 3-D data set has been recorded only as a roadmap, which has limited applicability in the cardiac area due to cardiac and respiratory motion.

Depiction of Instruments

Depicting instruments constitutes a significant parameter of MRI examinations. Distortions in the magnetic field can make metallic instruments cause incorrect coding and thus inaccurate local depiction of the instruments. This is not an issue for instruments made of plastic, ceramic, or fibrous composite materials, though direct depiction of these objects in an MR image places high demands on spatial resolution.

In principle, a distinction is made between passive and active tracking techniques of depicting instruments during MRI examinations:

- *Passive visualization:* Passive visualization depicts the instrument directly in the MR image as a part of this image. It is thus, in principle, an "anatomical" depiction of the instrument.
- *Active visualization:* Active visualization, on the other hand, takes advantage of the physics of MR imaging technology—the spatial positions of small coils attached to an instrument are recorded in 2-D or 3-D space and then projected actively onto an MR image. In addition to constructing the active instrument, it is also necessary to establish a receiving channel for the micro coils and to program dedicated software for this purpose.

Passive Instrument Visualization with Susceptibility Markers

Rubin et al. examined the imaging qualities of conventional catheters using MRI in 1990. These catheters caused only very minor signal disruptions in the MR image, which were insufficient for detecting the catheter with any degree of certainty. Thus, the authors doped polyethylene catheters with a ferromagnetic material.[91] This resulted in susceptibility artifacts in the MR image. These artifacts are caused when a substance with a significantly different magnetizability (aka susceptibility) compared to the surrounding tissues is depicted in an MR image. Since the susceptibility artifacts exceed the physical dimensions of the catheter, they were significantly easier to localize in the MR image. One drawback is that the scope of signal obliteration depends on the orientation of the catheter to the main magnetic field.

Bakker solved this problem by placing local markers on catheters in 1996.[92] These markers, composed of dysprosium oxide, also trigger susceptibility artifacts (▶ Fig. 3.64). Because of local distribution, this signal obliteration retains only a slight dependency on the catheter's orientation to the main magnetic field. As soon as a catheter with large artifacts is directed into a smaller vessel, the underlying anatomy is immediately blanketed and covered by the artifact.[93] In principle, it would be ideal to be able to control the artifact size based on the size of the examined vessels. This need has led to the development of the concept of field inhomogeneity.

Passive Visualization with the Principle of Field Inhomogeneity

The principle of field inhomogeneity is based on incorporating a loop from an insulated guide wire into a catheter.[94] When even a minor direct current is transmitted through this wire, it creates a small magnetic field that triggers a local inhomogeneity in the MRI device's main magnetic field. This leads to signal loss, the size of which depends on the strength of the direct current and the manner of coiling the wire, meaning it can be controlled externally.[95]

Active Visualization

In the event that vessels have helical courses, it is necessary to continually adapt the sectional plane in order to visualize the tip of the catheter. This drawback in cross-sectional imaging technology cannot be balanced out by thickening the depicted cross-section, since that can make it impossible to differentiate the borders of the vessel under certain circumstances.

Actively visualizing instruments offers another approach to solving this issue. In the simplest form of active visualization, a *micro coil* is fixed to the tip of the instrument. This coil is connected to the MRI scanner as a receiving coil. The micro coil's position can be determined using MRI in 2-D or 3-D space.[96] After the coil's position is projected onto the anatomical MR image, the tip of the catheter can then be guided appropriately. Once the micro coil's position is known, this knowledge can also be used to place an imaging sectional plane with great precision.[97] The number of micro coils can be increased, though determining the positions of various micro coils takes additional time. This enables examiners to depict not just an instrument's tip, but also its course.[98]

The development of multiple *parallel receiving channels* for MRI scanners also enabled additional progress in the field of active visualization technology, in the form of both in vitro[97] and in vivo[99] real-time depiction of background anatomy in conjunction with real-time depiction of micro coil position. The first approaches to implementing the technology of cross-sectional tracing have also been described using passive susceptibility markers[100] that, unlike active visualization technologies, do not result in any of the safety issues listed below.

In addition to the clearly categorizable technologies described here, there are numerous other technologies for visualizing instruments, which will not be detailed here.

> **Note**
>
> In particular, special emphasis should be placed on technology involving fiducial markers.[101] These technologies involve mounting configured micro coils with antennae on the instruments and then using the former—without establishing their own connection to the MRI scanner—to visualize instruments.

Safety Aspects

With regard to the safety aspects associated with MRI technology, one must comply with the generally accepted safety guidelines for strong magnetic fields. This means that ferromagnetic materials cannot be used for interventional MRI procedures. Adequate protection from noise, particularly during real-time sequences, is another important safety aspect. This affects primarily patients under sedation or narcosis. These patients are susceptible to overall warming of the body due to MR measurements. For this reason, there is a report regarding hyperthermia in children after MR exams performed under general anesthesia.

Heating phenomena caused by electrical conductors are important, particularly for interventional MRI. These involve primarily metallic materials which, while not ferromagnetic, conduct electricity very well due to their metallic properties. There is a chance that the electrical conductor will begin to resonate with the irradiated stimulation pulses and thus will begin to function as an antenna. Then, the energy transmitted via the radio frequency pulses will be collected by the conductor, causing an increase in heat. This resonance relies on very complex border conditions (including the position and orientation of the electrical conductor and the length and shape of the body in MR). Though the energy used for stimulation purposes during the MR sequence (indicated as "specific absorption rate") is a decisive factor for the degree of heating, if resonance occurs, even a small quantity of irradiated energy can cause a significant temperature increase. While examining a catheter for active visualization of a 0.5 T MRI, Wildermuth found no significant temperature increase. When examining at 1.5 T, however, he determined a temperature increase of 20°.[102] In vitro examinations of guide wires showed temperature increase of up to 50°.[103] Initial in vivo experiments conducted on pigs, using nitinol commercial guide wires, resulted in a temperature increase of 35° despite the cooling effects of blood flow in the aorta. In one case, when the animal was touched with an external wire tip, flying sparks were generated in repeated instances (▶ Fig. 3.65).[104] Various approaches for solving the issue of wire heating have been described. To this end, safety measures were built into the wires,[105] or electrically conductive components were replaced by photo-optic elements[106] or laser fibers.[107] One significant issue for these approaches was that they necessitated miniaturizing the instruments. Using transformers along the course of the electrical conductor is one possible solution to this problem.[108] In addition, developing non-metallic materials could avoid heating, provided that these materials allow manufacturers to produce wires with similar flexion and torsion properties compared to metallic wires.[109]

3.5.3 Pediatric Cardiology Applications

MRI-Guided Cardiac Interventions in Animal Trials

Numerous preparatory experimental works have dealt with the feasibility of performing MRI-guided interventions.

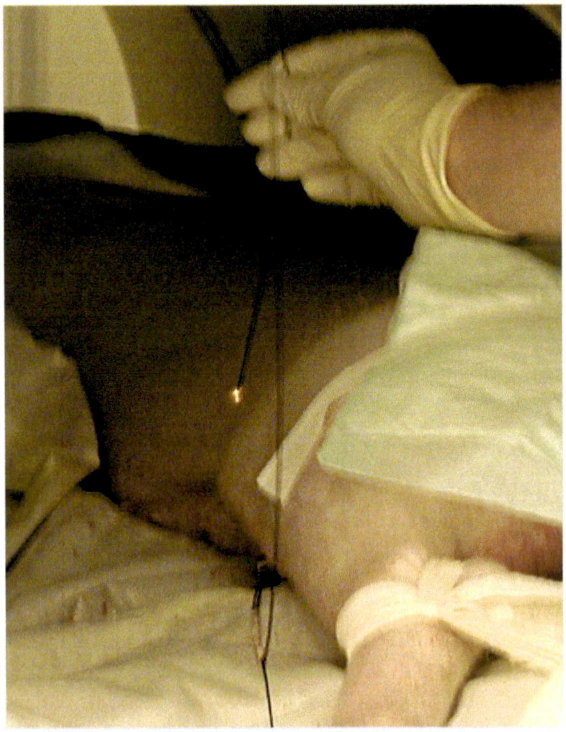

Fig. 3.65 Heating of a nitinol wire. During ongoing MR measurement, bending the tip of a commercially available nitinol wire when touching the pig caused sparks to form on the end of the wire.

These works have, on the one hand, led to improvements in real-time MR imaging. It was also necessary to test various implants. In addition to excellent anatomical and functional depiction of the heart, it is becoming increasingly possible to depict implants, such as heart valves, occlusion devices, and stents.[93,104,110,111] These devices are often made of metal and thus can cause the aforementioned susceptibility artifacts. In some cases, these artifacts can contribute to the visibility of implants and instruments in MR images,[112,113] but may also hinder performing the intervention in other instances.[83,114] Depending on which scientific emphasis was set for experimental works and when the experiments were conducted, the safety aspects were disregarded, meaning that it was often not possible to directly transfer the results of the experiments to everyday clinical settings.

Catheter Guidance for Probing the Cardiac Chambers and Vessels

Within the scope of animal trials, right and left heart catheter exams were performed to assess pressures and flow rates successfully with the help of active catheter visualization.[115] Even probing[93] and stenting[84] coronaries were possible in animal trials under real-time MRI guidance. In principle, both active and passive visualization techniques could be used in the cardiac region. The complex anatomy suggests that the combination of both techniques would be helpful, especially for cardiac interventions.

Combined MRI and fluoroscopic images were another option that was tested.[116] Initial works substantiate the feasibility of MRI guidance for performing electrophysiological exams in animal trials.[117] Complying with the safety aspects of the wires used is of particular importance during these trials. The option to record intracardiac signals during simultaneous MRI measurements also constitutes a technological issue. This can, however, be solved by using dedicated filter plates and by the use of measurement devices outside the radio frequency cage. Passive catheter visualization[77,118] has also proven the feasibility of MRI-guided radio frequency ablation as a possible component of electrophysiological exams.

One significant advantage of MRI for guiding radio frequency ablation is the option to immediately monitor the degree of heating effect. Thus, the good contrast in soft tissues allows MRI to examine a complete transmural ablation.[118] Just as a catheter can be furnished with a radio frequency probe and observed during MRI, it is possible to use MRI catheter guidance within the heart's chambers in order to apply substances to the myocardium.[119] In these cases, it is of particular interest to identify the areas affected by infarction as precisely as possible, since this allows the injection to be directed specifically into the infarction's marginal areas.

Balloon Dilatation and Stent Placement under MRI Guidance

Performing MR-guided balloon dilatations and stent placements in the periphery was among the first published works on the topic of vascular MRI interventions.[99,120] Various technologies were used to passively visualize balloon catheters. This allows a balloon to be filled with carbon dioxide,[121] which causes direct signal loss and susceptibility artifacts in the MR image. Solutions with high gadolinium concentrations have a similar effect in the MR image,[122] which is based on destructive signal interference caused by susceptibility artifacts. In both cases, the depicted size of the balloon in the MR image can differ from the physical dimensions of the balloon, since susceptibility artifacts cause destructive signal interference that exceeds the instrument's true dimensions (▶ Fig. 3.66a). It is particularly important to take this into account when using a balloon to determine the size of septal defects. Thus, additional experiments have been performed regarding this topic. Using an approximately 10% gadolinium solution causes an increase "only" in T1 time, without leading to susceptibility artifacts (▶ Fig. 3.66b).

The metal from stents can cause pronounced susceptibility artifacts that, while allowing simple localization of the stent in the MR image, also make it

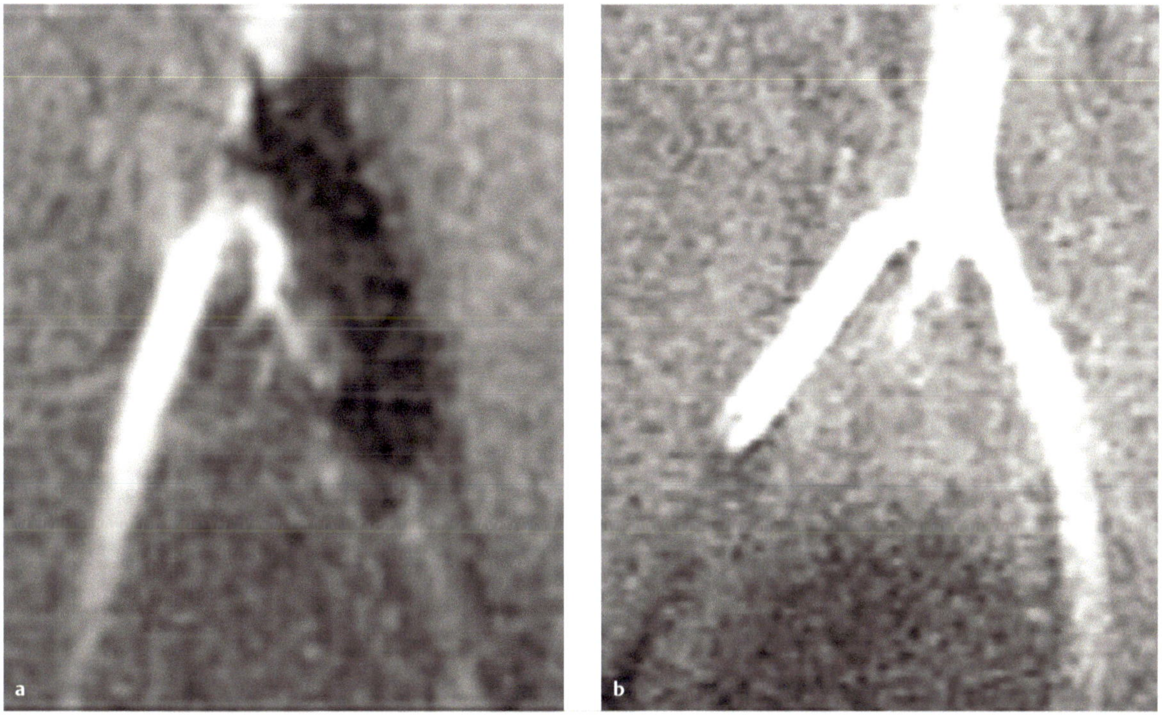

Fig. 3.66 MRI depiction of a balloon with radial k-space sampling.
a The balloon was filled with a high concentration of gadolinium solution within the left iliac artery of a pig.
b The balloon was filled with a gadolinium solution diluted with table salt at a 1:100 ratio within the right iliac artery of a pig. Note the lack of signal distal to the balloon due to the lack of blood flow after the balloon is inflated.

impossible to depict the surrounding anatomy.[114] Reports have been made regarding the experimental development of artifact-free metal stents.[93,123] Under MR guidance, the iliac arteries,[120] aorta, vena cava, carotids,[124] and coronaries[84] were furnished with a specially selected stent. Works regarding the placement of pulmonary stents and pulmonary valve carrying stents,[125] as well as stent PTA for aortic isthmus stenoses,[124] were of particular interest within the field of pediatric cardiology. The scope of these works demonstrated that, even after placing the stent, MRI allowed reliable flow measurement. Using blood pool contrast agents improved depiction of the shunt.[110] The experimental placement of aortic valves under MR guidance has been described both via transapical access[126] and via the groin.[127] One potential benefit of MR guidance is that the anatomy, including the outlets of the coronary arteries, can be depicted "online" and without injecting contrast agent.

Septal Puncture, Occlusion Device Placement, and Helical Embolization

Real-time depiction of the heart's anatomy now allows differentiation between the individual chambers and the septa. Consequently, it is logical to attempt to use MR guidance for interventions such as septal puncture and occlusion device placement. To this end, it was also necessary to modify and develop new, dedicated instruments that would be simple to distinguish in MR images for passive visualization, but would also cause no large artifacts that would render it impossible to distinguish their release or distinguish the underlying anatomy.[104] Subsequently, atrial septal occlusion devices were placed using real-time MR guidance in animal trials (▸ Fig. 3.67).[113,115,122] A measuring balloon was used during these interventions to successfully measure the size of the ASD. MRI-guided punctures of the atrial septum, either with a needle[128] or a laser, have also been performed successfully.[129] Numerous cardiac interventions can, on principle, also be performed using only ultrasound guidance.[130] This technology also has the benefit of no radiation exposure. TEE should be performed under sedation for cardiac interventions, such as closure of a septal defect. MR-guided interventions, on the other hand, can be performed on compliant patients without the need for sedation. This is of significant to patient management and comfort. Due to the fusion of X-ray and MR images, there is now the option to optimize interventional strategies for closing septal defects.[131]

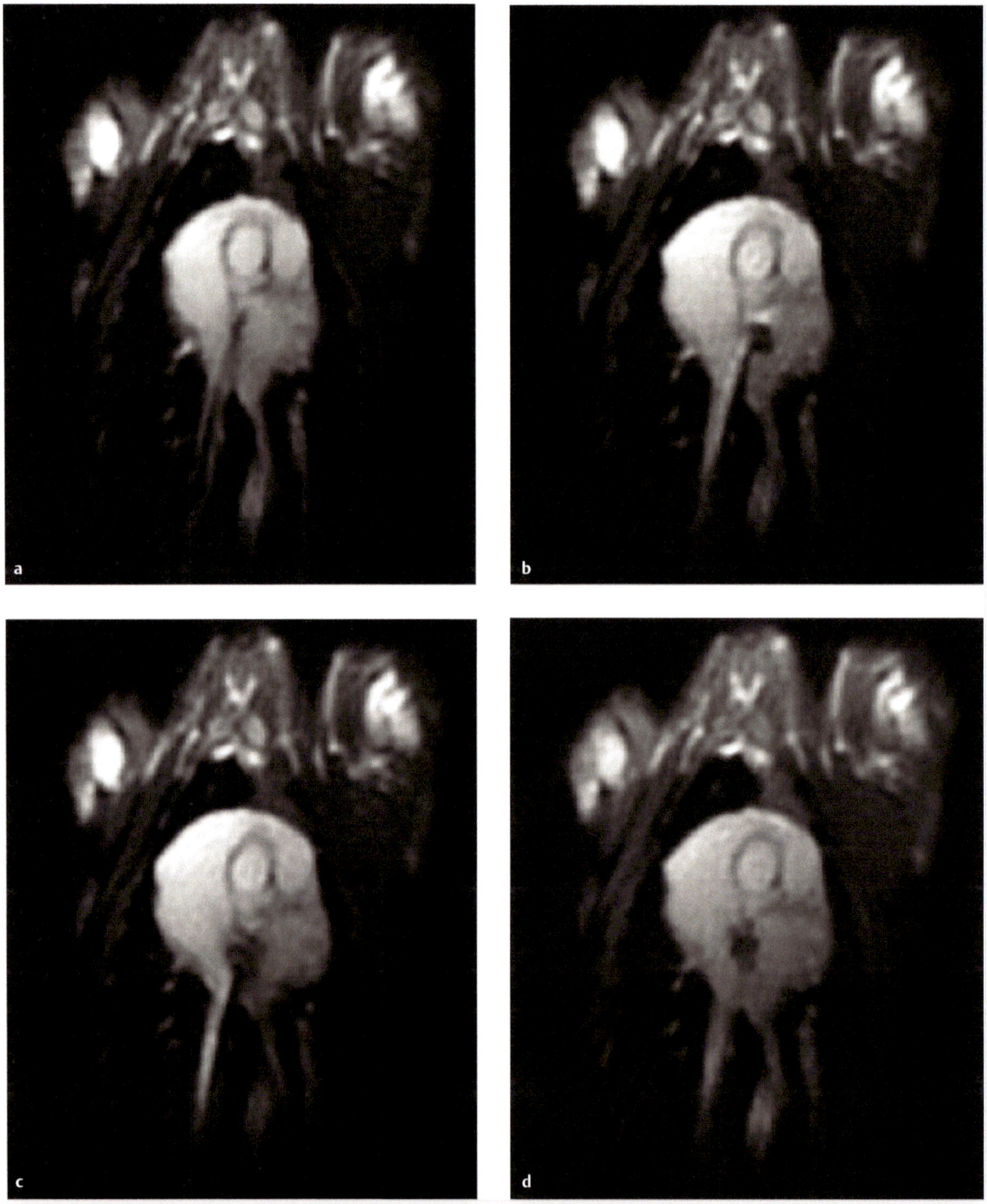

Fig. 3.67 Placement of atrial septal occlusion devices under real-time MRI guidance.

a Real-time MR images (SSFP), acquired using radial k-space sampling, depict the passage of an atrial septal occlusion device through the atrial septum.

b The first half of the occlusion device is then released within the left atrium.

c The second half of the occlusion device is released within the right atrium.

d After the occlusion device is disconnected, it orients itself parallel to the atrial septum.

Magnetic Resonance Imaging-Guided Patient Cardiac Interventions

The first MRI-guided cardiac catheterizations for patients used passive visualization techniques.[132] This allowed flow-directed catheters to be visualized by filling their balloons with carbon dioxide.[121] Due to the fact that not all necessary measurement instruments are MRI-compatible and MRI-safe, these types of measurements are performed by medical centers with proven expertise, and still require too many modifications to commercially available machines to gain traction in a broader clinical setting. Razavi et al. published the first individual case studies regarding MRI-guided cardiac catheter exams on human subjects.[132] The workgroup demonstrated that angiography equipment being available immediately adjacent to the MRI led to a significant decrease in radiation exposure. No additional fluoroscopy was required in 12 of 40 cases. Using these results, Razavi et al. convincingly verified the options for reducing radiation exposure caused by interventional MRI. The first systematic clinical use occurred in 2005 for patients with aortic coarctation, whereby a balloon angioplasty was performed using solely MRI guidance (▶ Fig. 3.68).[133]

Additional benefits of interventional MRI became apparent due to the differences between various measurement techniques for determining pulmonary vascular resistance. Thus, the results measured using the Fick principle differed from the values gleaned using the MRI phase contrast technique—primarily in cases of higher oxygen saturation, in which the Fick principle is known to be less precise. A work published at that same time also proved the higher efficacy of MRI with respect to thermodilution.[131] Pursuant works demonstrate that MRI-guided cardiac catheter exams also allow the ventricular pressure–volume ratio to be determined (▶ Fig. 3.69). To this end, ventricular pressure is measured via small catheters and synchronized with measured ventricular volume values determined via cine MRI. In physiology, pressure–volume ratios are considered the decisive value for determining cardiovascular function. These ratios allow examiners to derive integrated parameters of global ventricular function, myocardial contractility, and diastolic compliance.[134] In these cases, performing combined pressure, volume, and blood flow measurements is not very technically intensive and is only minorly invasive. Unlike for interventional procedures, no specially equipped MRI laboratories are necessary.

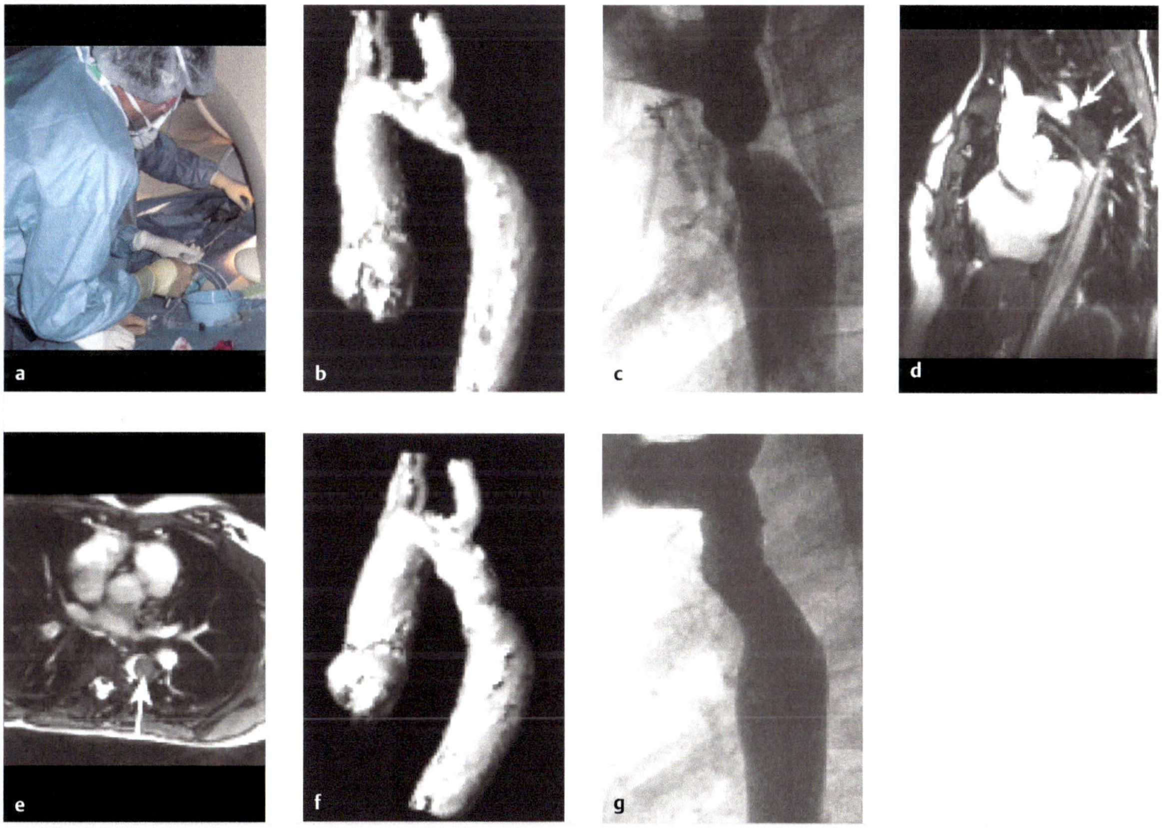

Fig. 3.68 Balloon angioplasty of a male patient with aortic coarctation.

a Operating situation.
b 3-D MRI before the intervention. Note the narrowing near the isthmus.
c Traditional X-ray angiogram before the intervention.
d MR-guided angioplasty: lateral projection.
e MRI-guided angioplasty: transverse slice.
f 3-D MRI after the intervention.
g Traditional X-ray angiogram after the intervention.

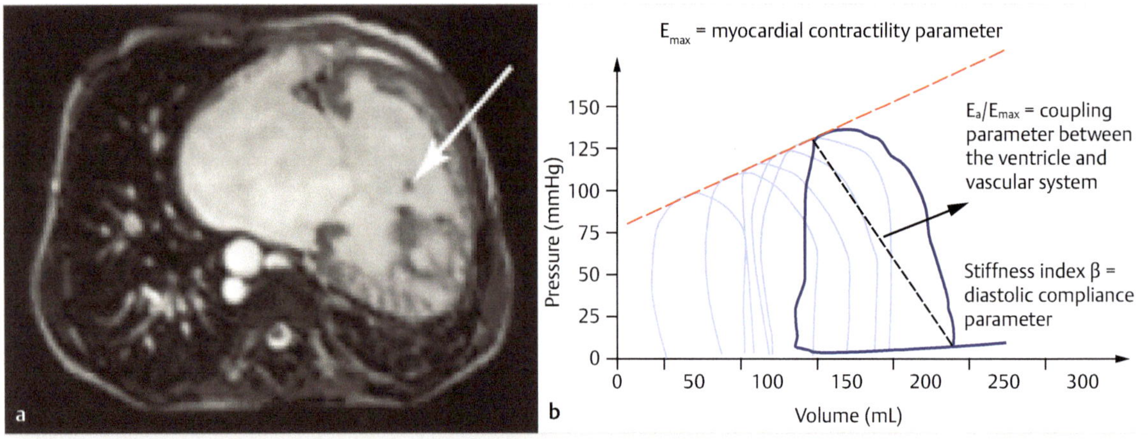

Fig. 3.69 MRI-guided cardiac catheter exam with determination of the ventricular pressure–volume ratio.
a The catheter for measuring pressure is depicted on the MR image as a small, circled artifact (arrow).
b Pressure–volume ratio measured via MRI for evaluating a case of combined systolic–diastolic heart failure.

References

[1] Eichstädt H, Felix R, Zeitler E, Eds. Herz—Große Gefäße. Diagnostik mit bildgebenden Verfahren. Berlin: Springer; 1996: 448

[2] Rice MJ, McDonald RW, Reller MD, Sahn DJ. Pediatric echocardiography: current role and a review of technical advances. J Pediatr. 1996; 128(1):1–14

[3] Schumacher G, Hess J, Bühlmeyer K, Eds. Klinische Kinderkardiologie. 3. Aufl. Berlin: Springer; 2001: 588

[4] Wilkenshoff U, Kruck I. Handbuch der Echokardiographie. Berlin: Blackwell Publishing; 2002: 223

[5] Gutberlet M. Angeborene Herzfehler. In: Hosten N, Lemke AJ, Felix R, Hrsg. Kernspintomographie. Landsberg: Ecomed; 1999

[6] Gutberlet M, Abdul-Khaliq H, Grothoff M, et al. Evaluation of left ventricular volumes in patients with congenital heart disease and abnormal left ventricular geometry. Comparison of MRI and transthoracic 3-dimensional echocardiography. RoFo Fortschr Geb Rontgenstr Nuklearmed. 2003; 175(7):942–951

[7] Vogel M, Gutberlet M, Dittrich S, Hosten N, Lange PE. Comparison of transthoracic three dimensional echocardiography with magnetic resonance imaging in the assessment of right ventricular volume and mass. Heart. 1997; 78(2):127–130

[8] Takuma S, Cardinale C, Homma S. Real-time three-dimensional stress echocardiography: a review of current applications. Echocardiography. 2000; 17(8):791–794

[9] Raedle-Hurst TM, Mueller M, Rentzsch A, Schaefers HJ, Herrmann E, Abdul-Khaliq H. Assessment of left ventricular dyssynchrony and function using real-time 3-dimensional echocardiography in patients with congenital right heart disease. Am Heart J. 2009; 157 (4):791–798

[10] Biamino G, Kruck I. Quantitative Methoden der M-Mode-, 2D- und Doppler-Echokardiographie. Berlin: Boehringer Mannheim; 1987

[11] Hatle L. Noninvasive assessment of valve lesions with Doppler ultrasound. Herz. 1984; 9(4):213–221

[12] Gutberlet M, Hosten N, Vogel M, et al. Quantification of morphologic and hemodynamic severity of coarctation of the aorta by magnetic resonance imaging. Cardiol Young. 2001; 11(5):512–520

[13] Beckmann S, Haug G. Streßechokardiographie interaktiv. Darmstadt: Steinkopff; 1998: 156

[14] Barasch E, Wilansky S. Dobutamine stress echocardiography in clinical practice with a review of the recent literature. Tex Heart Inst J. 1994; 21(3):202–210

[15] Orlandi C. Pharmacology of coronary vasodilation: a brief review. J Nucl Cardiol. 1996; 3(6 Pt 2):S27–S30

[16] Wei K. Approaches to the detection of coronary artery disease using myocardial contrast echocardiography. Am J Cardiol. 2002; 90 10A:48J–58J

[17] Nagel E, Lehmkuhl HB, Klein C, et al. Influence of image quality on the diagnostic accuracy of dobutamine stress magnetic resonance imaging in comparison with dobutamine stress echocardiography for the noninvasive detection of myocardial ischemia. Z Kardiol. 1999; 88(9):622–630

[18] Schiller NB, Shah PM, Crawford M, et al. Recommendations for quantitation of the left ventricle by two-dimensional echocardiography. American Society of Echocardiography Committee on Standards, Subcommittee on Quantitation of Two-Dimensional Echocardiograms. J Am Soc Echocardiogr. 1989; 2(5):358–367

[19] Parish V, Valverde I, Kutty S, et al. Dobutamine stress MRI in repaired tetralogy of Fallot with chronic pulmonary regurgitation: a comparison with healthy volunteers. Int J Cardiol. 2013; 166 (1):96–105

[20] Cheng SC, Dy TC, Feinstein SB. Contrast echocardiography: review and future directions. Am J Cardiol. 1998; 81 12A:41G–48G

[21] Becher H, Tiemann K. Improved endocardium imaging using modified transthoracic echocardiography with the second harmonic frequency (tissue harmonic imaging). Herz. 1998; 23(8):467–473

[22] Kasprzak JD, Ten Cate FJ. New ultrasound contrast agents for left ventricular and myocardial pacification. Herz. 1998; 23(8):474–482

[23] Malhotra V, Nwogu J, Bondmass MD, et al. Is the technically limited echocardiographic study an endangered species? Endocardial border definition with native tissue harmonic imaging and Optison contrast: a review of 200 cases. J Am Soc Echocardiogr. 2000; 13 (8):771–773

[24] Wilkenshoff UM, Hatle L, Sovany A, Wranne B, Sutherland GR. Age-dependent changes in regional diastolic function evaluated by color Doppler myocardial imaging: a comparison with pulsed Doppler indexes of global function. J Am Soc Echocardiogr. 2001; 14(10):959–969

[25] Wilkenshoff UM, Sovany A, Wigström L, et al. Regional mean systolic myocardial velocity estimation by real-time color Doppler myocardial imaging: a new technique for quantifying regional systolic function. J Am Soc Echocardiogr. 1998; 11(7):683–692

[26] De Boeck BW, Cramer MJ, Oh JK, van der Aa RP, Jaarsma W. Spectral pulsed tissue Doppler imaging in diastole: a tool to increase our insight in and assessment of diastolic relaxation of the left ventricle. Am Heart J. 2003; 146(3):411–419

[27] Abdul-Khaliq H, Schmitt B, Rentzsch A, et al. Evaluation of abnormal myocardial wall motions in patients with univentricular heart by tissue Doppler echocardiography. Z Kardiol. 2003; 92(4):319–325

[28] Sutherland GR, Di Salvo G, Claus P, D'hooge J, Bijnens B. Strain and strain rate imaging: a new clinical approach to quantifying regional myocardial function. J Am Soc Echocardiogr. 2004; 17(7):788–802

[29] D'hooge J, Heimdal A, Jamal F, et al. Regional strain and strain rate measurements by cardiac ultrasound: principles, implementation and limitations. Eur J Echocardiogr. 2000; 1(3):154–170

[30] Urheim S, Edvardsen T, Torp H, Angelsen B, Smiseth OA. Myocardial strain by Doppler echocardiography. Validation of a new method to quantify regional myocardial function. Circulation. 2000; 102 (10):1158–1164

[31] Kalender WA. Computed tomography. Fundamentals, system technology, image quality, applications. 3rd ed. Erlangen: Publicis; 2010

[32] Kalender WA, Seissler W, Klotz E, Vock P. Spiral volumetric CT with single-breath-hold technique, continuous transport, and continuous scanner rotation. Radiology. 1990; 176(1):181–183

[33] Flohr TG, McCollough CH, Bruder H, et al. First performance evaluation of a dual-source CT (DSCT) system. Eur Radiol. 2006; 16 (2):256–268

[34] Ertel D, Lell MM, Harig F, Flohr T, Schmidt B, Kalender WA. Cardiac spiral dual-source CT with high pitch: a feasibility study. Eur Radiol. 2009; 19(10):2357–2362

[35] European Commission. European guidelines on quality criteria for computed tomography. Report EUR 16262. Brussels, Belgium: European Commission; 1999

[36] International Commission on Radiological Protection (ICRP). Publication 103. The 2007 Recommendations of the International Commission on Radiological Protection. Ann ICRP. 2007; 37:2–4

[37] Bundesamt für Strahlenschutz (BfS). Bekanntmachung der aktualisierten diagnostischen Referenzwerte für nuklearmedizinische Untersuchungen; 2012. Im Internet: http://www.bfs.de/SharedDocs/Downloads/BfS/DE/fachinfo/ion/drw-nuklearmedizin.pdf?__blob=-publicationFile&v=1 (Stand: 19.07.2015)

[38] Deak PD, Smal Y, Kalender WA. Multisection CT protocols: sex- and age-specific conversion factors used to determine effective dose from dose-length product. Radiology. 2010; 257(1):158–166

[39] American Association of Physicists in Medicine (AAPM). Report no. 96. The measurement, reporting and management of radiation dose in CT. College Park, MD, USA: American Association of Physicists in Medicine; 2008

[40] Lell MM, May M, Deak P, et al. High-pitch spiral computed tomography: effect on image quality and radiation dose in pediatric chest computed tomography. Invest Radiol. 2011; 46(2):116–123

[41] Strahlenschutzkommission (SSK). Bildgebende Diagnostik beim Kind. Strahlenschutz, Rechtfertigung und Effektivität. Empfehlungen der Strahlenschutzkommission. 2006. Im Internet: http://www.ssk.de/SharedDocs/Beratungsergebnisse/2006/BildgebendeDiagnostik_-Kind.html (Stand: 18.06.2015)

[42] Kalender WA, Deak P, Kellermeier M, van Straten M, Vollmar SV. Application- and patient size-dependent optimization of x-ray spectra for CT. Med Phys. 2009; 36(3):993–1007

[43] Biglands JD, Radjenovic A, Ridgway JP. Cardiovascular magnetic resonance physics for clinicians: Part II. J Cardiovasc Magn Reson. 2012; 14:66

[44] Ridgway JP. Cardiovascular magnetic resonance physics for clinicians: part I. J Cardiovasc Magn Reson. 2010; 12:71

[45] Gutberlet M. Einsatz der Kernspintomographie in der Diagnostik und Verlaufskontrolle angeborener Herzfehler unter besonderer Berücksichtigung der Verwendung flusssensitiver Sequenzen und der Ventrikelfunktionsanalyse. Habilitationsschrift 2002. Im Internet: http://edoc.hu-berlin.de/habilitationen/gutberlet-matthias-2002-11-05/PDF/Gutberlet.pdf (Stand: 04.08.2015)

[46] Achenbach S, Barkhausen J, Beer M, et al. Konsensusempfehlungen der DRG/DGK/DGPK zum Einsatz der Herzbildgebung mit Computertomografie und Magnetresonanztomografie. RoFo Fortschr Geb Rontgenstr Nuklearmed. 2012; 184(4):345–368

[47] Fratz S, Chung T, Greil GF, et al. Guidelines and protocols for cardiovascular magnetic resonance in children and adults with congenital heart disease: SCMR expert consensus group on congenital heart disease. J Cardiovasc Magn Reson. 2013; 15:51

[48] Sommer T, Luechinger R, Barkhausen J, et al. Positionspapier der Deutschen Röntgengesellschaft (DRG) zu MR-Untersuchungen bei Patienten mit Herzschrittmachern. Fortschr Röntgenstr RöFo. 2015; 187:777–787

[49] Gutberlet M, Noeske R, Schwinge K, Freyhardt P, Felix R, Niendorf T. Comprehensive cardiac magnetic resonance imaging at 3.0 Tesla: feasibility and implications for clinical applications. Invest Radiol. 2006; 41(2):154–167

[50] Tsao J, Boesiger P, Pruessmann KP. k-t BLAST and k-t SENSE: dynamic MRI with high frame rate exploiting spatiotemporal correlations. Magn Reson Med. 2003; 50(5):1031–1042

[51] Hor KN, Baumann R, Pedrizzetti G, et al. Magnetic resonance derived myocardial strain assessment using feature tracking. J Vis Exp. 2011; 48(48):2356

[52] European CMR. Registry. Im Internet: www.eurocmr-registry.com/ (Stand: 06.08.2015)

[53] European Society of Cardiac Radiology. European MR/CT Registry. Im Internet: https://www.mrct-registry.org/ (Stand: 06.08.2015)

[54] Kellman P, Larson AC, Hsu LY, et al. Motion-corrected free-breathing delayed enhancement imaging of myocardial infarction. Magn Reson Med. 2005; 53(1):194–200

[55] Meharwal ZS, Trehan N. Vascular complications of intra aortic balloon insertion in patients undergoing coronary revascularization: analysis of 911 cases. Eur J Cardiothorac Surg. 2002; 21(4):741–747

[56] Tobin MJ. Pulmonary artery catheter problems. Appl Cardiopulm Pathophysiol. 1990; 3(3):279–285

[57] Mullins CE. Cardiac catheterization in congenital heart disease: pediatric and adult. Oxford: Blackwell; 2006: 217

[58] Knecht S, Nault I, Wright M, et al. Imaging in catheter ablation for atrial fibrillation: enhancing the clinician's view. Europace. 2008; 10 Suppl 3:iii2–iii7

[59] Ramcharitar S, Pugliese F, Schultz C, et al. Integration of multislice computed tomography with magnetic navigation facilitates percutaneous coronary interventions without additional contrast agents. J Am Coll Cardiol. 2009; 53(9):741–746

[60] Racadio JM, Babic D, Homan R, et al. Live 3D guidance in the interventional radiology suite. AJR Am J Roentgenol. 2007; 189(6): W357–64

[61] Rigatelli G, Zamboni A, Cardaioli P, et al. Three-dimensional rotational digital angiography in catheter-based congenital heart disease interventions. J Cardiovasc Med (Hagerstown). 2008; 9(4):432

[62] Diegeler A, Fröhner S, Dähnert I. Precise stent placement using the new Siemens Artis Zeego 3D rotation angiography in a stenosis of a Shelhigh pulmonary conduit. Innovations (Phila). 2010; 5(2):128–130

[63] Gerds-Li JH, Tang M, Kriatselis C, et al. Rapid ventricular pacing to optimize rotational angiography in atrial fibrillation ablation. J Interv Card Electrophysiol. 2009; 26(2):101–107

[64] Silvestry FE, Kerber RE, Brook MM, et al. Echocardiography-guided interventions. J Am Soc Echocardiogr. 2009; 22(3):213–231, quiz 316–317

[65] Eng MH, Salcedo EE, Quaife RA, Carroll JD. Implementation of real time three-dimensional transesophageal echocardiography in percutaneous mitral balloon valvuloplasty and structural heart disease interventions. Echocardiography. 2009; 26(8):958–966

[66] Steeg CN, Bierman FZ, Hordof AJ, Hayes CJ, Krongrad E, Barst RJ. "Bedside" balloon septostomy in infants with transposition of the great arteries: new concepts using two-dimensional echocardiographic techniques. J Pediatr. 1985; 107(6):944–946

[67] Trehan VK, Nigam A, Mukhopadhyay S, et al. Bedside percutaneous transseptal mitral commissurotomy under sole transthoracic echocardiographic guidance in a critically ill patient. Echocardiography. 2006; 23(4):312–314

[68] Weber HS, Mart CR, Myers JL. Transcarotid balloon valvuloplasty for critical aortic valve stenosis at the bedside via continuous transesophageal echocardiographic guidance. Catheter Cardiovasc Interv. 2000; 50(3):326–329

[69] Beitzke A, Stein JI, Suppan C. Balloon atrial septostomy under two-dimensional echocardiographic control. Int J Cardiol. 1991; 30(1):33–42

[70] Ewert P, Berger F, Daehnert I, et al. Transcatheter closure of atrial septal defects without fluoroscopy: feasibility of a new method. Circulation. 2000; 101(8):847–849

[71] Ewert P, Deutsches Herzzentrum Berlin, Berlin, Deutschland. Persönliche Mitteilung. 2010

[72] Kretschmar O, Universitätskinderspital Zürich, Schweiz. Persönliche Mitteilung. 2010

[73] Springer T, Dähnert I. Bedside percutaneous balloon angioplasty of severe recoarctation under sole transthoracic echocardiographic guidance in a critically ill high frequency ventilation dependent infant. Unveröffentlichter Fallbericht

[74] Sekar P, Hornberger LK. The role of fetal echocardiography in fetal intervention: a symbiotic relationship. Clin Perinatol. 2009; 36(2):301–327, ix

[75] Daehnert I, Ewert P, Berger F, Lange PE. Echocardiographically guided closure of a patent foramen ovale during pregnancy after recurrent strokes. J Interv Cardiol. 2001; 14(2):191–192

[76] Bouzas-Mosquera A, Rueda F, Aldama G, et al. Perventricular pulmonary valvuloplasty under echocardiographic guidance. Int J Cardiol. 2008; 130(3):e102–e104

[77] Grothoff M, Piorkowski C, Eitel C, et al. MR imaging-guided electrophysiological ablation studies in humans with passive catheter tracking: initial results. Radiology. 2014; 271(3):695–702

[78] Kos S, Huegli R, Bongartz GM, Jacob AL, Bilecen D. MR-guided endovascular interventions: a comprehensive review on techniques and applications. Eur Radiol. 2008; 18(4):645–657

[79] Saikus CE, Lederman RJ. Interventional cardiovascular magnetic resonance imaging: a new opportunity for image-guided interventions. JACC Cardiovasc Imaging. 2009; 2(11):1321–1331

[80] NRPB. Guidelines on patient dose to promote the optimisation of protection for diagnostic medical exposure. Report of an Advisory Group on Ionising Radiation 1999; 10 (1)

[81] Adam G, Bücker A, Glowinski A, Nolte-Ernsting C, Neuerburg J, Günther RW. Interventional MR tomography: equipment concepts. Radiologe. 1998; 38(3):168–172

[82] Bücker A, Neuerburg JM, Adam GB, et al. MR-gesteurte Spiralembolisation von Nierenarterien in einem Tiermodell. Rofo Fortschr Rontgenstr. 2003; 175(2):271–274

[83] Mahnken AH, Chalabi K, Jalali F, Günther RW, Buecker A. Magnetic resonance-guided placement of aortic stents grafts: feasibility with real-time magnetic resonance fluoroscopy. J Vasc Interv Radiol. 2004; 15(2 Pt 1):189–195

[84] Spuentrup E, Ruebben A, Schaeffter T, Manning WJ, Günther RW, Buecker A. Magnetic resonance-guided coronary artery stent placement in a swine model. Circulation. 2002; 105(7):874–879

[85] Pipe JG, Ahunbay E, Menon P. Effects of interleaf order for spiral MRI of dynamic processes. Magn Reson Med. 1999; 41(2):417–422

[86] Spielman DM, Pauly JM, Meyer CH. Magnetic resonance fluoroscopy using spirals with variable sampling densities. Magn Reson Med. 1995; 34(3):388–394

[87] Spuentrup E, Buecker A, Stuber M, Kühl HP. Images in cardiovascular medicine. Visualization of anomalous coronary artery in the presence of arrhythmia using radial balanced fast field echo coronary magnetic resonance angiography. Circulation. 2003; 107(23):e214

[88] Spuentrup E, Mahnken AH, Kühl HP, et al. Fast interactive real-time magnetic resonance imaging of cardiac masses using spiral gradient echo and radial steady-state free precession sequences. Invest Radiol. 2003; 38(5):288–292

[89] Rasche V, de Boer RW, Holz D, Proksa R. Continuous radial data acquisition for dynamic MRI. Magn Reson Med. 1995; 34(5):754–761

[90] Bücker A, Adam G, Neuerburg JM, et al. Real-time MRI with radial k-radial scanning technique for control of angiographic interventions. RoFo Fortschr Geb Rontgenstr Nuklearmed. 1998; 169(5):542–546

[91] Rubin DL, Ratner AV, Young SW. Magnetic susceptibility effects and their application in the development of new ferromagnetic catheters for magnetic resonance imaging. Invest Radiol. 1990; 25(12):1325–1332

[92] Bakker CJ, Hoogeveen RM, Weber J, van Vaals JJ, Viergever MA, Mali WP. Visualization of dedicated catheters using fast scanning techniques with potential for MR-guided vascular interventions. Magn Reson Med. 1996; 36(6):816–820

[93] Buecker A, Spuentrup E, Ruebben A, et al. New metallic MR stents for artifact-free coronary MR angiography: feasibility study in a swine model. Invest Radiol. 2004; 39(5):250–253

[94] Glowinski A, Adam G, Bücker A, Neuerburg J, van Vaals JJ, Günther RW. Catheter visualization using locally induced, actively controlled field inhomogeneities. Magn Reson Med. 1997; 38(2):253–258

[95] Glowinski A, Kürsch J, Adam G, Bücker A, Noll TG, Günther RW. Device visualization for interventional MRI using local magnetic fields: basic theory and its application to catheter visualization. IEEE Trans Med Imaging. 1998; 17(5):786–793

[96] Ackerman JL, Offutt MC, Buxton RB, et al. Rapid 3-D tracking of small RF coils. Montreal, Canada: Proc SMRM 5th Annu Meeting; 1986

[97] Rasche V, Holz D, Köhler J, Proksa R, Röschmann P. Catheter tracking using continuous radial MRI. Magn Reson Med. 1997; 37 (6):963–968

[98] Kocaturk O, Kim AH, Saikus CE, et al. Active two-channel 0.035' guidewire for interventional cardiovascular MRI. J Magn Reson Imaging. 2009; 30(2):461–465

[99] Buecker A, Adam GB, Neuerburg JM, et al. Simultaneous real-time visualization of the catheter tip and vascular anatomy for MR-guided PTA of iliac arteries in an animal model. J Magn Reson Imaging. 2002; 16(2):201–208

[100] Patil S, Bieri O, Jhooti P, Scheffler K. Automatic slice positioning (ASP) for passive real-time tracking of interventional devices using projection-reconstruction imaging with echo-dephasing (PRIDE). Magn Reson Med. 2009; 62(4):935–942

[101] Kuehne T, Fahrig R, Butts K. Pair of resonant fiducial markers for localization of endovascular catheters at all catheter orientations. J Magn Reson Imaging. 2003; 17(5):620–624

[102] Wildermuth S, Erhart P, Leung DA, Göhde S, Schoenenberger A, Debatin JF. Active instrumental guidance in interventional MR tomography: introduction to a new concept. RoFo Fortschr Geb Rontgenstr Nuklearmed. 1998; 169(1):77–84

[103] Konings MK, Bartels LW, Smits HF, Bakker CJ. Heating around intravascular guidewires by resonating RF waves. J Magn Reson Imaging. 2000; 12(1):79–85

[104] Buecker A, Spuentrup E, Schmitz-Rode T, et al. Use of a nonmetallic guide wire for magnetic resonance-guided coronary artery catheterization. Invest Radiol. 2004; 39(11):656–660

[105] Ladd ME, Quick HH. Reduction of resonant RF heating in intravascular catheters using coaxial chokes. Magn Reson Med. 2000; 43 (4):615–619

[106] Fandrey S, Weiss S, Muller J. Development of an active intravascular MR device with an optical transmission system. IEEE Trans Med Imaging. 2008; 27(12):1723–1727

[107] Weiss S, Kuehne T, Brinkert F, et al. In vivo safe catheter visualization and slice tracking using an optically detunable resonant marker. Magn Reson Med. 2004; 52(4):860–868

[108] Weiss S, Schaeffter T, Brinkert F, Kühne T, Bücker A. Ein Verfahren zur sicheren Visualisierung und Lokalisierung von Kathetern für MR-geführte intravaskuläre Prozeduren. Z Med Phys. 2003; 13 (3):172–176

[109] Krämer NA, Krüger S, Schmitz S, et al. Preclinical evaluation of a novel fiber compound MR guidewire in vivo. Invest Radiol. 2009; 44 (7):390–397

[110] Kuehne T, Saeed M, Moore P, et al. Influence of blood-pool contrast media on MR imaging and flow measurements in the presence of pulmonary arterial stents in swine. Radiology. 2002; 223(2):439–445

[111] Kuehne T, Saeed M, Reddy G, et al. Sequential magnetic resonance monitoring of pulmonary flow with endovascular stents placed across the pulmonary valve in growing Swine. Circulation. 2001; 104(19):2363–2368

[112] Buecker A, Spuentrup E, Grabitz R, et al. Magnetic resonance-guided placement of atrial septal closure device in animal model of patent foramen ovale. Circulation. 2002; 106(4):511–515

[113] Buecker A, Spuentrup E, Grabitz R, et al. Real-time-MR guidance for placement of a self-made fully MR-compatible atrial septal occluder: in vitro test. RoFo Fortschr Geb Rontgenstr Nuklearmed. 2002; 174 (3):283–285

[114] Meyer JM, Buecker A, Schuermann K, Ruebben A, Guenther RW. MR evaluation of stent patency: in vitro test of 22 metallic stents and the possibility of determining their patency by MR angiography. Invest Radiol. 2000; 35(12):739–746

[115] Schalla S, Saeed M, Higgins CB, Martin A, Weber O, Moore P. Magnetic resonance–guided cardiac catheterization in a swine model of atrial septal defect. Circulation. 2003; 108(15):1865–1870

[116] Rhode KS, Hill DL, Edwards PJ, et al. Registration and tracking to integrate X-ray and MR images in an XMR facility. IEEE Trans Med Imaging. 2003; 22(11):1369–1378

[117] Nazarian S, Kolandaivelu A, Zviman MM, et al. Feasibility of real-time magnetic resonance imaging for catheter guidance in electrophysiology studies. Circulation. 2008; 118(3):223–229

[118] Lardo AC, McVeigh ER, Jumrussirikul P, et al. Visualization and temporal/spatial characterization of cardiac radiofrequency ablation lesions using magnetic resonance imaging. Circulation. 2000; 102(6):698–705

[119] Lederman RJ, Guttman MA, Peters DC, et al. Catheter-based endomyocardial injection with real-time magnetic resonance imaging. Circulation. 2002; 105(11):1282–1284

[120] Buecker A, Neuerburg JM, Adam GB, et al. Real-time MR fluoroscopy for MR-guided iliac artery stent placement. J Magn Reson Imaging. 2000, 12(4):616–622

[121] Kuehne T, Yilmaz S, Schulze-Neick I, et al. Magnetic resonance imaging guided catheterisation for assessment of pulmonary vascular resistance: in vivo validation and clinical application in patients with pulmonary hypertension. Heart. 2005; 91(8):1064–1069

[122] Rickers C, Jerosch-Herold M, Hu X, et al. Magnetic resonance image-guided transcatheter closure of atrial septal defects. Circulation. 2003; 107(1):132–138

[123] Bücker A, Spuentrup E, Ruebben A, et al. Artifact-free in-stent lumen visualization by standard MR angiography using a new metallic MRI stent. Circulation. 2002; 105:1772–1775

[124] Kuehne T, Weiss S, Brinkert F, et al. Catheter visualization with resonant markers at MR imaging-guided deployment of endovascular stents in swine. Radiology. 2004; 233(3):774–780

[125] Kuehne T, Saeed M, Higgins CB, et al. Endovascular stents in pulmonary valve and artery in swine: feasibility study of MR imaging-guided deployment and postinterventional assessment. Radiology. 2003; 226(2):475–481

[126] McVeigh ER, Guttman MA, Lederman RJ, et al. Real-time interactive MRI-guided cardiac surgery: aortic valve replacement using a direct apical approach. Magn Reson Med. 2006; 56(5):958–964

[127] Kuehne T, Yilmaz S, Meinus C, et al. Magnetic resonance imaging-guided transcatheter implantation of a prosthetic valve in aortic valve position: Feasibility study in swine. J Am Coll Cardiol. 2004; 44 (11):2247–2249

[128] Raval AN, Karmarkar PV, Guttman MA, et al. Real-time MRI guided atrial septal puncture and balloon septostomy in swine. Catheter Cardiovasc Interv. 2006; 67(4):637–643

[129] Elagha AA, Kocaturk O, Guttman MA, et al. Real-time MR imaging-guided laser atrial septal puncture in swine. J Vasc Interv Radiol. 2008; 19(9):1347–1353

[130] Silvestry FE, Kerber RE, Brook MM, et al. Echocardiography-guided interventions. J Am Soc Echocardiogr. 2009; 22(3):213–231, quiz 316–317

[131] Ratnayaka K, Raman VK, Faranesh AZ, et al. Antegrade percutaneous closure of membranous ventricular septal defect using X-ray fused with magnetic resonance imaging. JACC Cardiovasc Interv. 2009; 2(3):224–230

[132] Razavi R, Hill DL, Keevil SF, et al. Cardiac catheterisation guided by MRI in children and adults with congenital heart disease. Lancet. 2003; 362(9399):1877–1882

[133] Krueger JJ, Ewert P, Yilmaz S, et al. Magnetic resonance imaging-guided balloon angioplasty of coarctation of the aorta: a pilot study. Circulation. 2006; 113(8):1093–1100

[134] Schmitt B, Steendijk P, Lunze K, et al. Integrated assessment of diastolic and systolic ventricular function using diagnostic MRI-catheterization: validation in pigs and application in a clinical pilot study. JACC Cardiovasc Imaging. 2009; 2(11):1271–1281

Suggested Readings

Bakker CJ, Bos C, Weinmann HJ. Passive tracking of catheters and guidewires by contrast-enhanced MR fluoroscopy. Magn Reson Med. 2001; 45 (1):17–23

Hor KN, Gottliebson WM, Carson C, et al. Comparison of magnetic resonance feature tracking for strain calculation with harmonic phase imaging analysis. JACC Cardiovasc Imaging. 2010; 3(2):144–151

Kouwenhoven M, Bakker CJG, Hartkamp MJ, et al. Current MR angiographic imaging techniques: a survey. In: Lanzer P, Rösch J, eds. Vascular diagnostics. Heidelberg: Springer; 1994: 375–398

Strother CM, Unal O, Frayne R, et al. Endovascular treatment of experimental canine aneurysms: feasibility with MR imaging guidanc Radiology. 2000; 215(2):516–519

Zhang Q, Wendt M, Aschoff AJ, Zheng L, Lewin JS, Duerk JL. Active MR guidance of interventional devices with target-navigation. Magn Reson Med. 2000; 44(1):56–65

4 Clinical Pictures

4.1 Shunt Defects

4.1.1 Atrial Septal Defect

Philipp Beerbaum, Joachim Lotz, Michael Steinmetz

Definition

The term "atrial septal defect" refers to various morphological and embryological defects of the atrial septum that in isolation, comprise a total of 5–10% of all congenital heart defects.[1] ASD often occurs in conjunction with other cardiovascular defects. Atrial septal defects should be distinguished from open PFO. Fetal atrial communication persists in approximately one-third of all children. Its clinical significance results primarily from the likelihood of paradoxical embolism of thrombi occurring from the venous area into the left systemic arterial area, and then into the aortic branches. Thrombi of this type can lead to strokes or peripheral embolisms.

Classification

The following three, most common types, will be described in detail (▶ Fig. 4.1):

- *Secundum ASD:* ASD II also known as fossa ovalis defect (approximately 70% of all ASDs), occurs in the central portion of the atrial septum with no connection to the atrioventricular valves (▶ Fig. 4.1, ▶ Fig. 4.2)
- *Primum ASD:* ASD I also known as partial AVSD, comprises approximately 15–20% of all ASDs. This type of defect is situated caudally and is connected to the atrioventricular valves (▶ Fig. 4.1, ▶ Fig. 4.3)
- *Sinus venosus ASD:* SVD comprising approximately 10–15% of all ASDs
  - superior: most common form (▶ Fig. 4.1); near the connection to the superior vena cava
  - inferior: less common; also known as "coronary sinus ASD" (▶ Fig. 4.1);[2] near the connection to the inferior vena cava

Coronary sinus defect (also known as unroofed coronary sinus) is an uncommon defect type (3–5% of all ASDs).

> **Note**
>
> SVD often occurs in conjunction with PAPVR (see Partial Pulmonary Venous Anomalies) (▶ Fig. 4.4 and ▶ Fig. 4.5). Thus, once SVD has been established, it is crucial to always search for concurrent PAPVR.

Hemodynamics

An ASD allows passage of blood between the left and right atrium, also known as a "shunt." The direction and shunt volume result from the varying compliance (elasticity) of the left and right ventricles. The right ventricle is less

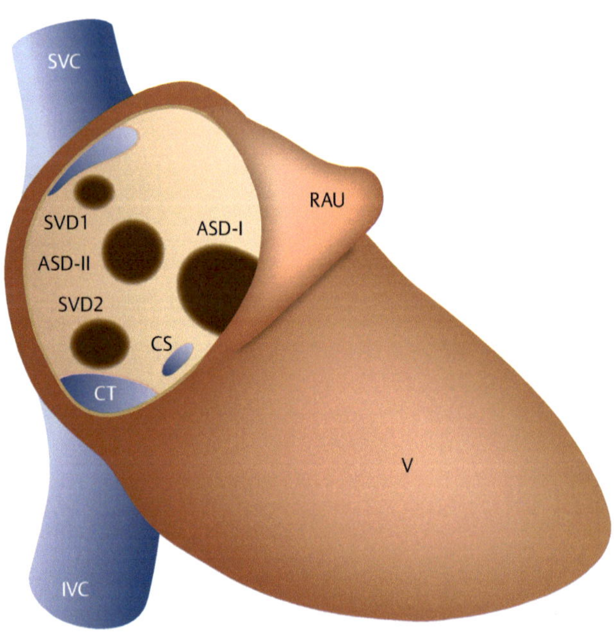

Fig. 4.1 Various forms of ASD. Schematic depiction.
ASD I = primum atrial septal defect (incl. atrioventricular septal defect)
ASD II = secundum atrial septal defect (aka fossa ovalis defect)
CS = coronary sinus (entrance)
CT = crista terminalis
IVC = inferior vena cava
RAU = right auricle
SVC = superior vena cava
SVD1 = type 1 sinus venosus defect (superior sinus venosus defect)
SVD2 = type 2 sinus venosus defect (inferior sinus venosus defect)
V = ventricle

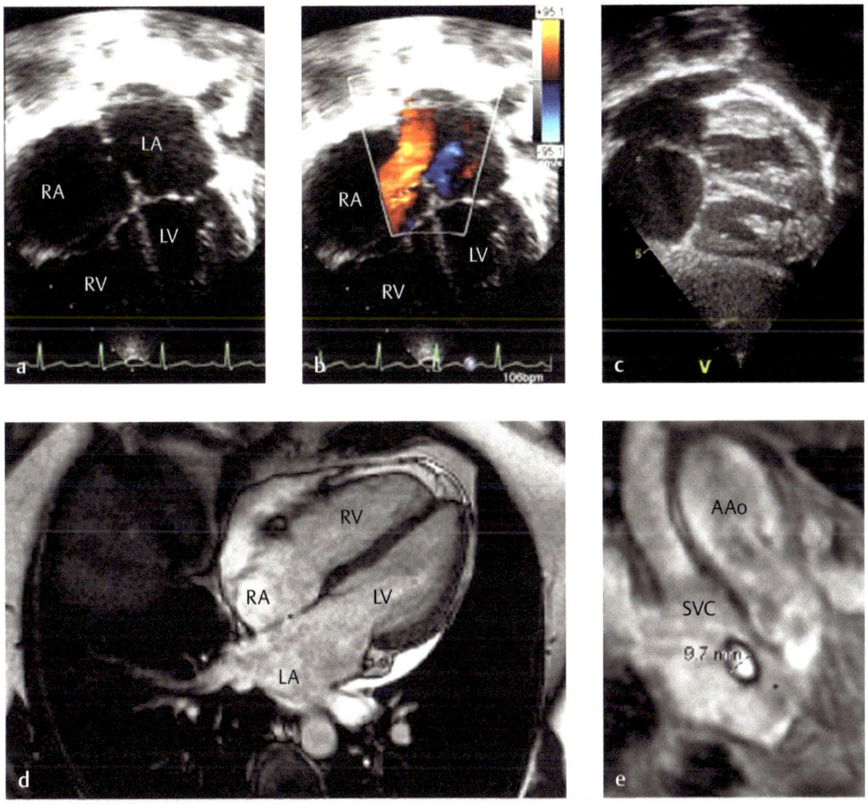

Fig. 4.2 Large ASD II. Two patients (**a**, **b**: patient 1; **c–e**: patient 2). Each asterisk indicates an ASD.
AAo = ascending aorta
LA = left atrium
LV = left ventricle
RA = right atrium
RV = right ventricle
SVC = superior vena cava

a 2-D echo, 4-chamber view, without color Doppler.
b 2-D echo of the same patient, 4-chamber view, with color Doppler. The left–right shunt is clearly visible.
c 2-D echo of a different patient with ASD II (see **d** and **e**), 4-chamber view.
d SSFP cine MRI, 4-chamber view, of the patient from **c** with clearly visible ASD II. Minor pericardial effusion is also visible near the atrioventricular valve in the left ventricle.
e Tangential SSFP cine MRI, parallel to the septum, for the patient from **c** and **d**. The size of the defect (approximately 10 mm) can be measured based on this slice.

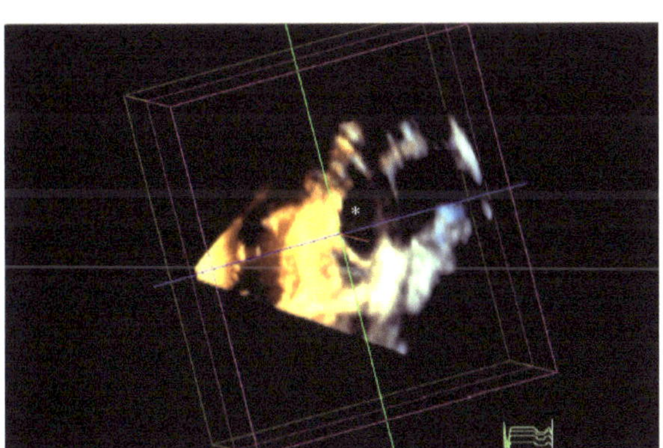

Fig. 4.3 Large, valve-adjacent ASD I. 3-D TEE; view from left atrium. The asterisk indicates the site of the ASD.

muscular and thus more elastic during diastole (meaning it demonstrates higher compliance) than the left ventricle. The reason for this is the low right ventricular afterload, since pulmonary arteriolar resistance comprises only approximately 10–15% of systemic arteriolar resistance, which is significant to the afterload of the left ventricle.

The left–right shunt that generally results from this phenomenon occurs primarily during late ventricular diastole and early ventricular systole. Depending on the size of the shunt, this increases or decreases volume load in the right atrium and right ventricle (▶ Fig. 4.6), in addition to the pulmonary vessels (arteries and veins), which dilate accordingly (▶ Fig. 4.7).

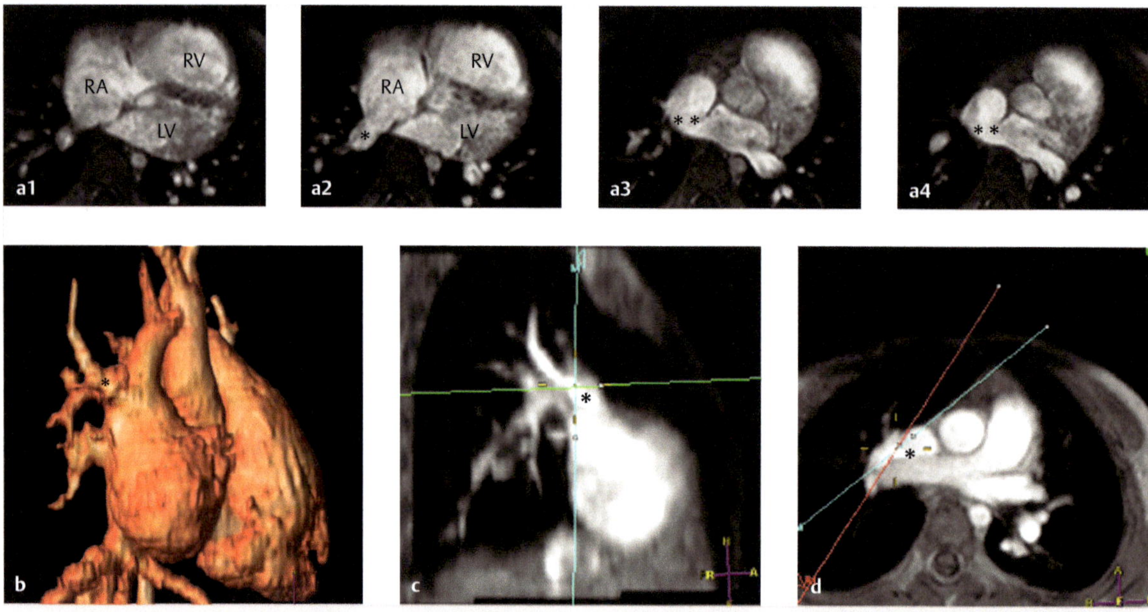

Fig. 4.4 SVD with concurrent PAPVR of a right superior pulmonary vein to the superior vena cava and right atrium. The single asterisk marks the right superior pulmonary vein. The PAPVR is especially easy to visualize using a 3-D whole heart MRI sequence (**a**). Both in MRI and MDCT (▶ Fig. 4.5), a 3-D data set offers the opportunity to depict the surface via volume rendering (**b**), as well as to create precise reconstructions using multiplanar reformats in various orientations (**c**, **d**).

LV = left ventricle
RA = right atrium
RV = right ventricle

a 3-D whole-heart MRI sequence with transverse reconstruction at four different levels to visualize the PAPVR (asterisk) and SVD (double asterisk).
b MRI, volume rendering.
c MRI, coronal multiplanar reformat.
d MRI, transverse multiplanar reformat.

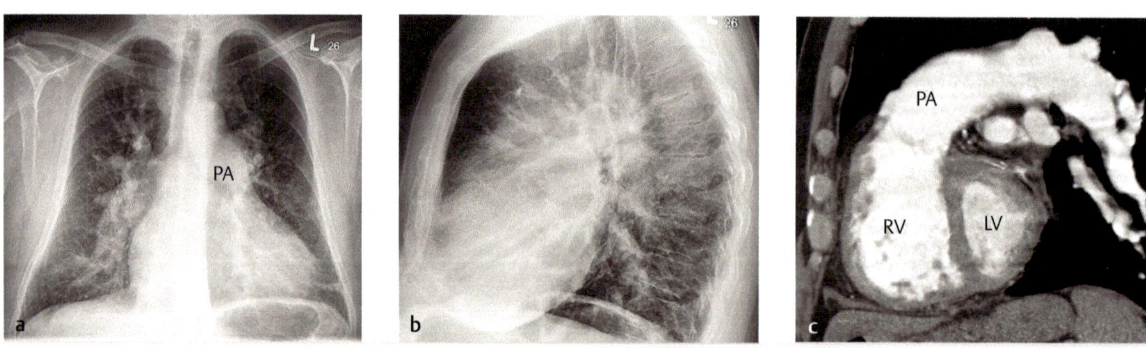

Fig. 4.5 Superior SVD accompanied by PAPVR. Sixty-five-year-old man. The thoracic X-ray (**a**) in p.-a. projection clearly depicts the enlargement of the right atrium and the significantly enlarged pulmonary arteries and veins (primarily on the right side, in this instance). The thoracic X-ray in lateral projection (**b**), in particular, shows the clear enlargement of the right ventricle and RVOT, as well as the pulmonary artery ("narrowing" of the retrosternal space) and pulmonary veins (▶ Table 4.1). Enlargement of the right ventricle with volume overload can also be identified easily using CT short-axis reconstruction (**c**) of the pulmonary artery. The volume overload of the right ventricle is clearly depicted by the flat curvature of the interventricular septum. The 3-D MDCT data set depicts the ASD (double asterisk), and the anomalous pulmonary venous connection to the superior vena cava (asterisk), using various angled multiplanar reconstructions (**d–g**).

RV = right ventricle
Ao = aorta
LA = left atrium
LV = left ventricle
PA = pulmonary artery
RA = right atrium
RAU = right auricle
RPA = right pulmonary artery
RV = right ventricle
SVC = superior vena cava

a P.-a. thoracic X-ray.
b Lateral thoracic X-ray.
c Short-axis reconstruction (75% of the RR interval) of the retrospectively gated MDCT data set (64 rows).

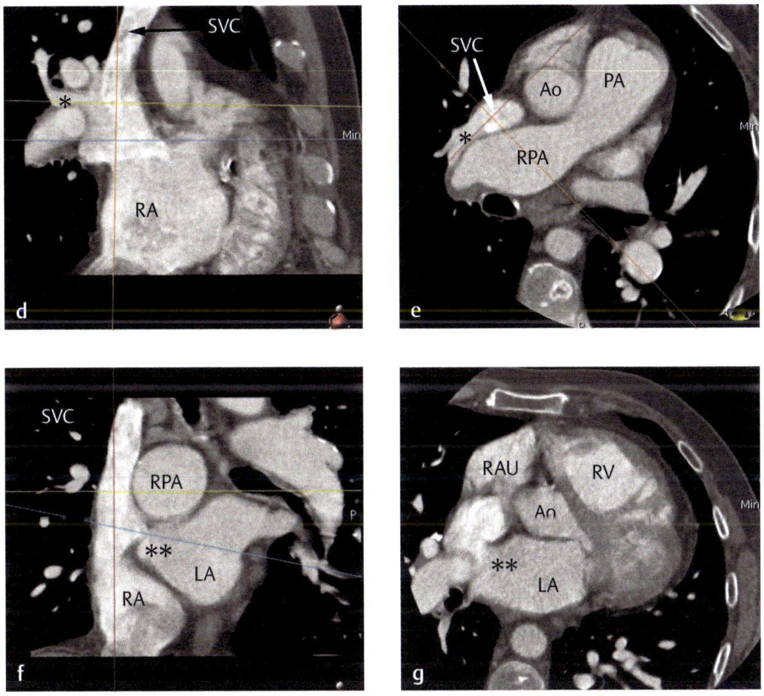

Fig. 4.5 (*Continued*) **Superior SVD accompanied by PAPVR.**

RV = right ventricle
Ao = aorta
LA = left atrium
LV = left ventricle
PA = pulmonary artery
RA = right atrium
RAU = right auricle
RPA = right pulmonary artery
RV = right ventricle
SVC = superior vena cava

d Multiplanar reconstruction of the 3-D MDCT data set (coronal cross-sectional orientation) through the anomalously connected pulmonary veins (asterisk). The colored lines represent the sectional planes for reconstructing **e**, **f**, and **g**.

e Multiplanar reconstruction of the 3-D MDCT data set in transverse cross-sectional orientation (planning cross-section, see yellow line in **d**). The orange line corresponds to the planning cross-section for the coronal reconstruction (**f**) to depict the superior SVD.

f Multiplanar reconstruction of the 3-D MDCT data set for the coronal reconstruction of the superior SVD (double asterisk). This sectional plane corresponds to the orange line in **d** and **e**.

g Angled transverse multiplanar reconstruction, running through the SVD, of the 3-D MDCT data set. The sectional planes used for reconstruction are marked as blue lines in **d** and **f**.

On the other hand, the left atrium retains this additional shunt volume after it passes through the lungs again. The left atrium is able to "decompress" due to the defect and is thus, in effect, not subject to volume overload (▸ Table 4.1). Throughout the course of the patient's life, the relative difference between ventricular compliance continues to increase, meaning that the left ventricle becomes increasingly inelastic as the patient ages. If an ASD is already present, this decreasing elasticity further exacerbates the left–right shunt.[3] Correspondingly, thoracic X-ray in p.-a. view depict both increased pulmonary vascular markings and a dilated pulmonary segment. The right atrium's dilation is also expressed in the form of pronounced right atrial contour (▸ Fig. 4.7a). In contrast, this dilation of the right ventricle and the RVOT are visible when taking images from lateral positions, primarily in the retrosternal area (▸ Fig. 4.7 b and d).

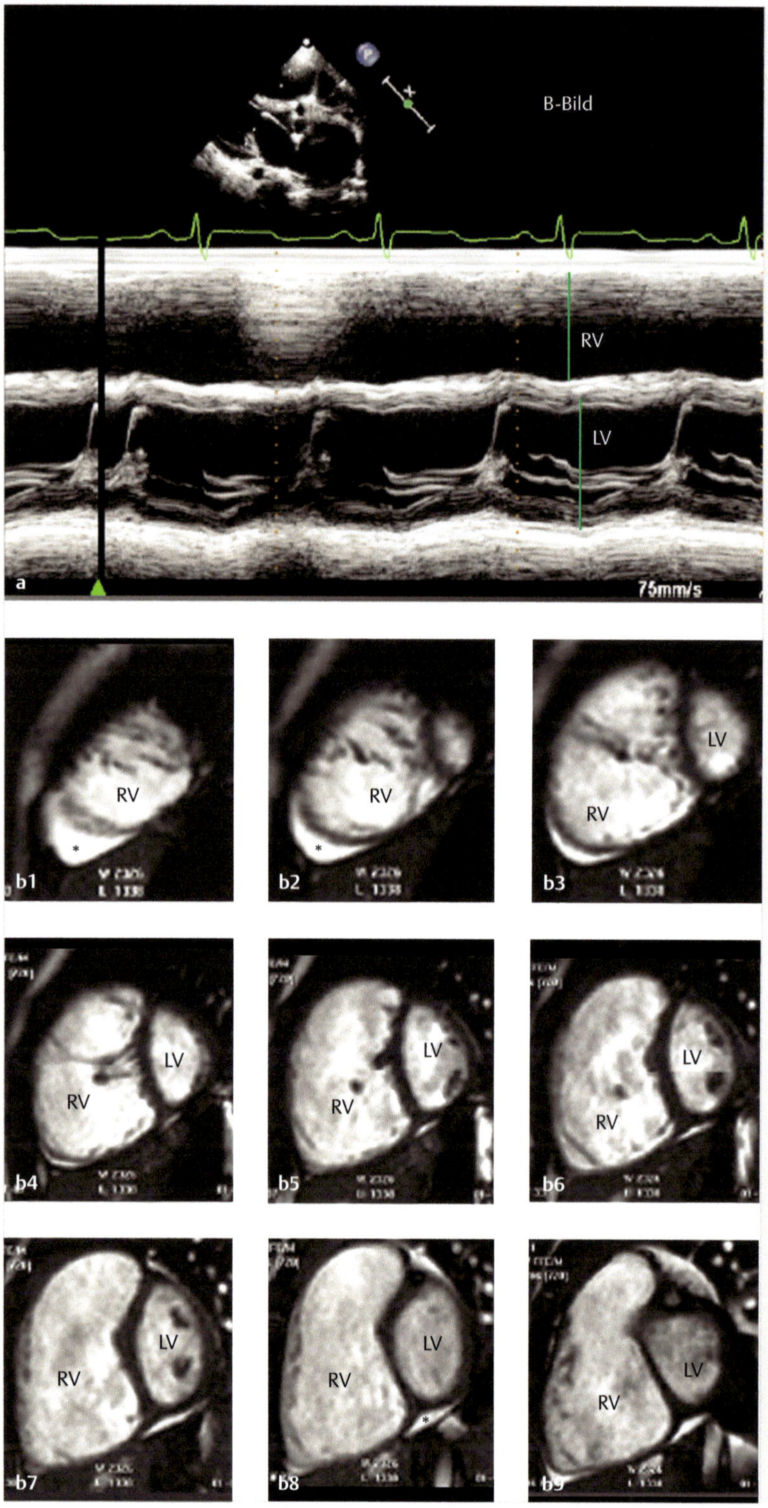

Fig. 4.6 Right ventricular volume overload caused by an ASD. Right ventricular volume overload caused by an ASD is already visible adjacent to the transducer using a 2-D TTE along the parasternal long axis, even in a B-mode image (**a**). Precise quantification is possible during M-mode, based on the end diastolic and end systolic diameters of the right ventricle. The left ventricular parameters can also be communicated in this fashion. Due to the complex right ventricular geometry, MRI (**b**) using the slice summation method (Simpson's method) still offers significant advantages compared to echocardiography. The end diastolic short-axis slices via the complete right and left ventricle using cine MRI and SSFP sequences for the same patient depict the significantly dilated right ventricle due to pronounced volume overload through the resulting left–right shunt.

LV = left ventricle

RV = right ventricle.

a 2-D-TTE, parasternal long axis (B image, M-mode).

b 2-D SSFP cine MRI.

Clinical Issues

With the exception of bicuspid aortic valve and mitral valve prolapse syndrome, ASD is the most common heart defect diagnosed in adults (▶ Fig. 4.5 and ▶ Fig. 4.7). In part, this is due to the fact that the right ventricle initially handles the excess volume load well and under these conditions can also increase cardiac output.

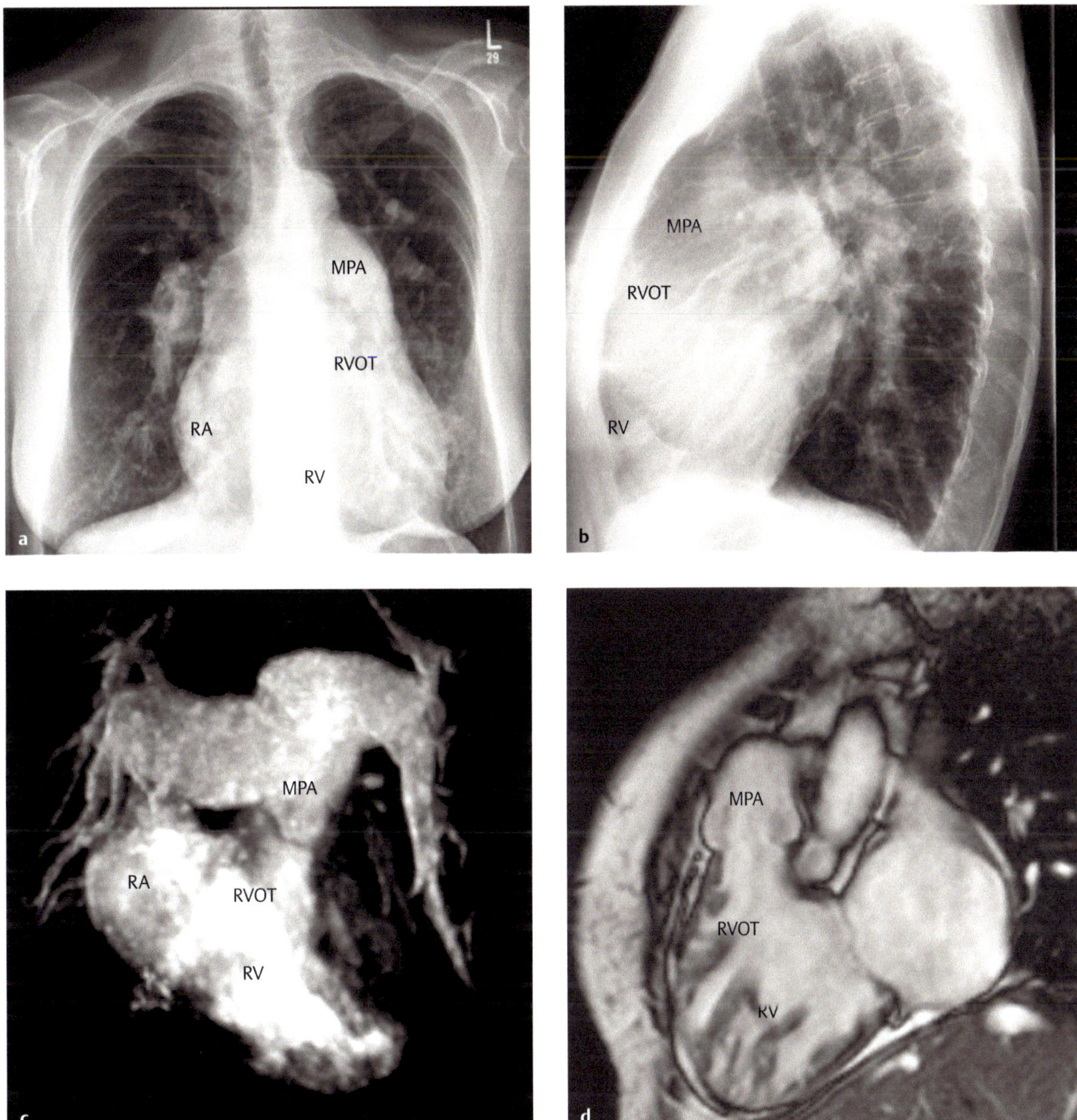

Fig. 4.7 ASD accompanied by dilation of the pulmonary vessels. Thoracic X-rays (**a**, **b**) of an adult male patient with significant dilation of the main pulmonary artery (MPA) and branches, right atrium, right ventricle, and RVOT, as well as a volume overload in the lungs. The MIP reconstruction of a contrast-enhanced MRA (**c**) and right ventricular long axis of an SSFP cine MRI sequence during systole (**d**) depicts the dilated right ventricle of the same patient, and the significantly dilated right and left pulmonary arteries.

MPA = main pulmonary artery (truncus pulmonalis)
RA = right atrium
RV = right ventricle
RVOT = right ventricular outflow tract

a P.-a. thoracic X-ray.

b Lateral thoracic X-ray.

c MIP reconstruction of a contrast-enhanced MRA, ventral view.

d SSFP cine MRI sequence during systole, right ventricular long axis, with approximate lateral projection corresponding to **b**.

Natural Progression and Indication for Treatment

Without treatment, clinical symptoms such as right ventricular heart failure, cardiac rhythm disorders, or progressive pulmonary arterial hypertonia[4] will begin to manifest. The indication for ASD closure is a result of studies on the natural progression of defects diagnosed later in life.[4,5] This data reveals that heart failure with exertional dyspnea and predominantly atrial, often difficult-to-treat tachycardic rhythm disorders occur with increasing frequency after age 30. After closure of a defect, these disorders are often irreversible. The indication for treatment is more frequently determined based on the extent of right ventricular volume load than on shunt ratio (Q_p:Q_s ratio) alone.[6]

Table 4.1 Volume load of the various cardiovascular compartments in a case of ASD.

Cardiovascular compartment	Volume load
Right atrium	+ +
Right ventricle	+ +
Pulmonary arteries	+ +
Pulmonary veins	+ +
Left atrium	-
Left ventricle	-
Aorta and conduit arteries	-
Systemic veins	-

Treatment Options and Preinterventional Diagnostics

Catheter-based interventional closure has become possible for the majority of type II ASDs, and is widely regarded as the treatment of choice (▶ Fig. 3.16 and ▶ Fig. 3.17). All other types are treated surgically, which yield exceptional results. Categorizing the efficacy of various imaging procedures is based primarily on their ability to classify the ASD type precisely, and to determine the defect's size and the dimensions of its margins compared to the surrounding cardiovascular structures. Additional diagnostic tasks include quantifying shunt volume, determining the volume's effects on right and left ventricular function, and the morphological depiction of concurrent defects, such as anomalous pulmonary venous connections (▶ Table 4.2). Precise, noninvasive quantification of shunt volume by determining the Q_p:Q_s ratio—meaning the cardiac output measured in the pulmonary artery (index "P") and aorta (index "S" = systemic artery)—is one application of MRI flow measurement (▶ Fig. 4.8).[7,8]

Postoperative and Postinterventional Issues

Rhythm disorders and, in extremely rare cases, cyanosis concurrent with inferior ASD (occasionally with the option to shunt the lower caval vein into the left atrium) are among the issues that may occur after surgical or interventional ASD corrections.[9]

Table 4.2 Preinterventional imaging diagnostics for an ASD.

Imaging methods	Focus	Value
2-D, 3-D TTE	• Defect size and margins • Left–right shunt, qualitative • Right heart dilatation • Ruling out pulmonary and systemic venous anomalies	+ + +
2-D, 3-D TEE	see TTE	+ + +
Cardiac MRI	• Quantifying the left–right shunt • Quantifying ventricular dilation and function • Measuring the defect (phase contrast method) • Anatomy of pulmonary and systemic veins	+ + + (Backup method)
MDCT	Backup method in cases of unclear echocardiographical findings and contraindication against cardiac MRI; may be helpful in cases of pulmonary parenchymatic comorbidity or to prove the existence of concurrent vascular defects, such as anomalous pulmonary venous connections	+ + (Backup method)
Invasive (diagnostic) cardiac catheter examination	• Measuring pressure and resistance (if indicated), pharmacological testing • In rare cases: invasive measurement of diastolic left ventricular functional parameters (e.g., left ventricular end diastolic diameter) in the event of suspected elevated risk of pulmonary edema after closure of an ASD • Ruling out pulmonary and systemic venous anomalies	+ + + (in cases of pulmonary hypertonia and suspected left ventricular restriction)

ASD, atrial septal defect; MDCT, multidetector computed tomography; MRI, magnetic resonance imaging; TEE, transesophageal echocardiography; TTE, transthoracic echocardiography.

Goals and Relative Value of Diagnostic Imaging

TTE is generally sufficient for preoperative diagnostics in children.[7] For adults, a thoracic X-ray may also be ordered due to morphological signs suggesting an ASD that are typically visible via imaging (▸ Fig. 4.7). TEE plays a central role for older children and adults. Clinical practice has shown that especially for these older patients with ASDs cardiac MRI is selected more and more frequently as the first-choice method.[10,11] For younger children, however, tomographic procedures are used only rarely, and generally only as a backup method for echocardiography or for postinterventional follow-up exams (▸ Table 4.2 and ▸ Table 4.3). MRI has a special role, and CT has a backup role for visualizing a PAPVR within the scope of an SVD (▸ Fig. 4.4). In particular, preparing multiplanar reformats of a 3-D MRA or of an MDCT data set (▸ Fig. 4.5) facilitates preoperative planning. One particular strength of MRI is its ability to measure shunt volume noninvasively (▸ Fig. 4.8) via flow measurement (using the phase contrast technique) in the aorta and pulmonary artery to calculate Q_p:Q_s ratios.

Table 4.3 Postinterventional imaging diagnostics in cases of ASD.

Imaging methods	Value
TTE	+
TEE	+++
Cardiac MRI	++
MDCT	+
Invasive cardiac catheter diagnostics	+

ASD, atrial septal defect; MDCT, multidetector computed tomography; MRI, magnetic resonance imaging; TEE, transesophageal echocardiography; TTE, transthoracic echocardiography.

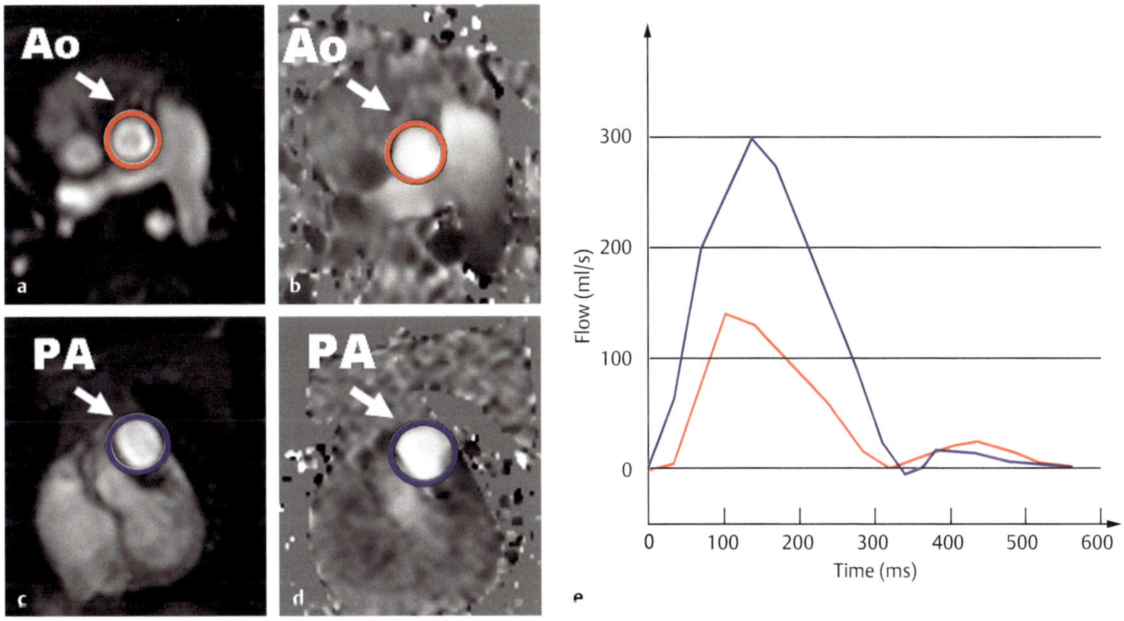

Fig. 4.8 Determining shunt volume using MRI.
Ao = aorta
PA = pulmonary artery

- **a** Through-plane MRI flow measurement (perpendicular to the course of the vessel) in the aorta, anatomical modulus image.
- **b** Phase image of the aorta, indicating flow velocity and direction. Cranial flow is coded in a pale color in the phase image. The red circle indicates the point of flow measurement in the aorta for the red flow curve in **e**.
- **c** Through-plane MRI flow measurement (perpendicular to the course of the vessel) in the pulmonary artery; anatomical modulus image.
- **d** Phase image of the pulmonary artery, indicating flow velocity and direction. Cranial flow is coded in a pale color in the phase image. The blue circle indicates the location of flow measurement in the pulmonary artery for the blue flow curve in **e**.
- **e** Corresponding flow volume curves in the aorta (red) and pulmonary artery (blue) for a male patient with pronounced left–right shunt (Q_p/Q_s ratio greater than 2).

4.1.2 Ventricular Septal Defect

Philipp Beerbaum, Joachim Lotz, Michael Steinmetz

Definition

The term "ventricular septal defect" encompasses various morphological and embryological defects of the interventricular septum. Comprising a total of 15–20% of all congenital heart defects, VSDs are the most common. This does not include VSD that is very commonly concurrent with complex heart defects (especially cyanotic ones). Thus, VSD occurs in isolation in 90% of cases.[12] Classification is based on morphological criteria and takes into account the division of the ventricular septum into a pars membranacea and a pars muscularis. Also note that the tricuspid valve and its septal leaflet attach to the septum somewhat closer to the cardiac apex (provided no atrioventricular canal resulting from an endocardial cushion defect is present), which results in the ability to create a connection between the left ventricle and right atrium near this "atrioventricular septum."

Classification

In principle, all membranous and muscular parts of the ventricular septum could be affected by a VSD. From a morphological or topographical perspective, the ventricular septum possesses an inlet segment near the cardiac base, a right ventricular trabeculated section that includes the apex cordis, and an outlet segment near the outflow tract toward the outlets of the great arteries (▶ Fig. 4.9).

The trabeculated segment of the muscular ventricular septum can be further subdivided into the central, marginal, and apical portions (▶ Fig. 4.14). This is significant to the extent that ventricular septal defects are generally described based on their anatomical position and their topographic and anatomical spatial relations (e.g., their position with respect to the atrioventricular valves or great arteries), since this type of classification results in various strategies for interventional treatment.

Classification of a VSD (▶ Fig. 4.9):

- *Type A:* Perimembranous (or subaortic) VSDs occurs (▶ Fig. 4.10 and ▶ Fig. 4.11) immediately inferior to the aortic valve in 70% of cases. Larger perimembranous or paramembranous VSDs are not limited to just the membranous portion, but also extend to the inlet septum, trabeculated septum (▶ Fig. 4.12), or outlet septum.
- *Type B:* A subpulmonary VSDs (▶ Fig. 4.13) are located in the supracristal portion of the membranous ventricular septum and thus in the outlet septum. This defect is not infrequently complicated by the right coronary aortic cusp prolapsing into the VSD (▶ Fig. 4.13), which can lead to progressive aortic valve insufficiency.

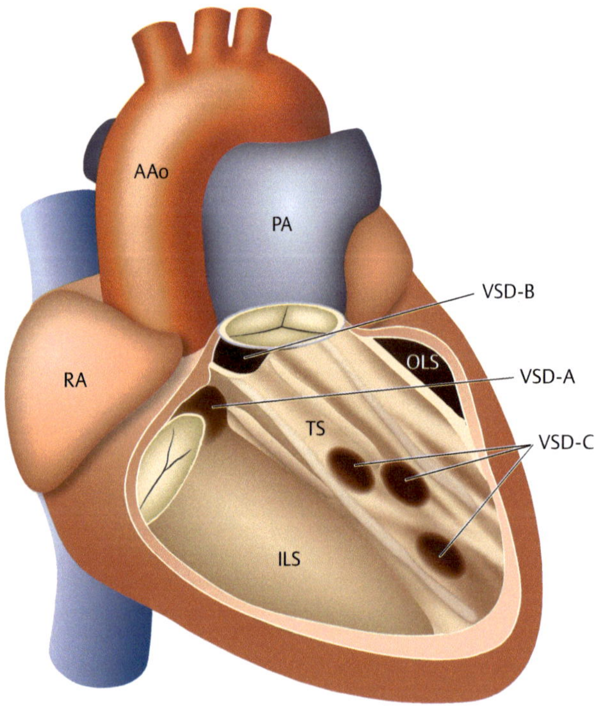

Fig. 4.9 Various types of VSDs. Schematic depiction. View from the right ventricle. In addition to subclassification as muscular or primarily membranous VSDs, it is also useful, from a clinical perspective, to describe VSDs based on their location in the inlet, trabecular, or outlet septum.
AAo = ascending aorta
ILS = inlet septum
OLS = outlet septum
PA = pulmonary artery
RA = right atrium
TS = trabeculated septum (trabeculated area)
VSD-A = type A ventricular septal defect (perimembranous or subaortic ventricular septal defect)
VSD-B = type B ventricular septal defect (subpulmonary or infundibular VSD)
VSD-C = type C ventricular septal defect (muscular ventricular septal defect).

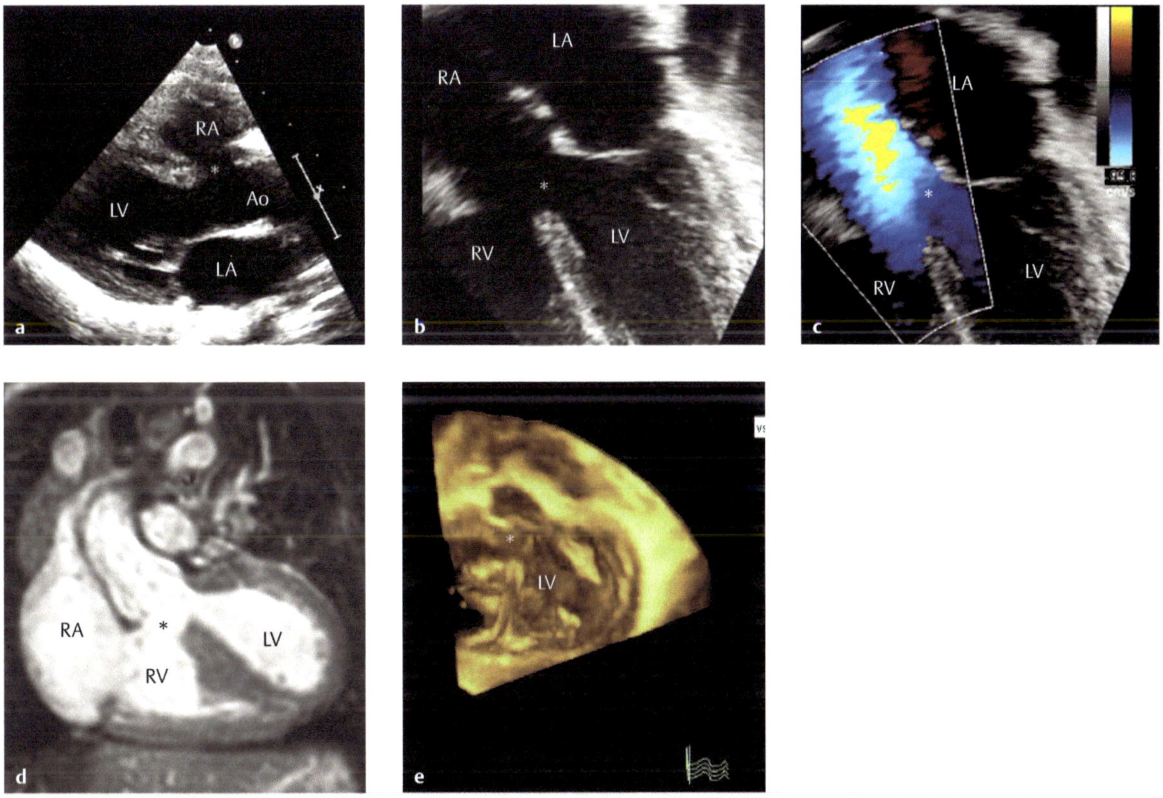

Fig. 4.10 Malalignment VSD as a special form of a subaortic or perimembranous VSD (type A).
Ao = aorta
LA = left atrium
LV = left ventricle
RA = right atrium
RV = right ventricle
a 2-D TTE depiction, parasternal long axis. Isolated malalignment VSD in the anterior outlet septum (**a–c**, asterisk) resulting from a conotruncal defect.
b Four-chamber view, without color Doppler.
c Four-chamber view, with color Doppler.
d Coronal slices through the defect (**d**, **e**, asterisk) and LVOT using an SSFP cine MRI sequence during systole.
e 3-D echo depiction.

- *Type C:* A muscular VSDs (approx. 10% of all VSDs) are fully surrounded by muscle and can occur anywhere in the muscular portion of the interventricular septum (▶ Fig. 4.14). Hybrid forms can also occur.

Note

- An inlet VSD (▶ Fig. 4.12) affects the same section of the septum as the VSD portion in cases of complete AVSD.
- Membranous VSDs (types A and B) constitute 90% of all VSDs.

Special forms:

- Atrioventricular canal VSD (approximately 6% of all VSDs) is handled separately in Chapter 4.1.3, Atrioventricular Septal Defect.
- Malalignment VSD is categorized as a conotruncal defect (▶ Fig. 4.10).
- Gerbode VSD is a defect of the atrioventricular portion of the membranous septum. This results in a shunt between the left ventricle and right atrium. This may be due to the fact that the tricuspid valve and its septal leaflet attach a few millimeters further apically toward the membranous portion of the septum than the mitral valve on the other side of the ventricular septum. This disparity causes a hemodynamic change compared to other types of VSDs (see below and ▶ Table 4.4).

Hemodynamics

For patients with isolated VSDs, clinical symptoms depend both on the defect's size and the ratio of downstream pulmonary and systemic vessel resistance. The anatomical position of the VSD is, in contrast, less crucial.[12,13]

In normal situations with low pulmonary arteriolar resistance, a left–right shunt occurs primarily during systole. During the contraction phase, the pulmonary artery supplies it directly, thus causing no volume overload in

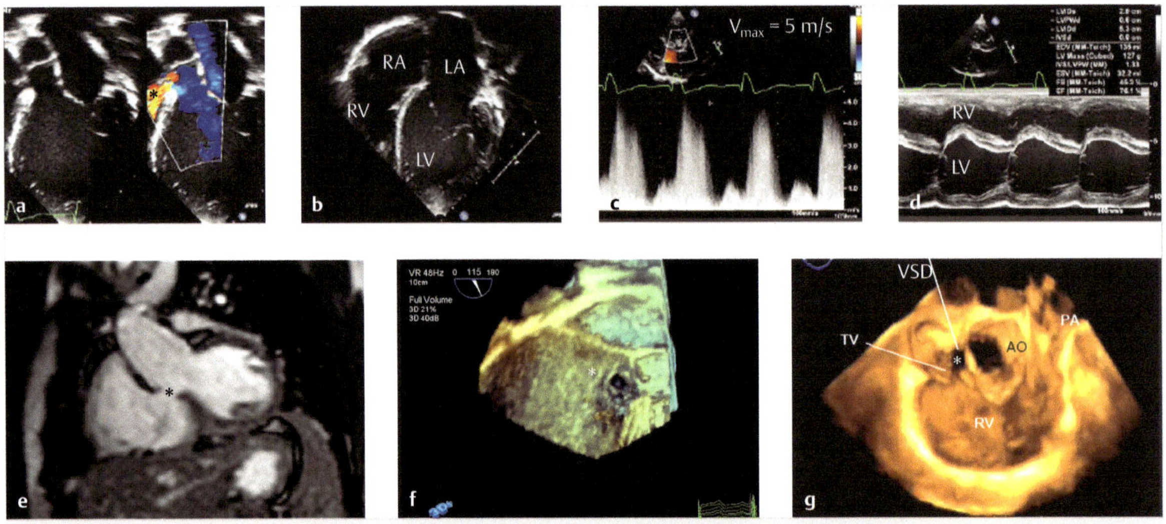

Fig. 4.11 Small, restrictive perimembranous or subaortic VSD (type A). The asterisk indicates the VSD (**a, e–g**).

Ao = Aorta
LA = left atrium
LV = left ventricle; PA = pulmonary artery; RA = right atrium
RV = right ventricle
VSD = ventricular septal defect
TV = tricuspid valve

a 2-D TTE with Doppler (right) and without Doppler (left).
b 2-D TTE, 4-chamber view.
c Spectral Doppler with flow acceleration to a maximum of 5 m/s near the restrictive perimembranous VSD.
d Enlarged left ventricular diameter and normal right ventricular diameters in echo M-mode. The right ventricle is thus not subject to the volume overload that typically occurs in cases of restrictive VSD (▸ Table 4.5).
e SSFP cine MRI, coronal slice orientation.
f 3-D TEE: reconstructions of the small, restrictive VSD with a TEE viewing angle of 115°.
g 3-D TEE: reconstructions of the small, restrictive VSD with a TEE viewing angle of 35°.

the right ventricle (▸ Fig. 4.11 and ▸ Fig. 4.13). Rather, this load is borne by the pulmonary vessels and left side of the heart. These cardiovascular structures can also dilate accordingly as a result of the volume overload (▸ Table 4.4).

A very small defect is restrictive, and the shunt is, consequently, rather minor. A larger VSD can still release pressure, but the shunt remains largely relevant, provided that pulmonary arteriolar resistance is normal. A large VSD can cause pressure between the ventricles to equalize. In cases of normal pulmonary arteriolar resistance, this leads to heart failure due to massive left–right shunt with critical reduction of systemic cardiac output. If anatomical stenoses of the RVOT, pulmonary valve, or pulmonary vessel bed are also present, the left–right shunt will malfunction less critically, and heart failure generally will not occur.

Long-term exposure of the pulmonary vessel bed to pressure and volume overload can develop into a progressive and ultimately irreversible increase in pulmonary arteriolar resistance. In the most extreme cases, this is known as "Eisenmenger syndrome." This can even cause shunt reversal with the development of cyanosis. This risk increases significantly after the first year of life. Thus, for cases of pressure-equalized VSDs, the defect should be closed beforehand.

Table 4.4 Volume load of the various cardiovascular compartments in a case of VSDs.

Cardiovascular compartment	Volume load
Right atrium	- (+) in exceptional cases: VSD of the atrioventricular septum (Gerbode defect with a shunt from the left ventricle to the right atrium)
Right ventricle	- (+) in exceptional cases: Gerbode defect (see above)
Pulmonary arteries	+ +
Pulmonary veins	+ +
Left atrium	+ +
Left ventricle	+ +
Aorta and conduit arteries	-
Systemic veins	-

VSD, ventricular septal defect.

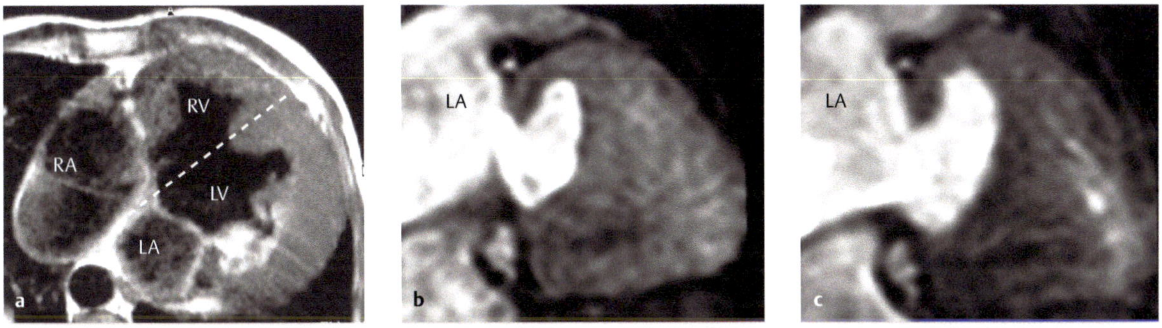

Fig. 4.12 Perimembranous VSD (type A) encompassing the membranous and trabecular portions of the septum.
LA = left atrium
LV = left ventricle
RA = right atrium
RV = right ventricle

a Transverse T1w, turbo SE image triggered during diastole with the planning slice (dotted line) for **b** and **c**.
b SSFP cine MRI during systole, section parallel to the VSD.
c SSFP cine MRI during diastole, section parallel to the VSD.

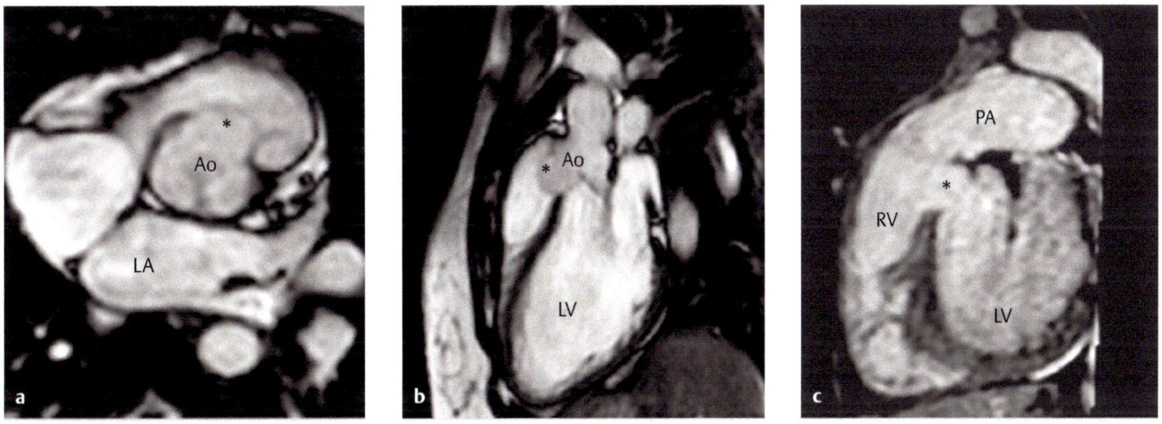

Fig. 4.13 Subpulmonary or infundibular VSD (type B) with prolapsed right coronary cusp. The SSFP cine MRI sequence and LVOT slice clearly show the right coronary cusp prolapsed into the RVOT (**a**, **b**, asterisks). The short-axis slice depicts the subpulmonary VSD (**c**, asterisk).
Ao = Aorta
LA = left atrium
LV = left ventricle
PA = pulmonary artery
RA = right atrium
RV = right ventricle

a SSFP cine MRI sequence, transverse section parallel to the valve.
b LVOT slice.
c Short-axis slice.

Note

Cases of Gerbode defect result in a special hemodynamic situation, since this syndrome causes volume overload in the right atrium and ventricle. In contrast, restrictive defects of the other portions of the septum (as already mentioned) do not cause volume overload of the right atrium and ventricle, even if a large shunt volume is present.

Clinical Issues

Small VSDs are often first diagnosed in adulthood. Due to dyspnea and limited exercise capacity, larger defects are often noted during infancy as signs of cardiac failure, often within the scope of bronchopulmonary infections.[12] Cyanosis does not occur until after shunt reversal (Eisenmenger syndrome).

Natural Progression and Indication for Treatment

Most patients with isolated, small- to medium-sized VSDs have a good prognosis, especially since spontaneous decreases in size up to full regression can occur in up to 50% of patients,[13] primarily in cases of muscular VSD. The indication for treatment is determined primarily by a shunt ratio (Q_p:Q_s ratio) of 1.5:1 to 2:1, and/or if pulmonary arterial pressure increases to half that of systemic values.[12]

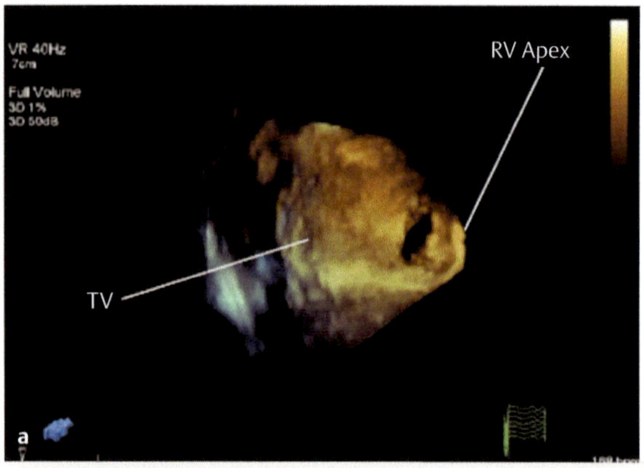

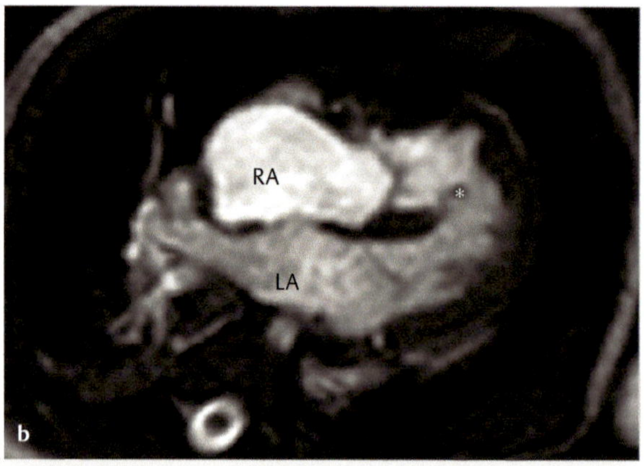

Fig. 4.14 Apical muscular VSD (type C).
LA = left atrium
RA = right atrium
RV = right ventricle
TV = tricuspid valve

a 3-D echo with view from the right ventricle.
b SSFP cine MRI, 4-chamber view (asterisk = VSD).

Symptomatic children with large VSDs receive surgical treatment within the first 6 months of life, while asymptomatic children with pressure-separating VSDs but relevant left–right shunt volume, are treated already as toddlers. Additional indications for surgery include pressure-separating defects without relevant shunts if the right coronary aortic cusp prolapses into the VSD, particularly in cases of subpulmonary VSD position (▶ Fig. 4.13), causing asymmetry of the aortic valve and aortic valve insufficiency.

Treatment Options and Preinterventional Diagnostics

Catheter interventional closure is primarily possible for muscular VSD, though it is fundamentally possible for cases of membranous VSD, as well. Especially in cases of Swiss cheese ventricular septum with multiple muscular VSDs, graduated treatment is often necessary. This entails a palliative surgical treatment by means of pulmonary artery banding, followed by a combined interventional surgical procedure, to be completed in tandem. For cases of large, isolated VSDs, surgical closure is the first-choice procedure and is generally performed from the right atrium from a trans-tricuspid view using a Dacron patch. Nowadays, trans-infundibular access is generally avoided.

Classifying the efficacy of the various imaging procedures prior to an intervention is based on the procedures' ability to precisely determine size, visualize the localization, and quantify shunt volume and its effects on left and right ventricular function. Fundamentally, the VSD can already be visualized well using echocardiography (▶ Fig. 4.10, ▶ Fig. 4.11, ▶ Fig. 4.13 and ▶ Fig. 4.14). 3-D echocardiography, in particular, is especially helpful for peri-interventional and perioperative planning. Not infrequently, TEE is the final, decisive diagnostic method for particular constellations, such as Gerbode defect or aortic valve prolapse in cases of subpulmonary VSD (▶ Fig. 4.13). Precise, noninvasive quantification of shunt volume by determining the Q_p:Q_s ratio remains within the domain of MRI flow measurement (▶ Fig. 4.8)[7,8] in cases of both ASD and VSD, provided no other valve defects are present. Shunt volume can also be estimated by comparing right and left ventricular SV as determined using volumetric analysis. This is, however, generally less precise than MR flow measurement. Estimating shunt volume by comparing right and left ventricular SV is also possible using retrospective ECG-triggered MDCT, but is only reasonable if the examination is necessary because of another indication (e.g., to assess the coronary arteries noninvasively) due to the high radiation exposure.[7]

Postoperative and Postinterventional Issues

Repeated imaging is only reasonable within the scope of concurrent defects or if a residual shunt is suspected (e.g., for quantification via MRI flow measurement). Residual defects can often be characterized in older children and adults using TEE, excellent results.

Goals and Relative Value of Diagnostic Imaging

Like in ASD patients, TTE is generally sufficient for assessing VSDs in preoperative diagnostics during childhood,[7] and can be supplemented by TEE. In cases of an inadequate acoustic window—particularly in adults—MRI visualization, MRI shunt quantification, and MRI ventricular volumetry are valuable diagnostic alternatives for cases of VSD, both for primary diagnosis and for follow-up exams.

4.1.3 Atrioventricular Septal Defect

Florentine Gräfe, Ingo Dähnert, Philipp Lurz

Definition

The term "atrioventricular septal defect" (formerly known as "endocardial cushion defect") encompasses congenital cardiac defects of the structures derived from the embryonic endocardial cushion, meaning from the atrioventricular septum and parts of the mitral and tricuspid valves. They constitute approximately 2–4% of all congenital heart defects.[12] Characteristics of these defects include a joint atrioventricular valve annulus (▶ Fig. 4.15) with either a single joint opening or two separate openings, a VSD of variable size, and an ASD I.[13]

In the most severe anomalies within this group, the primum septum and inlet ventricular septum are completely absent. This means that all chambers of the heart are connected, which was previously known as "total atrioventricular canal" (▶ Fig. 4.15).

Note

Trisomy 21 is present in 50% of patients with complete AVSD.

Classification

Signs of all AVSDs:

- Lack of membranous atrioventricular septum
- Joint atrioventricular valve annulus with joint or two separate openings
- Reduced distance between the atrioventricular valve and cardiac apex
- Superior displacement and lengthening of the LVOT

This is also known as a "goose-neck deformity" of the LVOT. In these cases, there is no fibrous aorto-mitral continuity. This stenosis or deformation of the LVOT is most pronounced during diastole, caused by the lack of atrioventricular border normally provided by the membranous septum.[14]

The following, most common types will be discussed in detail:

- *Complete AVSD* (most common type): A 4-leaflet or 5-leaflet atrioventricular valve (ostium commune) is present (with superior and inferior bridging leaflet), which extends to both ventricles via the septal defect (▶ Fig. 4.15). The division of the joined atrioventricular valve via both ventricles can be either balanced (▶ Fig. 4.16a, b and, c) or unbalanced (▶ Fig. 4.16a, b). This generally leads to hypoplasia in the contralateral ventricle.[15] The superior bridging leaflet may divide near the septum, resulting in a 5-leaflet joint atrioventricular valve. According to Rastelli, balanced, complete AVSD is further subclassified based on the degree of bridging of the anterior or superior bridging leaflet:
    - Type A (70% of cases) with further subdivision of the anterior leaflet into a superior bridging leaflet and a well-developed (right) anterior–superior leaflet; the left tendinous cords insert into the superior margin of the ventricular septum;

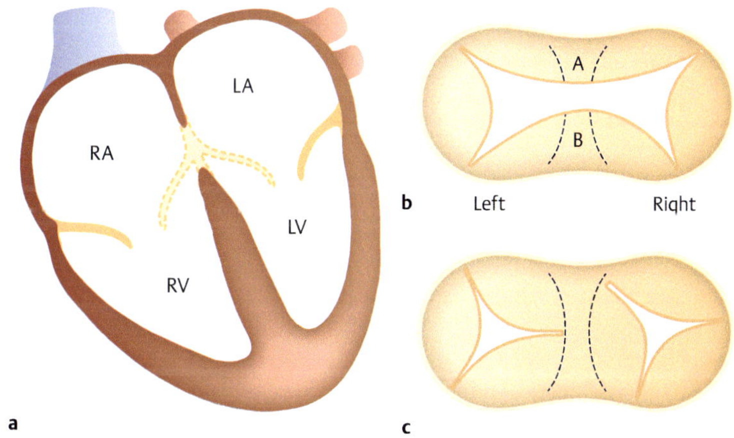

Fig. 4.15 Various forms of AVSD. Schematic depiction.
LA = left atrium
LV = left ventricle
RA = right atrium
RV = right ventricle

a The dotted line in the schematic 4-chamber view shows the absent atrioventricular septal and valve portions in a case of complete AVSD.

b Top view of a complete AVSD with joint 4-leaflet atrioventricular valve (ostium commune) without distinction between the superior and anterior bridging leaflet (A); B depicts the corresponding posterior and inferior bridging leaflet.

c Divided atrioventricular valve in a case of incomplete or partial AVSD. Two functionally separate atrioventricular valves are present, each communicating with one ventricle.

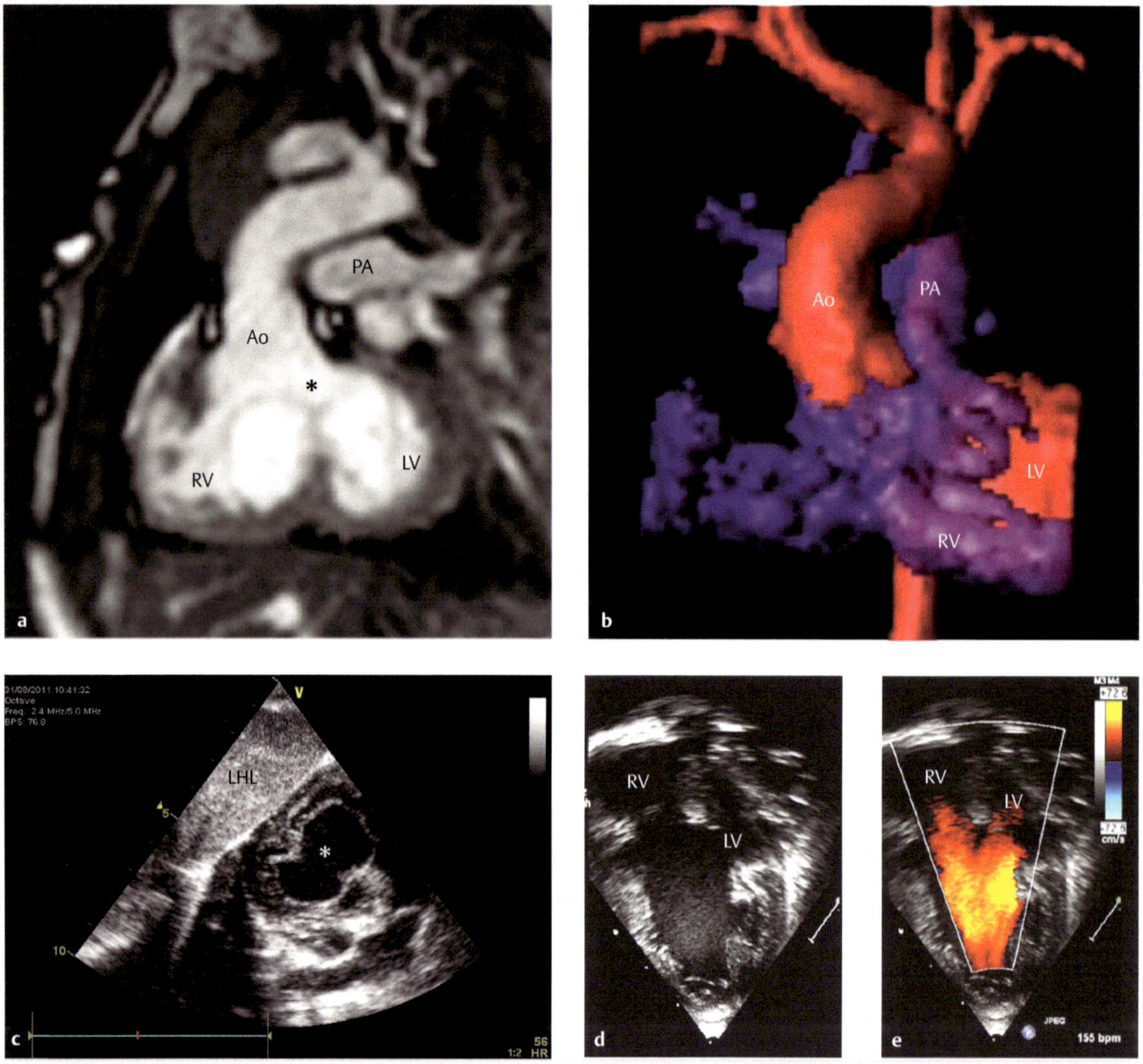

Fig. 4.16 DORV with concurrent AVSD. Various patients.
Ao = Aorta
LHL = left hepatic lobe
LV = left ventricle
PA = pulmonary artery
RV = right ventricle

a End diastolic cine MRI of an SSFP sequence near the joint atrioventricular valve, short axis. Top view of the opened valve. The joint anterior bridging leaflet (asterisk) can be easily distinguished.

b 3-D volume rendering reconstruction of an MRA in a DORV patient.

c Complete AVSD: Subcostal, short-axis slice of a TTE for a different patient, with depiction of the opened, butterfly-shaped joint atrioventricular valve (asterisk) in a case of complete atrioventricular canal.

d Unbalanced distribution of the joint atrioventricular valve in a case of complete AVSD and HLHS during ventricular filling in diastole, 2-D echo, and color Doppler TTE, apical 4-chamber view.

e Color Doppler TTE corresponding to **d**.

- Type B (15% of cases) with further subdivision of the anterior leaflet into a superior bridging leaflet extending far to the right, and a small anterior–superior leaflet; the left tendinous cords insert into the right papillary muscle;
- Type C (15% of cases) with no subdivision of the anterior leaflet; the bridging leaflet is large and extends to the right mural leaflet, while the anterior–superior leaflet is absent, resulting in complete bridging (► Fig. 4.15b).

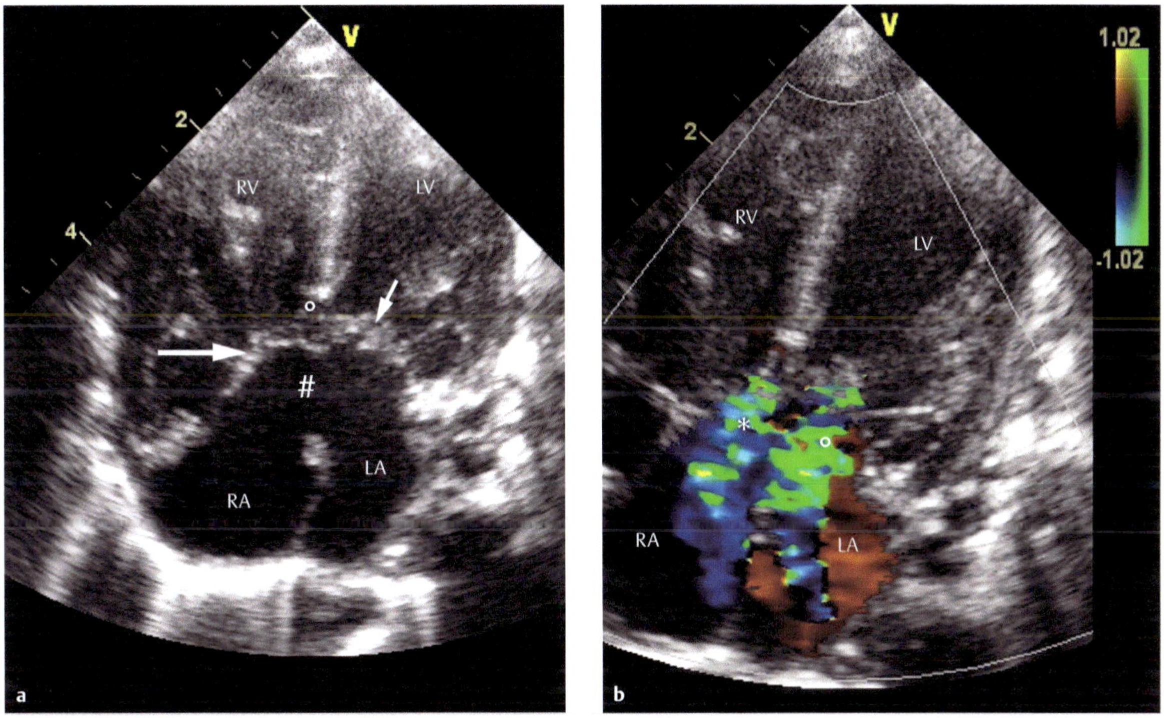

Fig. 4.17 Complete AVSD.
LA = left atrium
LV = left ventricle
RA = right atrium
RV = right ventricle

a Apical 4-chamber view in TTE. The large arrow indicates the joint atrioventricular valve, while the small circle indicates the VSD components (inlet area), the hatch mark is the ASD-I component (lack of septum primum), and the small arrow is the cleft in the anterior mitral leaflet.

b Apical 4-chamber view with color Doppler. Relevant insufficiency of the right (asterisk) and left segment (small circle) of the joint atrioventricular valve visible in color Doppler.

- *Partial AVSD* (second most-common type): ASD I with "cleft formation" in the anterior "mitral leaflet" is present near the atrioventricular valve (known as mitral cleft; ▶ Fig. 4.17).
- *Intermediate AVSD* (also known as transitional AVSD): The complete atrioventricular canal demonstrates restrictive or functionally closed VSD components caused by portions of the joined atrioventricular valve.[13]
- *AVSD:* This is a rare, special form of a muscular inlet VSD situated directly inferior to the atrioventricular valves.
- *Isolated mitral valve cleft:* This rare form can be considered the least severe form of AVSD with an intact septum.

Hemodynamics

The hemodynamics of complete AVSD are characterized by a generally large left–right shunt with pulmonary "recirculation." The shunt volume at the level of the ventricle thus depends primarily on pulmonary vascular resistance. The VSD is generally large and non-restrictive. Thus, few symptoms are usually present in newborns. With the drop in pulmonary vascular resistance at the age of 6–8 weeks, the left–right shunt increases at the level of the ventricle, which generally leads to early development of global congestive heart failure with pulmonary overflow and left ventricular volume overload (▶ Fig. 4.18). If untreated, AVSD can develop into a correspondingly early fixed pulmonary hypertension and triggering of Eisenmenger reaction.

The hemodynamic situation of a partial AVSD is similar to that of an ASD with volume overload occurring in the right ventricle and pulmonary arteries. Furthermore the extent of mitral valve regurgitation determines the hemodynamics. (▶ Fig. 4.19 and ▶ Table 4.5).

Clinical Issues

In cases of complete AVSD and large left–right shunt, global heart failure generally occurs within a few weeks (▶ Fig. 4.18). Within the first year of life, irreversible remodeling of the pulmonary vasculature due to the pulmonary overflow develops. Symptoms are generally less pronounced in cases of partial AVSD, and manifest heart failure rarely develops within the first year of life.

Natural Progression and Indication for Treatment

All AVSDs constitute an indication for surgery, regardless of the type of AVSD.[13]

Note

M!

For balanced forms, one should always attempt to enable complete biventricular correction by means of valve reconstruction.

For premature babies, very small children, or patients with concurrent illnesses, pulmonary banding can be performed as a palliative method before surgical correction. The development of a left atrioventricular valve insufficiency with enlargement of the cleft is unfavorable for reconstruction. Thus, the presence of left valve insufficiency (▶ Fig. 4.20) constitutes an indication for surgery, regardless of symptoms. In cases of unbalanced AVSDs, univentricular palliation must be performed.

Table 4.5 Volume load of individual cardiac compartments in a case of complete AVSD.

Cardiovascular compartment	Volume load
Right atrium	++
Right ventricle	++
Pulmonary arteries	++
Pulmonary veins	++
Left atrium	++
Left ventricle	++
Aorta and conduit arteries	-
Systemic veins	-

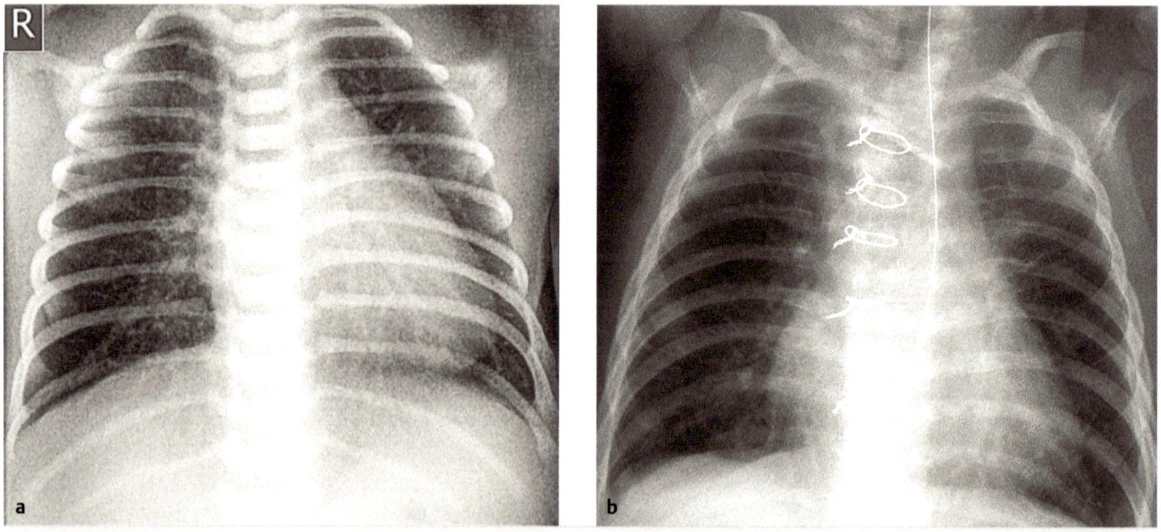

Fig. 4.18 Complete AVSD.
LA = left atrium
LV = left ventricle
RA = right atrium
RV = right ventricle

a Preoperative a.-p. thoracic X-ray of a newborn with complete AVSD, right aortic arch, persistent left superior vena cava, significantly increased pulmonary perfusion, and global cardiac enlargement.
b Suspended a.-p. thoracic X-ray of the same newborn, 3 months after surgery.

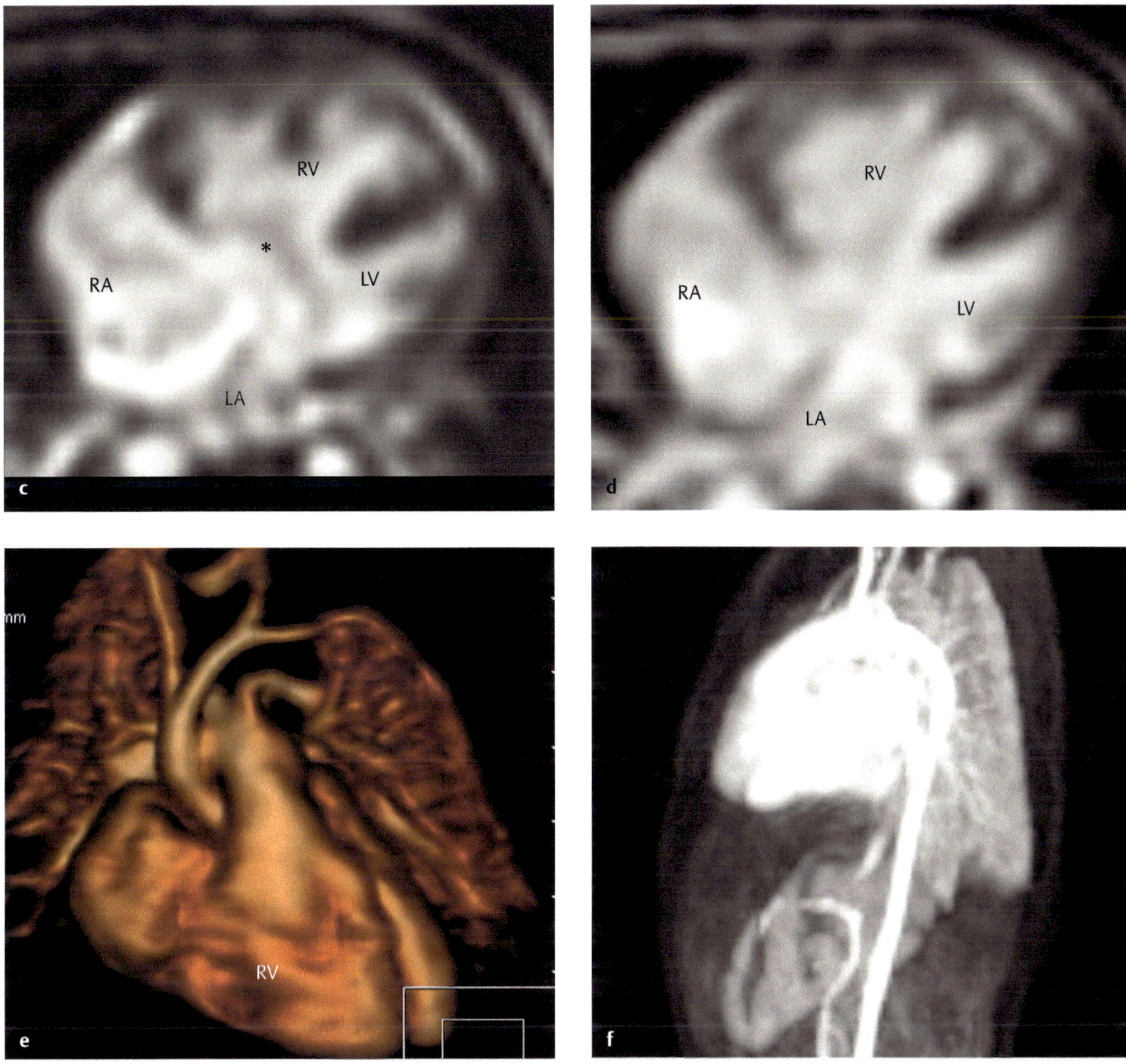

Fig. 4.18 (*Continued*) **Complete AVSD.**
LA = left atrium
LV = left ventricle
RA = right atrium
RV = right ventricle

c Preoperative cine MRI during systole with closed atrioventricular valve (asterisk) in the same newborn.
d Preoperative cine MRI during diastole with opened atrioventricular valve.
e 3-D reconstruction of the contrast-enhanced MRA of the aorta and pulmonary artery.
f 2-D reconstruction of the contrast-enhanced MRA of the aorta and pulmonary artery.

Preoperative Diagnostics

Particularly in cases of complete AVSD, thoracic X-ray (▶ Fig. 4.18) indicate significant cardiac enlargement with a prominent pulmonary segment and increased pulmonary vascular markings. These changes are, however, nonspecific. TTE is the initial method of choice, since it allows the atrioventricular valves and bridging leaflet to be depicted via the septal defect. The goose-neck deformity can be visualized in an LVOT cross-section. TEE is the predominant method used for larger children and adults. Cardiac MRI can be used in cases of a limited acoustic window (▶ Fig. 4.16 and ▶ Fig. 4.18), which also allows shunt volume to be calculated by determining the Q_p:Q_s ratio. CT plays no role in preinterventional diagnostics. Invasive levocardiography and dextrocardiography also allow pulmonary pressure to be measured, in addition to providing anatomical depictions. They have, however, been largely replaced by echocardiography and MRI in routine preoperative diagnostics, and are performed primarily for late-diagnosed AVSD in order to evaluate pulmonary vascular responsiveness (or after pulmonary banding was performed at a later date, on a case-by-case basis).

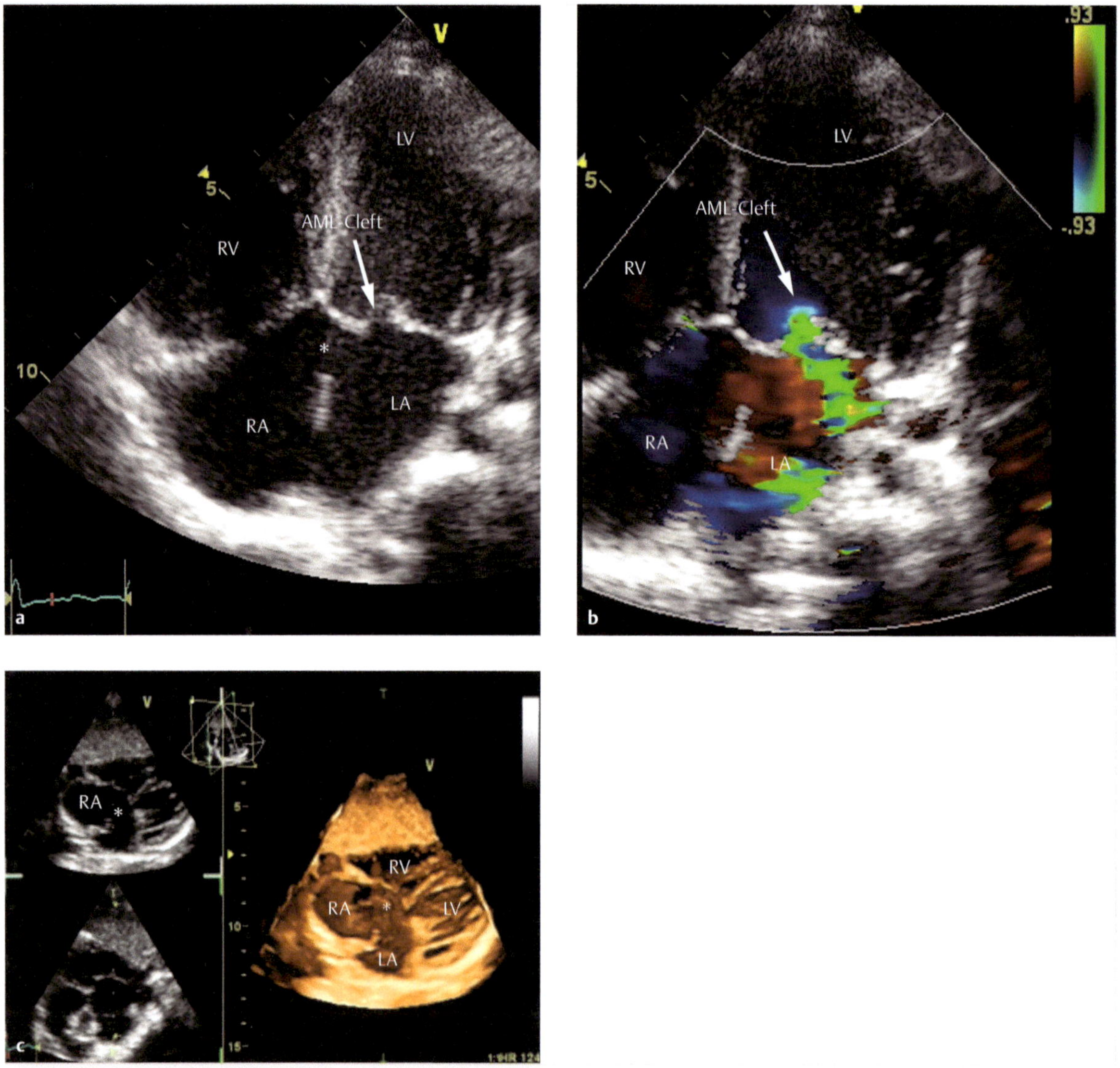

Fig. 4.19 Partial atrioventricular septal defect (ASD I) with absent septum primum and cleft in the anterior mitral leaflet. The asterisk indicates the absent septum primum, and the arrow indicates the cleft in the anterior mitral leaflet.

LA = left atrium
LV = left ventricle
RA = right atrium
RV = right ventricle

a TTE, apical 4-chamber view.
b Apical 4-chamber view with color Doppler: Mitral valve insufficiency is caused by the cleft in the anterior mitral leaflet.
c Real-time 3-D echocardiography of a partial atrioventricular septal defect (ASD I). The lack of septum primum is clearly visible (asterisk).

Postoperative Issues

The main perioperative and postoperative issues are generally transitory pulmonary vessel reactivity or hypertension, incomplete closure of the defect, atrioventricular blocking, and residual atrioventricular valve insufficiency. If the valves cannot be adequately reconstructed, the atrioventricular valve must be replaced.

Goals and Relative Value of Diagnostic Imaging

As mentioned previously, TTE is sufficient for preoperative diagnostics during childhood (▶ Table 4.6).[7] TEE is ideal after surgery and for adults. MRI can be useful in cases of limited acoustic window, either for visualizing concurrent defects or for quantifying shunt volume (▶ Table 4.7).

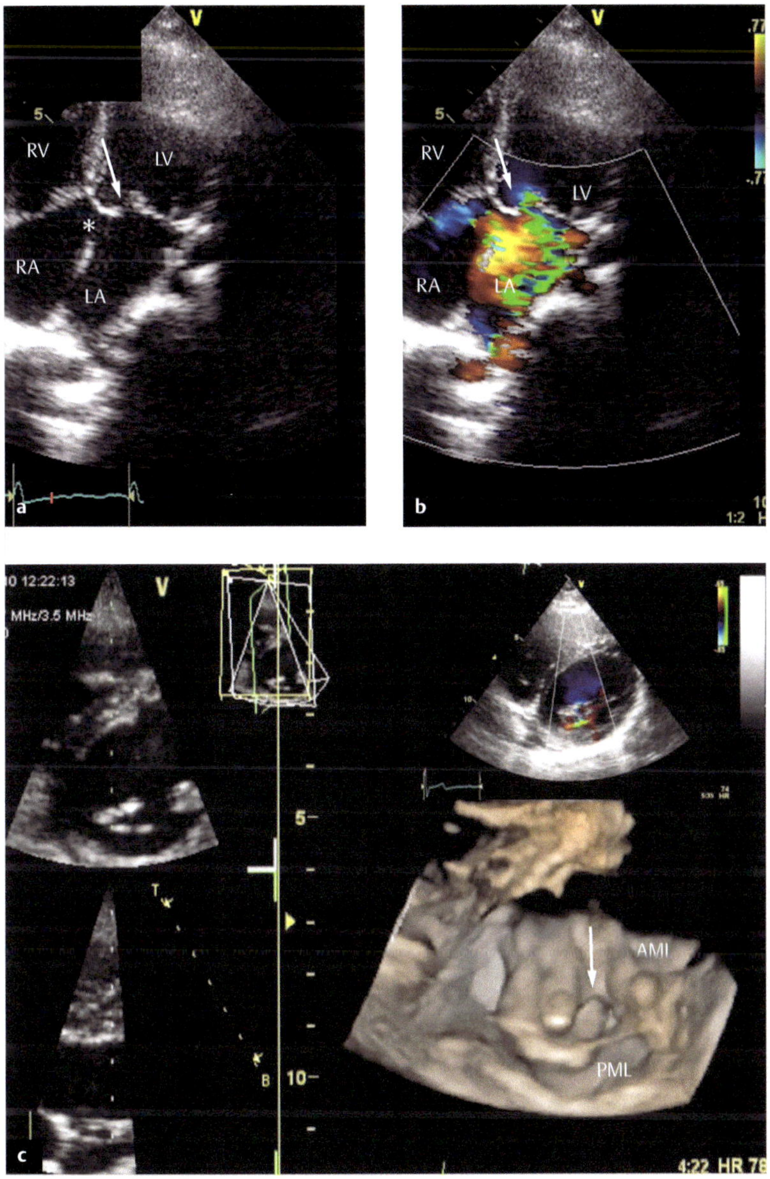

Fig. 4.20 Partial atrioventricular septal defect (ASD I) with absent septum primum and mitral valve insufficiency caused by a cleft in the anterior mitral leaflet. The asterisk indicates the location of the absent septum primum, and the arrow indicates the cleft in the anterior mitral leaflet.

AML = anterior mitral leaflet
LA = left atrium
LV = left ventricle
PML = posterior mitral leaflet
RA = right atrium
RV = right ventricle

- **a** 2-D TTE, apical 4-chamber view, without color Doppler.
- **b** 2-D TTE, apical 4-chamber view, with color Doppler.
- **c** Real-time 3-D echocardiography of the mitral valve with a cleft in the anterior mitral leaflet.

Table 4.6 Preoperative imaging diagnostics for AVSD.

Imaging methods	Focus	Value
2-D, 3-D TTE	• Defect size and margins • Anatomy and function of the atrioventricular valve • Ventricular balance • Ventricular function • Evaluating LVOT • Left–right shunt, qualitative • Right heart dilatation • Ruling out additional shunts (ASD II, additional VSD, PDA) • Ruling out pulmonary and systemic venous anomalies • Ruling out associated defects (e.g., aortic coarctation, tetralogy of Fallot, etc.)	+++
2-D, 3-D TEE	see TTE (can only be used in limited circumstances, since most patients are younger than 1 year)	+
Cardiac MRI	• Quantifying the left–right shunt • Quantifying ventricular dilation and function • Measuring the defect (phase contrast method) • Anatomy of pulmonary and systemic veins	++ (Backup method)
MDCT	Backup method in cases of unclear echocardiographical findings and contraindication against cardiac MRI; may be helpful in cases of pulmonary parenchymatic comorbidity or to prove the existence of concurrent vascular defects, such as anomalous pulmonary venous connections	++

ASD, atrial septal defect; AVSD, atrioventricular septal defect; LVOT, left ventricular outflow tract; MDCT, multidetector computed tomography; MRI, magnetic resonance imaging; PDA, patent ductus arteriosus; TEE, transesophageal echocardiography; TTE, transthoracic echocardiography; VSD, ventricular septal defect.

Table 4.7 Postoperative imaging diagnostics in a case of AVSD.

Imaging methods	Value
TTE	+++
TEE	++
Cardiac MRI	+++
MDCT	+
Invasive cardiac catheter diagnostics	+

MDCT, multidetector computed tomography; MRI, magnetic resonance imaging; TEE, transesophageal echocardiography; TTE, transthoracic echocardiography.

4.1.4 Patent Ductus Arteriosus

Philipp Beerbaum, Joachim Lotz, Michael Steinmetz

Definition

PDA (also known as patent ductus arteriosus) is the persistence of the fetal connection between the intrapericardial portion of the main pulmonary artery or proximal left pulmonary artery and the extrapericardial descending aorta immediately after the outlet of the left subclavian artery.[12] PDA is a common congenital heart defect, generally concurrent with other congenital defects in 5–10% of patients, though is more frequent in girls than in boys. From an embryological perspective, it develops from the distal portion of the left sixth aortic arch (▶ Fig. 4.21c; right aortic arch: ▶ Fig. 4.21a).[13] Approximately 60% of cardiac output flows through this arch. This duct normally closes within 72 hours after birth.

Classification

A clinical distinction is made between the following four forms of PDA[13]:

- Incidental finding in cases of complex defects (common)
- Isolated form in premature babies (common; ▶ Fig. 4.22)

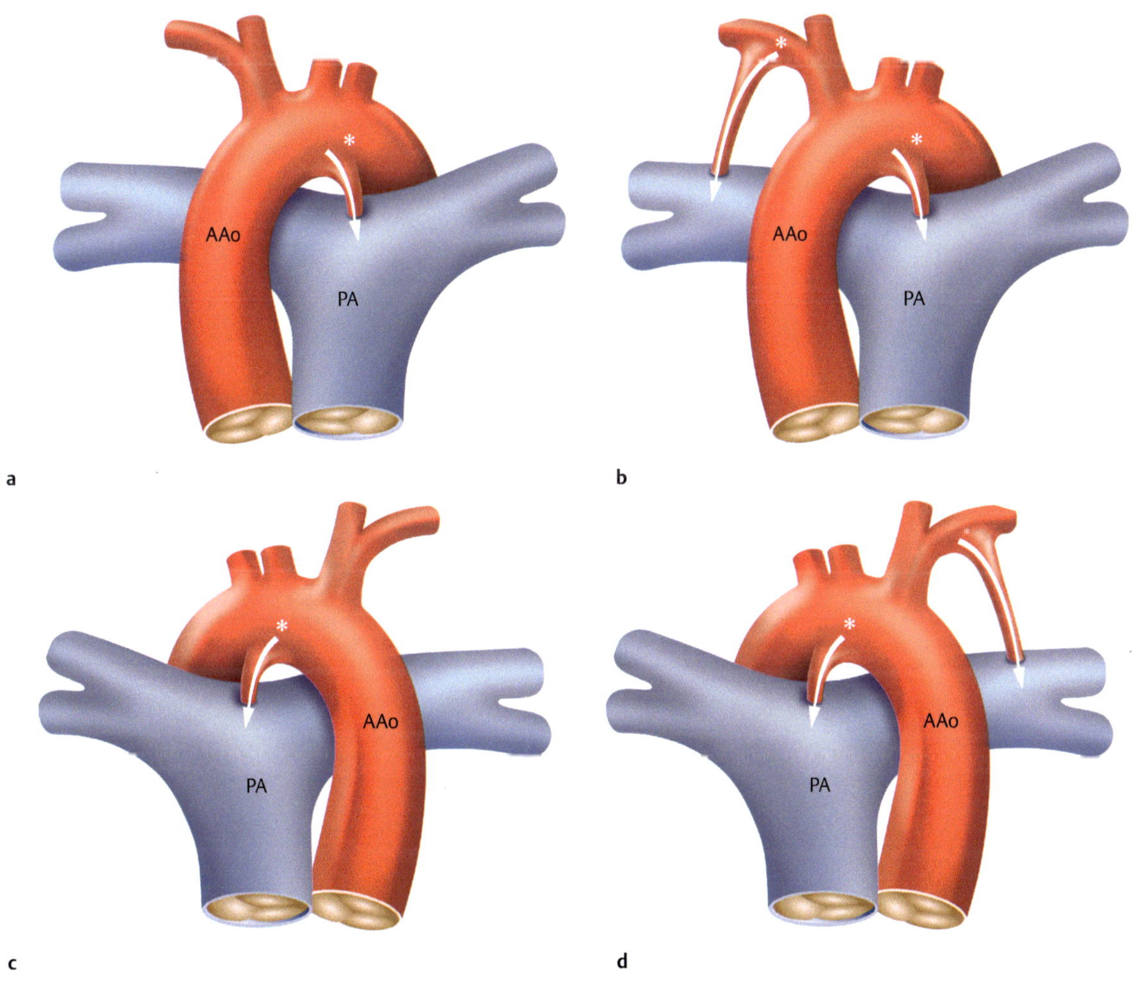

Fig. 4.21 Various forms of PDA. Schematic depiction. The asterisks indicate the PDA, and the arrows indicate the direction of blood flow. The course of the PDA is generally conical in the direction of the pulmonary artery.

AAo = ascending aorta
PA = pulmonary artery

a Left aortic arch.
b Left aortic arch, bilateral PDA (rare form).
c Right aortic arch.
d Right aortic arch, bilateral PDA (rare form).

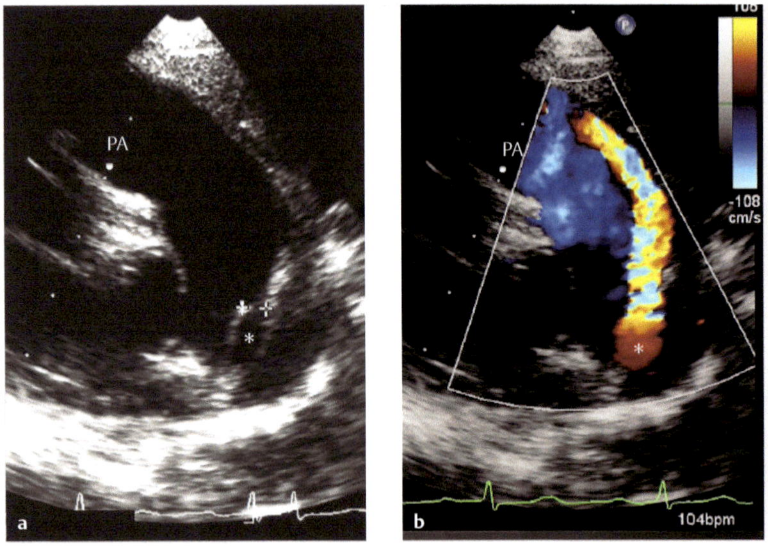

Fig. 4.22 PDA.
PA = pulmonary artery
a 2-D TTE depiction of a PDA (asterisk), short parasternal axis, near the pulmonary artery.
b The left–right shunt with flow acceleration can be depicted clearly using color doppler echocardiography.

- "Compensating" PDA in cases of ductal-dependent heart defects, such as HLHS (ductal-dependent systemic perfusion) or hypoplastic right heart syndrome (ductal-dependent pulmonary perfusion, e.g., in cases of pulmonary atresia)
- Isolated form in otherwise healthy children (rarer)

In very rare cases, a duct aneurysm can occur in a duct with isolated pulmonary (but not aortic) closure (▶ Fig. 4.23).

From pathological and anatomical perspectives, different variants are possible, including those dependent on the presence of a left or right aortic arch.[14] Bilateral PDA can also occur (▶ Fig. 4.21b and d), though only in extremely rare cases.

Hemodynamics

An isolated PDA causes a left–right shunt. In these cases, the shunt's size depends on the diameter of the PDA and the difference between systemic and pulmonary arteriolar resistance. If the PDA diameter is large enough, the left–right shunt generally increases in size during the first months of life.[13] In cases of a particularly large PDA with pressure equalization, if no closure between the aorta and pulmonary artery occurs within the first 6–12 months of life, there is a risk of progressive, often irreversible disorders of the pulmonary resistance vessels accompanied by increased pulmonary vessel resistance. This can lead to shunt reversal (also known as Eisenmenger syndrome). ▶ Table 4.8 depicts volume load.

Clinical Issues

Clinical signs of cardiac failure include a tendency toward infections, sweating, difficulty drinking, and growth disorders, and occur in early infancy solely in cases of extremely large PDA. Generally speaking, the concurrent illnesses remain predominant.

Table 4.8 Volume load of individual cardiac compartments in a case of PDA.

Cardiovascular compartment	Volume load
Right atrium	-
Right ventricle	-
Pulmonary arteries	++
Pulmonary veins	++
Left atrium	++
Left ventricle	++
Aorta (proximal to the PDA)	++
Systemic veins	-

Natural Progression and Indication for Treatment

If untreated, isolated PDA is associated with a 30% mortality rate.

> **Note**
>
> Spontaneous closure after the first weeks of life is extremely rare in mature newborns. Consequently, it is crucial to strive for interventional closure within the first months of life, even in asymptomatic patients.

Treatment must occur as soon as possible for symptomatic newborns. Since indomethacin is no longer effective for mature newborns, it cannot be used in treatment. Rather, a surgery or intervention is needed. Interventional closure using coils, spirals, or a shield system has become the treatment method of choice (▶ Fig. 4.24 and ▶ Fig. 4.25). Only very large PDAs or duct aneurysms generally require surgical closure (▶ Fig. 4.23).

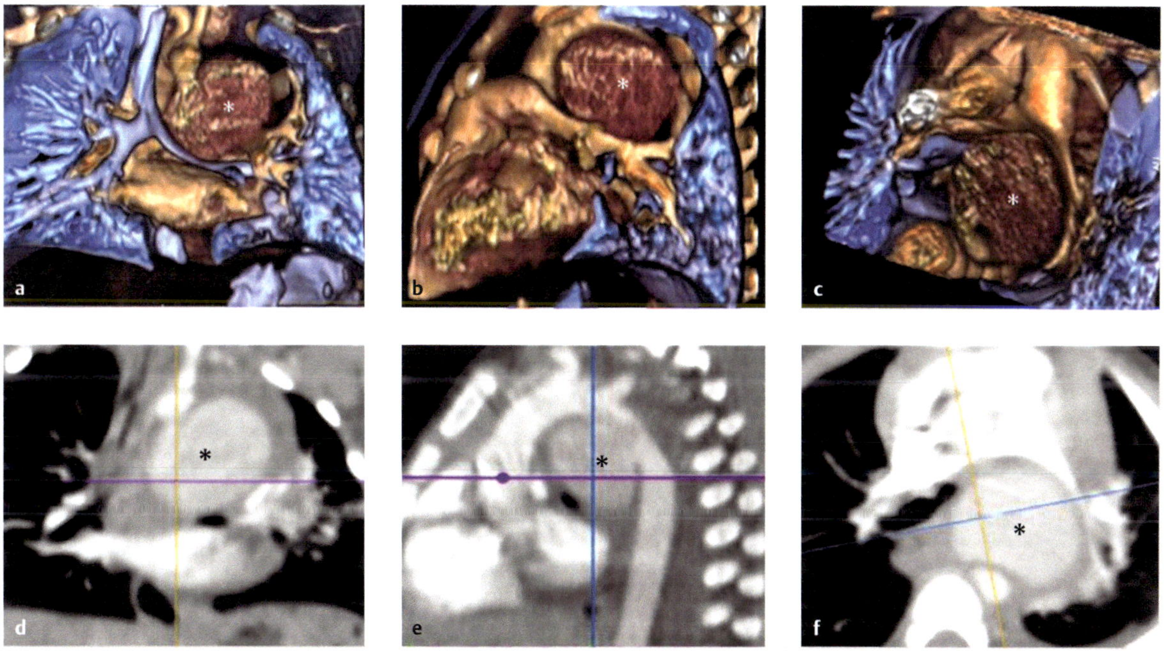

Fig. 4.23 Duct aneurysm. Two-month-old infant with acute respiratory decompensation within the scope of a pulmonary infection. Echocardiography findings raised suspicions of a duct aneurysm. A multi-row CT provided a complete anatomical depiction. The 3-D reconstructions showed a deviation of the trachea to the right and an obstruction in the left main bronchus (blue: air-filled space, reddish: blood-filled or contrast agent-filled vessels; the asterisk indicates the aneurysm). The left pulmonary artery, like the left main bronchus, is also compressed.

a Coronal 3-D reconstruction.
b Sagittal 3-D reconstruction.
c Transverse 3-D reconstruction.
d Coronal multiplanar 2-D reformat of the data set.
e Sagittal multiplanar 2-D reformat of the data set.
f Transverse multiplanar 2-D reformat of the data set.

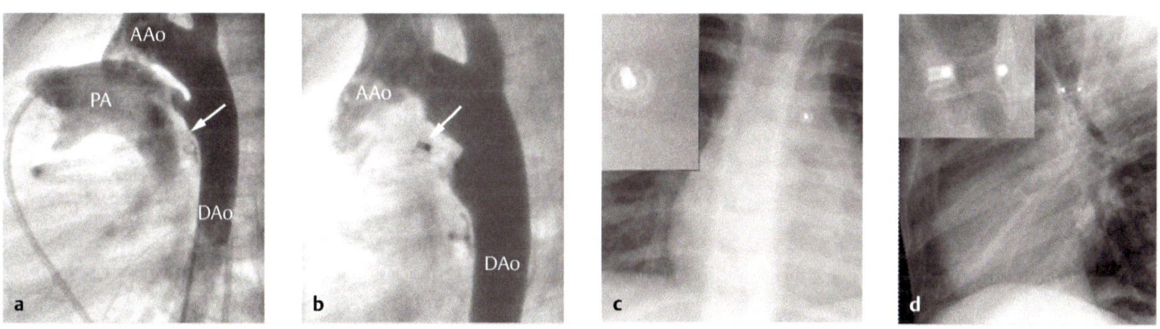

Fig. 4.24 PDA before and after closure with an Amplatzer™ duct occluder. 3.5-year-old girl.
AAo = ascending aorta
DAo = descending aorta
PA = pulmonary artery

a Angiogram of a large PDA running conically toward the pulmonary artery (arrow) before intervention.
b Angiogram after PDA closure using an Amplatzer™ duct occluder (arrow).
c P.-a. X-ray after closure of the PDA, occlusion device enlarged (insert).
d Lateral X-ray after closure of the PDA, occlusion device enlarged (insert).

Preinterventional Diagnostics

Generally speaking, PDA can be visualized clearly using Doppler echocardiography along a high (second-left intercostal area) parasternal short axis. This generally depicts three vessels in proximity to the main pulmonary artery branch: the PDA, and the left and right pulmonary arteries (▶ Fig. 4.22). Contrast-enhanced MRA also yields clear images (▶ Fig. 4.26a). In cases of a small PDA, a cine

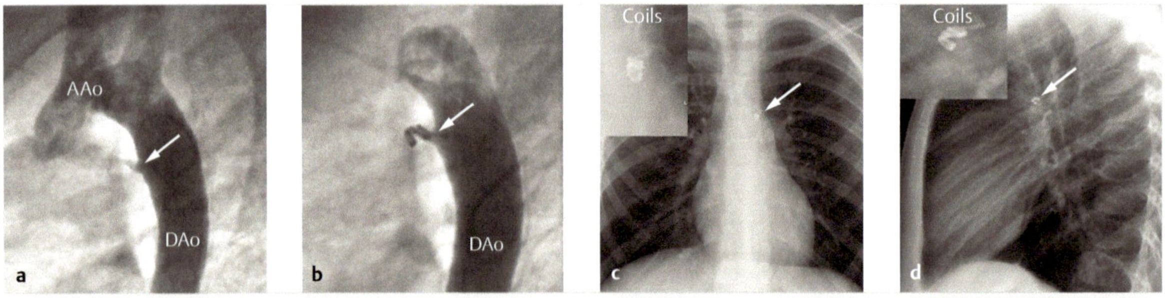

Fig. 4.25 PDA before and after closure with coils. Seven-year-old girl.
AAo = ascending aorta
DAo = descending aorta
a Angiogram of the small PDA (arrow) before intervention.
b Angiogram after closure with coils (arrow).
c P.-a. X-ray after PDA closure, coils enlarged (arrow and inset).
d Lateral X-ray after PDA closure, coils enlarged (arrow and inset).

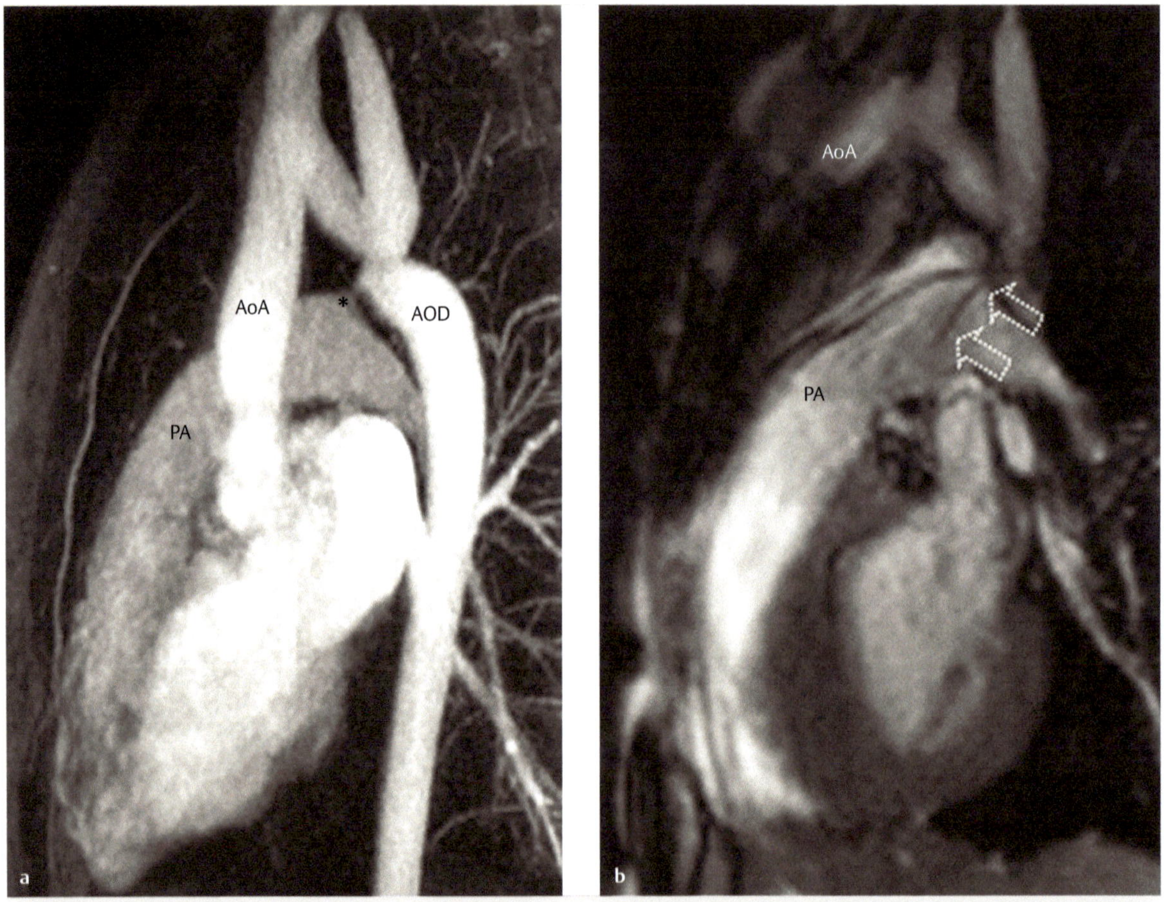

Fig. 4.26 Secondary PDA. Contrast-enhanced MRA with ancillary finding of a small PDA (**a**, asterisk) in a 12-year-old boy who had received an MRI to depict the aortic arch based on suspicion of an aortic coarctation. Two shunts were identified: a small, silent PDA which was also detected during the cine MRI due to dephasing caused by flow acceleration (**b**, arrows), and a small, perimembranous VSD (▶ Fig. 4.11).
a Contrast-enhanced MRA.
b Cine MRI using SSFP sequences, angled parasagittal section.

MRI through the pulmonary artery and aorta (▶ Fig. 4.26b), which allows the PDA to be detected due to MR dephasing caused by flow acceleration of the PDA via the left–right shunt, can also be helpful. MR flow measurement can be used for noninvasive shunt quantification in the ascending aorta, pulmonary artery, or distal to the PDA in the right and left pulmonary arteries. MDCT, likewise, can be used as a backup method (▶ Fig. 4.23).

Postoperative and Postinterventional Issues

A residual shunt can occur after surgical or interventional closure. Generally speaking, this can be evaluated via echocardiography. MRI using phase contrast technology is an alternative for quantifying any potential residual shunt.

Goals and Relative Value of Diagnostic Imaging

TTE is generally sufficient during childhood (▶ Table 4.9 and ▶ Table 4.10).[7]

Table 4.9 Preinterventional imaging diagnostics in a case of PDA.

Imaging methods	Focus	Value
2-D TTE	• Size and shape • Left–right shunt, qualitative • Dilatation of the aorta and pulmonary arteries • Ruling out concurrent defects	+ + +
2-D TEE	see TTE	+ +
Cardiac MRI	• Quantifying the left–right shunt • Quantifying ventricular dilatation and function • Measuring the defect (phase contrast method) • Anatomy of the aorta and pulmonary arteries	+ + (Backup method)
MDCT	Backup method in cases of unclear echocardiographical findings, where cardiac MRI is contraindicated	+
Invasive (diagnostic) cardiac catheter tests	• Measuring pressure and resistance (if indicated), pharmacological testing • In rare cases: invasive measurement of diastolic left ventricular functional parameters (e.g., left ventricular end diastolic pressure) in cases of suspected elevated risk of pulmonary edema after ASD closure • Ruling out pulmonary and systemic venous anomalies	+ + + (in cases of pulmonary hypertonia and suspected left ventricular restriction)

ASD, atrial septal defect; MDCT, multidetector computed tomography; MRI, magnetic resonance imaging; TEE, transesophageal echocardiography; TTE, transthoracic echocardiography.

Table 4.10 Postinterventional imaging diagnostics in a case of PDA.

Imaging methods	Value
TTE	+ + +
TEE	+ +
Cardiac MRI	+ +
MDCT	(+)
Invasive cardiac catheter diagnostics	+ + +

MDCT, multidetector computed tomography; MRI, magnetic resonance imaging; TEE, transesophageal echocardiography; TTE, transthoracic echocardiography.

4.1.5 Aortopulmonary Window (Aortopulmonary Septal Defect)

Florentine Gräfe, Ingo Dähnert, Philipp Lurz

Definition

APSD—also known as "aortopulmonary window," "aortopulmonary septal defect," and "aortopulmonary fistula"—is a very rare defect caused by an embryonic defect in the aortopulmonary septum. It can occur in isolation or concurrent with other congenital heart defects, such as coronary anomalies (in 50–66% of cases). This defect causes a connection of varying size between the ascending aorta and pulmonary artery (▶ Fig. 4.27). In these cases, two separate valve rings for the aortic and pulmonary valve are always present.

Classification

A rough distinction can be made between the proximal and distal types[13]:

- *Proximal defect* (62% of APSDs; ▶ Fig. 4.28, ▶ Fig. 4.29, and ▶ Fig. 4.30; also ▶ Fig. 4.27a): The APSD is located on the dorsal-lateral or posterior wall of the ascending aorta or the anterior-lateral wall of the pulmonary artery, meaning that the defect is directly cranial to the aortic and pulmonary valves.
- *Distal defect* (38% of APSDs; ▶ Fig. 4.31; also ▶ Fig. 4.27b): The APSD is located near the anterior wall of the right pulmonary artery. Very large defects may appear to be right pulmonary arterial outlets from the ascending aorta (hemitruncus). Unlike hemitruncus, however, a connection remains between the right pulmonary artery and the pulmonary arterial bifurcation.

Hemodynamics

Generally speaking, the APSD is large, meaning that it does not lead to pressure separation (restriction). In this respect, the APSD bears a pathophysiological resemblance to a large, window-like PDA. Nevertheless, it generally leads to earlier occurrence of heart failure (▶ Fig. 4.32), similar to cases of small children with large VSDs. If untreated, large APSDs can lead to fixed pulmonary hypertension and the Eisenmenger reaction. Volume load in cases of APSD is listed in ▶ Table 4.11.

Clinical Issues

Within the scope of pronounced left–right shunt with pulmonary overflowing, children generally exhibit a failure to thrive, recurrent pulmonary infections, and the clinical picture of heart failure (▶ Fig. 4.32).

Natural Progression and Indication for Treatment

Due to the poor prognosis for untreated defects (with the exception of small shunts), diagnosis is generally a sufficient indication for surgery.[13] A contraindication for surgical treatment only exists in cases where the Eisenmenger reaction has already occurred. For smaller defects, surgeons can also strive for interventional closure.

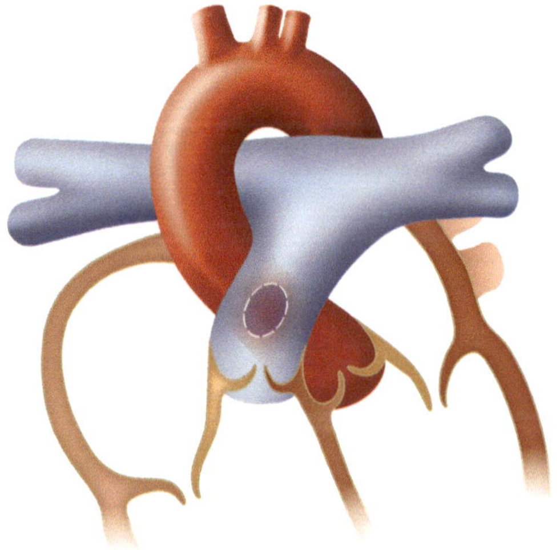

a

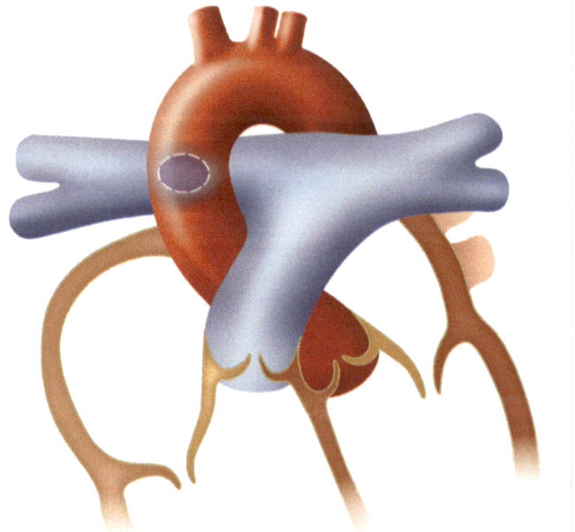

b

Fig. 4.27 Main types of APSD. Schematic depiction.
a Proximal (more common).
b Distal (less common) between the ascending aorta and right pulmonary artery.

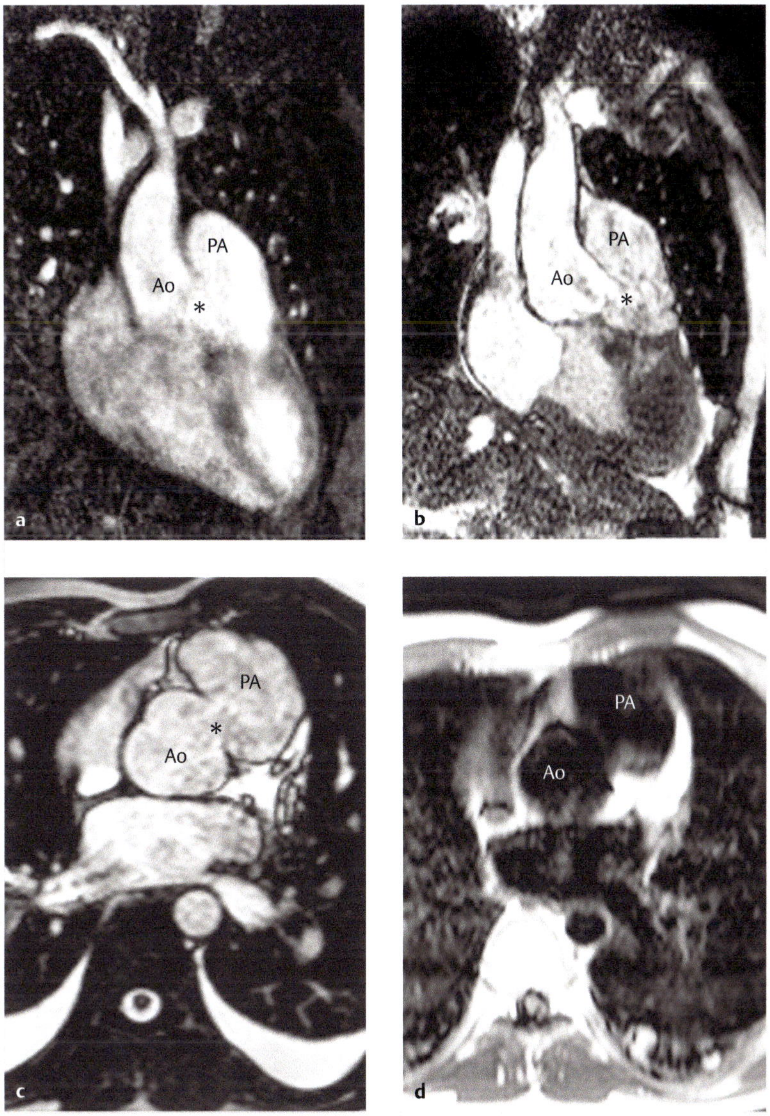

Fig. 4.28 Proximal APSD (asterisk). Twenty-three-year-old man.
Ao = aorta
PA = pulmonary artery

a MIP reconstruction of a contrast-enhanced MRA.
b Cine MRI with SSFP sequences, coronal orientation.
c Cine MRI with SSFP sequences, transverse orientation.
d ECG-triggered transverse black blood SE sequence.

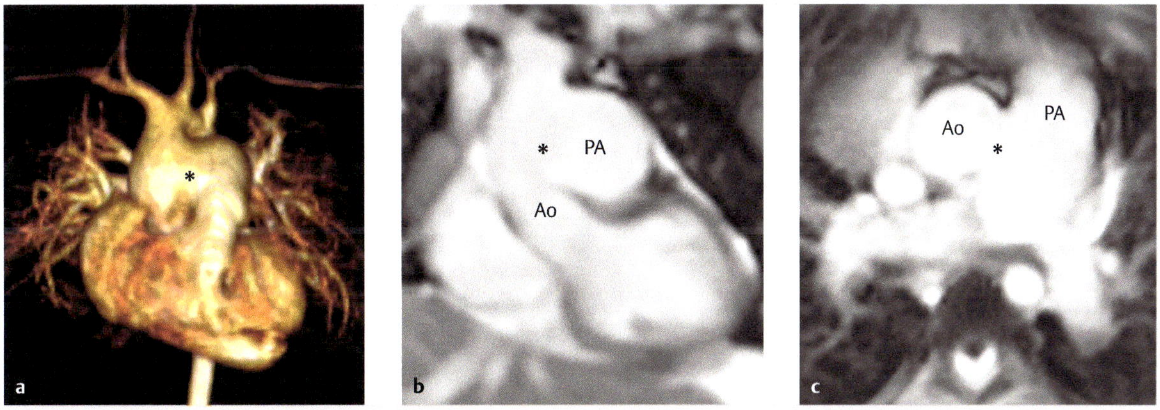

Fig. 4.29 Proximal APSD. Patient with large APSD (asterisk), pulmonary hypertonia, and bidirectional shunt.
Ao = aorta; PA = pulmonary artery

a MRI with 3-D reconstruction of a contrast-enhanced MRA.
b SSFP sequences, coronal slice near the APSD, depicting the very large defect.
c Corresponding axial slice.

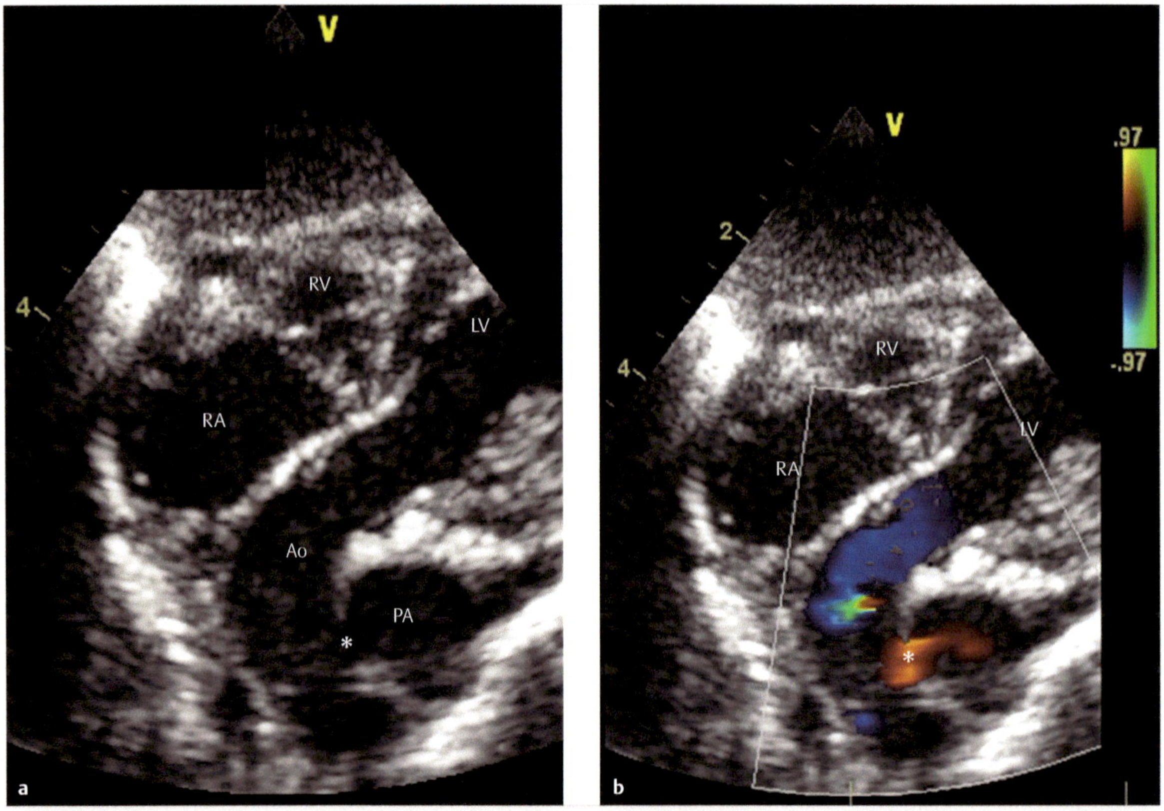

Fig. 4.30 Proximal APSD. Each asterisk indicates an APSD.
Ao = aorta
LV = left ventricle
PA = pulmonary artery
RA = right atrium
RV = right ventricle

a Subcostal 2-D echo slice depicting the great arteries.
b The left–right shunt is visible via the APSD as the red area (asterisk) on the color Doppler image.

Preinterventional and Preoperative Diagnostics

In general, TTE is adequate (▸ Fig. 4.30 and ▸ Fig. 4.31) for diagnostic purposes in children, especially in cases of proximal defects (▸ Fig. 4.30). In cases of distal defects, visualization can present difficulties. A cross-sectional imaging procedure, ideally an MRI, can be useful in such situations (▸ Fig. 4.28 and ▸ Fig. 4.29). In addition to visualization, MRI also allows absolute shunt quantification. MDCT is also, fundamentally, appropriate for visualizing defects, particularly if additional coronary and/or aortic anomalies are present or suspected.

Postoperative and Postinterventional Issues

Post-surgical prognosis is generally determined by concurrent defects and the degree of pulmonary hypertension. Similar to the closure of small defects, if the APSD is surgically treated within the first year of life—namely, before the onset of irreversible pulmonary changes—life expectancy is fully unaffected.[12]

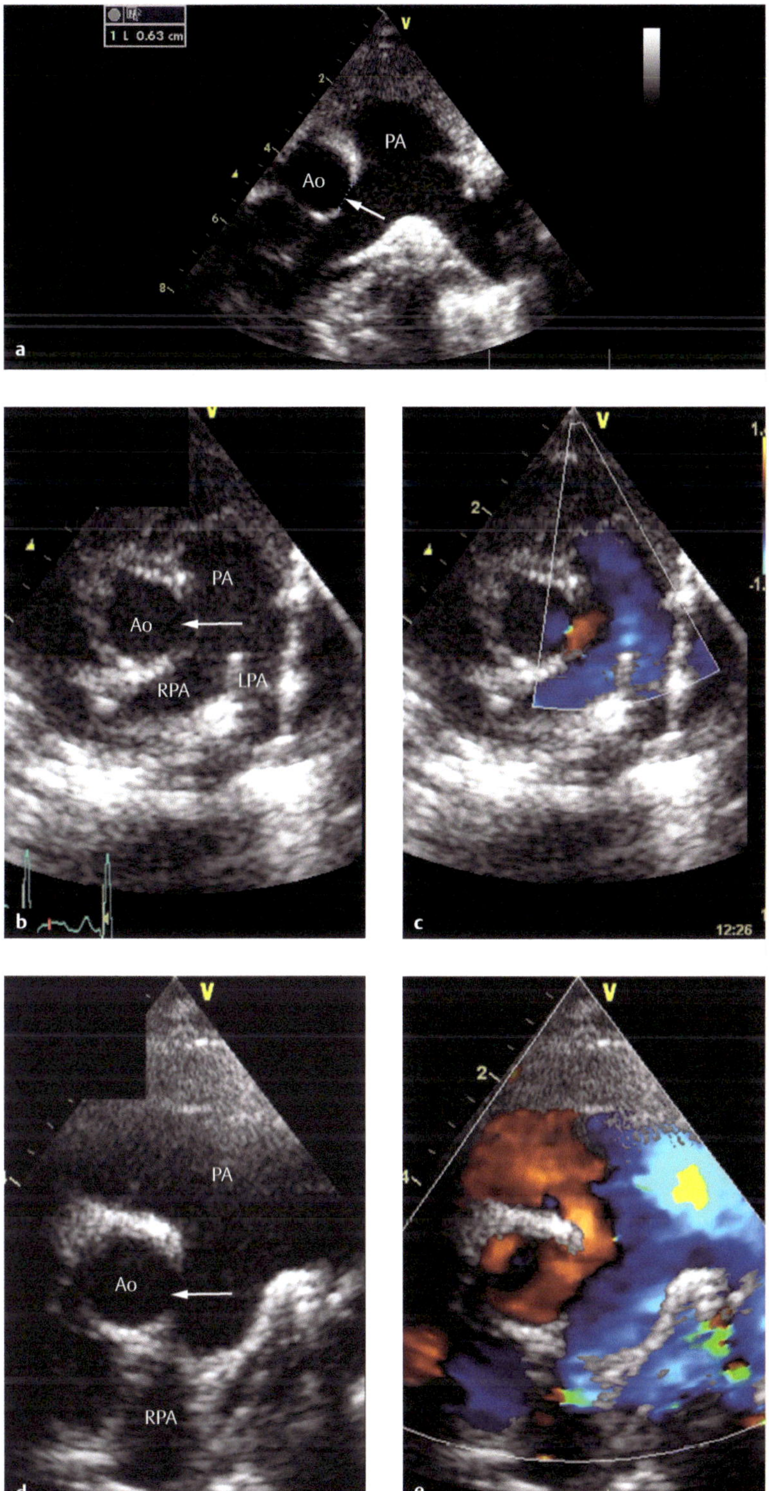

Fig. 4.31 Distal APSD. Each arrow indicates the position of an APSD. Doppler echocardiography exams, various patients.
Ao = aorta
LPA = left pulmonary artery
PA = pulmonary artery
RPA = right pulmonary artery

- **a** 2-D TTE image of the great vessels, short-axis parasternal view.
- **b** Great vessels, short-axis parasternal view, without color Doppler.
- **c** Great vessels, short-axis parasternal view, with color Doppler (the same patient as in **b**). The left–right shunt via the APSD is depicted in red on the image.
- **d** 2-D TTE image, parasternal short axis, without color Doppler.
- **e** 2-D TTE image, parasternal short axis, with color Doppler (the same patient as in **d**). The left–right shunt via the APSD is depicted in red on the image.

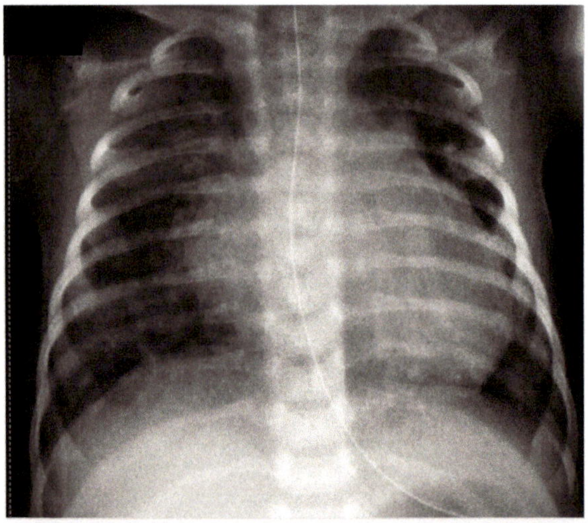

Fig. 4.32 APSD. Thoracic X-ray of a 4-week-old infant. Significantly enlarged heart, more pronounced on the left side. Considerable pulmonary hyperperfusion.

Goals and Relative Value of Diagnostic Imaging

TTE is generally sufficient during childhood (▸ Table 4.12 and ▸ Table 4.13).[7] Fluoroscopy can also be used to monitor peri-interventional catheter placement (▸ Fig. 4.33).

Table 4.11 Volume load for individual cardiac compartments in a case of complete APSD.

Cardiovascular compartment	Volume load
Right atrium	-
Right ventricle	-
Pulmonary arteries	++
Pulmonary veins	++
Left atrium	++
Left ventricle	++
Aorta and conduit arteries	-
Systemic veins	-

Table 4.12 Preinterventional or preoperative imaging diagnostics in cases of APSD.

Preinterventional/preoperative imaging methods for APSD	Focus	Value
2-D, 3-D TTE	• Defect size and position • Shunt, qualitative • Left heart dilation • Assessing right ventricular and pulmonary arterial pressure • Ruling out additional shunts • Assessing coronary anatomy • Ruling out pulmonary and systemic venous anomalies	+++
2-D, 3-D TEE	Refer to TTE (primarily helpful for proximal defects; can only be used in limited cases, since most patients are less than 1 year)	+
Cardiac MRI	• Quantifying the left–right shunt • Quantifying ventricular dilatation and function • Measuring the defect (phase contrast method) • Anatomy of pulmonary and systemic veins	+++ (Backup method)
MDCT	Backup method in cases of unclear echocardiographical findings and contraindication against cardiac MRI; may be helpful in cases of pulmonary parenchymatic comorbidity or to prove the existence of concurrent vascular defects, such as anomalous pulmonary venous connections	(+)
Invasive (diagnostic) cardiac catheter tests	• Measuring pressure and resistance (if indicated) and pharmacological testing of pulmonary vascular reactivity • Defect position and size in cases of distal defects • Ruling out pulmonary and systemic venous anomalies	++ (in cases of pulmonary hypertonia)

MDCT, multidetector computed tomography; MRI, magnetic resonance imaging; TEE, transesophageal echocardiography; TTE, transthoracic echocardiography.

Table 4.13 Postinterventional or postoperative imaging diagnostics in cases of APSD.

Imaging methods	Value
TTE	+++
TEE	+
Cardiac MRI	+++
MDCT	+
Invasive cardiac catheter diagnostics	++

MDCT, multidetector computed tomography; MRI, magnetic resonance imaging; TEE, transesophageal echocardiography; TTE, transthoracic echocardiography.

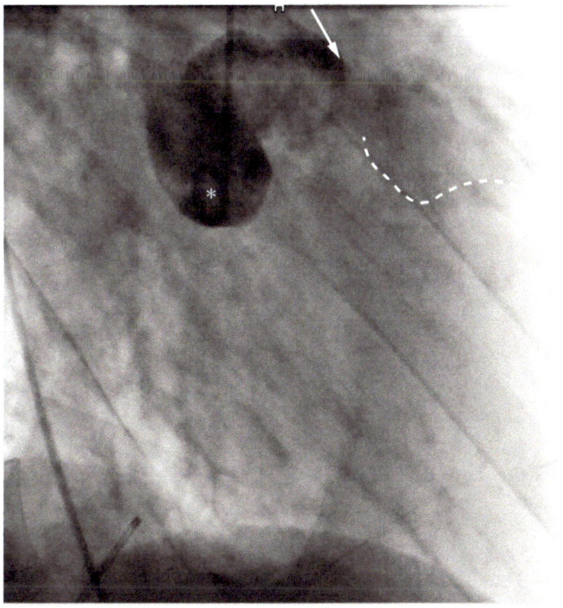

Fig. 4.33 APSD. A.–p. fluoroscopy of an adult male with APSD originating in the right coronary sinus (arrow). The pigtail catheter is positioned within the left coronary sinus of the aortic root (asterisk). The pulmonary root superior to the APSD is colorless (dotted line).

4.2 Right-Side Defects

4.2.1 Pulmonary Valve Stenosis

Samir Sarikouch, Matthias Grothoff, Erich Sorantin

Definition

Isolated pulmonary valve stenosis is the most common form of narrowed RVOT in cases of normal aortic origins (occurring in 80% of cases). It constitutes 6–8% of all congenital heart defects.[16] There are various clinical progressions based on the degree of stenosis, which are generally caused by adhesion of the tricuspid or bicuspid semilunar valves' commissures (▶ Fig. 4.34).

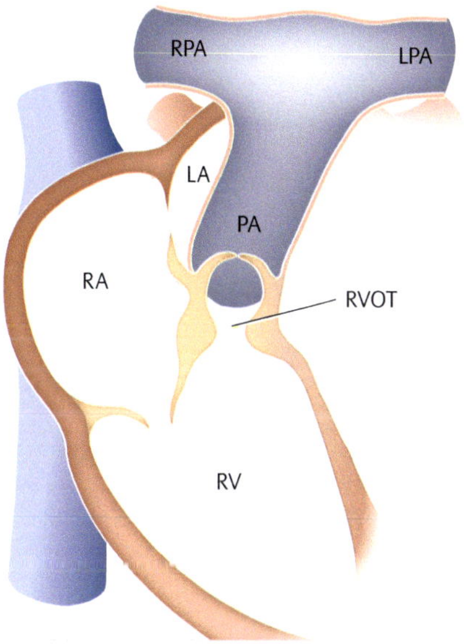

Fig. 4.34 Isolated valvular or infundibular pulmonary stenosis. Schematic depiction. Note the thickened portions of the pulmonary valve forming a dome-like shape, and the narrowed RVOT.
LA = left atrium
PA = pulmonary artery
RA = right atrium
RV = right ventricle
RVOT = right ventricular outflow tract

Natural Progression and Clinical Issues

If a moderate-to-severe pulmonary valve stenosis (▶ Table 4.15) is present, blood flow into the lungs is reduced, resulting in the development of cyanosis and ductal-dependent pulmonary blood flow. This clinical picture is then described as "critical pulmonary stenosis." In these cases, hypoplasia of the corresponding hypertrophied right ventricle is often also present.

In contrast, if only a minor degree of stenosis is present, diagnosis often first occurs based on systolic heart murmur or when signs of right ventricular heart failure arise. Fully unremarkable clinical progressions can also occur, meaning corresponding diagnostics only occur based on pathological ECG findings.

Treatment Options and Preinterventional Diagnostics

Nowadays, interventional catheter therapy using balloon valvuloplasty (▶ Fig. 4.36) is performed in the vast majority of cases of symptomatic, isolated pulmonary valve stenosis, which can generally be quantified clearly via Doppler echocardiography (▶ Fig. 4.35; ▶ Table 4.15)–

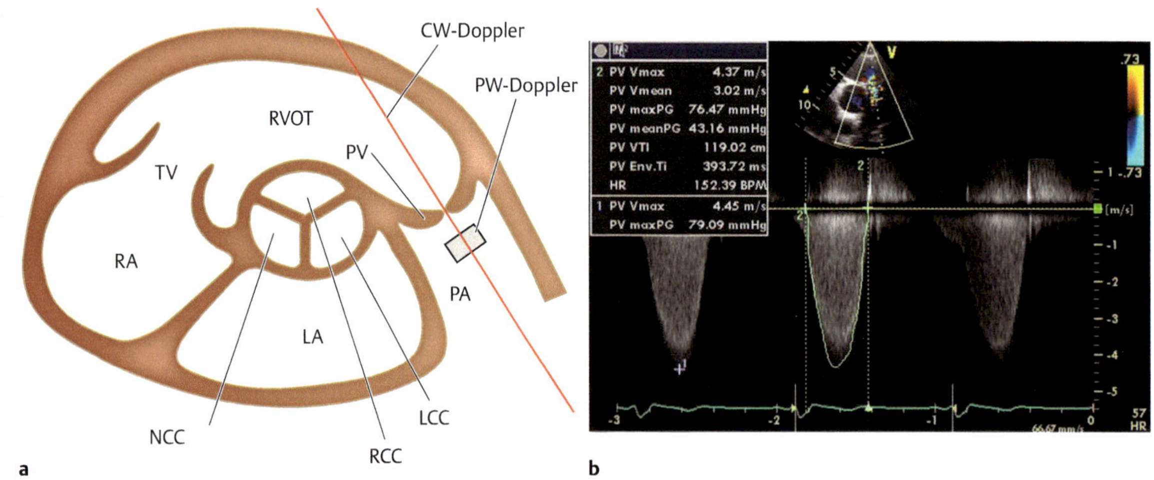

Fig. 4.35 Determining pressure gradient via the pulmonary valve.

PV = pulmonary valve
LA = left atrium
LCC = left coronary aortic leaflet
NCC = non-coronary aortic leaflet
PA = pulmonary artery
RA = right atrium
RCC = right coronary aortic leaflet
RVOT = right ventricular outflow tract
TV = tricuspid valve

a Schematic depiction of an echocardiographical doppler view (red line through the pulmonary valve). The position of the valvular stenosis and the pressure gradient can be determined via the pulmonary valve using PW Doppler.

b Echocardiographical doppler view in a male patient with high-grade stenosis of the pulmonary valve and a maximum measured flow velocity of 4.5 m/s. According to the Bernoulli equation, this results in a maximum estimated instantaneous pressure gradient of 79 mmHg via the pulmonary valve.

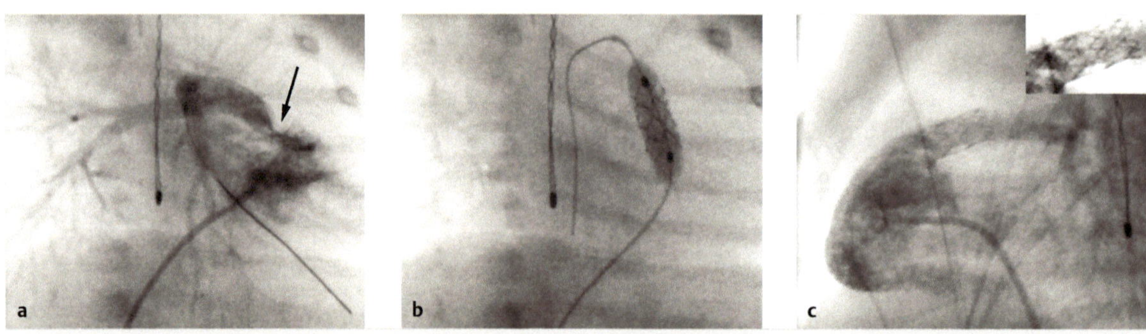

Fig. 4.36 Cardiac catheterization in a case of valvular or infundibular pulmonary stenosis.

a Direct cardiac catheterization in an underweight newborn with valvular or infundibular pulmonary stenosis within the scope of tetralogy of Fallot and recurrent hypoxic episodes, depicting a high-grade infundibular pulmonary stenosis (arrow).

b The balloon valvuloplasty with stent placement in the RVOT prevented further cyanosis until the final corrective surgery was performed. This figure shows stent dilatation in a.-p projection.

c The lateral projection after stent placement shows good preliminary results in the follow-up angiogram. Insert: enlarged view of stent.

meaning starting at a gradient of more than 3–40 mmHg in clinical practice. This can be performed even in newborns at very low risk. Surgical treatment is only used in very rare cases, often after unsuccessful balloon dilatation or in cases of pronounced dysplasia of the valve apparatus and/or associated subvalvular or supravalvular narrowing. This operation is often combined with narrow transannular patch plasty.[17]

Postoperative and Postinterventional Issues

Patients with pulmonary valve stenosis who were initially treated successfully using balloon valvuloplasty may develop new gradients or possess a residual gradient that must be monitored to assess the need for additional treatment. A residual peak gradient of less than 20–30 mmHg is generally well tolerated.[18] The prominent pulmonary segment, often first identifiable in the p.-a. thoracic X-ray, frequently remains present even after successful treatment (▶ Fig. 4.37).

Pulmonary valve insufficiency and the corresponding right ventricular volume overload occasionally occur after balloon dilatation. Much more commonly, they occur after surgical treatment. Consecutive right ventricular dilatation, which patients may tolerate well for years (▶ Fig. 4.37b and ▶ Fig. 4.45), can later lead to progressive tricuspid valve insufficiency and electrical instability, resulting in ventricular arrhythmia and right ventricular heart failure.

M!

Note

The main objective of imaging is determining the timing of the interventional or surgical pulmonary valve replacement, which should occur based on objective progression data.

Goals and Relative Value of Diagnostic Imaging

Both initial diagnosis of a congenital pulmonary valve stenosis and the indication for interventional or surgical treatment can generally be depicted very well using doppler echocardiography (▶ Fig. 4.35). MRI and MDCT play a large role, above all during postsurgical and postinterventional follow-up care. MRI is the method of choice for assessing right ventricular function, volume, and mass (▶ Table 4.14). It is also suitable for absolute quantification of pulmonary valve insufficiency (▶ Fig. 4.37) by means of calculating the regurgitation fraction:

$$RF = \frac{(\text{antegrade flow} - \text{retrograde flow})}{\text{antegrade flow}} \times 100$$

where

RF = regurgitation fraction in %

Antegrade and retrograde flow are indicated in ml.

Table 4.14 Focus of imaging diagnostics with the value of individual procedures for cases of pulmonary valve stenosis.

Clinical situation	Common diagnostic tasks	Imaging method of choice in light of practical clinical perspectives	Value of imaging method
Presurgical/preinterventional			
Ductal-dependent pulmonary blood flow	Duct size, right ventricular size, pulmonary valve diameter	Echocardiography	+++
		MRI	++
		MDCT	+
		Angiography/intervention	++
Antegrade pulmonary blood flow	Gradient through the pulmonary valve, right ventricular size, pulmonary valve diameter, ASD	Echocardiography	+++
		MRI	++
		MDCT	+
		Angiography/intervention	++
Postsurgical/postinterventional			
Minor residual stenosis, minor insufficiency	Right ventricular function	Echocardiography	++
		MRI	+++
		MDCT	+
		Angiography/intervention	-
Relevant residual stenosis	Right ventricular hypertrophy, assessing the degree of stenosis (primarily in cases of concurrent supravalvular stenosis)	Echocardiography	+++
		MRI	++
		MDCT	+
		Angiography/intervention	++
Relevant insufficiency	Quantifying pulmonary insufficiency, right ventricular size and function	Echocardiography	++
		MRI	+++
		MDCT	+
		Angiography/intervention	-

ASD, atrial septal defect; MDCT, multidetector computed tomography; MRI, magnetic resonance imaging.

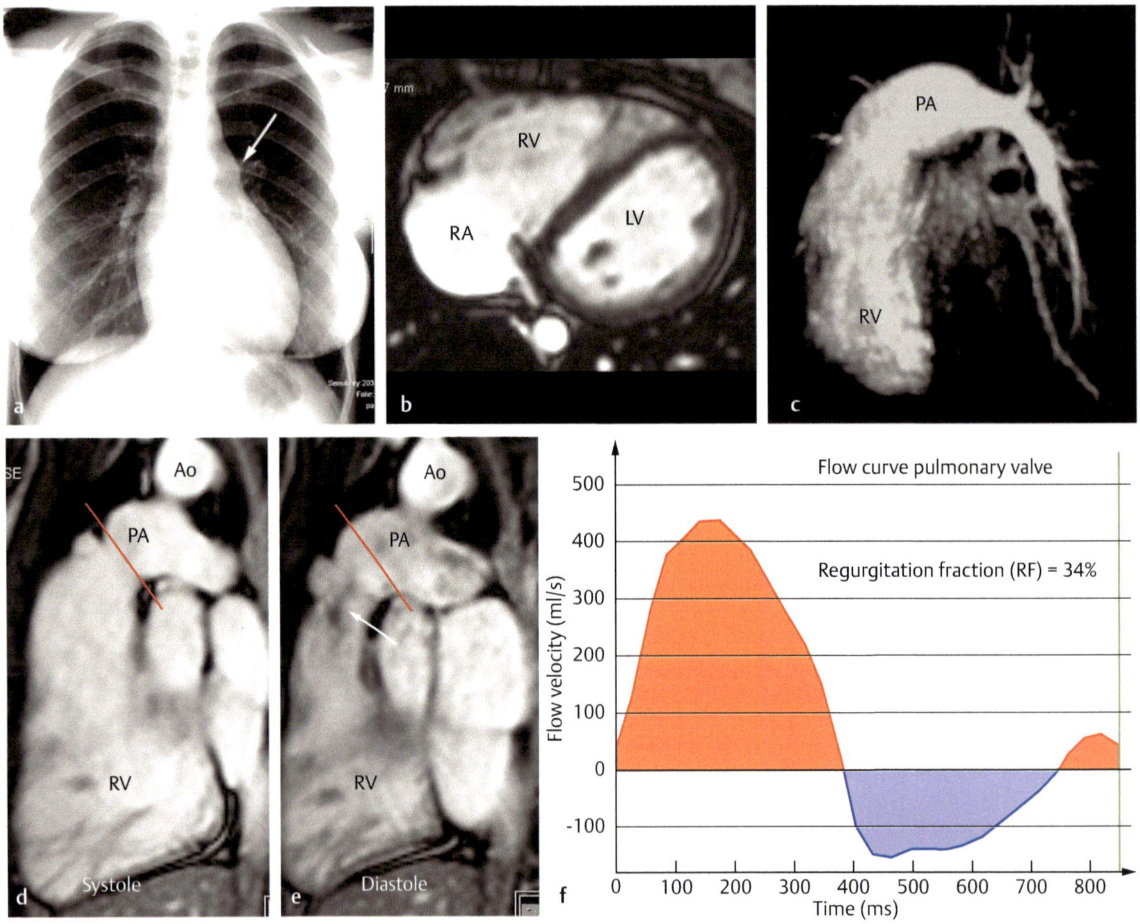

Fig. 4.37 Condition after a commissurotomy of a pulmonary valve stenosis. Various depictions of a 14-year-old girl's condition after a commissurotomy of a pulmonary valve stenosis during her first year of life. Now, only residual pulmonary valve insufficiency remains. Using MRI flow measurement in the "in-plane" (along the course of the vessel; **d**, **e**) and "through-plane" (perpendicular to the course of the vessel or cranial and parallel to the valve level; **d**, **e**, red line, cross-sectional plane for **g–i**) phase contrast techniques, pulmonary valve insufficiency can be quantified precisely as a regurgitation fraction in ml or in % (**f**; 34% in this case).

Ao = aorta
LV = left ventricle
PA = pulmonary artery
RA = right atrium
RV = right ventricle
SVC = superior vena cava

a P.-a. X-ray. The prominent pulmonary segment is still visible after surgery (arrow).

b The transverse SSFP cine MRI shows an enlarged right ventricle and a flattened interventricular septum resulting from volume overload (115 ml/m^2)

c The dilated pulmonary arteries can be recognized clearly in the lateral MIP reconstruction of a contrast-enhanced pulmonary MRA.

d Determining the sectional planes for **g–i** (systole) in the magnitude image of an in-plane image of the flow-sensitive GE sequence, in an angulated sagittal plane, through the pulmonary artery.

e Determining the sectional planes for **g–i** (diastole) in the magnitude image of an in-plane image of the flow-sensitive GE sequence, in an angulated sagittal plane, through the pulmonary artery. The arrow indicates early diastolic dephasing through the pulmonary valve due to pulmonary valve insufficiency.

f Flow curve through the pulmonary valve. Red indicates antegrade flow during systole, while blue indicates retrograde flow during diastole. The depicted interval corresponds to an RR interval of 882 ms, recorded based on heart rate.

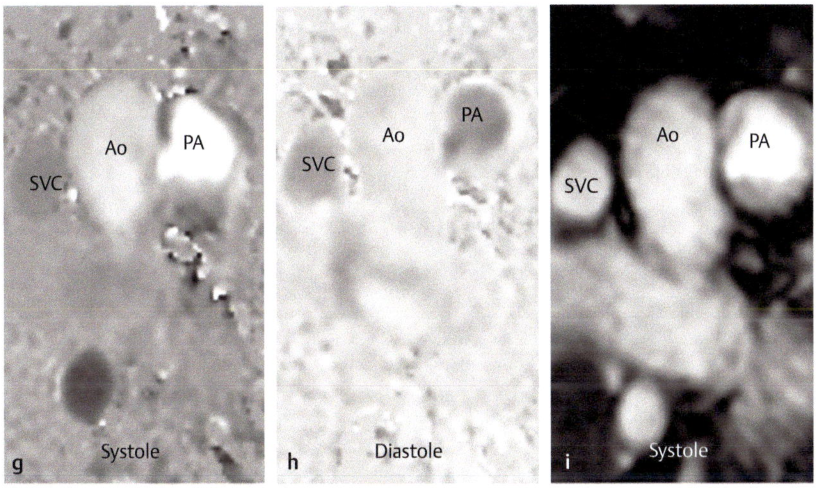

Fig 4.37 (*Continued*) **Condition after a commissurotomy of a pulmonary valve stenosis.**

Ao = aorta
LV = left ventricle
PA = pulmonary artery
RA = right atrium
RV = right ventricle
SVC = superior vena cava

g Phase image of the flow-sensitive GE sequence during systole. Cranial flow is light in color, while caudal flow is dark.
h Phase image of the flow-sensitive GE sequence during diastole. Retrograde flow in the pulmonary artery (caused by pulmonary valve insufficiency) is depicted in a dark color.
i Anatomical magnitude image of the flow-sensitive GE sequence during systole. Note the tricuspid pulmonary valve's opening during systole.

Table 4.15 Graduation of the pulmonary valve stenosis via invasive cardiac catheter pressure measurement, Doppler echocardiography, MR flow measurement, or determination of valve opening area.[7,13]

Parameter	Degree of severity of pulmonary valve stenosis			
	Minor (I)	Moderate (II)	Significant (III)	Severe (IV)
v_{max} (m/s)	<2.0	2.0–3.5	3.5–4.5	>4.5
Δp_{max} (mmHg)	<25	25–49	50–79	>80
Valve opening area (cm²/m² body surface area)	1.00–2.00	<1.00	<0.50	<0.25

Δp_{max}, maximum pressure gradient; v_{max}, maximum flow velocity.

MDCT allows concurrent changes to pulmonary structure and vascular changes caused by CTA (such as MAPCA and peripheral pulmonary stenosis) to be depicted (▸ Fig. 4.46). Vascular changes can also be depicted clearly using contrast-enhanced MRA (▸ Fig. 4.38). Dynamic visualization of the valve can also be performed via MDCT when using retrospective gating. Due to high radiation exposure, however, this method only comes into play in cases of inadequate acoustic windows and contraindications for MRI diagnostics.[7] MRI, in contrast, can be used as an alternative to echocardiography, while CT can only be used in certain cases, e.g., to assess a lung parenchyma. Likewise, a valve stenosis can be quantified noninvasively via Doppler echocardiography, MRI flow measurement, or valve planimetry (▸ Table 4.15; also ▸ Fig. 4.37).

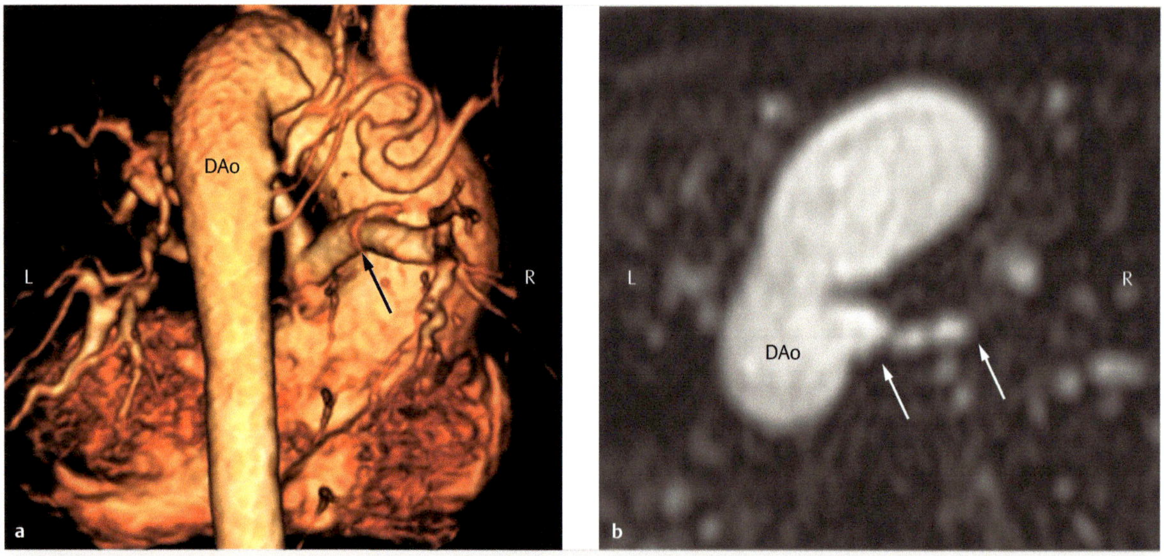

Fig. 4.38 MAPCA.
DAo = descending aorta

a 3-D depiction of multiple MAPCAs from a contrast-enhanced MRA, dorsal view, in a 32-year-old male patient. A particularly large aortopulmonary collateral from the descending aorta to the right lung is marked with an arrow.

b Axial multiplanar reformat of the large MAPCA to the right lung, in the same patient (arrow).

4.2.2 Tetralogy of Fallot

Samir Sarikouch, Matthias Grothoff, Erich Sorantin

Definition

In 1888, Etienne-Louis Arthur Fallot described a combination of pulmonary stenosis, large VSD, and right displacement of the aorta with concentric right ventricular hypertrophy (▶ Fig. 4.39).[19] Nowadays, anterior cephalic malrotation of the outlet septum is considered the main cause of this most common cyanotic defect, comprising up to 9% of all heart defects in international literature, and 2.5% of all cardiac defects in Germany in the 2006-07 year.[16]

Natural Progression and Clinical Issues

Similar to isolated pulmonary valve stenosis, the degree of stenosis of the RVOT determines the clinical symptoms, which can range from severe cyanosis with ductal-dependent pulmonary perfusion to the clinical picture of "pink Fallot." The commonly present infundibular (i.e., muscular) portion of an outflow tract stenosis (▶ Fig. 4.40) can lead to intermittent bouts of cyanosis, even in cases of minor or moderate pulmonary stenosis. The pulmonary arteries also demonstrate variable pathology. Stenoses, particularly those of the left pulmonary artery, are common and can lead to side differences in pulmonary perfusion (▶ Fig. 4.41). Hyperperfusion can also occur in certain pulmonary segments due to aortopulmonary collaterals (▶ Fig. 4.42).[20]

Treatment Options and Preinterventional Diagnostics

In cases of ductal-dependent pulmonary blood flow, catheter interventional procedures using balloon dilatation of valvular stenosis portions can be used (▶ Fig. 4.36). If cyanotic newborns cannot be treated using catheter procedures, either an aortopulmonary shunt is placed or early correction is performed. In cases of elective correction, generally during the first 6 months of life, the VSD is closed and the outflow tract stenosis is addressed by resecting the obstructing bundle of muscle in conjunction with a valvuloplasty. This procedure is commonly supplemented by a transannular patch due to the often-narrow valve rings. Like in cases of isolated pulmonary valve stenosis, preinterventional diagnostics fall within the domain of Doppler echocardiography (▶ Fig. 4.35 and ▶ Fig. 4.39d).

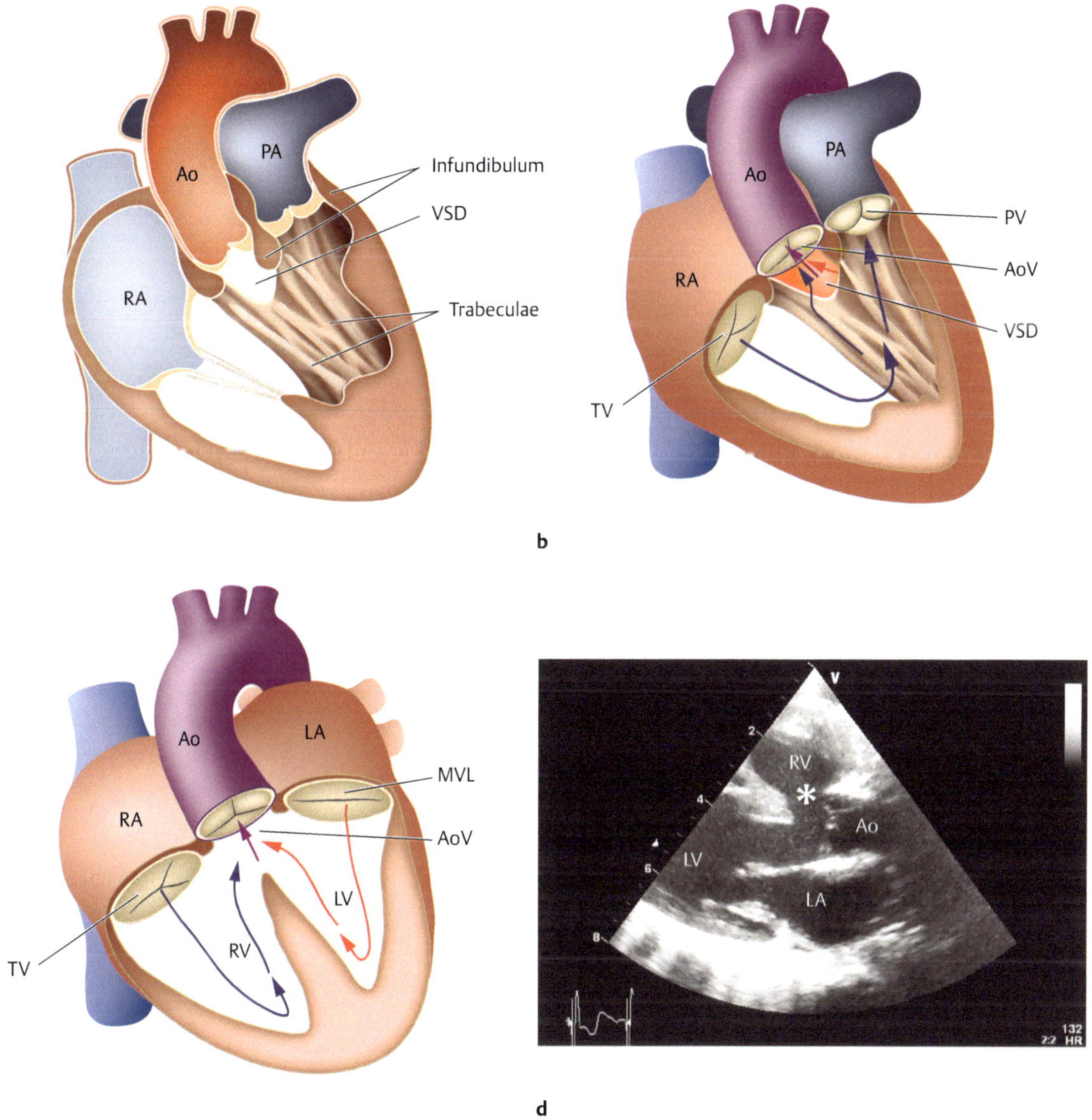

Fig. 4.39 Tetralogy of Fallot.

Ao = aorta
AoV = aortic valve
LA = left atrium
LV = left ventricle
MV = mitral valve
PA = pulmonary artery
PV = pulmonary valve
RA = right atrium
RV = right ventricle
TV = tricuspid valve
VSD = ventricular septal defect

a The schematic depiction of tetralogy of Fallot shows the aorta "overriding" the VSD, the pulmonary infundibular or pulmonary valve stenosis, and right ventricular hypertrophy. The trabecular segment of the right ventricle extends to the VSD.
b Schematic depiction of tetralogy of Fallot, view from the right ventricle, with color-coded blood flow (blue = deoxygenated, red = oxygenated, purple = mixed venous blood).
c Schematic depiction of tetralogy of Fallot in the indicated 4-chamber view.
d In the 2-D TTE, the aorta "overriding" the VSD (asterisk) is clearly visible seen along the parasternal long axis before surgical correction in a patient with tetralogy of Fallot.

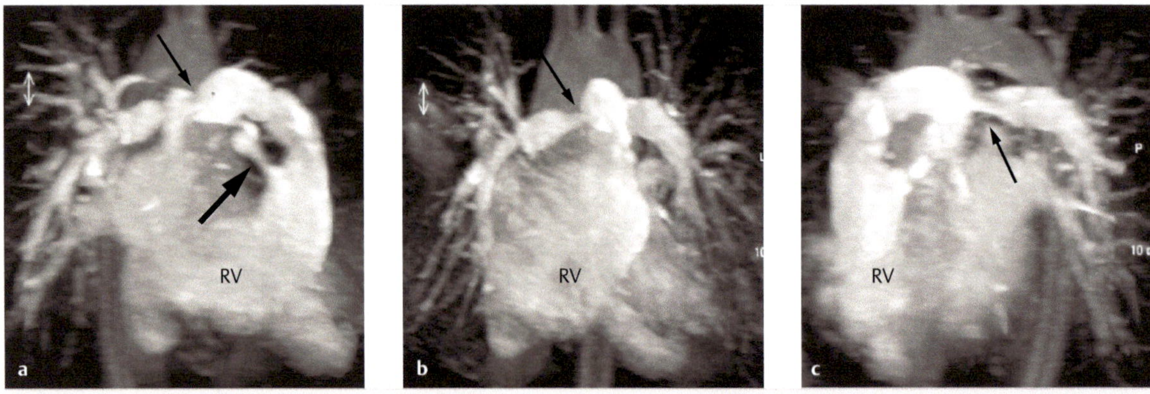

Fig. 4.40 Surgically corrected tetralogy of Fallot. 3-D MIP reconstruction from a contrast-enhanced MRA of a patient after surgical correction of tetralogy of Fallot using a valve-equipped conduit in the form of a prosthesis from the RVOT to the pulmonary bifurcation. The original subvalvular or infundibular pulmonary stenosis (**a**, thick arrow) is still visible in RAO projection. Multiple peripheral pulmonary stenoses (**a–c**, thin arrows) can also be seen in a.-p (**b**) and in LAO projection (**c**).
RV = right ventricle

a RAO projection.
b A.-p. projection.
c LAO projection.

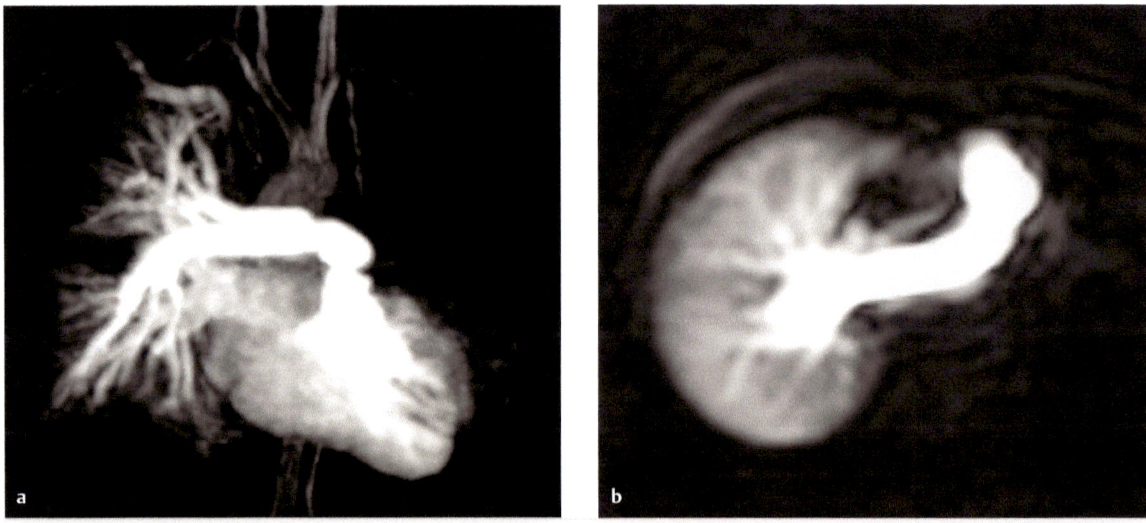

Fig. 4.41 Surgically corrected tetralogy of Fallot.

a 3-D MIP reconstruction from a contrast-enhanced MRA in a 9-year-old female patient after surgical correction of tetralogy of Fallot, with left pulmonary artery occlusion.
b The axial MR pulmonary perfusion image of the bolus track at the start of the contrast-enhanced MRA shows a lack of left-side pulmonary perfusion.

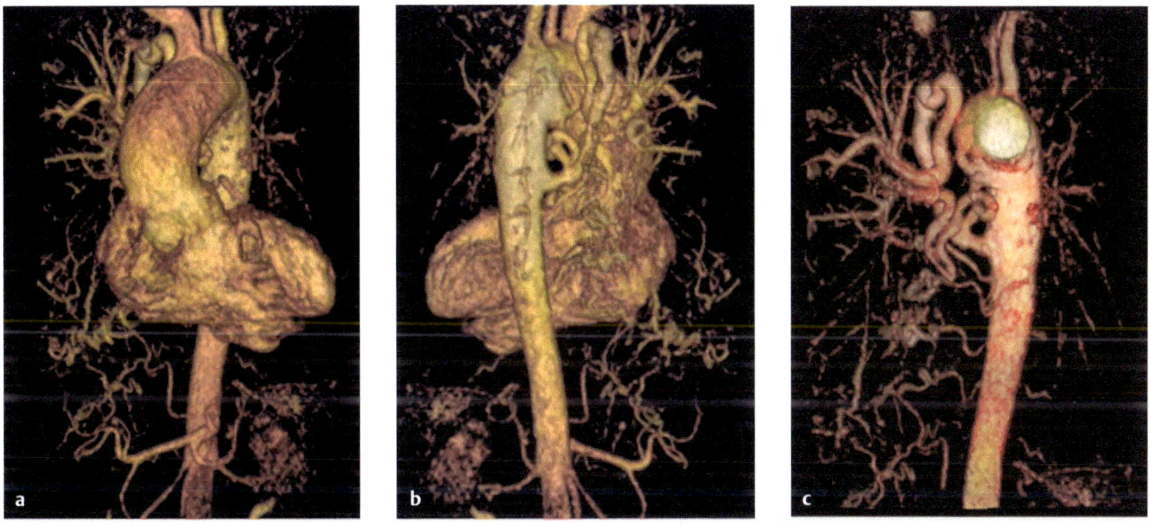

Fig. 4.42 Uncorrected tetralogy of Fallot. 3-D volume rendering reconstruction from a contrast-enhanced MRA in a 54-year-old woman with uncorrected tetralogy of Fallot, pulmonary atresia, and pulmonary perfusion exclusively via pronounced MAPCAs.
a A.-p. projection.
b Dorsal projection.
c A.-p. projection after "virtual" removal of the ventricle and the ascending aorta in post-processing.

Postoperative and Postinterventional Issues

During surgical correction of RVOT stenosis, a dilemma arises between moderate widening of the outflow tract with the risk of a relevant residual gradient, and considerable expansion using a patch (▶ Fig. 4.43 and ▶ Fig. 4.44), which carries the risk of significant pulmonary valve insufficiency. Higher perioperative mortality in cases of significant residual gradients leads to increased use of transannular patches. Similar to isolated pulmonary valve stenosis, right ventricular volume overload is generally well tolerated, sometimes for decades. The timing for a secondary pulmonary valve replacement has changed in recent years due to multiple studies for adult patients, where no regression of a right ventricular dilatation beyond 170–180 ml/m² could be proven.[71] In cases of right ventricular dilatation, a pronounced tricuspid valve insufficiency may develop, which will then require further treatment (▶ Fig. 4.45).

Pulmonary arterial stenoses are common after surgery (▶ Fig. 4.40, ▶ Fig. 4.41, and ▶ Fig. 4.43), and the use of foreign materials during primary correction renders them more common. Today, they remain within the domain of catheter interventional treatment. They are generally well managed via balloon dilatation and stent implantation.[20,22]

Goals and Relative Value of Diagnostic Imaging

Like in cases of isolated pulmonary valve stenosis, Doppler echocardiography is the initial method of choice for diagnostic purposes and for determining indication for surgery (▶ Table 4.16). In cases where the peripheral pulmonary arterial branches can only be assessed on a limited basis through the pulmonary parenchyma or where MAPCAs are present, MRI and MDCT imaging procedures using contrast-enhanced angiography (▶ Fig. 4.46; also ▶ Fig. 4.38 and ▶ Fig. 4.42) can be helpful before electing to use an invasive cardiac catheter. The main focus of tomographic procedures, especially MRI, is postoperative use. Monitoring progression requires consistent assessment of right ventricular function, volume, and muscle mass with respect to residual stenosis and pulmonary valve insufficiency (▶ Fig. 4.37) in order to be able to determine indications for additional surgery. In the meantime, specific reference values for the expected ventricular sizes and dimensions of the great vessels (in both cases, based on the patient's age and sex) are available for these heart defects.[23–25]

Newer interventional procedures, such as transcatheter valve replacement (▶ Fig. 4.44), require precise preinterventional assessment of the ventricle that underwent previous surgical treatment, RVOT, valve annulus, and the pulmonary valve, itself. This can occur via MRI or MDCT (▶ Fig. 4.43), especially if there is a contraindication against MRI (e.g., if an implantable cardioverter defibrillator [ICD] is present).

Table 4.16 Focus of imaging diagnostics with the value of individual procedures for tetralogy of Fallot.

Clinical situation	Common diagnostic tasks	Imaging method of choice	Value of imaging method
Preoperative (generally infants)			
Ductal-dependent pulmonary blood flow	Gradient and morphology of pulmonary stenosis (infundibular, valvular, supravalvular), aortopulmonary collaterals	Echocardiography	+++
		MRI	++
		MDCT	++
		Angiography/intervention	++
Antegrade pulmonary blood flow	Pulmonary stenosis gradient and morphology (infundibular, valvular, supravalvular), dimensions of the left and right pulmonary arteries, aortopulmonary collaterals	Echocardiography	+++
		MRI	+++
		MDCT	++
		Angiography/intervention	+
Postoperative			
Minor residual stenosis, minor insufficiency, residual shunt via the VSD	Morphological assessment of supravalvular stenoses, right ventricular function, shunt quantification	Echocardiography	++
		MRI	+++
		MDCT	+
		Angiography/intervention	+
Relevant residual stenosis	Right ventricular hypertrophy	Echocardiography	+++
		MRI	++
		CT	+
		Angiography/intervention	++
Relevant insufficiency	Right ventricular size and function, pulmonary insufficiency, tricuspid valve insufficiency	Echocardiography	++
		MRI	+++
		CT	+
		Angiography/intervention	+

CT, computed tomography; MDCT, multidetector computed tomography; MRI, magnetic resonance imaging; VSD, ventricular septal defect.

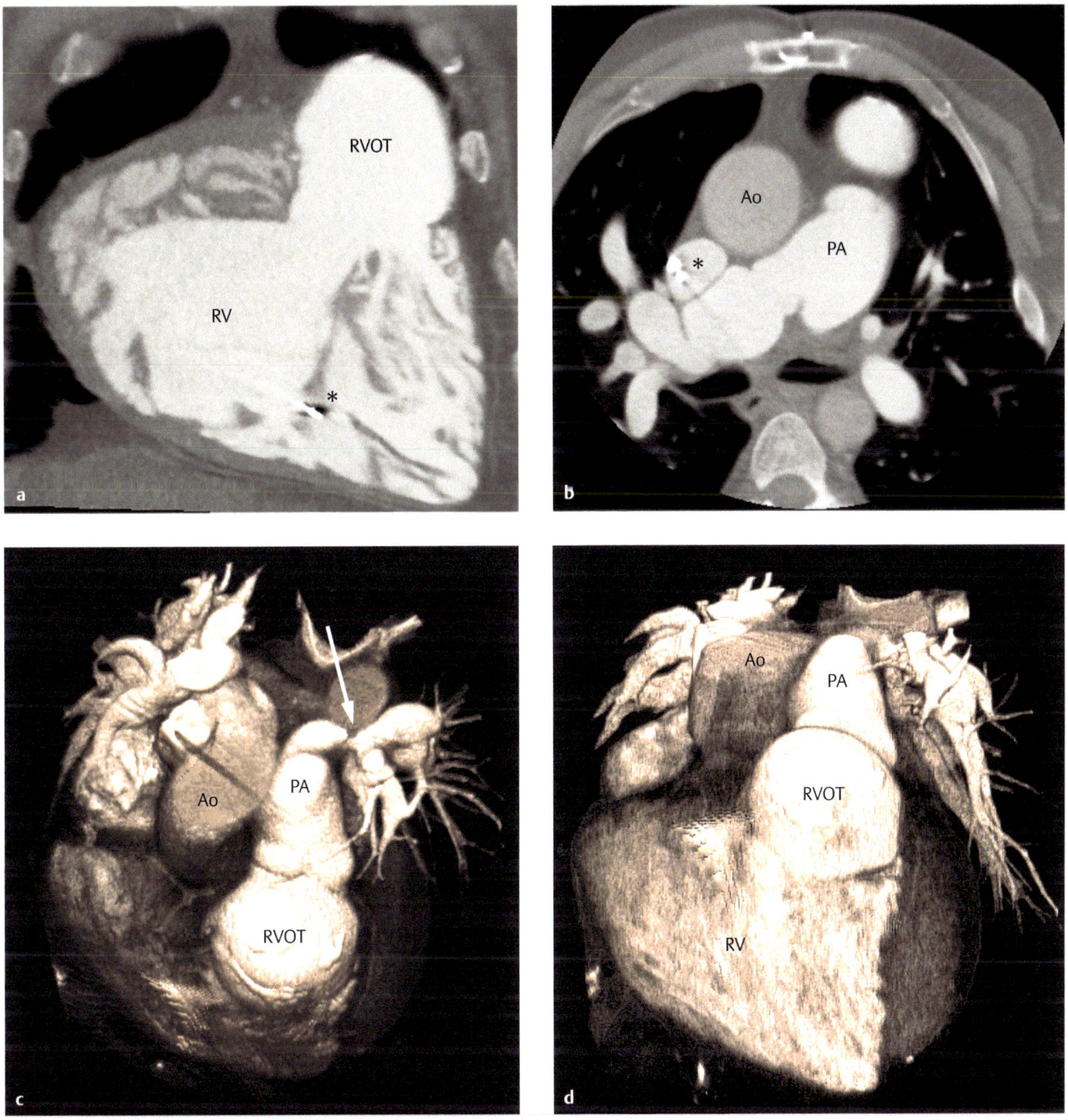

Fig. 4.43 Condition after corrective surgery for a case of tetralogy of Fallot in adulthood, and implantation of an ICD. Fifty-six-year-old male patient. The asterisk indicates the position of the ICD that was implanted due to ventricular tachycardia. Originally, a Blalock–Taussig shunt was placed.

Ao = aorta
PA = pulmonary artery
RV = right ventricle
RVOT = right ventricular outflow tract

a Angulated coronal reconstruction (RAO equivalent) through the dilated RVOT from an ECG-triggered MDCT data set (320 rows).

b The transverse images depict significant stenosis of the right pulmonary artery.

c 3-D volume rendering of the same data set, cranial view. Significant RVOT expansion after patch placement and high-grade stenosis of the left pulmonary artery (arrow). The reconstructions (**c**, **d**) each occurred during diastole in the 75% RR interval.

d Corresponding images for **c**, ventral view.

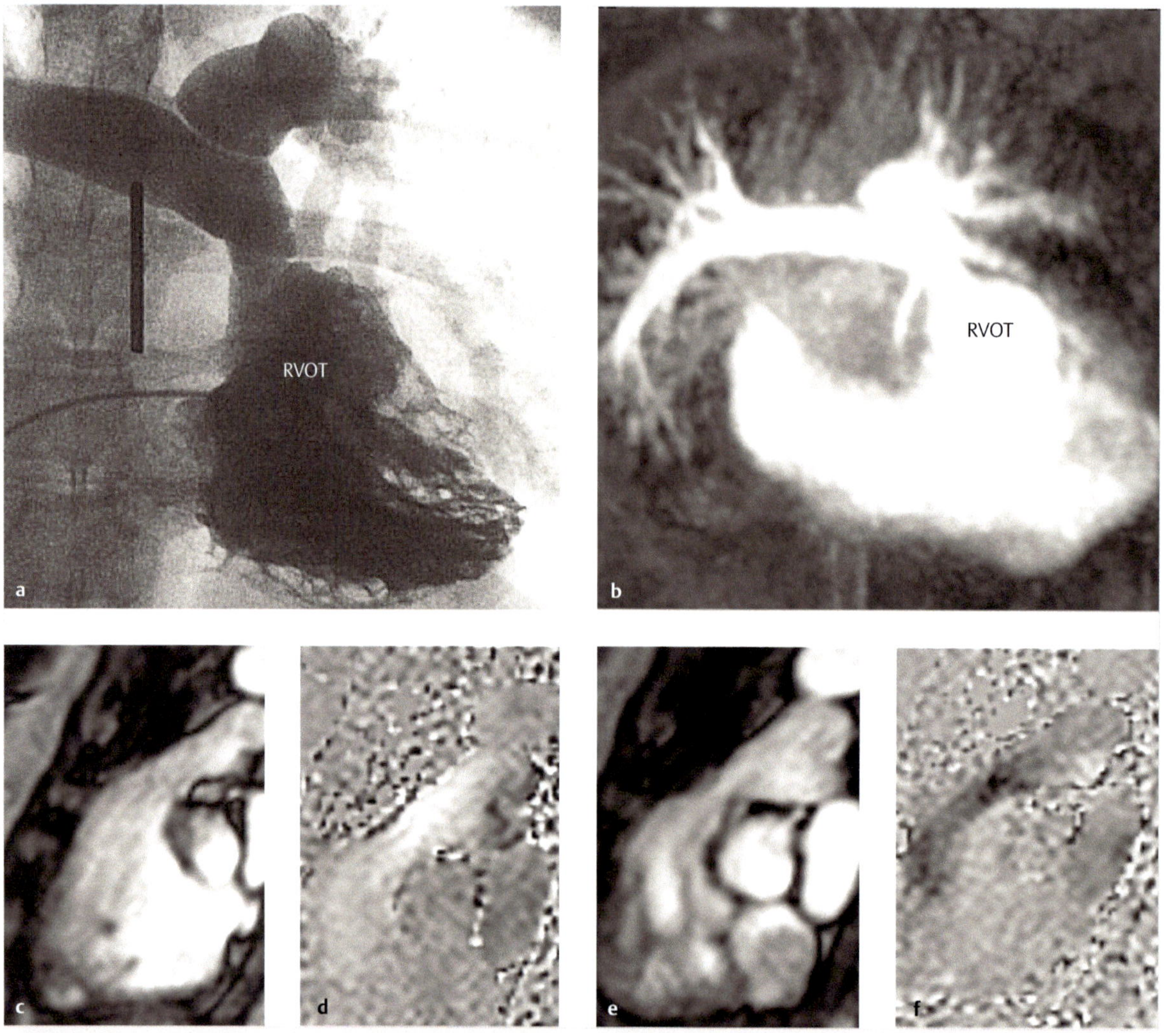

Fig. 4.44 High-grade restenosis of a xenograft in the pulmonary position after correcting tetralogy of Fallot. Nineteen-year-old female patient with high-grade residual stenosis of a xenograft in the pulmonary position, after surgical correction of tetralogy of Fallot, before a planned transcatheter pulmonary valve replacement (Melody valve). Magnitude and phase images of a flow-sensitive MRI GE sequence (**c–f**) show flow acceleration via the stenosed pulmonary valve to a maximum of 4 m/s, in terms of a maximum estimated instantaneous pressure gradient of 64 mmHg and a holodiastolic regurgitation fraction of 39%.
RVOT = right ventricular outflow tract

a Right ventriculography (RAO: right ventricular ejection fraction = 42%, right ventricular EDV = 126 ml/m^2).
b 3-D MIP of a contrast-enhanced MRA. Pronounced RVOT enlargement after patch plasty.
c Magnitude image of a flow-sensitive MRI GE sequence through the RVOT and the pulmonary artery of the same patient during systole.
d Phase image of a flow-sensitive MRI GE sequence through the RVOT and pulmonary artery of the same patient during systole.
e Magnitude image of a flow-sensitive MRI GE sequence through the RVOT and pulmonary artery of the same patient during diastole.
f The phase image of a flow-sensitive MRI GE sequence through the RVOT and pulmonary artery of the same patient during diastole clearly depicts diastolic regurgitation.

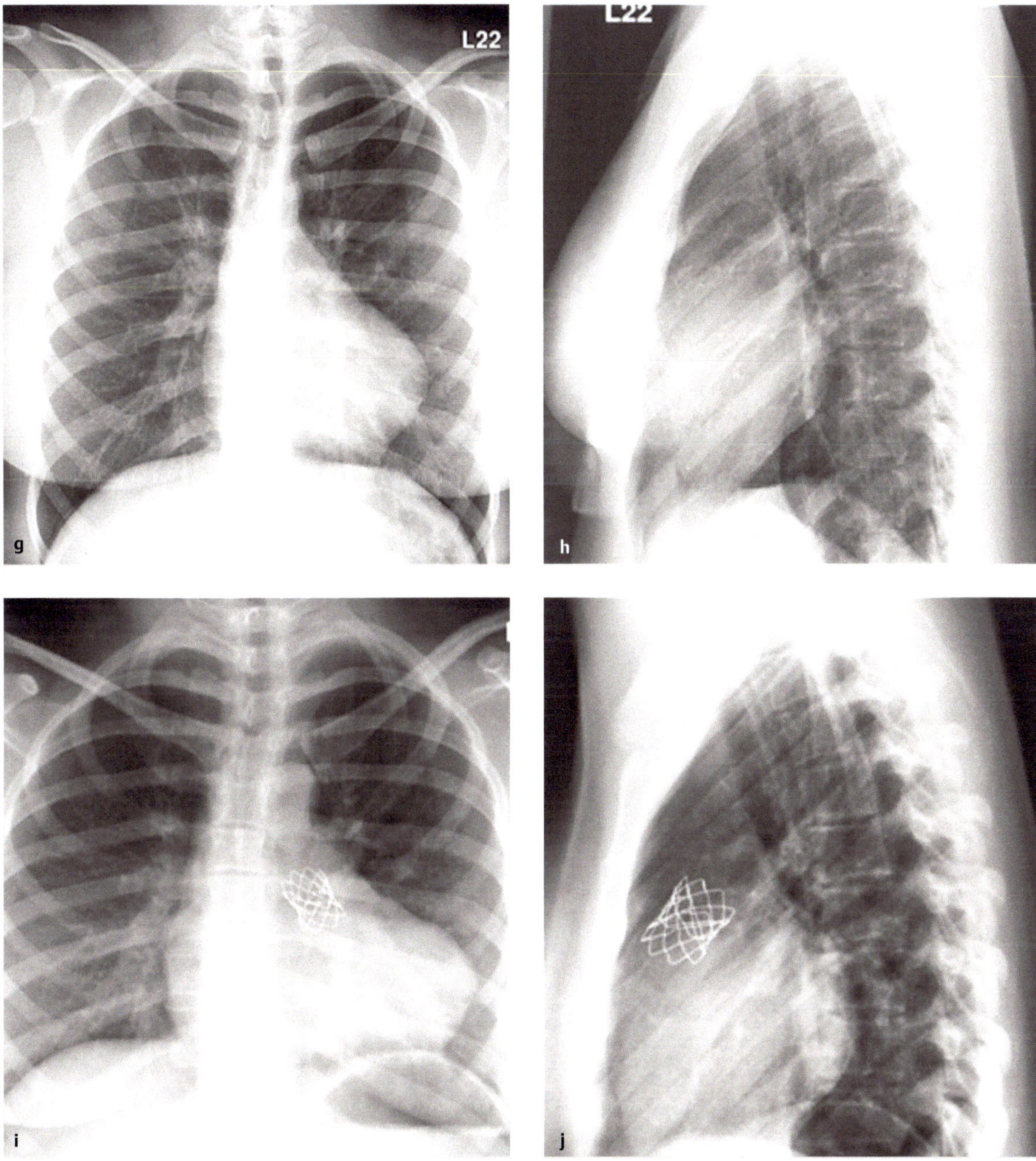

Fig 4.44 (*Continued*) **High-grade restenosis of a xenograft in the pulmonary position after correcting tetralogy of Fallot.**
RVOT = right ventricular outflow tract

g P.-a. thoracic X-ray before pulmonary valve implantation.
h Lateral thoracic X-ray before pulmonary valve implantation.
i P.-a. thoracic X-ray after transcatheter pulmonary valve implantation.
j Lateral thoracic X-ray after transcatheter pulmonary valve implantation.

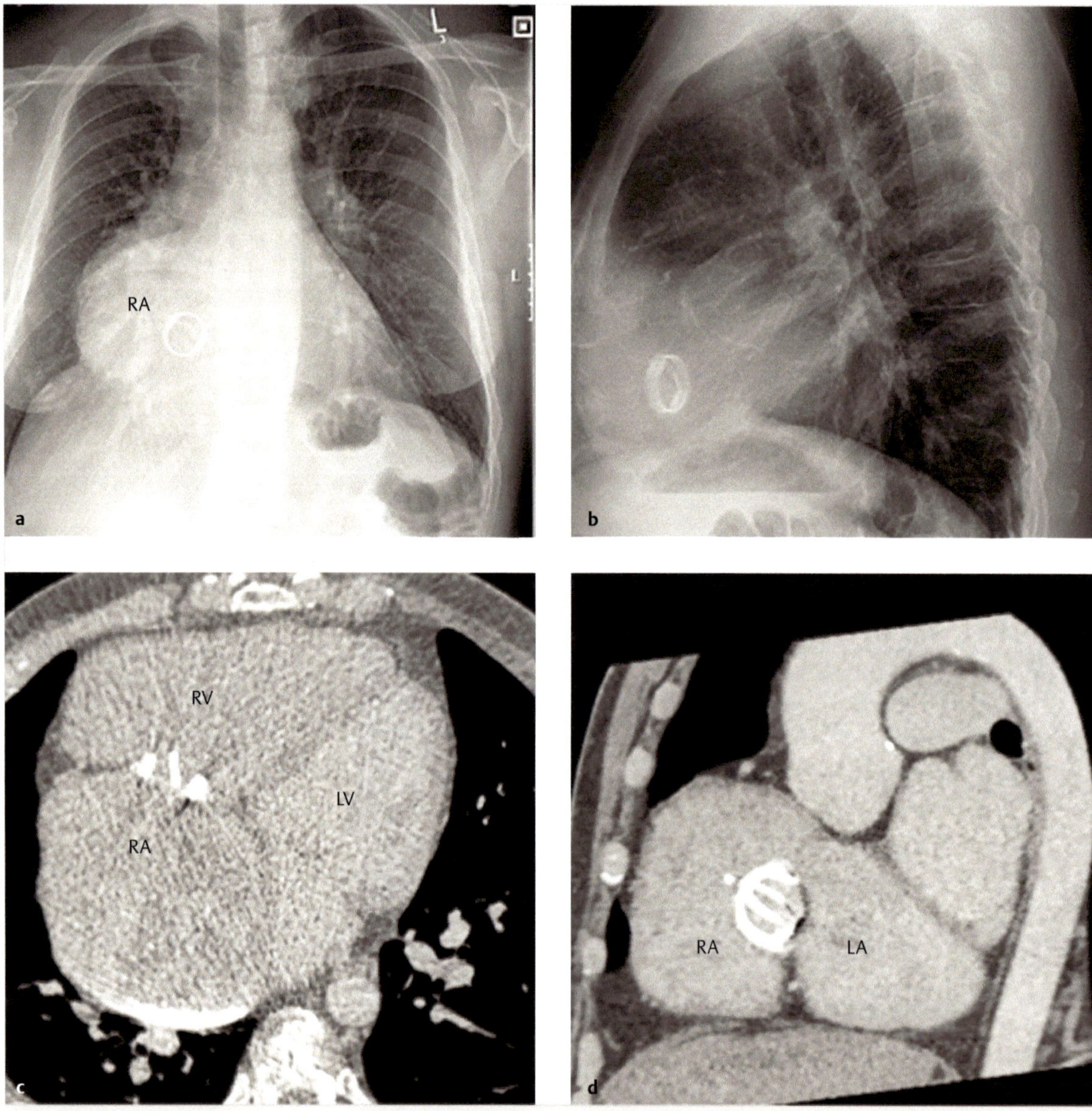

Fig. 4.45 Condition after tricuspid valve replacement, 30 years after surgical correction of tetralogy of Fallot. Fifty-one-year-old male patient after mechanical tricuspid valve replacement. Significantly enlarged right atrium and right ventricle.

LA = left atrium
LV = left ventricle
RA = right atrium
RV = right ventricle

a P.-a. thoracic X-ray.
b Lateral thoracic X-ray.
c Transverse reconstructions from an ECG-triggered MDCT data set (diastolic reconstruction in the 75% RR interval).
d Corresponding angulated sagittal reconstruction near the tricuspid valve replacement. The valve segments opened during diastole are clearly visible.

4.2.3 Pulmonary Atresia with Ventricular Septal Defect and Intact Ventricular Septum

Samir Sarikouch, Matthias Grothoff, Erich Sorantin

Definition

Pulmonary atresia with VSD (approx. 1% of all heart defects[16]) can be described as an extreme variant of tetralogy of Fallot, in which complete closure of the RVOT to the lungs occurs (▶ Fig. 4.42 and ▶ Fig. 4.46). The aorta is displaced similarly to cases of tetralogy of Fallot, and the VSD is generally large. Pulmonary perfusion occurs via the ductus arteriosus or multiple aortopulmonary collaterals, the MAPCAs.[26]

In cases of pulmonary atresia with intact ventricular septum (approx. 0.5–1.0% of all heart defects[16]), complete closure of the RVOT to the lungs also occurs. The blood in the right ventricle cannot drain through a ventricular septal defect. Thus, significant hypoplasia of the right ventricle's greatly thickened walls often occurs in this situation (▶ Fig. 4.47). Associated anomalies of the tricuspid valve are common. Connections may also arise between the right ventricle (which is subjected to significant pressure overload) and the coronary arteries, which further complicates surgical treatment.[27] In both situations, additional atrial septal defects are often present.

Natural Progression and Clinical Issues

The lack of antegrade pulmonary perfusion is common in both types of heart defects. Clinical status after birth is determined primarily based on the type of pulmonary perfusion and the location of the central pulmonary arteries. If a fairly normal pulmonary arterial system is present and pulmonary perfusion occurs mostly via the ductus arteriosus, the duct is held open using prostaglandin. If, as is generally the case, multifocal pulmonary circulation occurs via individual MAPCAs (▶ Fig. 4.42), attempts to hold open the ductus arteriosus are generally unsuccessful. This causes differing pulmonary circulation in the different pulmonary lobes, resulting in the development of heart failure and increased resistance in these pathological vessels.

> **Note**
>
> In cases of pulmonary atresia with intact ventricular septum (▶ Fig. 4.47a), an adequate atrial shunt is of great importance, since this is the only way to reintroduce systemic blood into circulation.

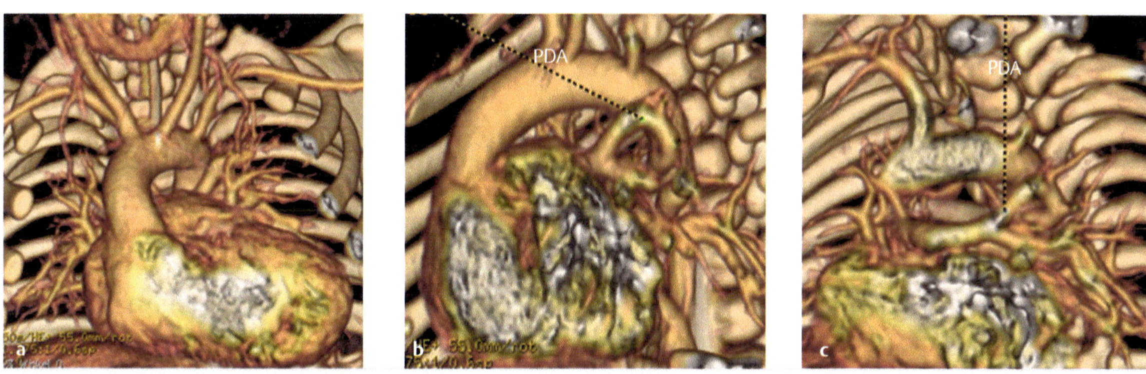

Fig. 4.46 Tetralogy of Fallot and pulmonary atresia. 3-D volume rendering from a non ECG-triggered MDCT data set (acquired using 64 rows) in a newborn with heterotaxia and tetralogy of Fallot accompanied by pulmonary atresia.
PDA = patent ductus arteriosus

a The a.-p depiction shows the left aortic arch and a lack of RVOT.
b Left-lateral projection with a PDA.
c Native peripheral pulmonary vascular system, posterior view (after removing the spinal column and ribs).

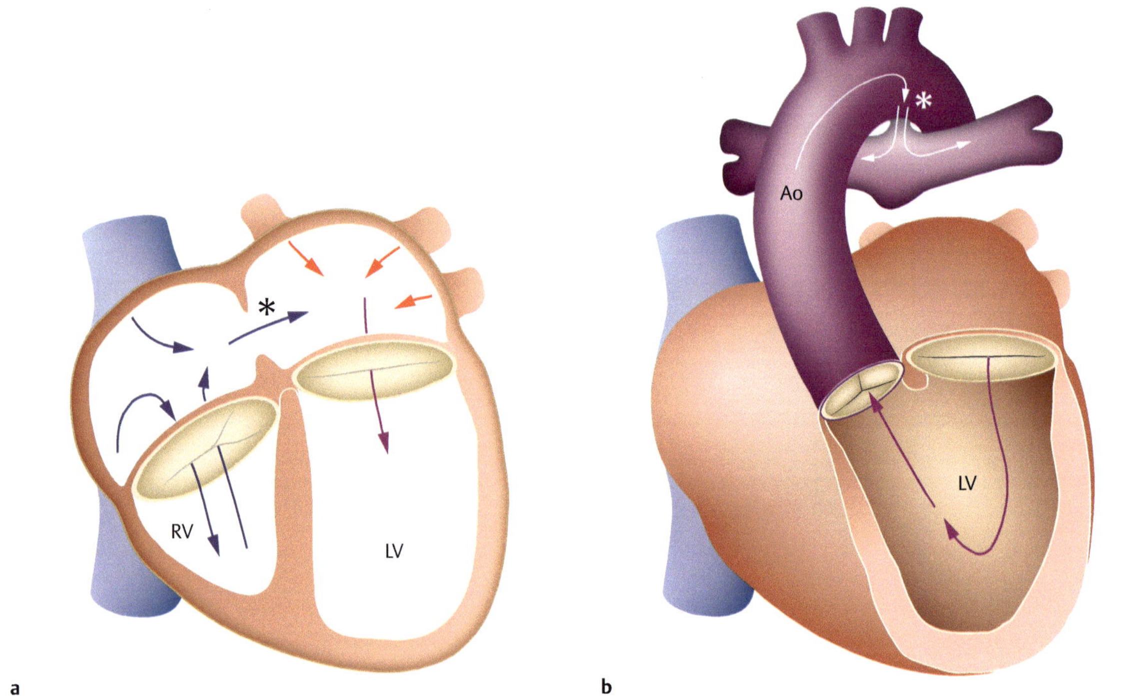

Fig. 4.47 Pulmonary atresia without VSD. Schematic depiction.
Ao = aorta
LV = left ventricle
RV = right ventricle

a Hypoplastic right ventricle with regurgitation via the tricuspid valve and a large ASD (asterisk).
b Pulmonary atresia and filling by mixed venous blood through a PDA.

Treatment Options and Preinterventional Diagnostics

For both types of heart defects, if a membranous pulmonary atresia is present, there is a possibility of antegrade, catheter interventional or surgical opening, provided that the central pulmonary arteries are normal. The presence of a right ventricle that is adequately large or capable of development is a prerequisite for these procedures. Particularly for cases of pulmonary atresia with intact ventricular septum, pronounced hypoplasia in the right ventricle renders biventricular correction impossible. As a result, treatment must take the form of definitive palliation in the sense of Fontan circulation. The sections on HLHS and univentricular heart address this topic in greater detail. If an adequately large ventricle is present, biventricular correction is desirable. If multiple MAPCAs are present, they must be combined surgically (i.e., unifocalized) in order to ensure antegrade pulmonary perfusion after implanting a conduit (valve-equipped [▶ Fig. 4.48] or valve-less) and in order to be able to close the VSD.

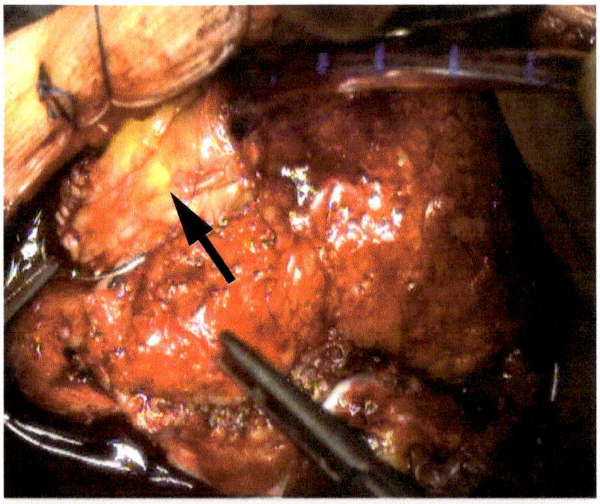

Fig. 4.48 Secondary pulmonary valve replacement using a decellularized homograft (arrow) in a case of pulmonary atresia. The anastomosis on the ventricular side is not yet complete. (With the gracious permission of Dr. Thomas Breymann, Medical School of Hannover.)

Table 4.17 Focus of imaging diagnostics with the value of individual procedures in cases of pulmonary atresia.

Clinical situation	Common diagnostic tasks	Imaging method of choice	Value of imaging method
Preoperative			
Ductal-dependent unifocal pulmonary perfusion	Pulmonary atresia morphology (infundibular, membranous), central pulmonary arteries, ventricular size	Echocardiography	+++
		MRI	++
		CT	++
		Angiography/intervention	++
Multifocal pulmonary perfusion	Aortopulmonary collateral topography, ventricular size	Echocardiography	+++
		MRI	++
		CT	++
		Angiography/intervention	++
Pulmonary atresia in cases of intact ventricular septum	Ventricular size, coronary fistula	Echocardiography	+++
		MRI	++
		CT	++
		Angiography/intervention	++
Postoperative			
Increased right ventricular pressure	Pulmonary arterial stenoses, residual MAPCA	Echocardiography	++
		MRI	+++
		CT	++
		Angiography/intervention	++
Relevant conduit stenosis	Right ventricular hypertrophy	Echocardiography	++
		MRI	+++
		CT	++
		Angiography/intervention	++
Relevant insufficiency	Right ventricular size and function, pulmonary valve insufficiency, tricuspid valve insufficiency	Echocardiography	++
		MRI	+++
		CT	+
		Angiography/intervention	++

CT, computed tomography; MAPCA, major aortopulmonary collateral arteries; MRI, magnetic resonance imaging.

Postoperative and Postinterventional Issues

Stenosis of the consolidated pulmonary arteries often occurs after unifocalization and biventricular correction. In some cases, certain pulmonary areas receive both antegrade perfusion and perfusion from the residual MAPCAs (i.e., double perfusion). Individual pulmonary segments can only be supplied with blood by aortopulmonary collaterals, which elevates the risk of developing pulmonary arterial hypertonia in these areas.[28]

After biventricular correction, cardiac function for the right chamber is determined by frequent pressure elevation due to the newly created central pulmonary vascular system, the sometimes abnormally formed peripheral pulmonary vascular system, and the function of the implanted conduit. The persistence of significant MAPCAs can cause volume overload in the left ventricle.

Goals and Relative Value of Diagnostic Imaging

Doppler TTE is the primary method of choice in preoperative diagnostics, including in cases of pulmonary atresia with and without VSD (▸ Table 4.17). In order to assess aortopulmonary collaterals, additional imaging is often necessary. Imaging procedures can be performed in vasively if interventional measures or additional parameters that can only be acquired via invasive procedures are scheduled, or by means of contrast-enhanced MRA and CTA. If appropriate protocols are used, radiation exposure from CTA can be lower than that from an invasive cardiac catheter examination. The significance of noninvasive cross-sectional imaging becomes most apparent in postoperative follow-up examinations. In this regard, MRI is at the forefront of assessing biventricular volumes, function, muscle mass, and of quantifying residual insufficiency.

4.2.4 Absent Pulmonary Valve

Samir Sarikouch, Matthias Grothoff, Erich Sorantin

Definition

Absent pulmonary valve, a rare congenital disorder, nearly always occurs exclusively in conjunction with tetralogy of Fallot. Only the rudiments of a pulmonary valve have formed, resulting in pronounced pulmonary valve insufficiency (which is even detectable in utero) leading to sometimes massively oversized central pulmonary arteries (▶ Fig. 4.49). Chromosomal anomalies, such as microdeletion 22q11 or DiGeorge syndrome, can be detected in some patients.[29]

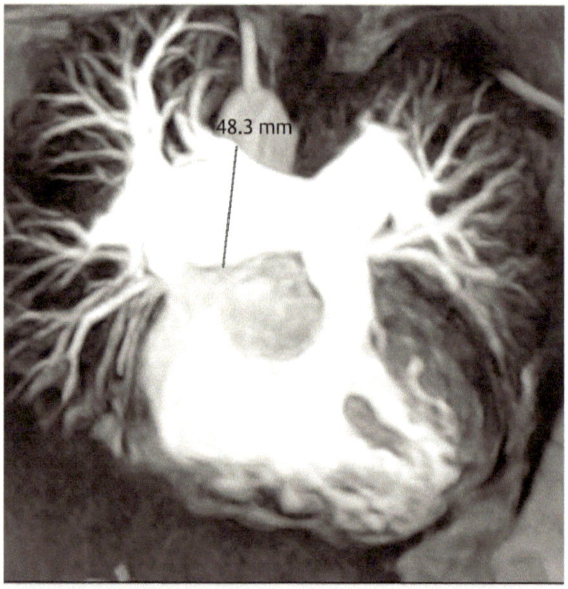

Fig. 4.49 Absent pulmonary valve. 3-D MIP reconstruction of a contrast-enhanced MRA of the pulmonary arteries in an 18-year-old female patient with an absent pulmonary valve. Continual dilatation of the peripheral pulmonary arterial branches, to a maximum of 48.3 mm near the right pulmonary artery, after a corrective surgery in childhood and a secondary pulmonary valve replacement using a decellularized homograft.

Natural Progression and Clinical Issues

An impression of the trachea or bronchus, generally combined with malacia of the bronchial tree, often occurs as a result of this massive enlargement of the central pulmonary arterial segments. Severe obstructive crises can result, requiring continued artificial ventilation.[30] If no serious impairment of the airways is present, heart failure due to pulmonary flooding generally occurs within the first 6 months of life.

Treatment Options and Preinterventional Diagnostics

Impressions of the airways with a persistent need for artificial respiration necessitate surgical treatment in newborns. These treatments not only reduce volume load in the pulmonary arteries by closing the VSD, but also allow the pulmonary valve to be replaced. Surgical reduction of the expanded pulmonary arteries often occurs in conjunction with suspensionplasty in order to decompress the airways.

In cases of mild respiratory involvement, surgical correction is performed within the first 6 months of life, similar to tetralogy of Fallot. Doppler echocardiography, alone, is generally sufficient for determining the diagnosis. In order to assess the impression of the airways, another, more in-depth cross-sectional imaging diagnostic method is used—primarily MDCT with the option for multiplanar reformatting.

Postoperative and Postinterventional Issues

Malacia of the trachea and central bronchi generally persists after surgery and improves at varying rates. Despite surgical reduction of the pulmonary arteries, intraluminal treatment may be required. The airways often remain the focus of postoperative imaging diagnostics. Over time, volume overload in the right chamber after surgical correction without replacement of the pulmonary valve can necessitate a secondary replacement. In cases of primary pulmonary valve replacement, the degeneration of largely biological implants leads to RVOT stenosis, which will later require valve replacement surgical or interventional procedures (▶ Fig. 4.44).

Table 4.18 Focus of imaging diagnostics with the value of individual procedures in cases of absent pulmonary valve.

Clinical situation	Common diagnostic tasks	Imaging method of choice	Value of imaging method
Preoperative			
Need for artificial respiration	Extent and topography of airway compression in relation to the pulmonary arteries	Echocardiography	++
		MRI	++
		CT	+++
		Angiography	+
Heart failure	Right and left ventricular size and function	Echocardiography	++
		MRI	+++
		CT	+
		Angiography	-
Postoperative			
Bronchomalacia	Persistent impression through the pulmonary arteries	Echocardiography	+
		MRI	++
		CT	+++
		Angiography/intervention	+
Neopulmonary valve stenosis	Right ventricular hypertrophy	Echocardiography	+++
		MRI	++
		CT	+
		Angiography/intervention	+
Relevant pulmonary valve insufficiency	Right ventricular size and function, tricuspid valve insufficiency	Echocardiography	++
		MRI	+++
		CT	+
		Angiography/intervention	+

CT, computed tomography; MRI, magnetic resonance imaging.

Goals and Relative Value of Diagnostic Imaging

In addition to primary diagnosis, which can generally be performed via echocardiography, assessing pulmonary arterial size (▶ Fig. 4.49) and their relationship to the trachea and bronchus are the focus of preoperative diagnostics. In addition to MRI, MDCT with the option for multiplanar reformatting can also be used (▶ Table 4.18). In addition to the graduation of residual pulmonary valve insufficiency, right ventricular function, and muscle mass and restenosis near the valve carrying conduit, assessing the respiratory tract and its anatomical relationship to the pulmonary arteries remains an important component of postoperative follow-up care. MRI can be used to this end, with excellent results.

4.2.5 Ebstein's Anomaly

Nicole Nagdyman, Matthias Gutberlet

Definition

Ebstein's anomaly, named after Dr. Wilhelm Ebstein, is an extremely rare congenital heart defect (comprising approximately 0.5% of all congenital heart defects)[31,32] in which the septal and possibly also posterior tricuspid leaflets are displaced apically into the right ventricle (▶ Fig. 4.50). This leads to division of the right ventricle into a basal "atrialized" (non-functional) right ventricle that enlarges the right atrium, and a smaller apical (but functional) right ventricle.

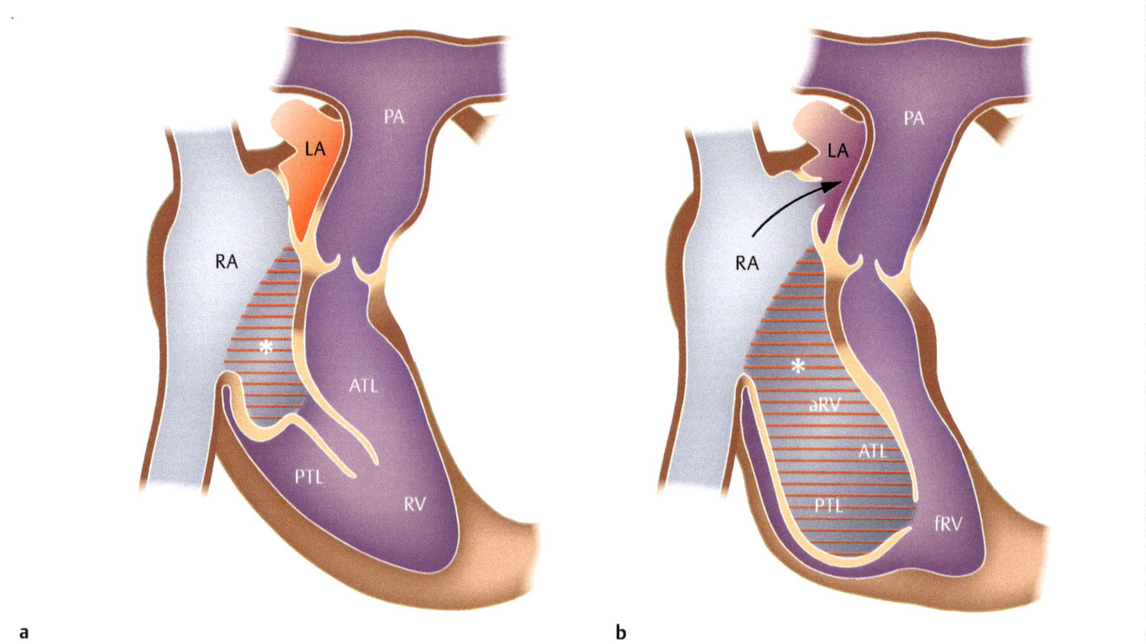

Fig. 4.50 Ebstein's anomaly in varying degrees of severity. Schematic depiction.

aRV = atrialized right ventricle (atrialized, non-functional right ventricle)
ATL = anterior tricuspid leaflet
fRV = functional right ventricle (functional, smaller right ventricle)
LA = left atrium; PA = pulmonary artery
PTL = posterior tricuspid leaflet
RA = right atrium

a Mild form. Minor displacement of the posterior tricuspid leaflet and lengthening of the anterior tricuspid leaflet with the correspondingly atrialized right ventricle (cross-hatched surface, indicated with an asterisk).
b Severe form with concurrent ASD (arrow). Pronounced adhesion of the posterior tricuspid leaflet and subsequent severe diminishment of the functional segment of the right ventricle.

Individual tricuspid leaflets are dysplastic and may possess narrow attachments, with varying degrees of distinctiveness, to the ventricular septum or right ventricular wall. The anterior leaflet is usually elongated (▸ Fig. 4.51; also ▸ Fig. 4.50b), but generally originates near the atrioventricular sulcus. Both genetic predisposition and the concurrent myocardial fibrosis have been described in detail.[33]

Natural Progression and Clinical Issues

Ebstein's anomaly spans a broad clinical spectrum and ranges from cases diagnosed prenatally (with death in utero)[34] to initial manifestations occurring in 80-year-old patients.[35] Ebstein's anomaly occurs predominantly in cases of situs solitus, but also with ccTGA in rare cases. In these instances, the anterior leaflet is often smaller and possesses an additional cleft in 30% of cases.

The hemodynamic effects of Ebstein's anomaly are determined by the size and pumping capacity of the right ventricle, as well as the concurrent valve malfunction, namely tricuspid valve insufficiency. It can, however, also lead to functional stenosis or even atresia. An ASD (▸ Fig. 4.50b) or PFO (▸ Fig. 4.50a) occurs in about 80% of patients.[36] In cases of pronounced tricuspid valve insufficiency or limited right ventricular function, a right–left shunt with cyanosis can occur via the defect (▸ Fig. 4.50b).

Accessory conduction tracts are generally localized around the opening of the malformed valve[37] (e.g., within the scope of Wolff–Parkinson–White syndrome) and are visible in about 20% of patients with Ebstein's anomaly.

Right ventricular dilatation can lead to impairment of the interventricular septum and, subsequently, diastolic disruption of left ventricular filling with a subsequent reduction in left-side pumping capacity. This is depicted in dynamic images as diastolic bulging (▸ Fig. 4.51, ▸ Fig. 4.52, ▸ Fig. 4.53, ▸ Fig. 4.54e, and ▸ Fig. 4.51d).

Under certain circumstances, severe forms of Ebstein's anomaly can be associated with mortality in newborns.[38] Due to the postnatal increase in pulmonary vascular resistance, not much blood flows through the circulatory system, tricuspid valve insufficiency is exacerbated, and patients present with pronounced cyanosis, right heart failure, and limited systemic cardiac output. Tricuspid valve insufficiency causes progressive heart failure that can be associated with hepatomegaly, edema formation, and metabolic acidosis.

Mild forms are often discovered by accident. Moderate forms show the start of limited exercise capacity during adolescence or adulthood, or in cases of concurrent ASD, cyanosis while at rest or when subjected to stress.

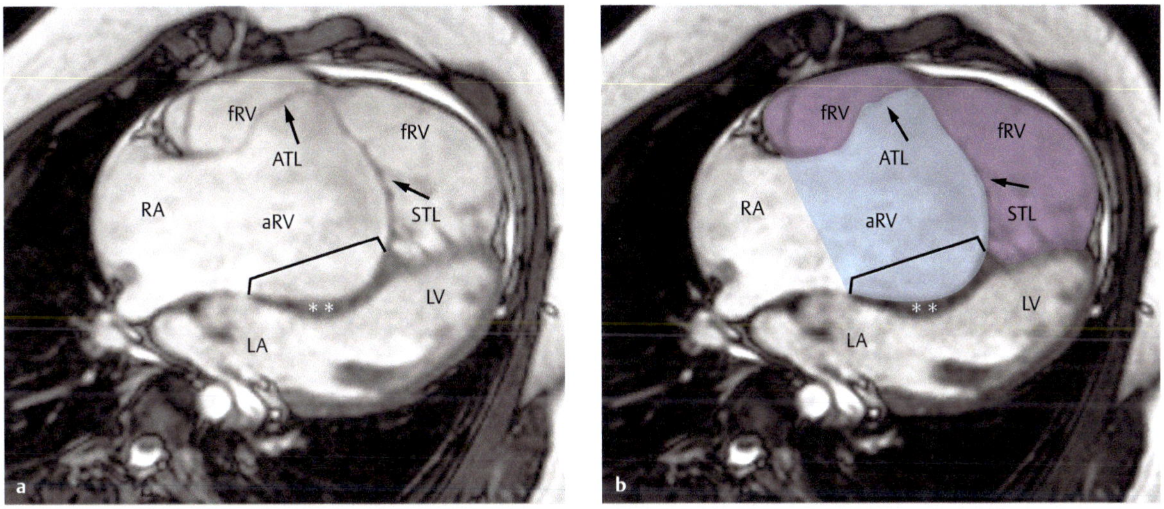

Fig. 4.51 Ebstein's anomaly. The arrows indicate the anterior and septal tricuspid leaflet, respectively.

aRV = atrialized right ventricle (atrialized, non-functional right ventricle)
ATL = anterior tricuspid leaflet
fRV = functional right ventricle (functional, smaller right ventricle)
LA = left atrium
LV = left ventricle
RA = right atrium
STL = septal tricuspid leaflet

a MRI of an adult male patient with no surgical treatment, SSFP cine sequence, 4-chamber view. Significant apical displacement of the septal tricuspid leaflet (distance indicated in square brackets) with pronounced diastolic bulging (double asterisk) in the left ventricle. Though the anterior tricuspid leaflet attaches to the anatomical annulus fibrosus, it is significantly extended and possesses endocardial adhesions near the free wall of the massively enlarged right ventricle.

b Severe case of Ebstein's anomaly, planimetric image. The atrialized portions are light blue and only the very small, functional portion of the right ventricle is depicted in purple.

Various classification systems, such as Carpentier's surgical classification[39] or newborn echocardiographical classification,[38] were developed in order to adapt treatment strategies based on the illness's severity.

Treatment Options and Preinterventional Diagnostics

Patients with mild forms of Ebstein's anomaly often need no treatment for years or even decades, while patients with moderate forms benefit from medication treatment for heart failure once they begin to display signs of limited exercise capacity.

Critically ill newborns with severe forms of Ebstein's anomaly may, under certain circumstances, require prostaglandin E in order to improve pulmonary circulation via the ductus arteriosus and, if needed, supplementary mechanical respiration or catecholamine therapy. It may be necessary to perform a palliative surgery with a final option to separate circulation by a FONTAN operation.[40]

Generally accepted indications for surgery:

- Limited exercise capacity corresponding to NYHA class III
- Pronounced cyanosis
- Development of paradoxic embolisms
- Cardiothoracic ratio of more than 0.65 in X-rays

Various tricuspid valve reconstruction procedures that include reduction (plication) of the atrialized right ventricle have also been described.[39,41,42] Sebening et al. developed a technique that encompassed forming a monocuspid valve while retaining the atrialized ventricular segment[43]—similar to the surgical method developed by Hetzer et al.[44]—in which the atrialized ventricular segment also remains untouched. It is intended to reduce the anatomical tricuspid valve opening, so that the most mobile leaflet (usually the elongated anterior leaflet) finds a contralateral structure for systolic valve closure. In severe cases, a bidirectional shunt or Fontan tunnel can be placed in order to reduce right ventricular overload.[40] The cone technique established by Da Silva et al. is growing more popular.[45] This technique involves removing the anterior leaflet and then mobilizing the septal and posterior portions and plicating the right ventricle in order to construct a new valve apparatus composed entirely of the body's own leaflet tissue.

Patients with symptomatic Wolff–Parkinson–White syndrome should receive an electrophysiological examination with ablation of the accessory tracts. In these cases, however, the success rate is lower, and the risk of recurrence in patients with Ebstein's anomaly is higher than in patients with structurally unremarkable hearts.

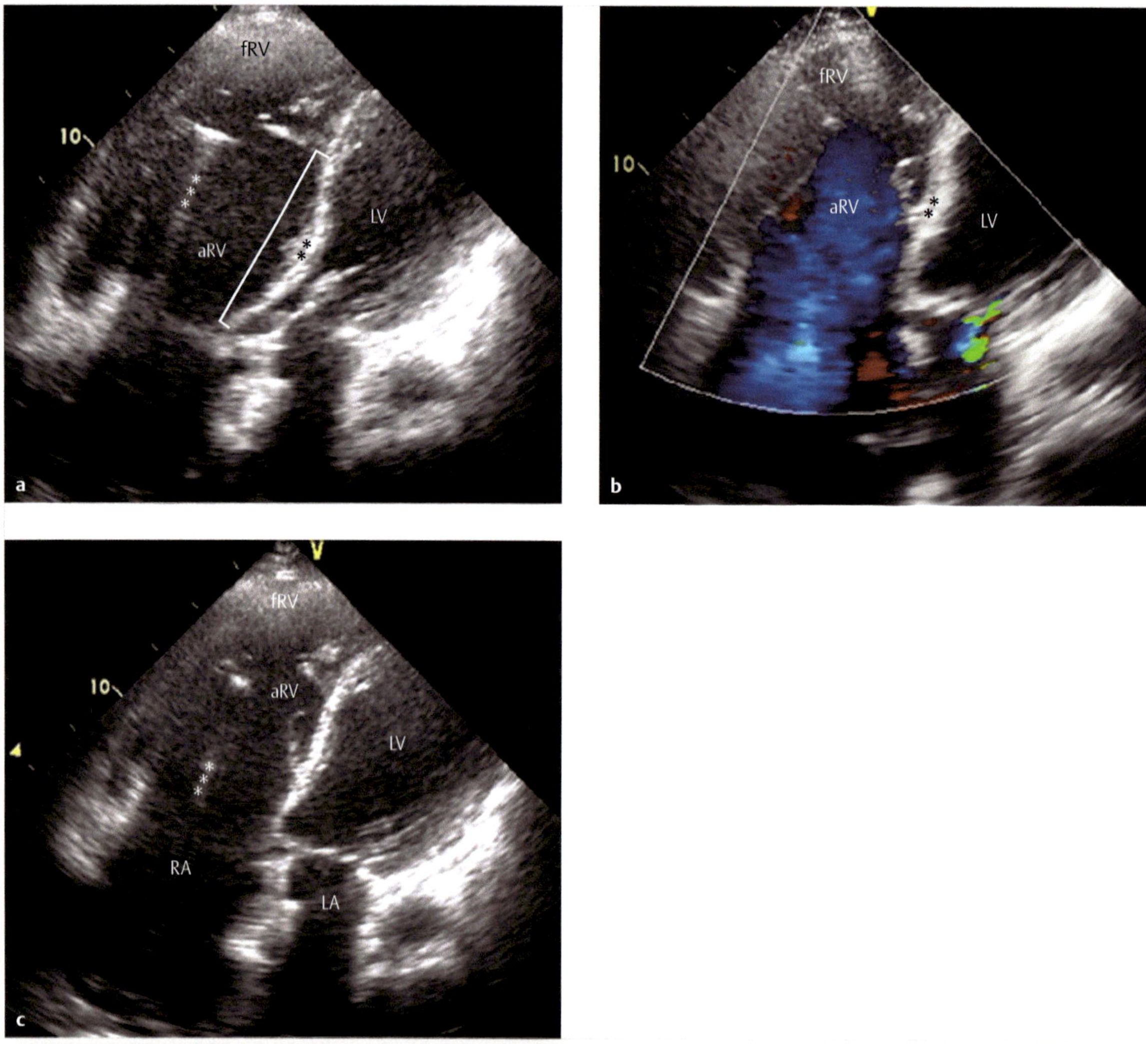

Fig. 4.52 Severe case of Ebstein's anomaly. The triple asterisk indicates the position of a pacemaker lead in the right ventricle.

aRV = atrialized right ventricle (atrialized, non-functional right ventricle)
fRV = functional right ventricle
LA = left atrium
LV = left ventricle
RA = right atrium

a 2-D TTE during diastole, apical 4-chamber view, in a 59-year-old male patient with Ebstein's anomaly and an implanted pacemaker, with no previous surgical correction. Significant apical displacement of the septal tricuspid leaflet (square brackets) with diastolic bulging (**a**, **b**, double asterisk) of the interventricular septum into the left ventricle. Large atrialized right ventricle and relatively small, functional right ventricle.

b Using color Doppler during systole, the 2-D TTE of the same patient shows a pronounced tricuspid valve insufficiency jet (blue) in the atrialized segment of the right ventricle and into the right atrium.

c No septal bulging is visible during systole.

Patients with intermittent or chronic atrial flutter may also benefit from a maze procedure within the scope of valvular surgery. The goal of this surgery, just like interventional ablation, is to interrupt repeated events; switch off spontaneously active, rapidly "firing," stimulation-causing centers; and to reinstate normal pathways and coordinated activation of the atrial muscle tissue.

Note

Since progressive heart failure is a significant risk factor for postoperative fatality, nowadays it seems more beneficial to document and operate on patients during NYHA stage II, before a significant drop in cardiac performance.

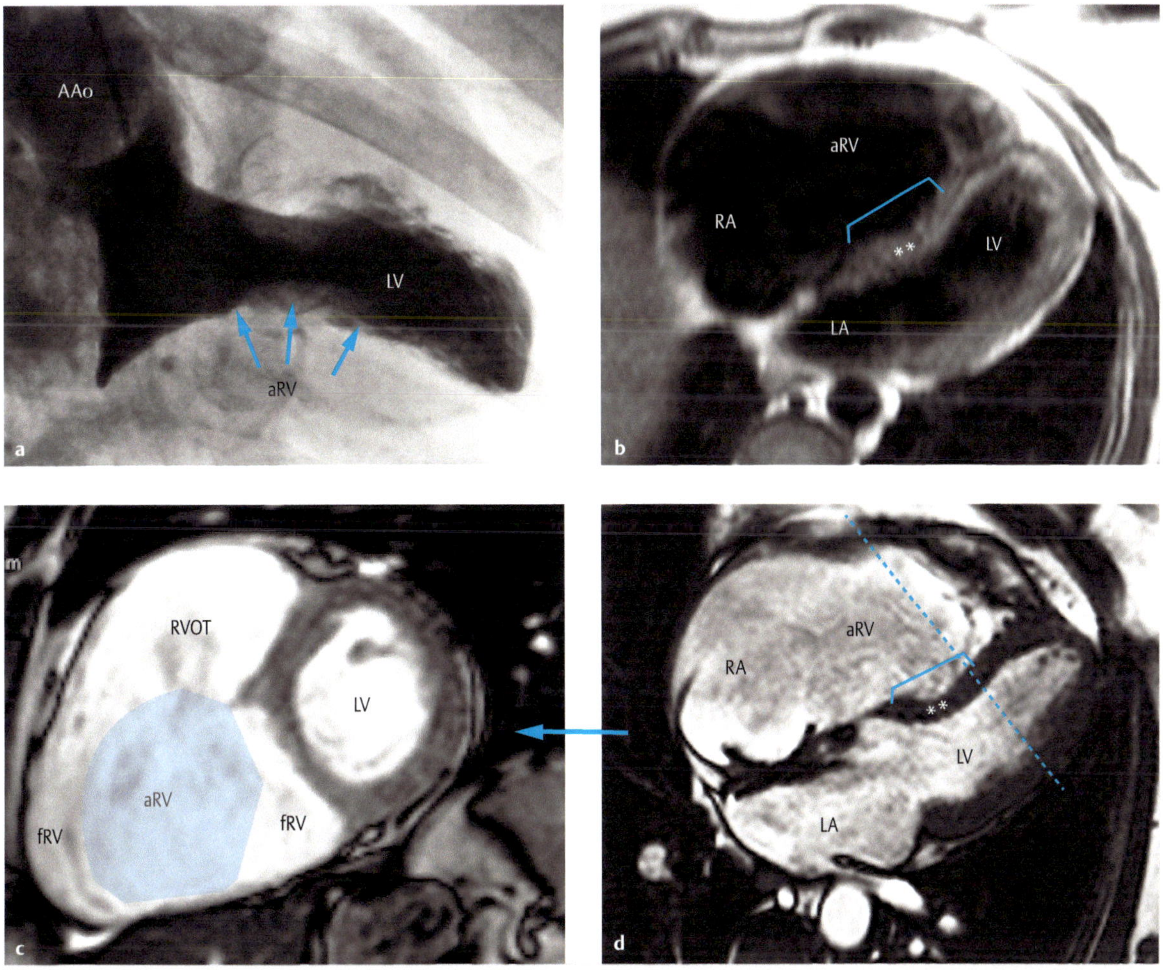

Fig. 4.53 Severe case of Ebstein's anomaly. Forty-two-year-old female with Ebstein's anomaly and no prior surgical treatment. Left ventricle, displaced left dorsally by the atrialized right ventricle during diastole (**a**, arrows). Evidence of diastolic bulging (**b**, **d**, double asterisk) and sectional plane (**d**, dotted line) for the short-axis slice in **c**. The atrialized right ventricular segment and its relation to the functional right ventricle and RVOT is marked schematically (light blue area) in the mid-ventricular short-axis slice (**c**). The square brackets in **b** and **d** indicate the apical displacement of the septal tricuspid leaflet.

AAo = ascending aorta
aRV = atrialized right ventricle (atrialized, non-functional right ventricle)
fRV = functional right ventricle (functional, smaller right ventricle)
LA = left atrium
LV = left ventricle
RA = right atrium
RVOT = right ventricular outflow tract

a Levocardiogram of an invasive cardiac catheter examination during diastole, RAO projection.
b Transverse MRI SE image.
c SSFP cine MRI sequence, mid-ventricular short axis.
d SSFP cine MRI sequence during diastole, 4-chamber view

Postoperative Issues

In the phase immediately after surgery, right ventricular function may initially be so severely limited that catecholamine treatment is unavoidable.

One Mayo Clinic study with a large patient population described right ventricular functional disorders, primarily cardiac rhythm disorders, which resulted in a large rehospitalization rate over the long term.[46] Reoperations for the tricuspid valve are relatively common, both after reconstruction and after successful valve replacement. It remains to be seen whether the cone technique will improve this application.

Goals and Relative Value of Diagnostic Imaging

Echocardiography is the simplest and most widely used procedure (▶ Table 4.19) for diagnosing Ebstein's anomaly (▶ Fig. 4.52). Diagnosis often occurs prenatally via fetal echocardiography. The 4-chamber view in 2-D echocardiography makes it possible to assess the apical displacement of the tricuspid leaflet, its adherence to the wall, and the size of the right ventricle. Special indices allow examiners to assess the extent of the anomaly.[47] Furthermore, an ASD or PFO can be visualized. Color Doppler sonography allows the insufficiency to be depicted, while simple Doppler sonography allows the tricuspid valve stenosis to be visualized (▶ Fig. 4.52b). Shunts (and their orientation) in the atrial region can also be depicted clearly.

3-D ECG can be used to visualize the precise morphology of the tricuspid leaflet or to conduct functional analyses.[48,49]

TEE is used primarily before and after heart surgery. This method emphasizes visualizing the surgically usable leaflet, namely its size, mobility, attachments, and fenestrations. Cardiac and tricuspid valve function (residual insufficiency, ruling out stenosis) are assessed using TEE both during and after surgery.

An invasive *cardiac catheter examination* (▶ Fig. 4.53a) should not be performed until there is suspicion of additional anomalies that cannot be explained via echocardiography or MRI, and is helpful as an electrophysiological examination in the presence of symptomatic accessory pathways.

Table 4.19 Value of individual diagnostic procedures in assessing various aspects of Ebstein's anomaly.

Findings	Echocardiography			P.-a. + thoracic X-ray, lateral	MRI with flow measurement	MDCT, ECG-triggered	Cardiac catheter
	TTE	TEE	3-D				
Morphology of the tricuspid valve apparatus							
Dysplasia and dislocation	high	high	high	-	high	moderate	moderate
Wall adherences	high	high	high	-	high	high	moderate
Tricuspid valve function							
Insufficiency	high	high	moderate	-	high	moderate	moderate
Stenosis	high	high	-	-	high	moderate	high
Size of cardiac compartments							
Right atrium	high	high	high	moderate	high	high	moderate
Right ventricle (including atrialized ventricle)	moderate	high	moderate to high	moderate	high	high	moderate
Left ventricle (including paradoxical septal motion)	high	high	high	moderate	high	high	high
Left atrium	high	high	high	moderate	high	high	moderate
Function of cardiac compartments							
Right ventricle	moderate	high	high	–	high	moderate	high
Left ventricle	high	high	high	–	high	moderate	high

CT, computed tomography; MRI, magnetic resonance imaging; TEE, transesophageal echocardiography; TTE, transthoracic echocardiography.

> **Note**
>
> In cases of cyanosis while at rest or under stress in mild cases of tricuspid valve insufficiency, interventional closure of the ASD (▶ Fig. 4.54) should be discussed. During the intervention, however, it must be ensured that the closure will not in any way impair ventricular function.

The *X-ray examination* depicts the characteristic, Franconian wine bottle shape of the heart's silhouette (▶ Fig. 4.54a and b), which develops primarily as a result of right atrial dilatation. A cardiothoracic ratio of more than 0.65 is associated with worse prognoses.[50]

In recent years, *MRI* has gained a great deal of traction as a noninvasive procedure in preoperative diagnostics (▶ Table 4.19).[51,52] In cases of very complex 3-D anatomy, MRI yields accurate information regarding the size and function of the atrialized and functional segments of the right ventricle, as well as extremely helpful information on the morphology of the displaced tricuspid leaflets (▶ Fig. 4.51 and ▶ Fig. 4.53). As a result, MRI has become a crucial information source for surgical planning. In addition, it is possible to perform absolute quantification of tricuspid valve insufficiency and shunt volume in cases of concurrent ASD or PFO, using a combination of volumetric analysis of the right atrium and ventricle, and MRI flow measurement using the phase contrast technique.[53-55] Planning the cine MRI sequence in transverse slices is especially helpful for precise planimetric analysis of the atrialized and functional segments of the right ventricle (▶ Fig. 4.51).

CT is used only rarely in patients with Ebstein's anomaly, both due to radiation exposure and to the generally good image quality yielded by echocardiography and MRI examinations.[56] In patients that are difficult to image and for whom MRI examinations are contraindicated (such as those with cardiac pacemakers), CT remains a viable alternative (▶ Fig. 4.54). Volumetric and functional analysis of the right ventricle can also be performed in conjunction with MDCT, though this results in worse temporal resolution.

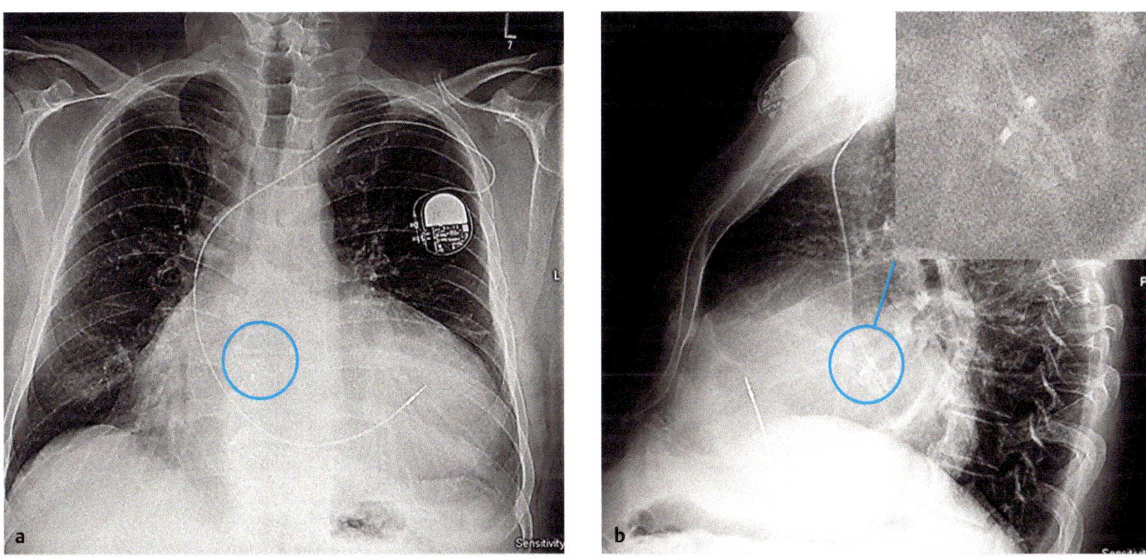

Fig. 4.54 Ebstein's anomaly with concurrent ASD. Fifty-nine-year-old female patient with no previous surgical treatment, with Ebstein's anomaly and an ASD that was closed using an atrial occlusion device (**a**, **b**, blue circle). Multiplanar reformats of a MDCT data set are visible in **c–f**. The triple asterisk (**e**, **f**) indicates the occlusion device. In addition, artifacts of the pacemaker lead in the right ventricle are visible in each reformat (**c–f**, asterisk). The atrialized portion (light blue area) and functional segment of the right ventricle (pale red area) are marked schematically in all orientations (**c–e**).

aRV = atrialized right ventricle (atrialized, non-functional right ventricle)
fRV = functional right ventricle (functional, smaller right ventricle)
LA = left atrium
LV = left ventricle
RA = right atrium

a P.-a. X-ray. Typical "Bocksbeutel" (Franconian wine bottle) shape of the heart caused by enlargement of the right atrium and ventricle.
b Lateral X-ray. Enlarged depiction of the atrial septal occlusion device.

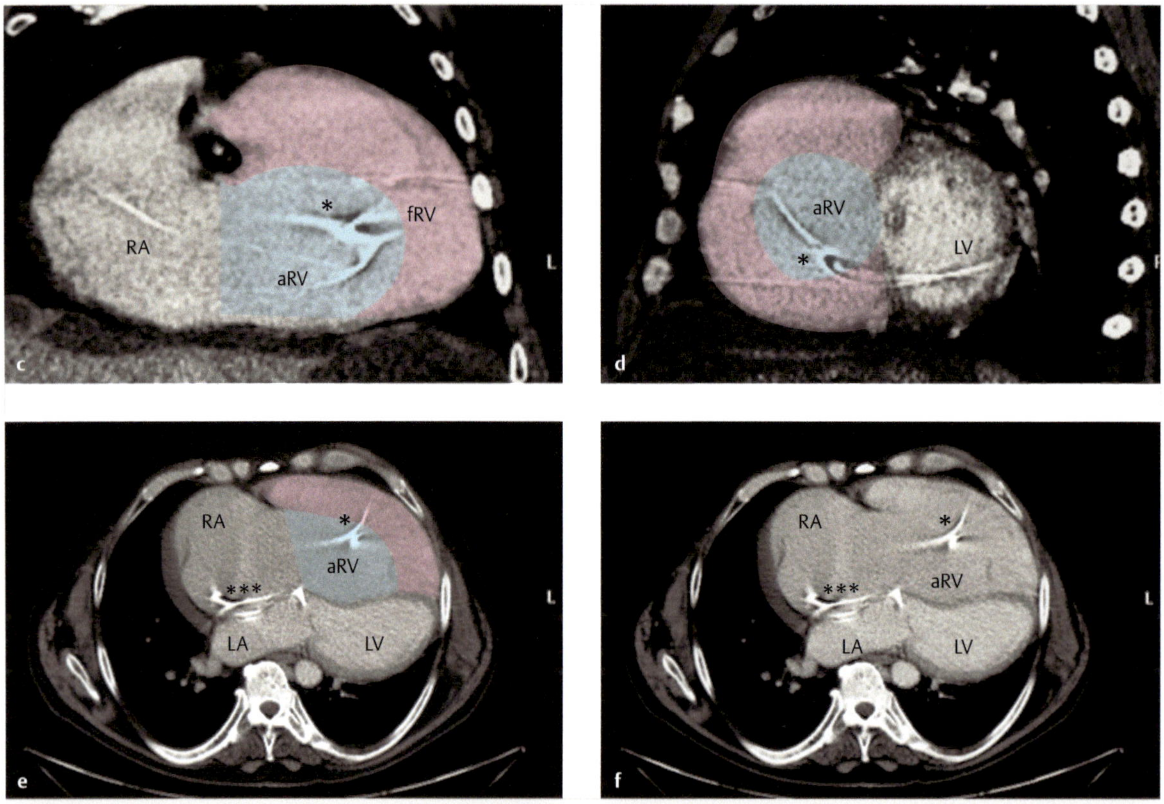

Fig 4.54 (*Continued*) **Ebstein's anomaly with concurrent ASD.**

aRV = atrialized right ventricle (atrialized, non-functional right ventricle)
fRV = functional right ventricle (functional, smaller right ventricle)
LA = left atrium
LV = left ventricle
RA = right atrium

c Coronal reformat from an MDCT data set.
d Sagittal reformat from an MDCT data set.
e Transverse reformat from an MDCT data set marking the atrialized, non-functional right ventricle and the functional, smaller right ventricle.
f Transverse reformat from an MDCT data set during diastole, without marking. Significant bulging of the interventricular septum into the left ventricle is visible.

4.3 Left-Side Defects

4.3.1 Subaortic Stenosis, Valvular Aortic Stenosis, and Supravalvular Aortic Stenosis

Joachim Lotz, Joachim G. Eichhorn, Michael Steinmetz

Definition

Stenoses near the LVOT can take the form of subvalvular, valvular, or supravalvular aortic stenoses (▶ Fig. 4.55). Aortic coarctation is a special form of aortic stenosis. These stenoses are similar, in that they lead to increased afterload in the left ventricle. They can occur in isolation or in conjunction with other defects.

Classification

Subvalvular Aortic Stenosis

In cases of isolated subvalvular aortic stenosis, a fibrous membrane or fibromuscular ring is generally located below the aortic valve (▶ Fig. 4.56; also ▶ Fig. 4.55a). In rare cases, muscular bulging occurs in isolation near the septum, accessory mitral valve tissue, or a malformed mitral valve apparatus as a result of subaortic stenosis. In cases of HOCM, muscular subaortic stenoses can also occur due to asymmetrical septal hypertrophy with potential obstruction near the LVOT.

Shone's complex, defined as a combination of subaortic stenosis with an abnormal mitral valve and an aortic coarctation, should be regarded as a special form of subaortic stenosis.

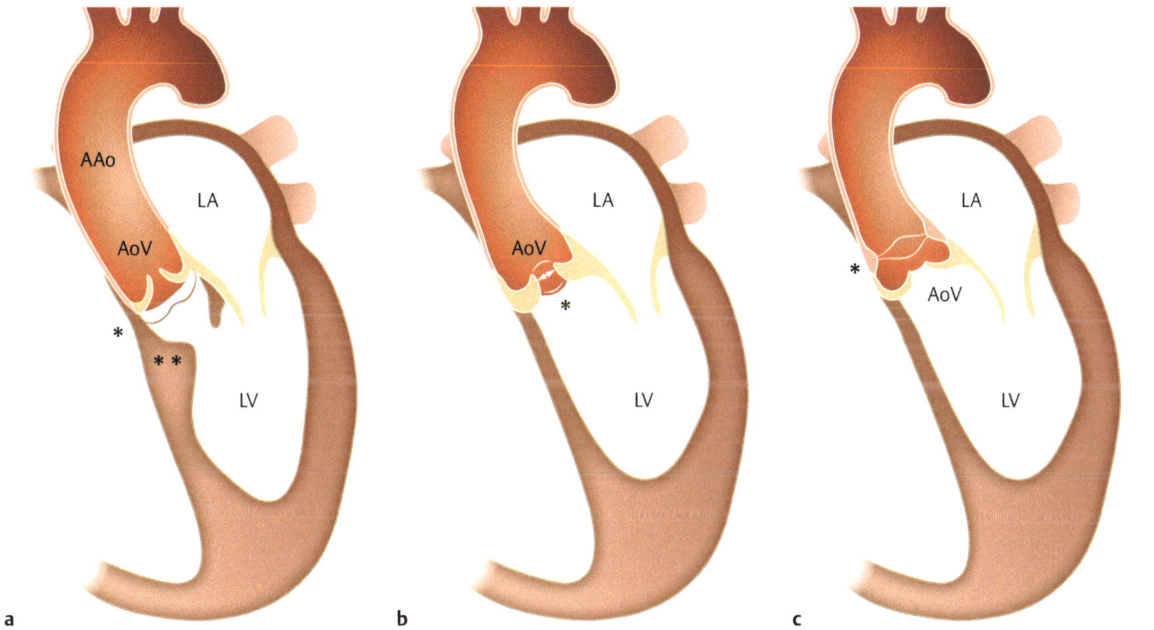

Fig. 4.55 Various forms of aortic stenoses. Schematic depiction.

AAo = ascending aorta
AoV = aortic valve
LA = left atrium
LV = left ventricle.

a Subvalvular stenosis with subvalvular membrane (asterisk) and subvalvular muscular bulge (double asterisk) in the LVOT.
b Valvular aortic stenosis (asterisk) with thickened semilunar valve.
c Supravalvular aortic stenosis with supravalvular membrane (asterisk).

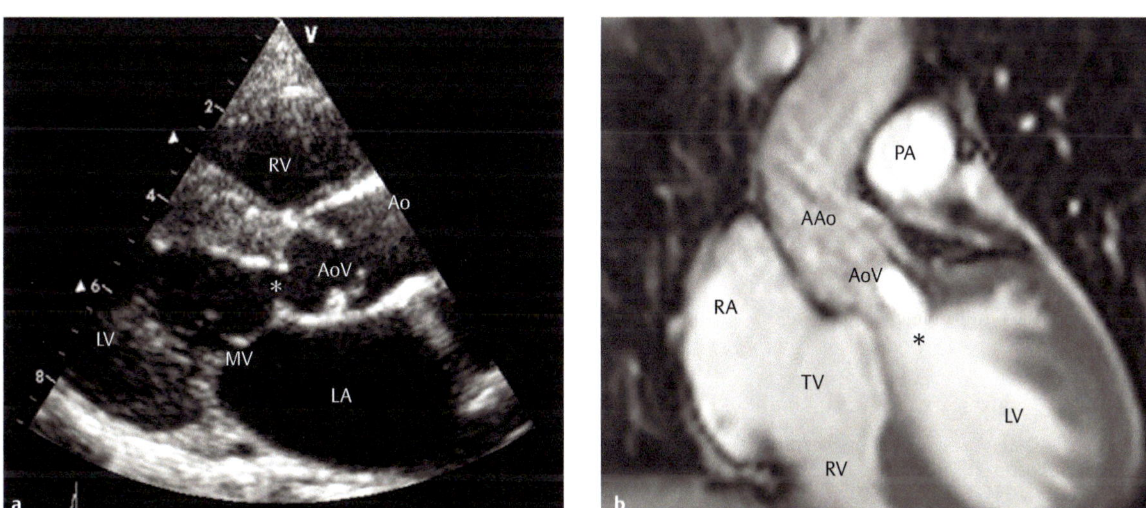

Fig. 4.56 Subvalvular aortic stenosis. Two different patients.

AAo = ascending aorta
AoV = aortic valve
LA = left atrium
LV = left ventricle
MV = mitral valve
PA = pulmonary artery
RA = right atrium
RV = right ventricle
TV = tricuspid valve

a 2-D TTE image, parasternal long axis, of a patient with subvalvular aortic stenosis (asterisk), clearly depicting the bilateral subvalvular membrane in the LVOT, inferior to the opening aortic valve.
b SSFP cine MRI, coronary section, of another patient with subvalvular aortic stenosis (asterisk), depicting both the subvalvular membrane and dephasing jet during systole, rendered visible by flow acceleration in the LVOT.

Subvalvular aortic stenoses are often components of complex cardiac abnormalities (DORV, malalignment VSD, etc.). Thirty-seven percent of patients with an isolated subvalvular aortic stenosis also possess a perimembranous VSD. Corrective surgeries (e.g., in cases of VSD, AVSD, complex defects) can also cause a secondary subaortic stenosis to form.

Aortic Valve Stenosis

In aortic valve stenosis (▶ Fig. 4.55b) the aortic valve generally opens incompletely due to congenital or acquired thickening or merging of individual cusps. An undersized valve ring is another potential cause. Congenital or functional bicuspid valves that do not open fully due to merging of the commissures (raphe formation) remain the most common cause (▶ Fig. 4.57 and ▶ Fig. 4.58).

A distinction is made between the following forms (▶ Fig. 4.58):

- true bicuspid valve with only two sinuses, and generally two semilunar valves of the same size, and
- the much more common "bicuspidalized" aortic valve which, from an anatomical perspective, possesses three sinuses and three semilunar valves, two of which are merged via a thickening (known as a raphe), meaning that these valves are generally of two different sizes.

Pathological and anatomical specimens also show a rudimentary third cusp, even when imaging apparently bicuspid valves.

Bicuspid aortic valve often occurs in conjunction with an aortic coarctation. Monocuspid valves can also occur. The cusps may also thicken in cases of congenital or acquired valve dysplasia (e.g., after rheumatic fever). This can also lead to valves being unable to open fully. In extreme cases, the valve cannot be defined, and appears perforated. The degree of severity of aortic stenosis is classified in accordance with ▶ Table 4.20.

> **Note**
>
> Aortic coarctation is often concurrent with a bicuspid aortic valve.

Critical aortic stenosis in newborns is its own independent entity. In these cases, systemic circulation perfusion remains dependent on the arterial duct, even postnatally. If untreated, critical aortic stenosis can lead to acute heart failure and left ventricular decompensation postnatally. Prenatally, it can lead to the development of endocardial fibroelastosis or hypoplastic left heart syndrome (HLHS).

Supravalvular Aortic Stenosis

Supravalvular aortic stenosis (▶ Fig. 4.59 and ▶ Fig. 4.60; also ▶ Fig. 4.55c) can occur in isolation or in conjunction with other defects. Most commonly, hourglass-shaped stenoses are found near the sinotubular junction, while more extensive stenoses, hypoplasia of the aorta as a whole, or membranous forms occur in rarer cases.

A histological examination nearly always reveals a change in media formation or collagen or elastic fibers, meaning that the aortic wall is less elastic and Windkessel function is limited. The distal segments of the commissures are affected, which may result in limited mobility. This can lead to coronary displacement or stenoses caused by atypical cusps. In certain cases, stenoses may also occur in the vessels originating from the aorta. A combination of subvalvular and supravalvular aortic stenoses is common. Various syndromes are associated with supravalvular aortic valve stenosis: Perhaps the best known is Williams–Beuren syndrome. Supravalvular aortic stenoses can, however, also occur in cases of genetic aortic disease (elastic gene mutation), in cases of genetic hypercholesterinemia, and other genetic disorders.[58]

Hemodynamics

An obstruction of the LVOT, aortic valve, or ascending aorta increases afterload in the left ventricle, leading to consecutive hypertrophy and, as it progresses, to limited contractility. This is directly dependent on the degree of stenosis and the pressure gradients that must be overcome in the left ventricle. In addition, flow acceleration and turbulence of the blood near and distal to the stenosis (▶ Fig. 4.61) can occur. These phenomena can be visualized clearly, particularly when using 4-D flow measurement.

Clinical Issues

Cases of isolated subvalvular or supravalvular aortic stenosis often do not present clinical symptoms for a long time. More severe stenoses can be associated with limited exercise capacity up to manifest heart failure with pulmonary edema. In rare cases, syncope or the symptoms of angina pectoris may occur. From an auscultatory viewpoint, a harsh crescendo systolic murmur can be heard with a maximum point above the second-left intercostal space and radiating into the carotid arteries.

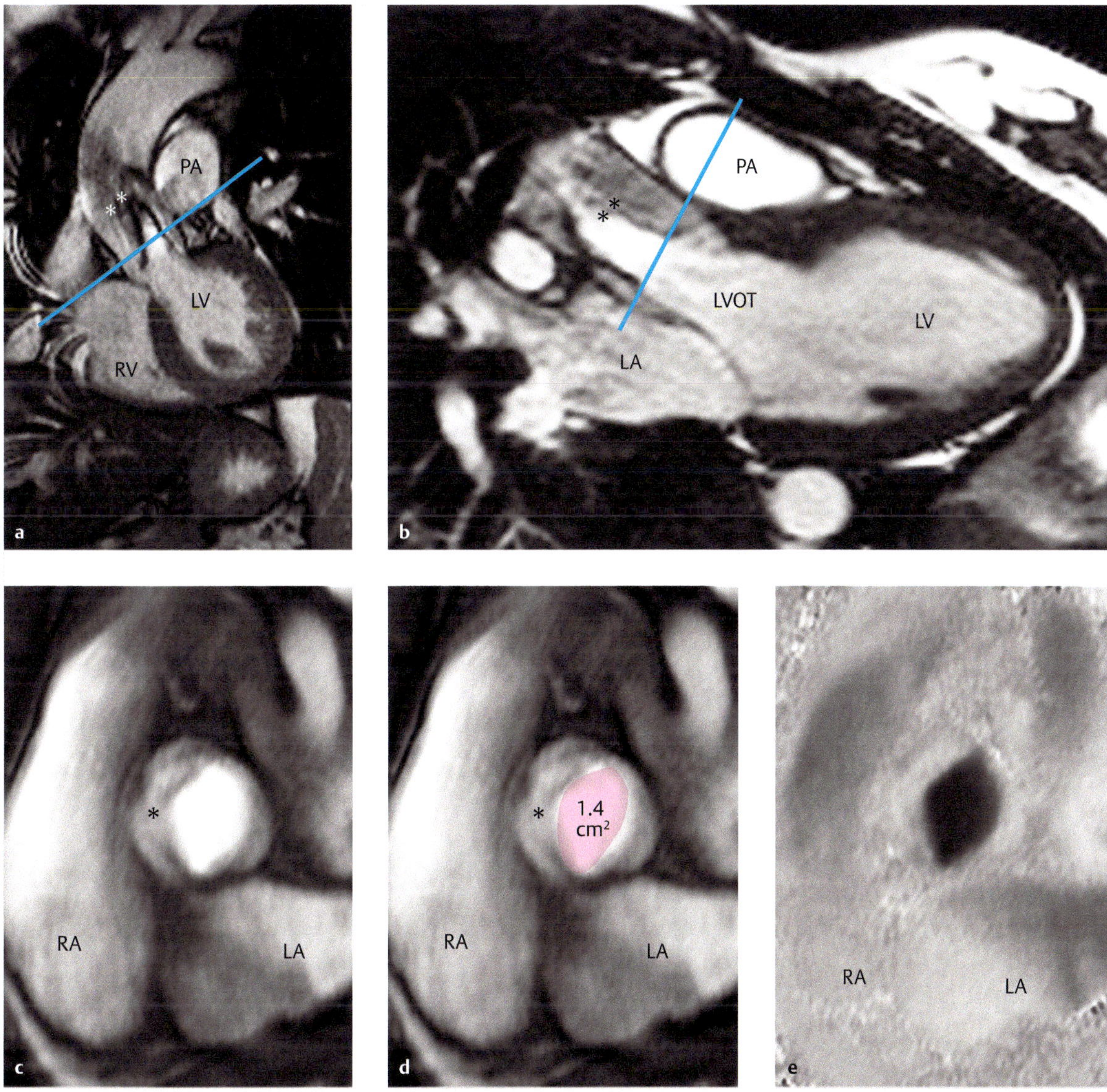

Fig. 4.57 Isolated, congenital "bicuspidalized" type 1 N/R aortic valve and moderate stenosis. (▸ Fig. 4.58). Twenty-five-year-old male patient. A maximum instantaneous pressure gradient of 30 mmHg was estimated using doppler echocardiography. The patient exhibited no clinical symptoms.

LA = left atrium
LV = left ventricle
LVOT = left ventricular outflow tract
PA = pulmonary artery
RA = right atrium

- **a** Coronal SSFP cine MRI during systole, with a fully opened aortic valve and signal loss caused by dephasing (double asterisk) in a case of turbulent flow due to flow acceleration. The blue line indicates the sectional plane for **c–e** for depiction and planimetric analysis of the aortic valve.
- **b** LVOT image corresponding to **a**. Here, the blue line also indicates the sectional plane for **c–e** for the depiction and planimetric analysis of the aortic valve.
- **c** Magnitude image of through-plane flow measurement (section in accordance with the blue lines in **a** and **b**) of the fully opened bicuspid aortic valve with a maximum valve opening area of 1.4 cm^2 (**d**). The three sinuses and the raphe (asterisk) between the right coronary and non-coronary cusp are visible in **c** and **d**.
- **d** The maximum valve opening area in systole is depicted as the red area in planimetric measurements. This can, in principle, also be performed in the phase image (**e**).
- **e** Phase image corresponding to **c**. Cranial flow is depicted in black. The maximum measured flow velocity in MRI was 3.1 m/s in the sense of an estimated maximum instantaneous pressure gradient of 38 mmHg.

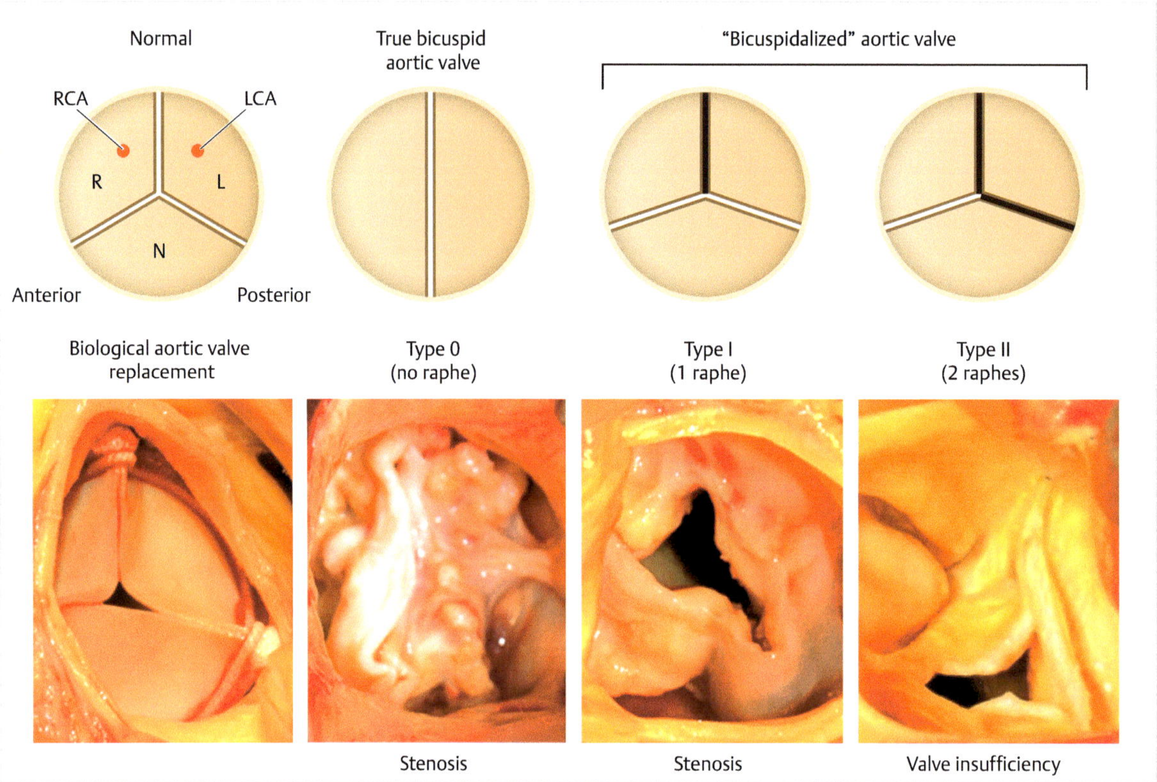

Fig. 4.58 Classification of bicuspid and "bicuspidalized" aortic valves. Schematic depiction of classification (top)[57] with the corresponding intraoperative examples and pathologies (bottom). Note: In cases of true bicuspid aortic valve, both valves are usually the same size and only two sinuses exist. In cases of "bicuspidalized" aortic valve, the semilunar valves are merged via one or two raphes (black) and possess three sinuses. (Intraoperative images with the gracious permission of Dr. E. Girdauskas, Cardiac Surgery Clinic, Bad Berka Central Hospital.)

L = left coronary cusp
LCA = left coronary artery
N = non-coronary cusp
R = right coronary cusp
RCA = right coronary artery

Table 4.20 Classification of the degree of severity of aortic valve stenosis. Classification based on pressure gradients can also be applied to subvalvular and supravalvular aortic stenoses.[61]

Degree of severity	Cardiac catheter peak gradient (mmHg)	CW Doppler v_{max} (m/s)	Bernoulli maximum instantaneous gradient (mmHg)	Bernoulli mean instantaneous gradient (mmHg)	Echo aortic valve orifice area (cm²)
Trivial					
Minor	< 30	< 3	< 36	< 25	> 1.5 (> 1 cm²/m²)
Moderate	30–50	3–4	36–64	25–40	1.0–1.5 (0.6–1.0 cm²/m²)
Severe	> 50	> 4	> 64	> 40	< 1.0 (< 0.6 cm²/m²)

CW, continuous wave.

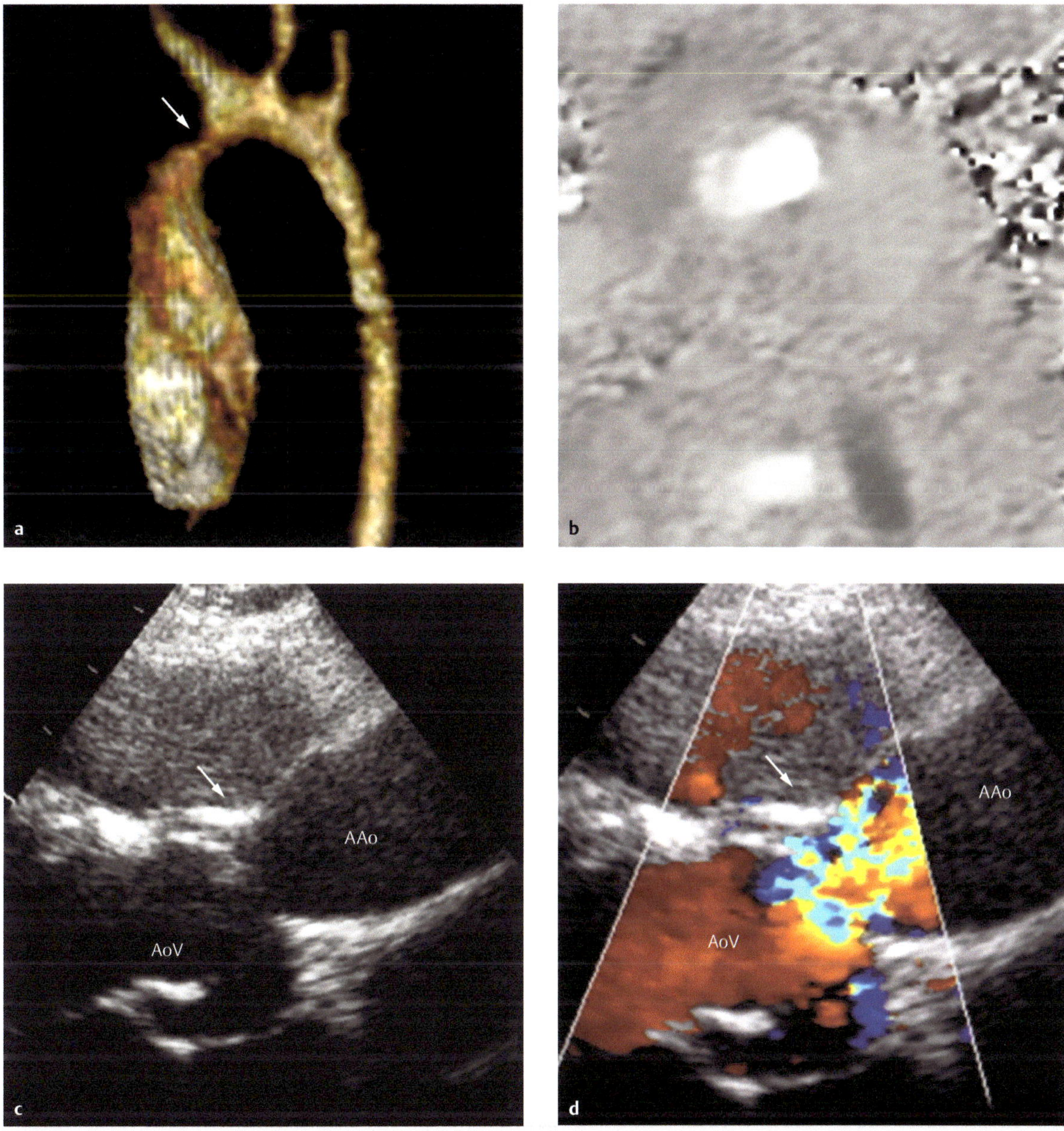

Fig. 4.59 Supravalvular aortic stenosis. Two patients. Two-month-old infant with hypoplastic aortic arches, condition after surgical reconstruction of the aortic arch (**a**, **b**). Residual stenosis near the ascending aorta (**a**, arrow). A 2-D TTE image, parasternal long axis, of another patient with supravalvular aortic stenosis (**c**, **d**) clearly shows the supravalvular membrane (arrows) and flow acceleration in color Doppler.

AAo = ascending aorta
AoV = aortic valve

a 3-D reconstruction of a contrast-enhanced MRA for a supravalvular aortic stenosis, angulated sagittal orientation, along the aortic arch.

b Through-plane acquisition of a phase contrast image, depicting slightly increased cranial flow in white. The maximum measured flow velocity was 2.5 m/s, corresponding to an estimated maximum instantaneous pressure gradient of 25 mmHg. Flow velocity was 1.1 m/s proximal to the stenosis in the ascending aorta.

c 2-D TTE depiction of a supravalvular aortic stenosis (arrow), parasternal long axis, without a color Doppler signal.

d 2-D TTE of a supravalvular aortic stenosis (arrow), parasternal long axis, with color Doppler signal and corresponding flow acceleration.

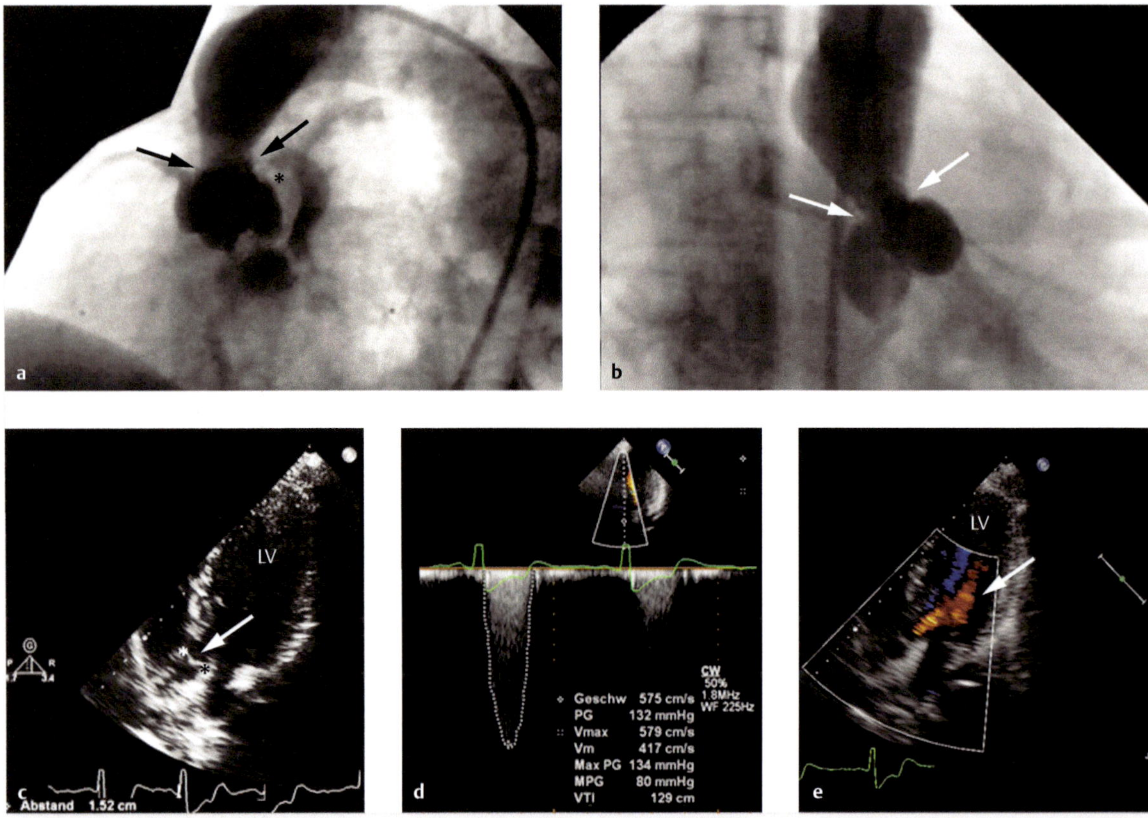

Fig. 4.60 Combined valvular and supravalvular aortic stenosis and left and right coronary artery origin stenoses. Seventeen-year-old female patient with a mutation in the elastin gene and dysplastic aortic valve syndrome. The arrows in **a** and **b** indicate the supravalvular aortic stenosis, and the asterisk in **a** indicates the origin stenoses in the left coronary artery.
LV = left ventricle

- **a** Cardiac catheter examination with angiography of the ascending aorta, LAO projection. The peak pressure gradient, measured invasively, corresponded to 100 mmHg.
- **b** Cardiac catheter examination with angiography of the ascending aorta, RAO projection.
- **c** Corresponding 2-D TTE image, 5-chamber view, depicting a small aortic valve with a diameter of 15 mm (arrow), corresponding to less than two standard deviations from the standard based on body surface area.
- **d** Significant flow acceleration to a maximum of 5.8 m/s in CW-Doppler, with an estimated mean pressure gradient of 80 mmHg and a maximum of 134 mmHg.
- **e** Color Doppler depiction (arrow) of the concurrent aortic valve insufficiency.

Natural Progression and Indication for Treatment

Pronounced subvalvular and supravalvular aortic stenoses are generally progressive. Less pronounced forms can, however, remain unchanged for many years.[59] They usually are not present at birth, but rather develop during the first few years of life. In rare cases, fetal or neonatal subaortic stenoses occur in conjunction with endocardial fibroelastosis and a hypoplastic left ventricle. Aortic valve insufficiency can also occur in conjunction with the initial stenoses, primarily in cases of progressive ectasia of the ascending aorta.

Indication for treatment is determined based on the guidelines of the Germany Association for Pediatric Cardiology[60,61] for cases of isolated subvalvular, valvular, or supravalvular aortic stenoses with a median Doppler gradient > 40 mmHg, a valve opening area < 1 cm^2, or a peak-to-peak pressure gradient (measured invasively) > 50 mmHg (▸ Table 4.20). Independent of gradients, treatment is indicated under the following conditions:

- development of complaints (i.e., heart failure, angina pectoris)
- progressive left ventricular dilation or reduced left ventricular function
- new or progressive aortic valve insufficiency
- ECG repolarization disorders

In cases of combined subaortic stenosis associated with other cardiac abnormalities, the overall findings are decisive when making treatment decisions.[60,61]

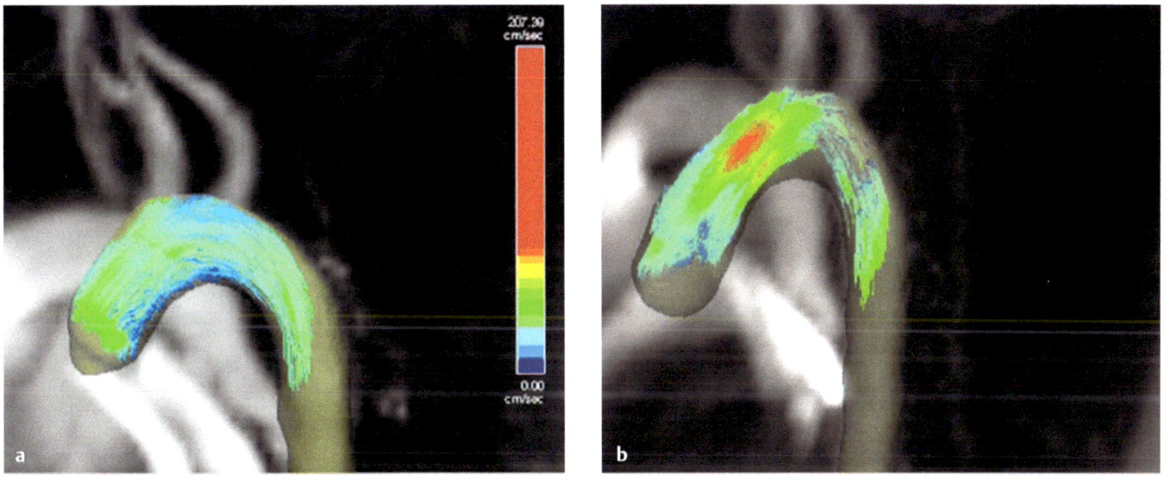

Fig. 4.61 Tricuspid and bicuspidalized aortic valve. 4-D MR flow measurement in an animal model.
a Normal tricuspid aortic valve.
b Bicuspidalized aortic valve. In addition to flow acceleration, turbulence is occurring near the ascending aorta.

Treatment Options and Diagnostics

In addition to echocardiography, cardiac MRI, or cardiac CT, diagnostic procedures—especially in cases of complex defects—include invasive cardiac catheter examinations (▶ Fig. 4.60). Morphology and valvular or ventricular function remain the focus[62] of these procedures. For noninvasive procedures, doppler echocardiography and MRI best address both topics. Both modalities can provide either planimetric estimates or indirect estimates of maximum instantaneous pressure gradients via the stenosis, with the help of flow measurement and the Bernoulli equation. If precise invasive pressure gradient measurement is needed, or if it is necessary to depict the coronaries or even to perform simultaneous treatment, then invasive cardiac catheter examinations are the method of choice (▶ Fig. 4.60).

In cases of subvalvular aortic stenosis, treatment consists of surgically resecting the fibrous ring, with or without myectomy. In rare cases, patch reconstruction of the LVOT (also known as the Konno procedure) is necessary in cases in which tunnel-shaped stenoses are present.[63] The risk of recurrence in cases of simple resection is 20% within 10 years.[64] Purely interventional treatment using balloon valvuloplasty has achieved good results thus far in cases of subvalvular aortic stenosis.[65]

Valvular and sometimes also supravalvular aortic stenoses, on the other hand, can often be treated using purely interventional procedures, such as balloon valvuloplasty.[66] In cases of valvular aortic stenoses, however, there is a risk of aortic valve insufficiency developing as a result of the intervention, itself. Traditional surgical treatment consists of aortic valve replacement. In these cases, both mechanical aortic valves (requiring lifelong anticoagulation treatment) and biological aortic valves (with limited durability) can be used. Biological valves present the choice between xenografts (e.g., valves from a pig), homografts (human aortic grafts), and autografts, in which the patient's own pulmonary valve is implanted in the aorta's place and the pulmonary valve is then replaced using a homograft or a conduit with a mechanical valve, also known as the Ross procedure.[67] In addition, the option for valve reconstruction may exist if certain prerequisites are met.[68]

Postoperative and Postinterventional Issues

Possible complications after surgical treatment of an aortic stenosis include the following:

- aortic valve insufficiency
- damage to the mitral valve, particularly to the anterior mitral leaflet, requiring mitral valve reconstruction or even replacement
- iatrogenic VSD
- cardiac rhythm disorders
- the development of left bundle branch block or atrioventricular block

During surgical treatment of the supravalvular aortic stenosis, coronary perfusion disorders may arise based on the need for coronary reimplantation. Stenosis of the valve-equipped conduit or of the homograft from the right ventricle to the pulmonary artery can result from a Ross procedure. This may be difficult to see with TTE, particularly in older patients, due to the retrosternal positioning. In these cases, MDCT and MRI offer the additional option of graduating the stenosis, e.g., via MR flow measurement as a good alternative to Doppler echocardiography.[7]

Goals and Relative Value of Diagnostic Imaging

The general goal of preinterventional and postinterventional imaging is assessing the degree of severity of the stenosis and acquiring as precise a description as possible of its morphology in order to classify the stenosis more accurately.[57] In addition, imaging is intended to assist with the description of close anatomical relationships with the mitral valve apparatus and with any other potentially associated defects, as well as with the assessment of hemodynamic effects (e.g., regarding left ventricular function and muscle mass).[7,69] Particularly in cases of valvular stenoses, valve morphology must be visualized precisely in order to be able to evaluate the possibility of valve reconstruction compared to valve replacement.

> **Note**
>
> Before a Ross procedure or replacement of the ascending aorta, the diameter of the aortic annulus, LVOT, ascending aorta (and pulmonary valve annulus for Ross procedures), RVOT, and main pulmonary artery should be determined for surgical planning purposes.

Within the scope of standard diagnostics, the position, morphology, and degree of severity of the stenosis can be evaluated using TTE, or TEE under poor imaging conditions. The dimensions of the LVOT and the aortic valve, as well as the involvement of the mitral valve or mitral valve apparatus in the stenosis, can generally be assessed clearly. Both left ventricular size and hypertrophy, as well as concurrent aortic valve insufficiency can also be clearly assessed (▸ Fig. 4.56a, ▸ Fig. 4.59c, d and ▸ Fig. 4.60c).

In addition, it is also possible to assess the pulmonary valve, RVOT, and pulmonary vascular bed in light of a Ross procedure. Doppler echocardiography allows us to estimate the maximum and mean gradients. Associated cardiac defects can also be described or ruled out, and the degree of aortic valve insufficiency can be assessed. The majority of patients, particularly young patients who can be imaged easily, can undergo surgery only after doppler TTE diagnostics have been performed.[59–62]

Particularly in cases of associated defects in which additional information is necessary (e.g., regarding the course of the coronaries for planned myectomies or septostomy, aortic valve replacement, Ross procedures, or ascending aorta replacement), as well as for postoperative patients,[7,13,69] cross-sectional imaging procedures such as MRI or MDCT can be used.

> **Note**
>
> In general, MRI and multi-slice CT are only class I3 indications,[7] meaning that their use is technically possible and validated, but is only indicated on a case-by-case basis.

A cardiac catheter examination may be necessary in order to determine pressure gradients via the stenosis with precision, or in cases of complex defects. Post-stenotic dilatation of the ascending aorta can be visualized and quantified using a cardiac catheter, MRI, or multislice CT (▸ Table 4.21).

4.3.2 Aortic Coarctation

Joachim Lotz, Joachim G. Eichhorn, Michael Steinmetz

Definition

Aortic coarctation is defined as more than 25–30% narrowing of the diameter of the aorta at the transition between the origin of the left subclavian artery and the distal aortic arch in the descending aorta (generally originating from the posterior wall opposite the duct opening), which is exacerbated by membrane-like thickening of the intima media (▸ Fig. 4.62 and ▸ Fig. 4.63). It comprises approximately 5–8% of all congenital heart defects, and is twice as common in men as in women.

Classification

The previous classification into preductal and postductal (or infantile and adult) aortic isthmus stenoses, which was once common, is generally no longer used. The stenosis is generally located opposite (or juxtaductal to) the ductus arteriosus (▸ Fig. 4.62). One exception is critical aortic coarctation in newborns, which can lead to emergency situations in cases of acute duct closure (see below).

Aortic coarctation is often associated with additional heart defects, most commonly with bicuspid aortic valve (in up to 85% of cases), and generally with aortic valve stenosis, PDA, VSD, and even additional arterial vascular anomalies, such as atypical origins of the right subclavian artery (lusoria artery) or origin stenosis of the left subclavian artery. Aortic coarctation commonly (in approximately 30% of cases) also develops in female patients with Turner syndrome (X0 chromosome).

Hemodynamics

In cases of critical aortic coarctation in newborns, perfusion in the lower half of the body depends on the persistence of the ductus arteriosus, which, as a right-left shunt, directs oxygen-depleted blood from pulmonary circulation into the descending aorta. Correspondingly, cyanosis (arterial oxygen saturation generally corresponding to 75–85%) then develops in the lower half of the body, whereas the upper half of the body (as measured on the right arm) experiences normal arterial oxygen saturation. Closing the PDA can, in acute situations, lead to increased afterload and consecutive left ventricular decompensation accompanied by heart failure and cardiogenic shock.

Table 4.21 Relative value of individual imaging procedures for assessing various aspects of aortic stenoses.[7,61]

Findings	Echocardiography			Thoracic X-ray, a.-p./lateral	MRI with flow measurement	MDCT, ECG-triggered	Cardiac catheter (angiography and hemodynamics)
	TTE	TEE	3-D				
Morphology of the valve apparatus and stenosis							
Bicuspid/tricuspid	moderate	high	high	-	high	high	moderate
Wall adherences	high	high	high	-	high	moderate	moderate
Aortic valve function							
Insufficiency	high	high	-	-	high	low	high
Stenosis	high	high	-	-	high	moderate	moderate
Graduation of stenosis							
Morphological	high	high	high	-	high	high	moderate
Functional	high	high	high	-	high	low	high
Left ventricular function and myocardial morphology							
Left ventricular function	high	high	high	-	high	moderate	high
Myocardial morphology	high	high	-	-	high	high	moderate
Left ventricular size	high	high	high	moderate	high	high	high
Morphology of the ascending aorta							
Post-stenotic dilatation	moderate	low	-	moderate	high	high	high

a.-p., anterior–posterior; ECG, electrocardiography; MDCT, multidetector computed tomography; MRI, magnetic resonance imaging; TEE, transesophageal echocardiography; TTE, transthoracic echocardiography.

Note

Even in cases of minor aortic coarctation, increased afterload and consecutive ventricular hypertrophy occurs in the left ventricle. Arterial hypertonia develops in the upper half of the body proximal to the stenosis, and—in cases of normal or decreased arterial blood pressure—in the lower half of the body distal to the stenosis. The resulting blood pressure gradient between the upper and lower extremities is an important diagnostic indication for the presence of an aortic coarctation.

In cases of persistent and hemodynamically relevant aortic coarctation, pronounced collateral circulation between the upper and lower halves of the body often develops. Typical collateral vessels, sometimes with reverse flow, are the internal mammary or internal thoracic arteries, the aortic intercostal arteries of the third–eighth intercostal area, and the left subclavian artery, which then dilate as a result of their increased internal flow (▶ Fig. 4.64 and ▶ Fig. 4.65). This phenomenon can be visualized clearly using different imaging modalities.

Clinical Issues

After the PDA has been closed, critical aortic coarctation in newborns leads inevitably to acute left ventricular heart failure with the development of tachydyspnea, tachycardia, a blue-gray skin discoloration, renal failure, and intestinal hypoperfusion, with risks ranging from the development of necrotic enterocolitis all the way up to cardiogenic shock.

Patients with non-critical aortic coarctation have a difference in blood pressure between their upper and lower extremities, as well as arterial hypertonia proximal to the stenosis. Based on severity, this leads to symptoms such as weakened femoral pulse and cold feet, the development of an intermittent claudication, headaches, and epistaxis. Furthermore, the chronic increased afterload causes left ventricular hypertrophy, which, depending on its severity, can lead to chronic heart failure.

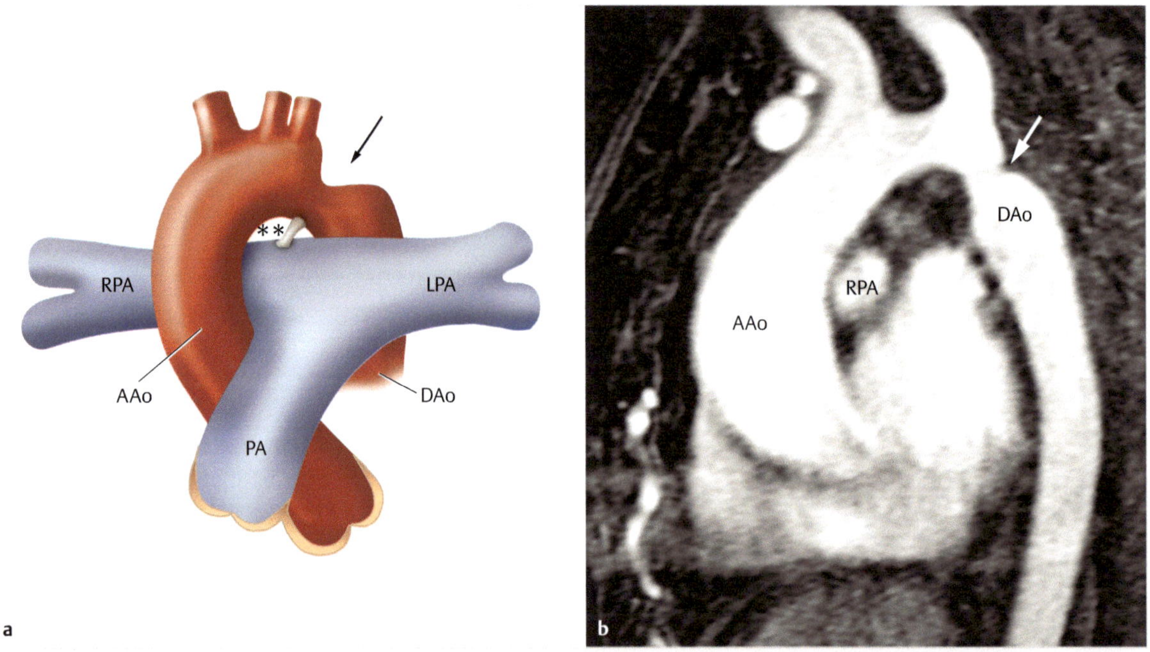

Fig. 4.62 Aortic coarctation. Moderate aortic isthmus stenosis near the transition between the origin of a typically dilatated left subclavian artery and the distal aortic arch in the descending aorta, through a membrane-like thickening of the intima media on the opposite (juxtaductal) posterior wall (arrow) superior to the ductus arteriosus.

AAo = ascending aorta
DAo = descending aorta
LPA = left pulmonary artery
PA = pulmonary artery
RPA = right pulmonary artery

a Schematic depiction.
b Parasagittal MIP reconstruction of a contrast-enhanced MRA.

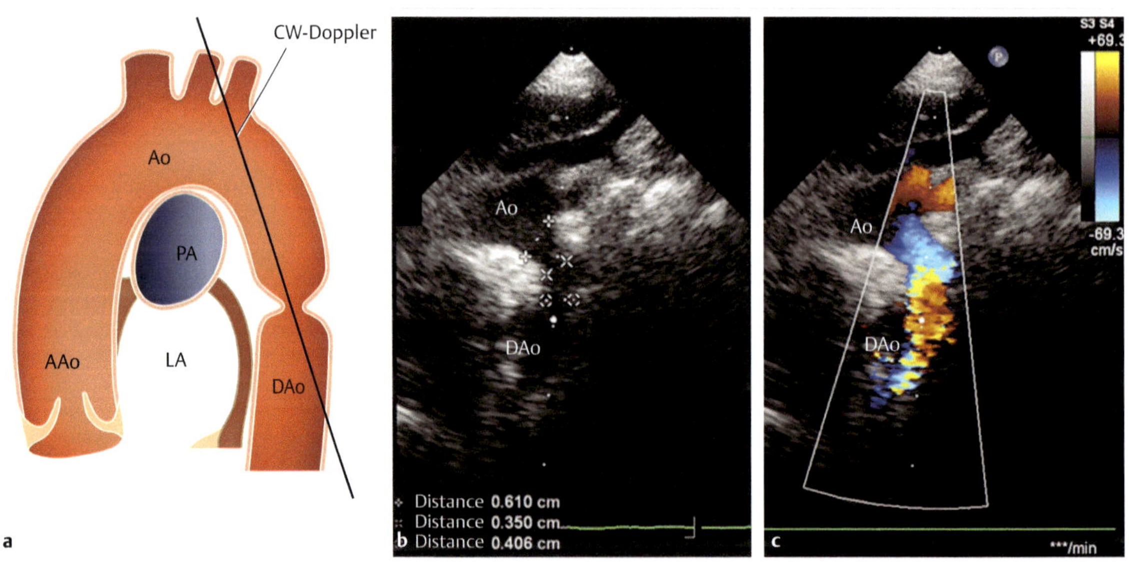

Fig. 4.63 Aortic coarctation.
AAo = ascending aorta
Ao = aorta
DAo = descending aorta
LA = left atrium
PA = pulmonary artery.

a Schematic depiction of the suprasternal view of an aortic coarctation in an infant, CW Doppler, for evaluating maximum instantaneous pressure gradients.
b Typical 2-D echo image, suprasternal long axis, with an angular course of the descending aorta and minor "ridge" pulling medially into the lumen of the descending aorta.
c Corresponding color Doppler image with minor flow acceleration near the isthmus.

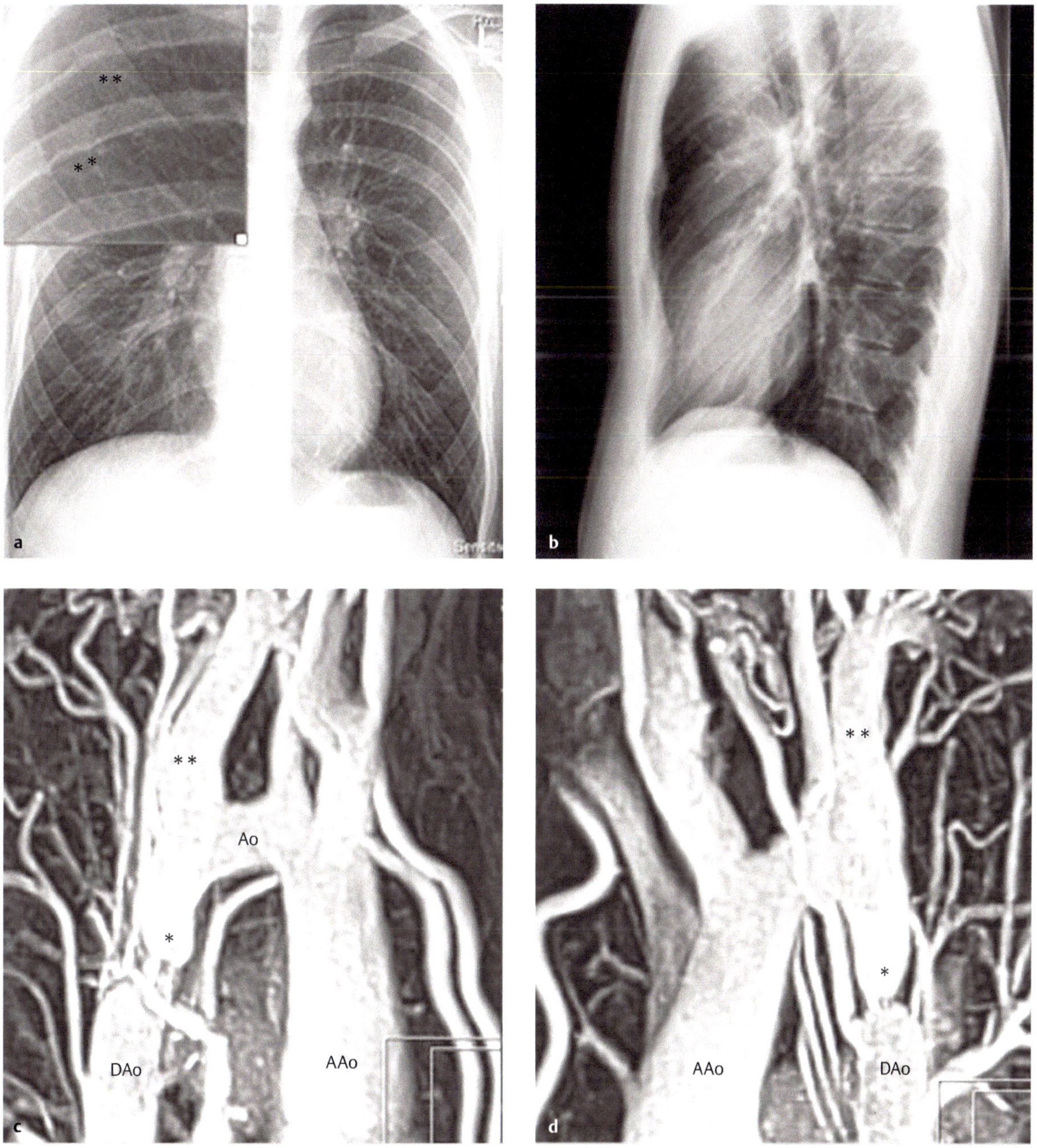

Fig. 4.64 Aortic coarctation with collateralization. Sixteen-year-old male patient with high-grade aortic coarctation (**c**, **d**, asterisks) and pronounced collateralization. The left subclavian artery dilated significantly by collateral flow is depicted in the MIP reconstruction (**c**, **d**, double asterisk).

AAo = ascending aorta
Ao = aorta
DAo = descending aorta

a Thoracic X-ray, p.-a. projection. The enhanced image depicts examples of typical rib notching (double asterisks) on the lower margin of the third–eighth dorsal ribs caused by intercostal collaterals.

b Thoracic X-ray, lateral view.

c Corresponding 3-D MIP reconstruction of a contrast-enhanced MRA, RAO projection.

d Corresponding 3-D MIP reconstruction of a contrast-enhanced MRA, lateral projection.

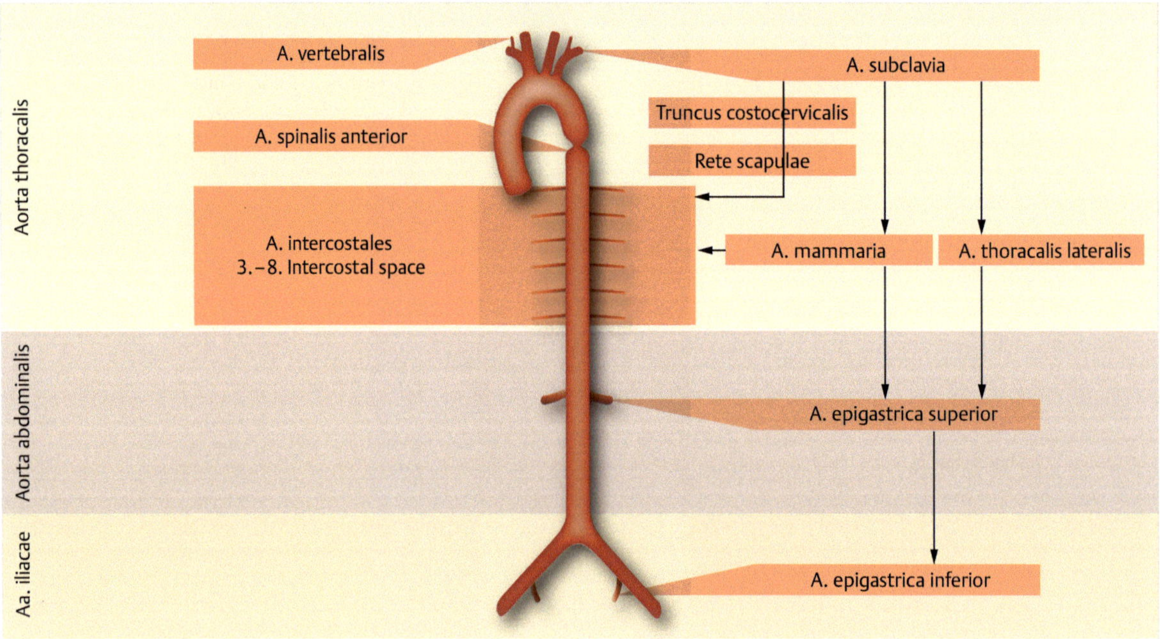

Fig. 4.65 Possible collateral flows in a case of aortic coarctation. Schematic depiction.

Natural Progression and Indication for Treatment

After the PDA is closed, critical aortic stenosis in a newborn is incompatible with life. Under these circumstances, there is always an indication for treatment, often on an emergent basis. If treatment cannot be performed immediately, the PDA must be held open using a prostaglandin E1 infusion, and catecholamine treatment should be initiated before the operation.

Depending on form, non-critical aortic coarctation may only cause arterial hypertonia, with the corresponding elevated risk of cardiovascular events. It may remain undiscovered until late into adulthood.

Indication for treatment exists in cases of a systolic blood pressure gradient of 20 mmHg between the upper and lower halves of the body. Treatment is also indicated if a systolic blood pressure gradient of less than 20 mmHg associated with arterial hypertonia (for children over the 97th blood pressure percentile by age) and a morphologically significant narrowing (stenosis or aortic diameter near the diaphragm of less than 0.8 mm)[70,71] are present.

Treatment Options and Preinterventional Diagnostics

For newborns and infants, surgical correction by means of a left lateral thoracotomy is the treatment method of choice. We strive to resect the stenosis and establish an end-to-end anastomosis, ideally without using foreign materials (▶ Fig. 4.66). Alternatively, a subclavian flap aortoplasty (▶ Fig. 4.67) or indirect dilatation using foreign materials (Goretex or Dacron) is performed. Nowadays, this surgical technique, known as a "Vossschulte patch aortoplasty," has largely been abandoned due to the aneurysms that commonly occur near the patch (▶ Fig. 4.68).

In very rare cases of elongated stenoses, tubular prosthetic conduits made of foreign materials are implanted. In cases of high-grade stenoses with a potentially poor prognosis for end-to-end anastomosis, extra-anatomical bypasses made of various materials may be placed (▶ Fig. 4.69).

During a subclavian flap aortoplasty, the aortic isthmus is dilatated via the left subclavian artery (▶ Fig. 4.67). The artery is disconnected, its origin is folded downward, and it is used as an enlargement patch (▶ Fig. 4.70). Then, the remaining distal subclavian artery is supplied via collateral circulation (▶ Fig. 4.70d). As a result of this intervention, however, the patient's left arm generally lags behind the right arm in terms of growth, and thus is somewhat shorter.

Aortic coarctation is often associated with hypoplasia of the aortic arch. It must be surgically enlarged via a median thoracotomy using a heart–lung machine and selective head perfusion, or supplied by means of a bypass from the ascending aorta to the descending aorta (▶ Fig. 4.68c).

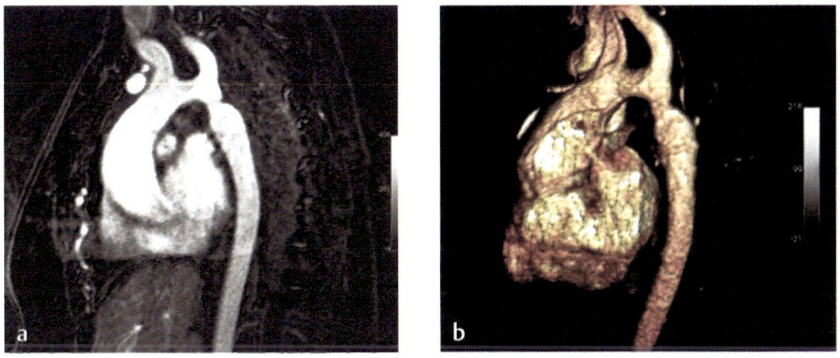

Fig. 4.66 Condition after surgical correction of an aortic coarctation by means of end-to-end anastomosis. Only minor residual or restenosis with minor post-stenotic dilatation of the ascending artery is visible.

a Parasagittal subtractive reconstruction from a contrast-enhanced MRA.

b 3-D reconstruction of the contrast-enhanced MRA using the volume rendering technique.

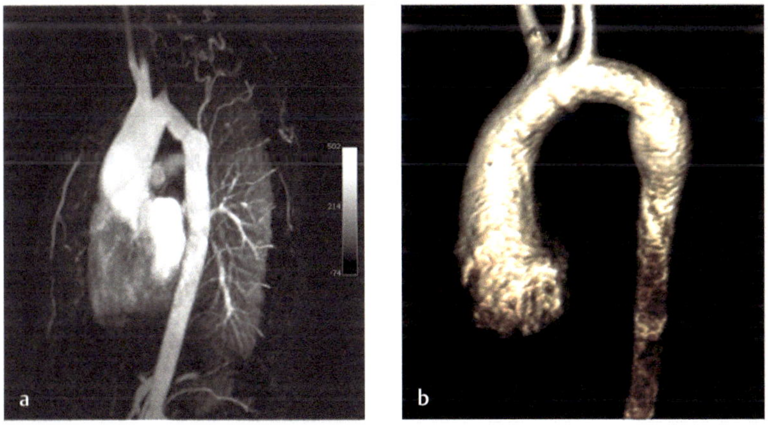

Fig. 4.67 Condition after performing a Waldhausen subclavian flap aortoplasty. The proximal left subclavian artery was used for the aortoplasty of an aortic coarctation. Thus, the proximal left subclavian artery is not depicted. No relevant residual stenosis is visible, but residual collaterals are visible in the MIP reconstruction (**a**). The descending aorta near the anastomosis demonstrates ectatic dilatation to a maximum of 2.5 cm.

a 3-D MIP reconstruction, lateral projection, of a contrast-enhanced MRA.

b 3-D volume rendering of a contrast-enhanced MRA.

Balloon angioplasty has become the treatment of choice for older children, adolescents, and adults, particularly for short stenoses. For adolescents and adults, this is generally combined with stent placement (▶ Fig. 4.71). The stenosis is often dilated gradually using balloons 2.5–3 times the diameter of the isthmus, though no larger than the diameter of the aorta near the diaphragm or of the pre-stenotic aortic arch.[72]

Postoperative and Postinterventional Issues

This surgery carries the risk of damaging the phrenic and recurrent nerves, resulting in unilateral paralysis of the diaphragm or vocal cords. In rare cases, the thoracic duct can also be damaged, leading to subsequent chylothorax. In even rarer cases, paraplegia of the lower extremities (also known as post-coartectomy syndrome) can occur. The restenosis rate after surgery is high, namely 5–10% in older children (▶ Fig. 4.66). For cases of critical aortic coarctation or aortic arch hypoplasia (▶ Fig. 4.68c), however, this rate is substantially higher.[73,74]

Catheter interventions carry the risk of damage near the arterial vascular access (bleeding, thrombosis, aneurysms). Dilatation can also cause the aorta to rupture or aneurysms or dissections to form, though only in rare cases. If a stent is placed, there is a risk of stent fracture, stent dislocation, or restenosis caused by neointima formation near the stent.

Over the long term, this can lead to restenosis, aneurysm formation, or persistent arterial hypertonia in a not inconsequential number of patients. Patients with associated bicuspid aortic valve have an elevated risk of restenosis or ectasia of the ascending aorta, and patients have an elevated risk of developing aneurysms near the surgical site after aortic arch or patch aortoplasty, particularly if foreign materials were used (▶ Fig. 4.68).[75,76]

Note

Arterial hypertonia is often still present immediately after aortic coarctation treatment and persists in up to 50% of patients without evidence of relevant residual stenosis or restenosis.

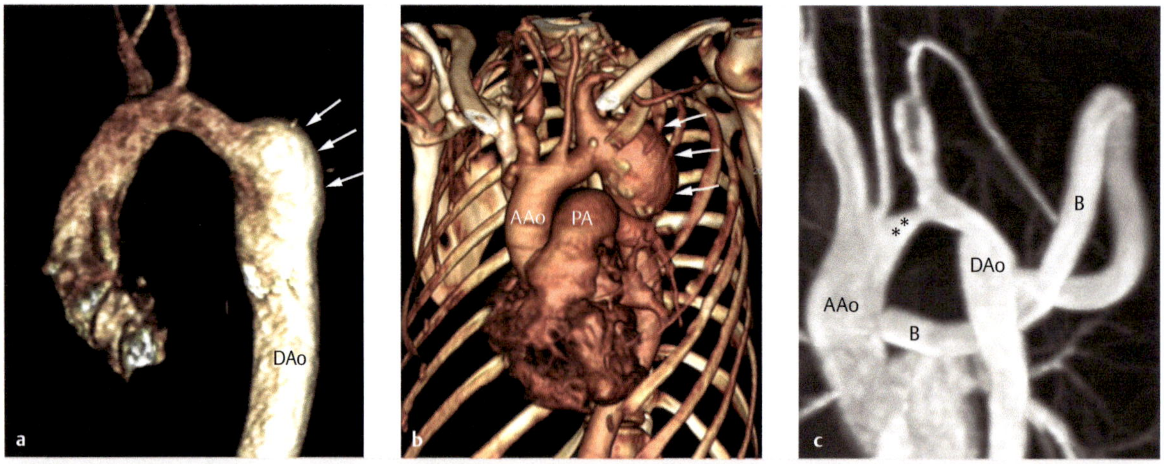

Fig. 4.68 Formation of an aneurysm after a Vossschulte patch aortoplasty. Depiction of the thoracic aorta of three different patients after placing an indirect aortoplasty patch made of foreign materials (Vossschulte patch aortoplasty). The 3-D volume rendering of a contrast-enhanced MRA (a), like the 3-D volume rendering of a CTA (b), shows a typical complication of this surgical technique, namely the development of an aneurysm (**a**, **b**, arrows) near the patch aortoplasty. In addition to the patient's condition after a Vossschulte patch aortoplasty, the 3-D MIP reconstruction of an MRA still depicts a hypoplastic aortic arch (**c**, double asterisk). For this reason, an extra-anatomical bypass of the ascending aorta was attached to the descending aorta, without any relevant residual restenoses or aneurysm formation.

AAo = ascending aorta
B = bypass
DAo = descending aorta
PA = pulmonary artery

a 3-D volume rendering of a contrast-enhanced MRA.
b 3-D volume rendering of a CTA.
c MIP reconstruction of a contrast-enhanced MRA.

The lack of elasticity in the aortic arch and associated hemodynamic changes are believed to be the cause of this persistent arterial hypertonia. Thus, consistent antihypertensive treatment should be given.[77]

Goals and Relative Value of Diagnostic Imaging

For infants and small children, *echocardiography* is the imaging method of choice due to the generally good acoustic window. In particular, this technique can be used to depict the degree of stenosis, a potentially open ductus arteriosus, left ventricular function, and associated defects. Ideally, the aortic arch is depicted via a suprasternal or jugular acoustic window (▶ Fig. 4.63) when using cranial extension, or from a right parasternal view.

For older children, adolescents, adults, and especially for patients with previous surgeries, echocardiographic depiction can be significantly restricted by the limited acoustic window. In these cases, *MRI* and particularly contrast-enhanced MRA (including 3-D reconstruction) are the modalities of choice (▶ Fig. 4.64c and d), followed by *multi-slice CT* (▶ Fig. 4.72; also ▶ Fig. 4.68b). Both of the former allow detailed depiction of the stenosis, collaterals, left ventricular function and mass, and associated defects, as well as aneurysms or restenosis in previously treated patients. Particularly after stent placement (▶ Fig. 4.70 and ▶ Fig. 4.71), multi-slice CT is superior to MRI if there is evidence of restenosis caused by neointima formation or stent fractures. Although performing an MRI after stent placement in the aorta is not contraindicated, and many stents (particularly nitinol ones) only generate minor artifacts, MRI quality near the stent is still limited. MRI can be used for precise quantification of an associated bicuspid aortic valve andO any stenoses it may have caused, as well as aortic valve insufficiency and ventricular function. MRI flow measurement is suited to determining the extent of collateralization of the aortic coarctation. In cases of very high-grade, subtotal stenoses, collateral flow can be significantly higher than that in the aorta immediately distal to the stenosis. This can be depicted well using 4-D flow measurement (▶ Fig. 4.72). This method can also be used to estimate the relevance of a restenosis.[78,79] In the future, new 4-D MRI flow measurement

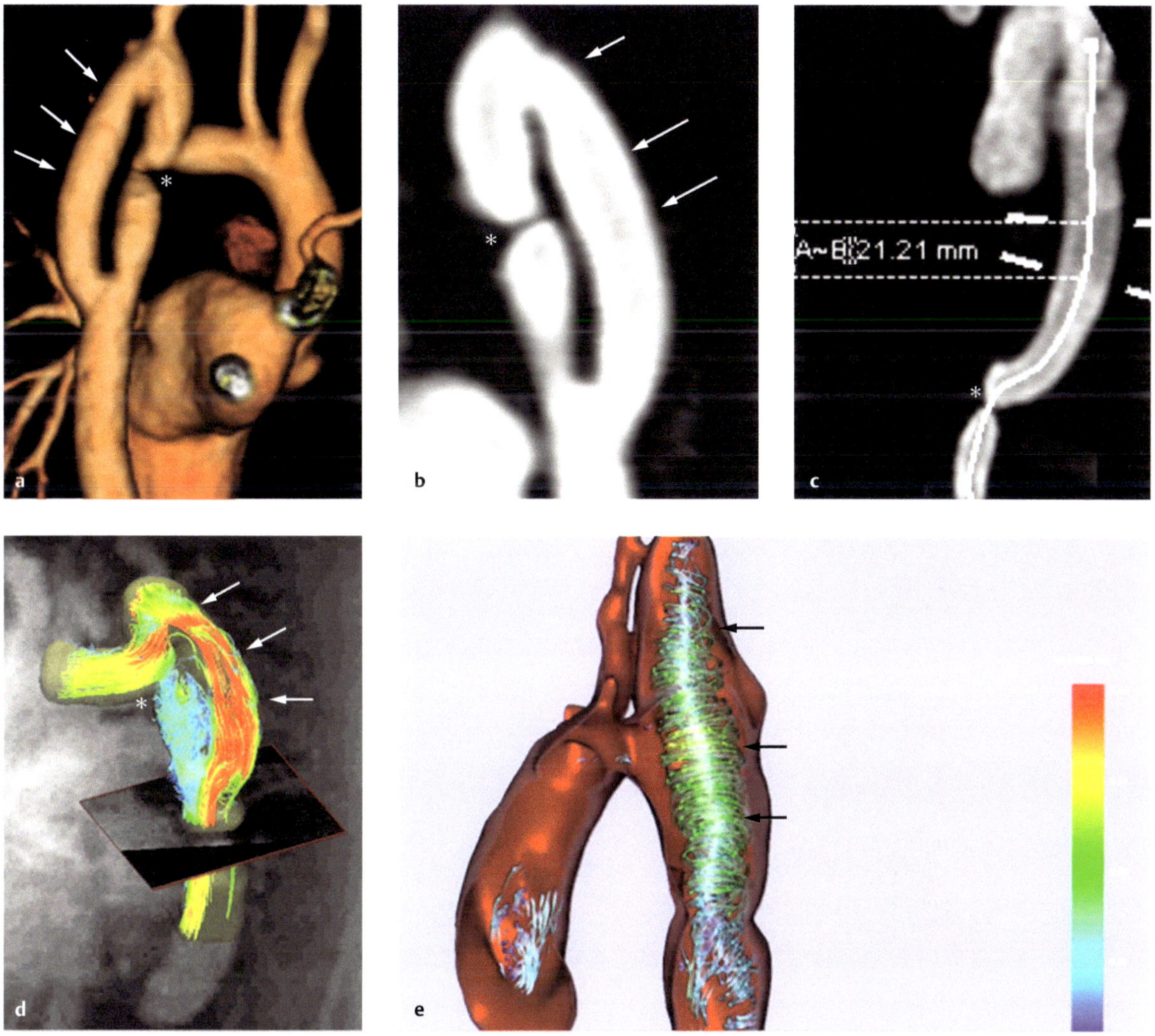

Fig. 4.69 Extra-anatomical bypass in a case of high-grade aortic coarctation. The images **a**, **b**, and **d** depict the non-resected, high-grade native aortic isthmus stenosis (**a, b, d**, asterisk) in a 29-year-old man. The aortic coarctation was treated using an extra-anatomical bypass (**a-e**, arrows) from the left subclavian artery to the descending aorta. Though normal maximum flow velocities (**d**) are visible in **d** and **e**, pronounced vortex formation (**e**) is also visible. The vortex formations in the bypass were calculated using 4-D MR flow measurement.

a 3-D volume rendering of a contrast-enhanced MRA.
b Sagittal MIP reconstruction of a contrast-enhanced MRA.
c Curved reformat, with centerline, of a contrast-enhanced MRA.
d Visualization of 4-D flow: here, the maximum flow velocities were depicted.
e Visualization of 4-D flow: here, the vortices (vortex formations) were depicted.

technologies[80] could also be helpful for planning optimal surgical techniques in order to restore physiological flow, if possible (▶ Fig. 4.69). Just like Doppler echocardiography, MRI also allows instantaneous pressure gradients to be estimated by determining maximum flow velocity in the stenosis by means of MRI flow measurement and the phase contrast technique, and by using the simplified Bernoulli equation. This correlates well to invasively measured pressure gradients, at least for minor-to-moderate stenoses.[78]

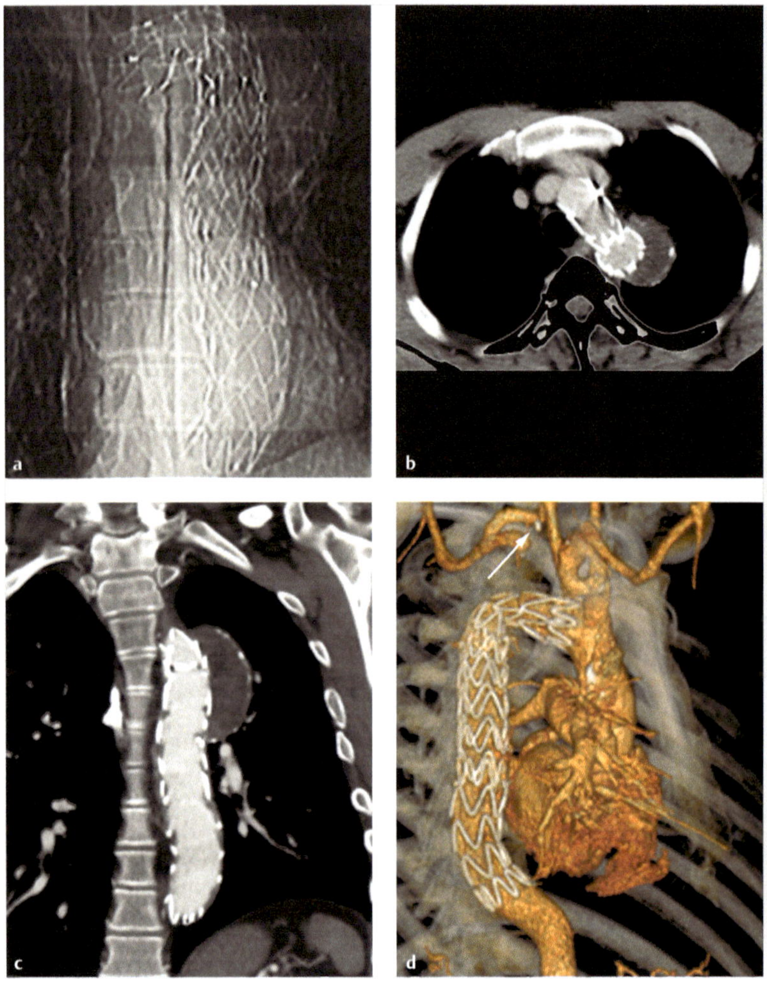

Fig. 4.70 Condition after subclavian flap aortoplasty. Forty-three-year-old male patient after an aortic coarctation operation with a Waldhausen subclavian flap aortoplasty and aneurysm formation, which was treated by placing a thoracic aortic stent. No stent fracture is detectable.

a CT topographic image in a.-p. orientation.
b Transverse reconstruction of a multi-slice CT data set.
c Coronal reconstruction of a multi-slice CT data set. The thrombosed aneurysm segment left lateral to the stent, which was caused by the stent, is clearly visible.
d 3-D volume rendering of a multi-slice CT data set. The surgically "disconnected" left subclavian artery, which is now supplied via the carotid-subclavian bypass (arrow), is clearly visible.

Note

M!

All tomographic procedures measure the diameter of the ascending aorta, the transverse and distal aortic arch, and the descending aorta distal to the stenosis. The length of the stenosis, as well as any potentially associated vascular anomalies (head and neck vessels, renal arteries) or collaterals are determined. This is decisive for treatment planning purposes.[62]

Often, the *thoracic X-ray* in p.-a. projection depicts an aortic coarctation in adults due to the typical rib notches, shallow recesses on the inferior margins of the third–eighth dorsal ribs (▶ Fig. 4.64a). Otherwise, heart size is generally normal and only enlarged in cases of critical aortic coarctation. X-rays depict signs of pulmonary obstruction. Due to this pre-stenotic enlargement of the left subclavian artery generally present near the aortic coarctation (▶ Fig. 4.64, ▶ Fig. 4.66, ▶ Fig. 4.72) and the post-stenotic enlargement of the descending aorta, X-ray or angiographic images depict a typical left-side "notch," the image of a double aortic knob. In principle, Doppler echocardiography and tomographic procedures are used for preoperative diagnostics. A postinterventional stent fracture, however, can also be recognized on a simple X-ray p.-a./lateral image (▶ Fig. 4.70a).

An invasive *cardiac catheter examination* is indicated for precise quantification and invasive measurement of the pressure gradient (▶ Table 4.22). Generally speaking, the decision to perform surgical or interventional treatment can occur noninvasively using Doppler echocardiography and/or MRI or multi-slice CT tomographic procedures. To that end, invasive diagnostics are usually only performed if an interventional treatment (namely, balloon angioplasty or stent placement) is also anticipated.[81] However, there are already initial case studies using MRI-guided aortic coarctation treatment with fluoroscopy as a backup.[82]

▶ Table 4.22 compares the relative value of imaging procedures.

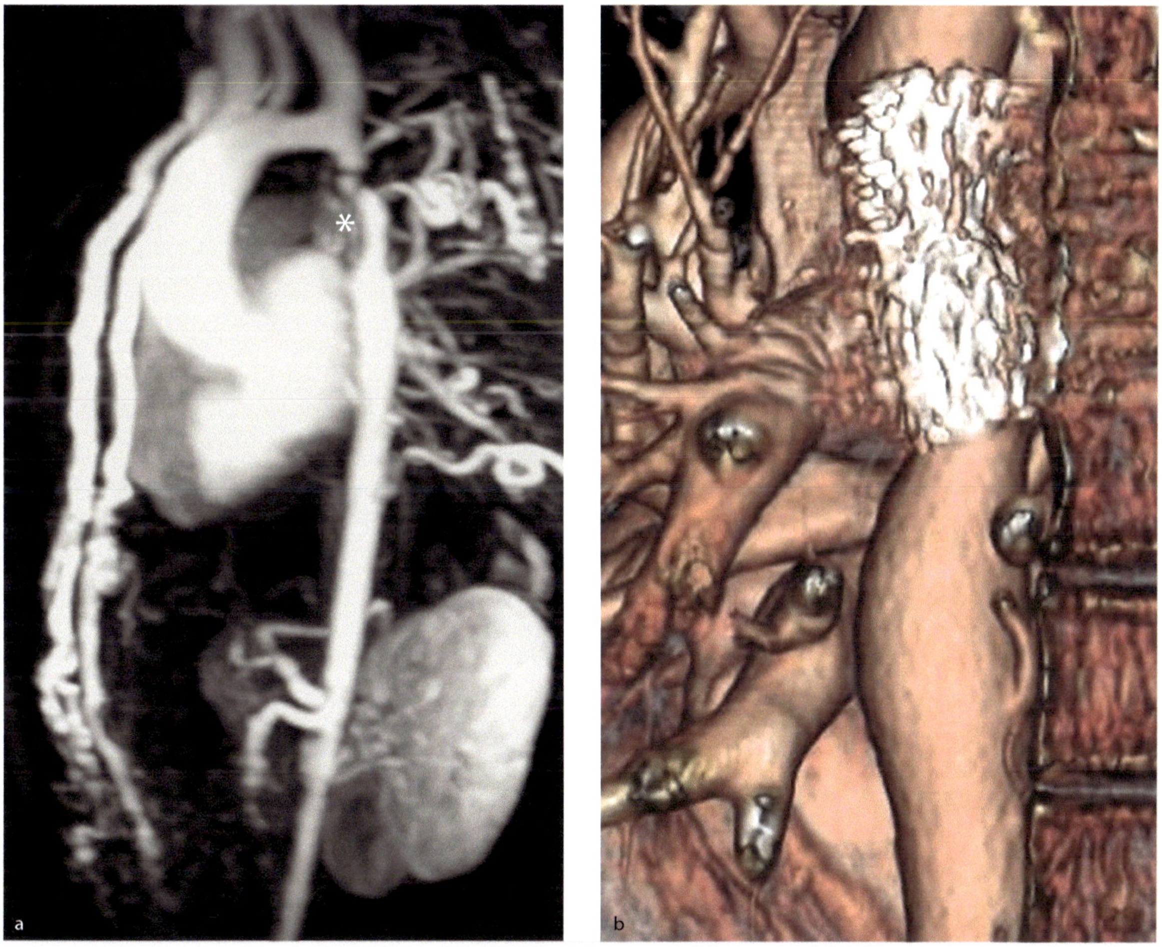

Fig. 4.71 Stent placement in a case of high-grade aortic coarctation. Thirty-nine-year-old female patient with high-grade aortic coarctation (**a**, asterisk) and pronounced collateralization via the mammarian and intercostal arteries.
a 3-D MIP reconstruction of a contrast-enhanced MRA before implantation.
b 3-D volume rendering from a CTA after stent implantation.

Table 4.22 Relative value of individual imaging procedures for assessing various aspects of aortic coarctation.

Findings	Echocardiography			Thoracic X-ray, p.-a./ lateral	MRI with flow measurement	MDCT ECG-triggered	Cardiac catheter (angiography and hemodynamics)
	TTE	TEE	3-D				
Aortic arch morphology	high	–	moderate	–	high	high	high
Associated cardiac defects	high	high	high	–	high	moderate	high
Isthmus stenosis graduation							
• **Morphological**	high	–	high	–	high	high	high
• **Functional**	high	–	–	–	high	low	high
Left ventricular function	high	high	high	–	high	moderate	high
Myocardial morphology	high	high	–	–	high	high	moderate

ECG, electrocardiography; MDCT, multidetector computed tomography; MRI, magnetic resonance imaging; TEE, transesophageal echocardiography; TTE, transthoracic echocardiography.

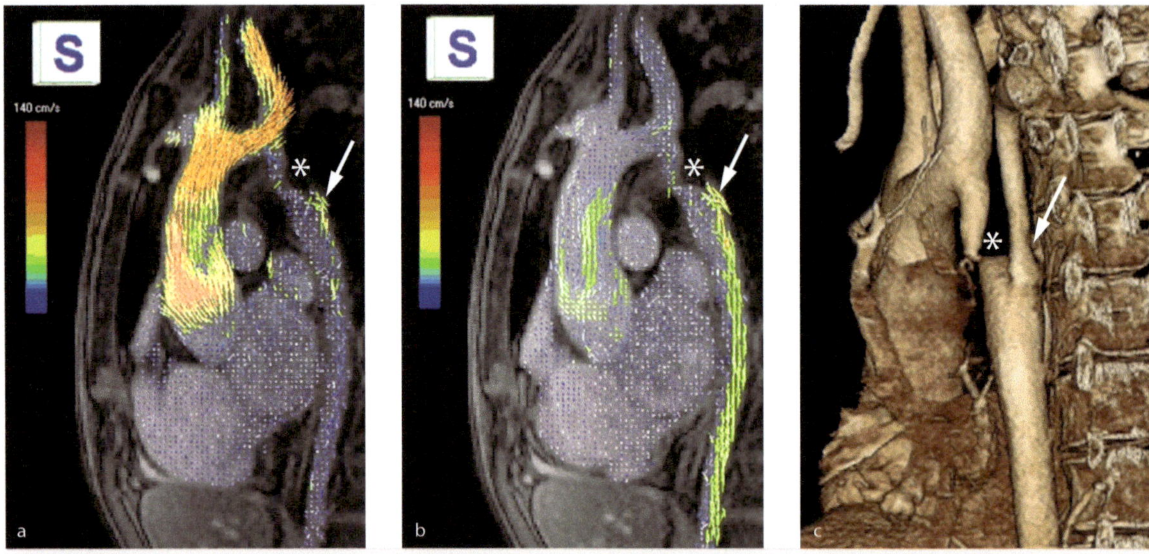

Fig. 4.72 High-grade aortic coarctation with collateral formation. Patient with high-grade, sub-total aortic coarctation (**a–c**, asterisks) and pronounced collateral formation. 4-D MR flow measurement reveals that no relevant flow via the stenosis can be demonstrated either during systole or diastole, though pronounced, primarily diastolic collateral flow is present (**a–c**, arrows).

a 4-D MR flow measurement with reconstruction of the maximum flow velocities during systole.
b 4-D MR flow measurement with reconstruction of the maximum flow velocities during diastole. During diastole, the descending aorta is supplied primarily by collateral flow.
c 3-D volume rendering reconstruction of a CTA, dorsal view.

M!

Note

The MRI and multi-slice CT tomographic procedures are each class I2 indications for diagnosing a coarctation, meaning the diagnostic precision is comparable to that of other diagnostic methods.[7]

4.3.3 Interrupted Aortic Arch

Joachim Lotz, Joachim G. Eichhorn, Michael Steinmetz

Definition

This rare congenital defect is characterized by a complete interruption between two segments of the aortic arch (interrupted aortic arch, IAA), which are, at most, still connected via residual connective tissue, but possess no vascular connection to one another (like in cases of aortic isthmus atresia). Unlike aortic coarctation, IAA is a rare congenital heart defect, comprising less than 0.1% of all heart defects. In theory, the aortic arch can be interrupted at any point (▸ Fig. 4.73), regardless of whether a left or right arch is present.[83]

Classification

The interruption is classified as one of three types based on its location from distal to proximal (▸ Fig. 4.73). Frequency is indicated using the system developed by Schumacher et al.:[83]

- *Type A:* Interruption distal to the origin of all head and arm vessels (approximately 40% of cases)
- *Type B:* Interruption between the left subclavian artery and the left carotid artery (approximately 55% of cases)
- *Type C:* Interruption between the left carotid artery and the brachiocephalic trunk (this is mirrored for right-side aortic arch, namely, between the right carotid artery and right subclavian artery; approximately 5% of cases)

An isolated form occurs only in about 3–4% of cases,[83,84] most of which are type A. Otherwise, a number of primarily left-side defects with concurrent PDA and VSD, bicuspid aortic valve and more complex defects such as TGA, truncus arteriosus, or even HLHS have been described.

Hemodynamics and Clinical Issues

"Ductal-dependent" systemic circulation is common to all types. In these cases, antegrade perfusion occurs via the descending aorta and thus all circulation in the lower body occurs solely via a PDA. Depending on the location of the interruption, the distal head and arm vessels may be supplied via the PDA and retrograde perfusion via the distal arch segment. Due to the left-right shunt through the PDA, affected children begin to display

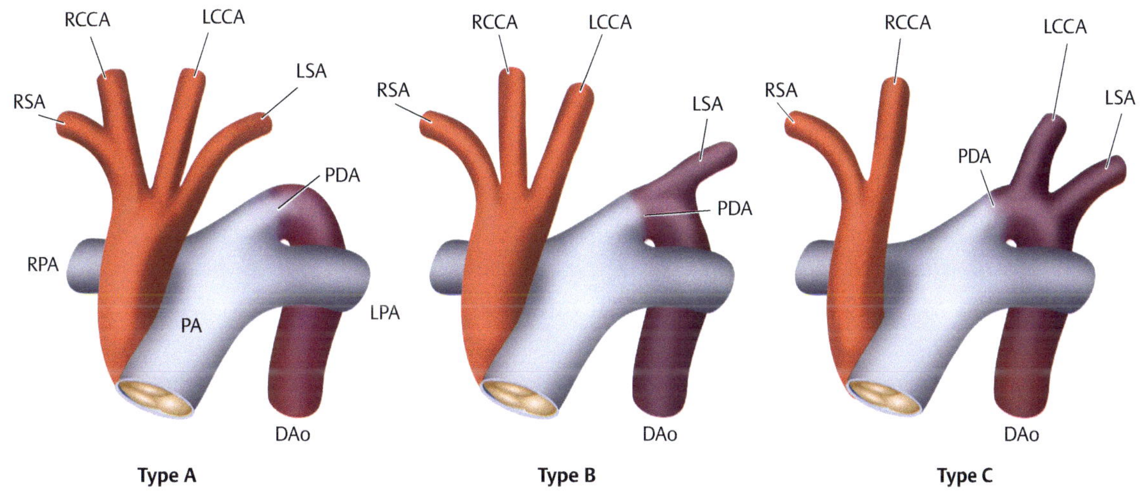

Fig. 4.73 Three most common types of IAA. Schematic depiction.
AAo = ascending aorta
DAo = descending aorta
LCCA = left common carotid artery
LPA = left pulmonary artery
LSA = left subclavian artery
MPA = main pulmonary artery (truncus pulmonalis)
PDA = patent ductus arteriosus
RCCA = right common carotid artery
RPA = right pulmonary artery
RSA = right subclavian artery

clinical symptoms caused by a difference in transcutaneously measured oxygen saturation (with a lower value in the lower extremities and a normal value in the right hand), provided that these measurements are taken during screenings. Physiologic closure of the PDA is fatal to these patients, and correlates to additional clinical symptoms. Nevertheless, an IAA can also first manifest itself clinically in adulthood.[84,85]

Treatment

Like in cases of HLHS, a prostaglandin E infusion can be used to enlarge the PDA or hold it open, though this is a temporary, emergency treatment. If possible, surgical treatment should occur as a single intervention in newborns (namely an end-to-end anastomosis, subclavian artery angioplasty, or prosthetic interposition), based on the concurrent defects and the length and localization of the interruption. As mentioned, the mortality rate remains high.[83]

Diagnostics and the Role of Imaging Procedures

Though fetal echocardiography can be used to diagnose this condition prenatally, the condition is not apparent in many patients until after birth, not infrequently after the patient has entered cardiogenic shock. In less severe cases with only partial ductal closure, symptoms may closely resemble those of a preductal aortic coarctation. In theory, it is also possible to use MRI for prenatal diagnosis.[86]

Thoracic X-rays often depict pronounced cardiomegaly caused by the pronounced right–left shunt. A diagnosis cannot, however, be determined using thoracic X-rays.

Final diagnosis is usually determined solely using TTE. The interruption can often be depicted clearly from a suprasternal view. In mild cases, a tomographic method is preferable to a cardiac catheter examination. Despite the radiation exposure,[84,85,87] CT is preferable to MRI in critically ill patients due to the speed of the former method (▶ Fig. 4.74). For hemodynamically stable children, MRI should be used in order to reduce radiation exposure.

In addition to diagnosing and classifying the IAA, it is beneficial to determine the course of the interruption or length of atresia, as well as its spatial relationship to airways (trachea and main bronchus) and to the esophagus prior to surgery. The often-variable origin of the left subclavian artery is important for preoperative planning.[83]

Postoperative management must include not just an assessment of cardiac function, but must also rule out or quantify any restenoses and assess their hemodynamic significance. If a larger distance must be bridged surgically (and the distal arch pulled far to the front), this can lead to bronchial compression. Thus, if clinical symptoms include airway obstruction, bronchial compression must be ruled out definitively.

The preoperative and postoperative value of the various imaging procedures depends on the concurrent illnesses paramount to the aortic coarctation (▶ Table 4.22).

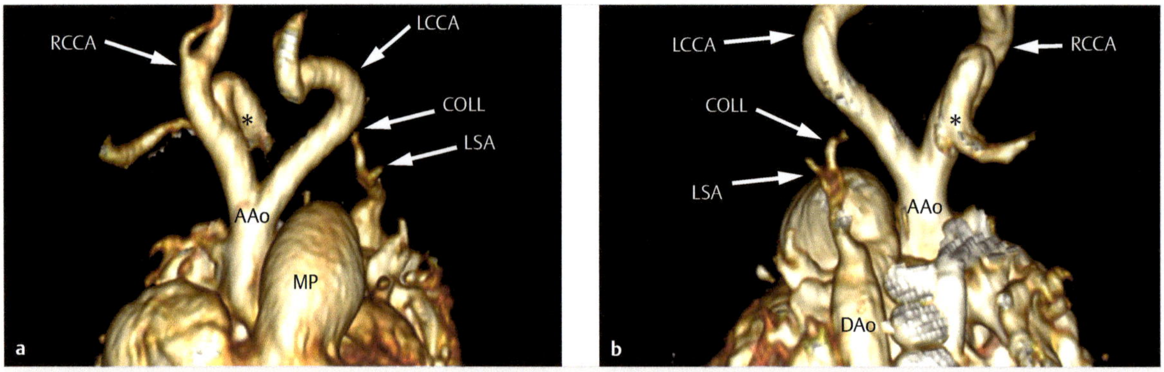

Fig. 4.74 Type A IAA. Two-week-old infant in overall poor clinical condition, with a systolic blood pressure difference > 35 mmHg between the upper and lower extremities.

AAo = ascending aorta
COLL = collaterals
DAo = descending aorta
LCCA = left common carotid artery
LSA = left subclavian artery
MPA = main pulmonary artery (truncus pulmonalis)
RCCA = right common carotid artery

a A.-p. 3-D reconstruction of a CTA. The ascending aorta is divided into the right and left common carotid arteries. The transverse and descending segments of the aortic arch are absent. The right subclavian artery (asterisk) originates dorsally to the right common carotid artery. The aorta continues as a descending aorta with collaterals supplied by cranial flow, which are supplied by the left vertebral and paravertebral arteries, left-dorsally to the ectatic pulmonary arterial stem.

b P.-a. 3-D reconstruction of a CTA. From a dorsal view, the descending aorta (which is supplied by the left vertebral arteries and paravertebral collaterals and has no direct connection to the ascending aorta) is clearly visible left-lateral to the spinal column. The ductus arteriosus, which ensures perfusion of the lower half of the body both prenatally and immediately postnatally, is closed after 14 days. This explains the delayed onset of clinical symptoms. The left subclavian artery originates from the collateral stem as a tiny vessel.

In the future, 4-D MRI will likely also provide additional insights into altered preoperative and postoperative hemodynamic situations in cases of IAA.[88]

4.4 Complex Defects

4.4.1 Transposition of the Great Arteries

Matthias Gutberlet, Christian Kellenberger

Definition

In cases of TGA, a discordant ventriculoarterial connection is present, in which the outflow tracts of the right and left ventricles run parallel to one another (▶ Fig. 4.75) rather than crossing (as occurs in normal anatomy).[83,89–91] Thus, the aorta originates partially or fully from the morphologic right ventricle, and the pulmonary artery, from the morphologic left ventricle, respectively.

In the case of a normal atrioventricular connection between the right atrium and the morphologic right ventricle, a developmental disorder of the embryonic conotruncus is present. These cases are described as complete transposition of the great arteries with intact interventricular septum (TGA IVS—often simplified to D-TGA), because the RVOT and thus also the ascending aorta are displaced to the right ("D" stands for "dextro-," ▶ Fig. 4.75).

Ventricular inversion is present if an anomalous atrioventricular connection between the morphologic right ventricle and morphologic left atrium also occurs. The TGA is then considered "congenitally corrected" and is thus also known as "congenitally corrected transposition" (ccTGA, colloquially often also called L-TGA),[91] since, in these cases of ventricular inversion, the ascending aorta generally (in up to 85% of cases[83]) originates left of the pulmonary artery from the left-displaced, morphologic right ventricle ("L" stands for "levo-,"; ▶ Fig. 4.76 and ▶ Fig. 4.77; also ▶ Fig. 4.75b). However, the correct nomenclature for this congenital heart defect is ccTGA.

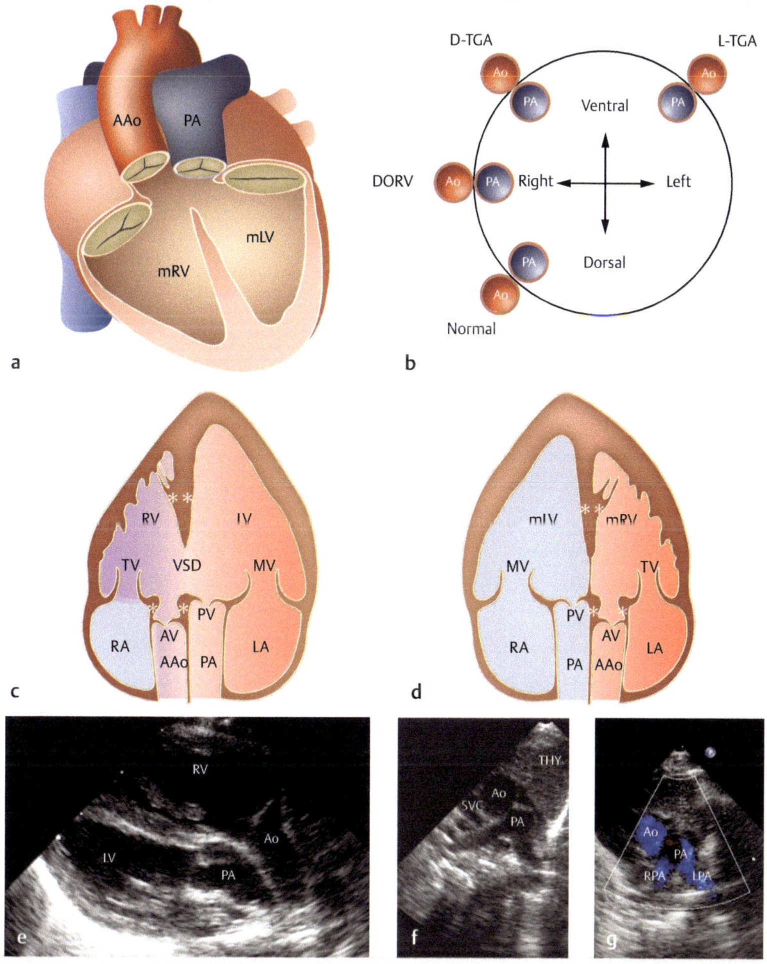

Fig. 4.75 Schematic depiction of the forms of TGA.
AAo = ascending aorta
Ao = aorta
AV = aortic valve
DORV = double outlet right ventricle
D-TGA = dextro-transposition of the great arteries
LA = left atrium
LPA = left pulmonary artery
L-TGA = levo-transposition of the great arteries
LV = left ventricle
mLV = morphologic left ventricle
mRV = morphologic right ventricle
MV = mitral valve
PA = pulmonary artery (truncus pulmonalis)
PV = pulmonary valve
RA = right atrium
RPA = right pulmonary artery
RV = right ventricle
SVC = superior vena cava
THY = thymus
TV = tricuspid valve
VSD = ventricular septal defect

a Schematic depiction of the parallel arrangement of the ventricular outflow tracts.

b Schematic depiction of the arrangement of the great vessels (aorta and pulmonary arteries) with respect to one another near the valve, showing various pathologies of the great vessels compared to normal clinical findings (normal).

c Schematic TTE depiction of the appearance of a TGA, or complete transposition of the great arteries. Note the muscular conus (**c**, **d**, asterisk) around the RVOT and the position of the aortic valve compared to the pulmonary valve. The double asterisks in **c** and **d** indicate the moderator band, which is defined as one of the numerous characteristics of the morphologic right ventricle.

d Schematic depiction of the appearance of a ccTGA, TTE image.

e TTE image of a newborn with TGA IVS, or complete transposition of the great arteries with intact interventricular septum. The connection of the aorta to the right ventricle and of the main pulmonary artery to the left ventricle are visible along the parasternal long axis. The outflow tracts do not cross one another.

f TTE image of the same newborn as in **e**. 2-D echocardiography image, suprasternal transthoracic view of the great vessels. Good acoustic window, thymus clearly visible. The right-anterior origin of the ascending aorta and the left-posterior origin of the main pulmonary artery branching into the right and left pulmonary arteries is visible in **f** and **g**.

g TTE image of the same newborn as in **e** and **f**. Color Doppler echocardiography.

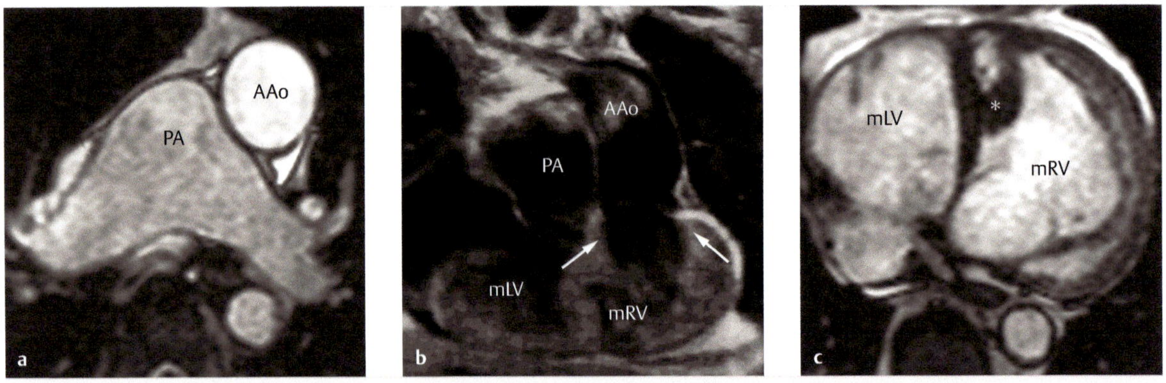

Fig. 4.76 L-TGA. MRI of a 40-year-old, previously asymptomatic male patient with ccTGA.
AAo = ascending aorta
mLV = morphologic left ventricle
mRV = morphologic right ventricle
PA = pulmonary artery

a SSFP cine. Transverse plane. The levoposition of the aorta compared to the pulmonary artery is visible the origin of the great vessels.
b Coronal plane of a black blood SE sequence. Typical parallel positioning of the ascending aorta and the main pulmonary artery, which originates from the right-displaced, morphologic left ventricle. The left-displaced, morphologic right ventricle is characterized by a muscular conus (white arrow).
c Moderator band (asterisk) and significant right ventricular trabeculation.

Note

In cases of ccTGA, the morphologic right ventricle and its tricuspid valve (▶ Fig. 4.77d) are located on the left side, except for in cases of situs inversus (▶ Fig. 4.78). The left-displaced aorta then originates from the morphologic right ventricle (▶ Fig. 4.76a,c and ▶ Fig. 4.77c,e). The morphologic right ventricle is supplied by the normal left atrium (▶ Fig. 4.77a). Morphological characteristics of the right ventricle include the following:

- Moderator band (▶ Fig. 4.76c, ▶ Fig. 4.77a, ▶ Fig. 4.78b)
- Subvalvular muscular conus (▶ Fig. 4.75c,d, ▶ Fig. 4.76b, ▶ Fig. 4.77b,c and, ▶ Fig. 4.78b)
- Significant trabeculation (▶ Fig. 4.76c, ▶ Fig. 4.77a,d, f and, ▶ Fig. 4.78b)
- A tricuspid valve (▶ Fig. 4.77d)

Natural Progression, Clinical Issues, and Hemodynamics

Complete Transposition of the Great Arteries (TGA IVS)

Nowadays, TGA is generally diagnosed in utero using fetal ultrasound.[6,7,83,89–91] TGA IVS is only compatible with life postnatally if an additional shunt is present. Thus, prostaglandin E can be administered postnatally so that the ductus arteriosus does not close. If an adequate shunt is no longer present, it is often necessary, under emergency conditions, to create one during an intervention using the Rashkind maneuver,[91,92] an atrial balloon septostomy, while employing X-ray or potentially also echocardiography monitoring.

Since 50% of children with TGA IVS often do not survive beyond age 2 even after an atrial septostomy, nowadays surgical correction is generally performed early. The arterial switch operation has a mortality rate of 1% and an excellent long-term prognosis.[93]

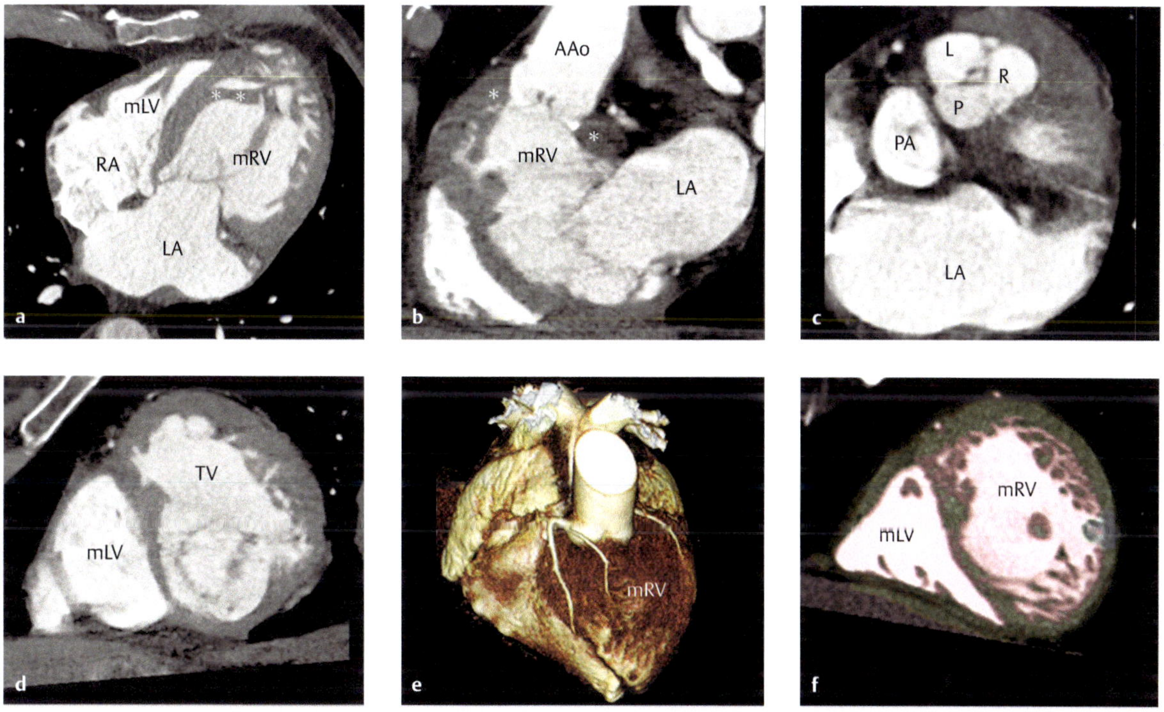

Fig. 4.77 L-TGA. Various reconstructions of a 4-D MDCT data set (64 rows), acquired using retrospective gating in a 72-year-old male patient with ccTGA and pronounced tricuspid valve insufficiency, before a potential tricuspid valve reconstructive procedure.

AAo = ascending aorta
L = left coronary semilunar valve
LA = left atrium
LAD = left anterior descending artery
LV = left ventricle
mLV = morphologic left ventricle
mRV = morphologic right ventricle
P = posterior semilunar valve
PA = pulmonary artery
R = right coronary semilunar valve
TV = tricuspid valve

a Reconstruction, 4-chamber view, depicting the moderator band (double asterisk) of the significantly dilated, left-displaced, morphologic “right” systemic ventricle with pronounced trabeculation.

b Long-axis reconstruction depicting the subaortic muscular conus (asterisk).

c The transverse reconstruction depicts the typical L-TGA position of the aorta and pulmonary artery to one another. Minor insufficiency of the tricuspid aortic valve is visible. As most commonly described,[83] the right coronary artery originates near the posterior semilunar valve and supplies the morphologic right ventricle on the left side and the left anterior descending artery (LAD) and the circumflex (CX) from the area to the left coronary semilunar valve (▶ Fig. 4.77e) and supply the morphologic left ventricle on the right side.

d The short-axis reconstruction depicts the left-displaced tricuspid valve, opened during diastole, from a direct frontal view.

e 3-D volume rendering depicting coronary supply of the left-displaced, morphologic right ventricle.

f The strong trabeculation of the morphologic right ventricle is most prominent in the short-axis reconstruction of a midventricular slice. The green area indicates the segmented muscle mass measured automatically by the software. Since not all trabeculae were recognized automatically, additional manual correction is necessary to accurately determine muscle mass.

Congenitally Corrected Transposition of the Great Arteries (ccTGA)

In cases of ccTGA, the morphologic right ventricle serves as a systemic ventricle. This later causes concentric right ventricular hypertrophy. As a result, patients with ccTGA can often remain completely asymptomatic until late into adulthood.[91,94–97] ccTGA can, however, lead to “right ventricular heart failure” (which corresponds clinically to left heart failure) at a much earlier age,[98] as well as cardiac rhythm disorders. In symptomatic patients, the typical treatment consists of treating heart failure. A double-switch operation—a procedure combining an arterial and atrial switch operation—may, however, become necessary.[97,99,100] In cases of pronounced heart failure, a heart transplant may be used as a last-resort option.

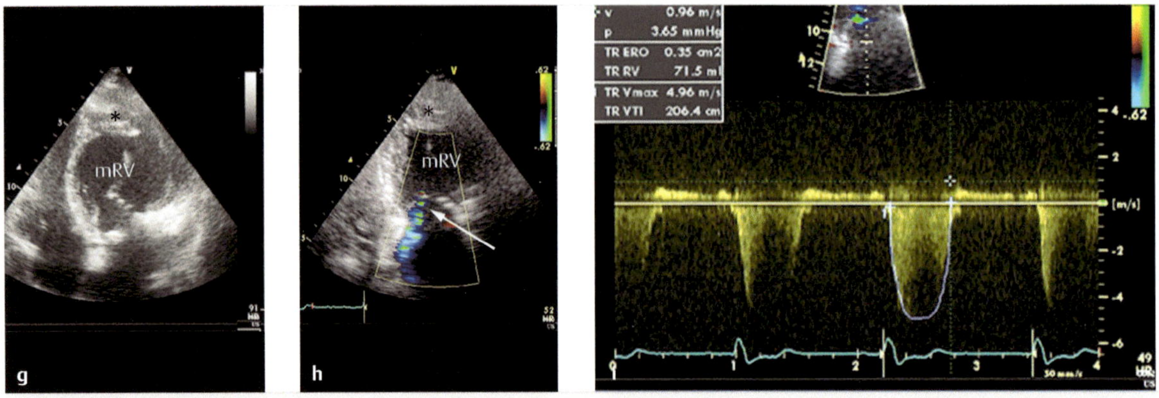

Fig 4.77 *(Continued)* **L-TGA.**

AAo = ascending aorta
L = left coronary semilunar valve
LA = left atrium
LAD = left anterior descending artery
LV = left ventricle
mLV = morphologic left ventricle
mRV = morphologic right ventricle
P = posterior semilunar valve
PA = pulmonary artery
R = right coronary semilunar valve
TV = tricuspid valve

g 2-D TTE, 4-chamber view, with the morphologic right ventricle meant to be identified using the moderator band (asterisk).
h A holosystolic insufficiency jet in a case of high-grade tricuspid valve insufficiency (arrow) is visible in color Doppler.
i Maximum flow velocity of 4.96 m/s through the tricuspid valve was determined using spectral Doppler.

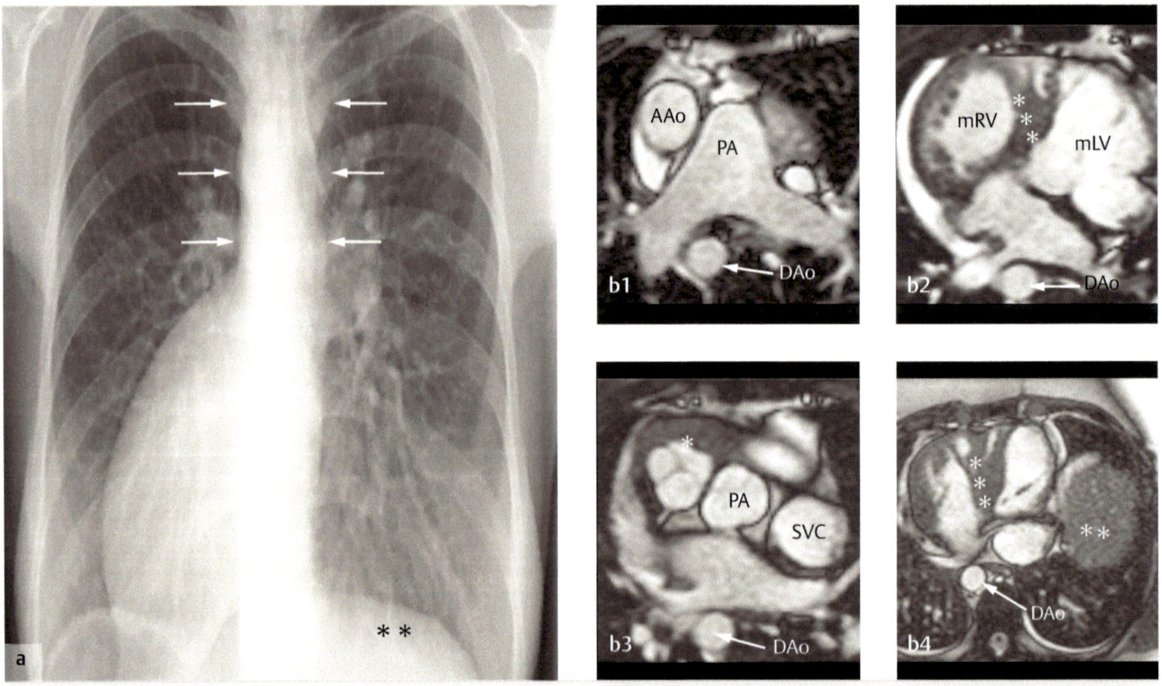

Fig. 4.78 ccTGA. Twenty-five-year-old female patient with situs inversus and ccTGA.

AAo = ascending aorta
DAo = descending aorta
mLV = morphologic left ventricle
mRV = morphologic right ventricle
PA = pulmonary artery
SVC = superior vena cava

a Narrow vascular band (arrow) in a traditional p.-a. thoracic X-ray, caused by the directly retrosternal and almost parallel position of the great vessels.
b Various axial slices from an SSFP cine MRI. Top left, the typical parallel position of the great vessels. Top right and bottom right, a prominent moderator band (triple asterisk). Bottom left, a muscular conus (asterisk) surrounding the aorta. Bottom right, a left-displaced liver (double asterisk, refer to the double asterisk in **a**).

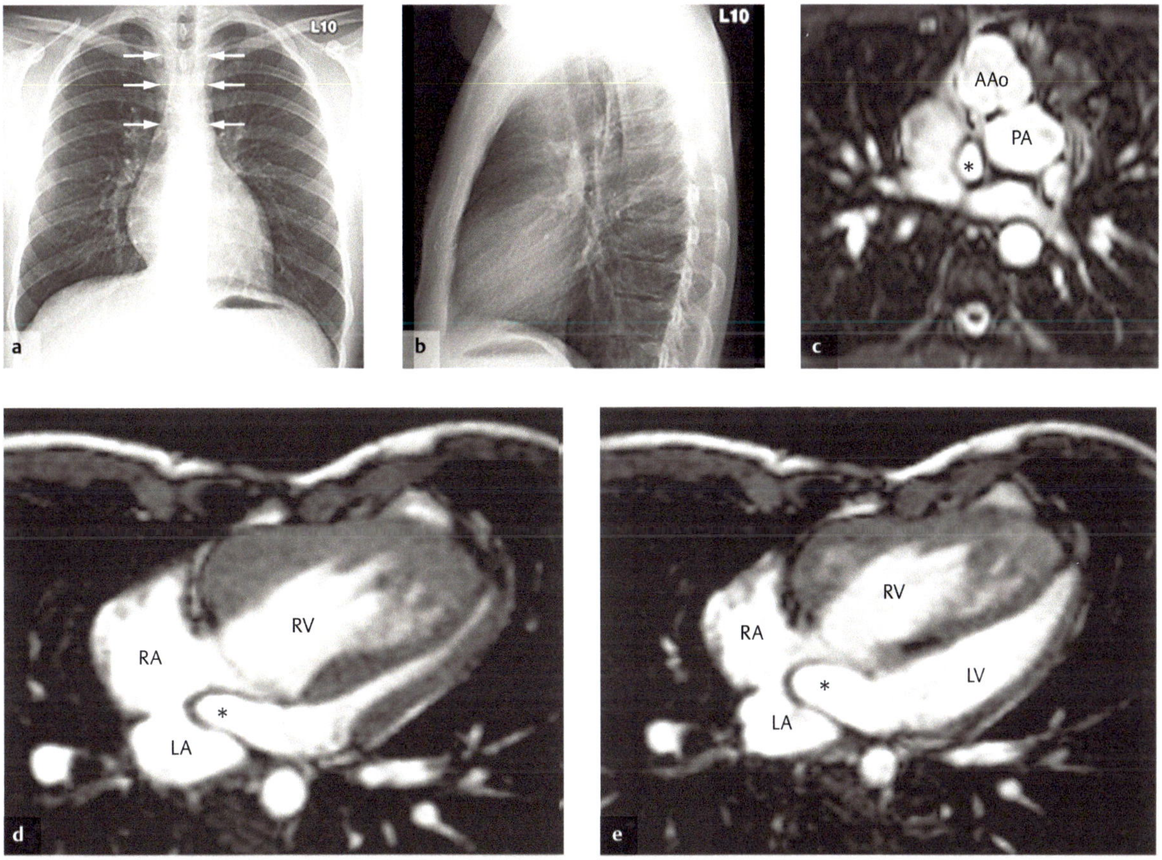

Fig. 4.79 Atrial switch operation for TGA IVS. Twenty-five-year-old male patient after an atrial switch operation for correcting complete transposition of the great arteries.

AAo = ascending aorta
LA = left atrium
LV = left ventricle
PA = pulmonary artery
RA = right atrium
RV = right ventricle

a Thoracic X-ray in p.-a projection, with a typical "narrow vascular band" (arrows).
b Thoracic X-ray, lateral projection.
c Cine MRI depiction of dextroposition of the ascending aorta and atrial tunnel (asterisk) using transverse SSFP sequences.
d Four-chamber-view of the cine MRI SSFP sequence during systole. Dyssynchrony of the right ventricle serving as a systemic ventricle, with significant hypertrophy, dilatation, and limited ventricular function (see **e**). Unremarkable appearance of the atrial tunnel (**d**, **e**, asterisks).
e Four-chamber view of the cine MRI SSFP sequence during diastole. The iatrogenic connection between the right and left atria caused by the formation of the venous atrial tunnel is clearly visible.

Treatment Options and Diagnostics

Atrial Switch Operation

Senning achieved physiological correction of TGA IVS in the atria via an atrial diversion (▶ Fig. 4.79, ▶ Fig. 4.80, ▶ Fig. 4.81, ▶ Fig. 4.82, ▶ Fig. 4.83, ▶ Fig. 4.84) for the first time in 1959. After Mustard's modifications[101] in the 1960s and 1970s, this remained the standard surgical procedure for correcting TGA IVS, in some cases well into the 1980s. Atrial diversion was achieved either by placing a GoreTex atrial tunnel (or venous baffle) (Senning method), or by using the body's own pericardium (Mustard method).

After an atrial switch operation, the right ventricle serves as a systemic ventricle with subsequent concentric hypertrophy, similar to cases of ccTGA. Over time, dilatation occurs, and "right ventricular heart failure" begins to develop (▶ Fig. 4.79d,e), which corresponds to left ventricular heart failure in a clinical sense.[91,102] Due to atrial manipulation during surgery, more than half of patients develop cardiac rhythm disorders within 10 years,[103] which often require pacemaker or ICD placement (▶ Fig. 4.81c, ▶ Fig. 4.82, ▶ Fig. 4.83, ▶ Fig. 4.84). Rarer complications, which nevertheless can be easily evaluated using noninvasive imaging techniques, include atrial tunnel leaks and stenoses. These occur most frequently near the anastomosis with the superior vena cava due to closer anatomical relationships, and usually can be treated successfully by means of stent implantation (▶ Fig. 4.81c, ▶ Fig. 4.82, ▶ Fig. 4.83, ▶ Fig. 4.84).

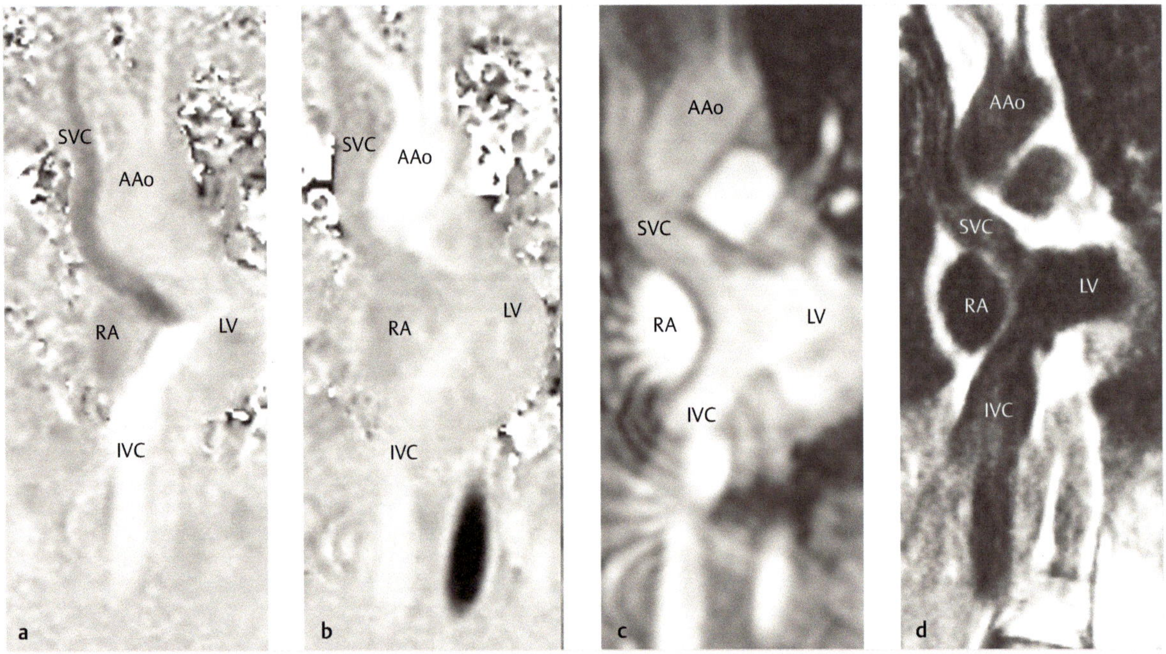

Fig. 4.80 Atrial switch operation for TGA IVS. Angulated coronal depiction of the atrial tunnel in a female patient with TGA IVS after an atrial switch operation, with various MRI sequences. Regular flow in the superior and inferior vena cavas (**a**, **b**) with no evidence of a baffle stenosis (**c**, **d**).

AAo = ascending aorta
IVC = inferior vena cava
LV = left ventricle
RA = right atrium
SVC = superior vena cava

a Phase image of the in-plane MRI sequence during diastole. Caudal flow is black, and cranial flow is pale in color.
b Phase image of MR flow measurement during systole. Caudal flow is black, and cranial flow is pale in color.
c Magnitude image of the MR flow measurement in the same orientation as (**a**,**b**,**d**).
d SE image (same sectional plane as **a–c**).

Arterial Switch Operation

Anatomical correction of TGA IVS is currently the surgical method of choice. During this procedure, both the ascending aorta and the main pulmonary artery are cut through cranial to the valve, swapped, and the coronary arteries are reinserted into the "neoaorta." Jatene's team first performed this procedure successfully in 1975.[104] Using this surgical technique, the pulmonary artery proximal to the bifurcation is cut through and then displaced ventrally, while the mobilized ascending aorta is displaced dorsally above the coronary origins, using the Lecompte maneuver.[105] This results in typical anatomy (▸ Fig. 4.85, ▸ Fig. 4.86, ▸ Fig. 4.87, ▸ Fig. 4.88, ▸ Fig. 4.89) with the neoaorta being "embraced" by the left and right pulmonary arteries.[89] This encourages stenoses to form in this area.

As a result of perioperative issues when relocating the coronary arteries, myocardial hypoperfusion can occur perioperatively, which can require immediate reoperation.[106,107] In rarer cases, stenoses of the reinserted coronary arteries can lead to ischemia later in life after an arterial switch operation. In these patients, symptoms of angina pectoris caused by myocardial ischemia, or even myocardial infarction, can occur (▸ Fig. 4.90b). Supravalvular stenoses of the left and right pulmonary arteries (▸ Fig. 4.87 and ▸ Fig. 4.88), as well as (usually) clinically insignificant aortic valve insufficiencies or dilatations or stenoses of the neoaorta (▸ Fig. 4.90a and ▸ Fig. 4.91) also occur more commonly,[89,107–109] though they can be visualized and quantified clearly using noninvasive diagnostic imaging methods.

Goals and Relative Value of Diagnostic Imaging

Thoracic X-ray

The characteristic signs of TGA in a traditional thoracic X-ray in p.-a. projection include the narrow vascular band[83] through the great vessels located immediately behind one another (or, in cases of ccTGA, directly retrosternal, and positioned side-by-side), causing a pronounced cardiac waist due to the lack of a pulmonary segment (▸ Fig. 4.78a, ▸ Fig. 4.79a,b, ▸ Fig. 4.81c and, ▸ Fig. 4.83a,d). All other findings are largely dependent upon additional concurrent malformations. The diagnosis, itself, cannot be determined solely using X-rays.

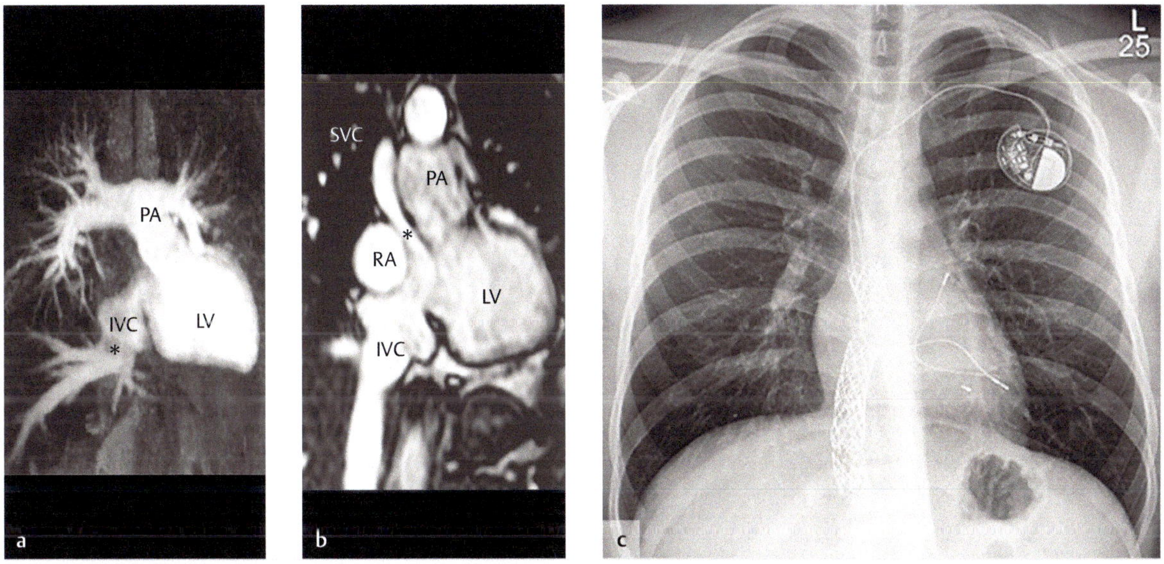

Fig. 4.81 Atrial switch operation for TGA IVS. Three different patients after an atrial switch operation to treat TGA IVS.

IVC = inferior vena cava
LV = left ventricle
PA = pulmonary artery
RA = right atrium
SVC = superior vena cava

a MIP of a contrast-enhanced MRA, RAO projection. Note the pulmonary arteries originating from the left ventricle and the inferior vena cava (asterisk) connecting to the left ventricle via the venous tunnel.

b Angulated coronal cine MRI SSFP sequence. Long-segment stenosis of the atrial tunnel is visible near the superior vena cava (asterisk).

c P.–a. thoracic X-ray. The depiction shows the stents in the superior and inferior vena cavas for treating atrial tunnel stenoses.

Doppler Echocardiography

Note

Doppler echocardiography is the key diagnostic method for TGA.

In infants, anatomical relationships can generally be assessed clearly via TTE before surgery.[7,83] The characteristic feature, namely the parallel placement of the great vessels or their lack of crossing, is visible in infants along the parasternal long axis (▶ Fig. 4.75e), but can also usually be seen from a subcostal (▶ Fig. 4.75f and g) or 4-chamber view (▶ Fig. 4.75c and d). If the invasive Rashkind maneuver is performed,[92] the coronary origins are generally also depicted in order to be able to recognize coronary origin abnormalities before surgery.

TTE is also the key method for depicting double discordance for ccTGA[6] and the common concurrent anomalies, particularly those of the atrioventricular valves (such as Ebstein's anomaly). Especially in adults, the acoustic window can be significantly impaired in its ability to assess the right ventricle, atrial tunnel (particularly near the superior vena cava) or the pulmonary arterial branches after an atrial or arterial switch operation.[6,7,83,90] At that point, either TEE or tomographic procedures must be used (▶ Table 4.23). The tricuspid valve insufficiency—commonly present as well after an atrial switch operation for treating TGA IVS (in which the right ventricle serves as the systemic ventricle) as in ccTGA (in which the morphologic right ventricle on the wrong side also serves as the systemic ventricle)—can often be assessed accurately using Doppler echocardiography (▶ Figs. 4.82 c and d).

Magnetic Resonance Imaging

Native Transposition of the Great Arteries Without Prior Surgical Treatment

If it is impossible to adequately assess the situation using echocardiography, consider using MRI (e.g., with the navigator technique) to depict the coronary origins (▶ Fig. 4.90a).[110] Regardless, spatial resolution in MRI is limited, especially for newborns and very small coronaries. Furthermore, deep sedation or even narcosis is generally needed due to the often long examination times.

In addition to echocardiography, MRI is the method of choice, particularly for classifying morphologic right ventricular anatomy (▶ Fig. 4.76, ▶ Fig. 4.78, and ▶ Table 4.23).[6,7,83,96,100,111–113] MRI is of particular importance for

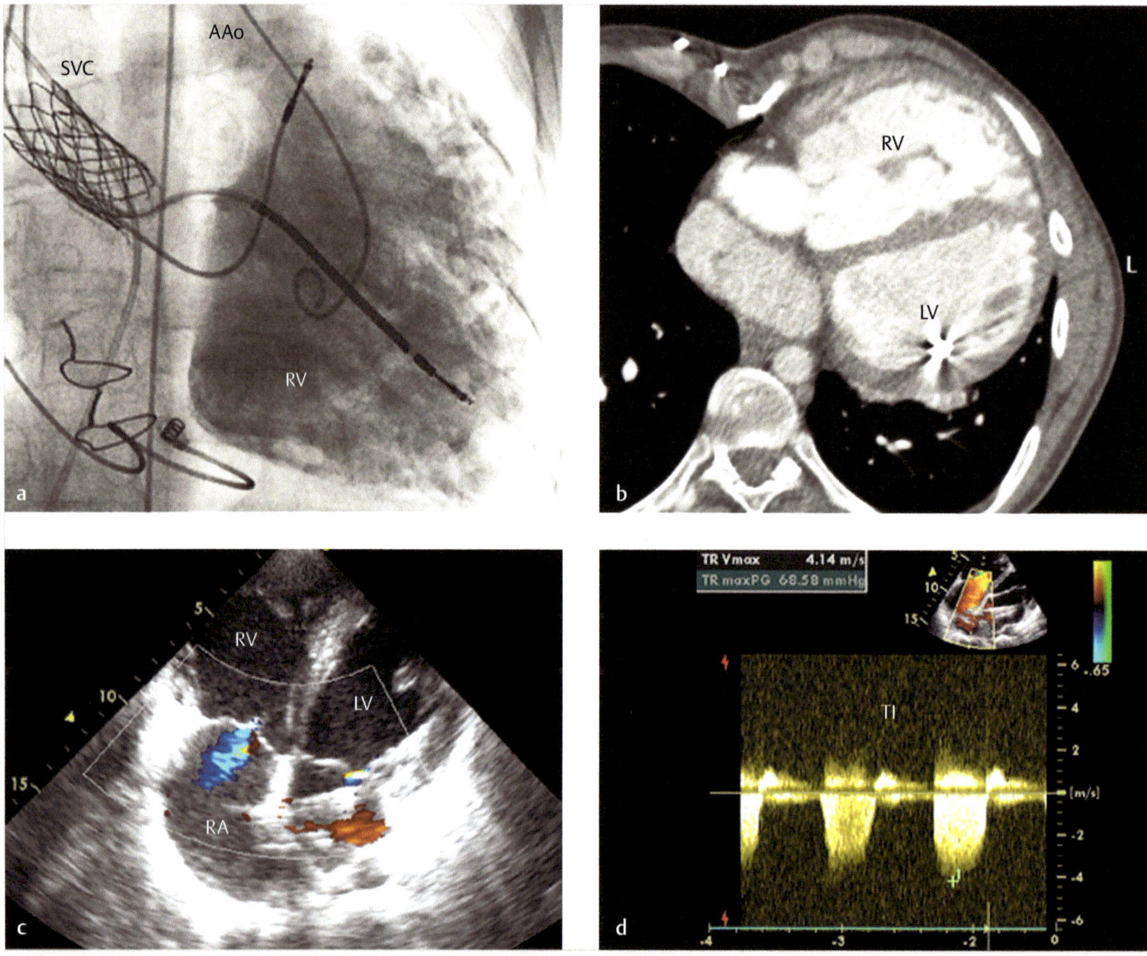

Fig. 4.82 Atrial switch operation for TGA IVS. Twenty-one-year-old male patient after an atrial switch operation to correct TGA IVS (▶ Fig. 4.83 and ▶ Fig. 4.84).

AAo = ascending aorta
LV = left ventricle
RA = right atrium
RV = right ventricle
SVC = superior vena cava
TI = tricuspid valve incompetence (tricuspid valve insufficiency)

a Levocardiogram of the significantly enlarged, hypertrophied right ventricle, which is serving as a systemic ventricle. Stent in the cranial segment of the atrial tunnel, pacemaker electrodes, and ICD.

b Transverse reconstructions of a multi-slice CT data set, with significantly enlarged right ventricle.

c Color Doppler echocardiography, 4-chamber view, depicting a holosystolic insufficiency jet (blue) of the tricuspid valve.

d Spectral Doppler depicting a maximum flow velocity of 4.14 m/s at the tricuspid valve, in the sense of a maximum pulmonary gradient of 68.58 mmHg.

recognizing concurrent anomalies and assessing right ventricular function and muscle mass.[91,98,114–116] This is crucial for follow-up exams, which are generally required throughout the patient's life in order to assess clinical progression (▶ Figs. 4.79d and e).[6] If flow measurement via doppler echocardiography is impossible, flow measurement via MRI could also be important for precise quantification of tricuspid valve insufficiency, which is considered a significant marker of prognosis both after atrial switch and in cases of ccTGA. Flow quantification of the tricuspid valve incompetence can be performed either via direct flow measurements at the tricuspid valve or, more accurately, by comparing flow measurements in the pulmonary artery and aorta or right and left ventricular volumetric analysis.

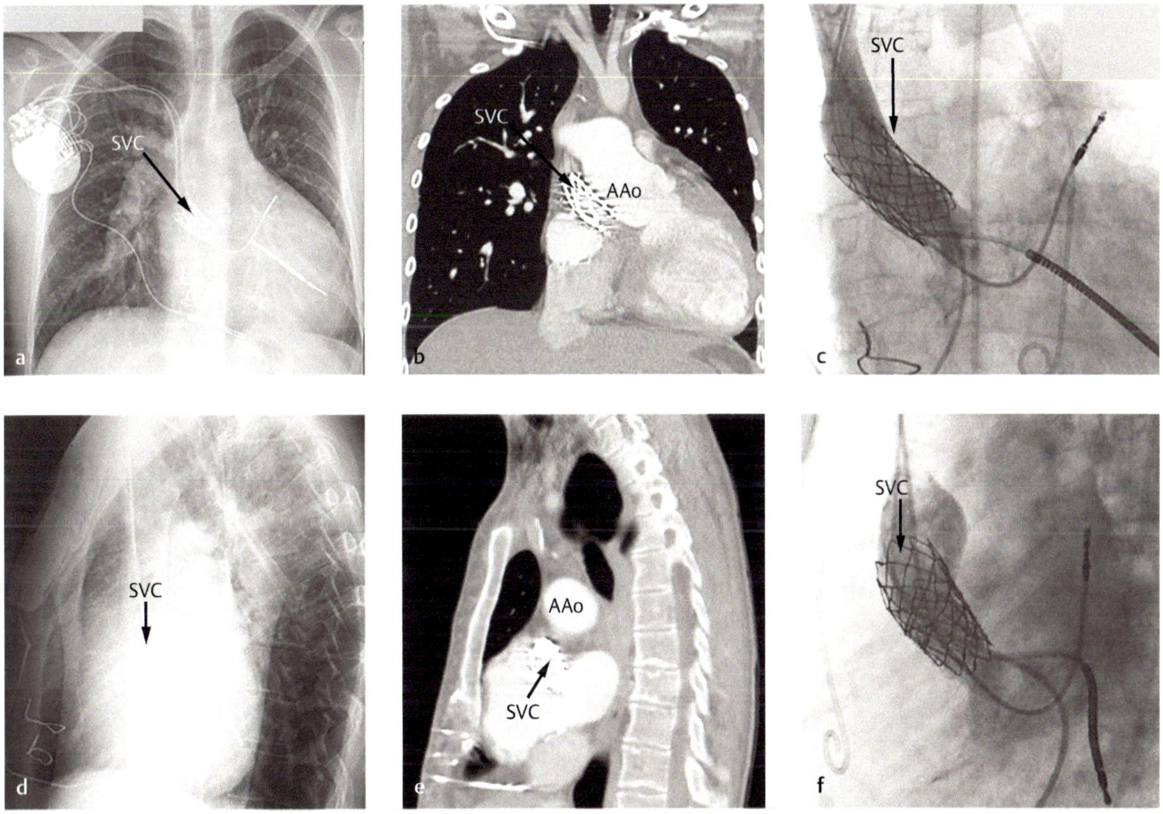

Fig. 4.83 Atrial switch operation for TGA IVS. Images of the same patient as in ▶ Fig. 4.82 and ▶ Fig. 4.84 are depicted.

AAo = ascending aorta
SVC = superior vena cava
a Thoracic X-ray, p.-a. projection.
b Coronal CT reconstruction corresponding to **a**.
c Interventional depiction of stent placement in the cranial anastomosis of the atrial tunnel with the superior vena cava.
d Thoracic X-ray, lateral projection.
e Lateral CT reconstruction corresponding to **d**.
f Follow-up image of the implanted stent.

Table 4.23 Relative value of individual imaging procedures for assessing findings in cases of ccTGA, both preoperatively and after atrial or arterial switch.

Diagnostic tasks	Thoracic X-ray	Echocardiography	MRI	Multi-slice CT	Nuclear medicine	Cardiac catheter
ccTGA:						
• **Anatomy**	+	+++	+++	++	–	++
• **Morphologic right ventricular function**	–	++	+++	++	+	++
• **Assessing tricuspid valve insufficiency**	–	++	++	–	+	+
Atrial switch:						
• **Anatomy/coronaries**	–	++	++	+++	–	+++
• **Baffle assessment**	–	++	+++	+++		++
• **Morphologic right ventricular function**	–	++	+++	++	+	++
• **Assessing tricuspid valve insufficiency**	–	++	++	–	+	+
Arterial switch:						
• **Coronary arteries**	–	+	++	+++	–	+++
• **Pulmonary arterial branches**	–	++	+++	+++	–	+++
• **Neoaortic insufficiency**	–	++	+++	–	+	++

CT, computed tomography; ccTGA, congenitally corrected transposition.

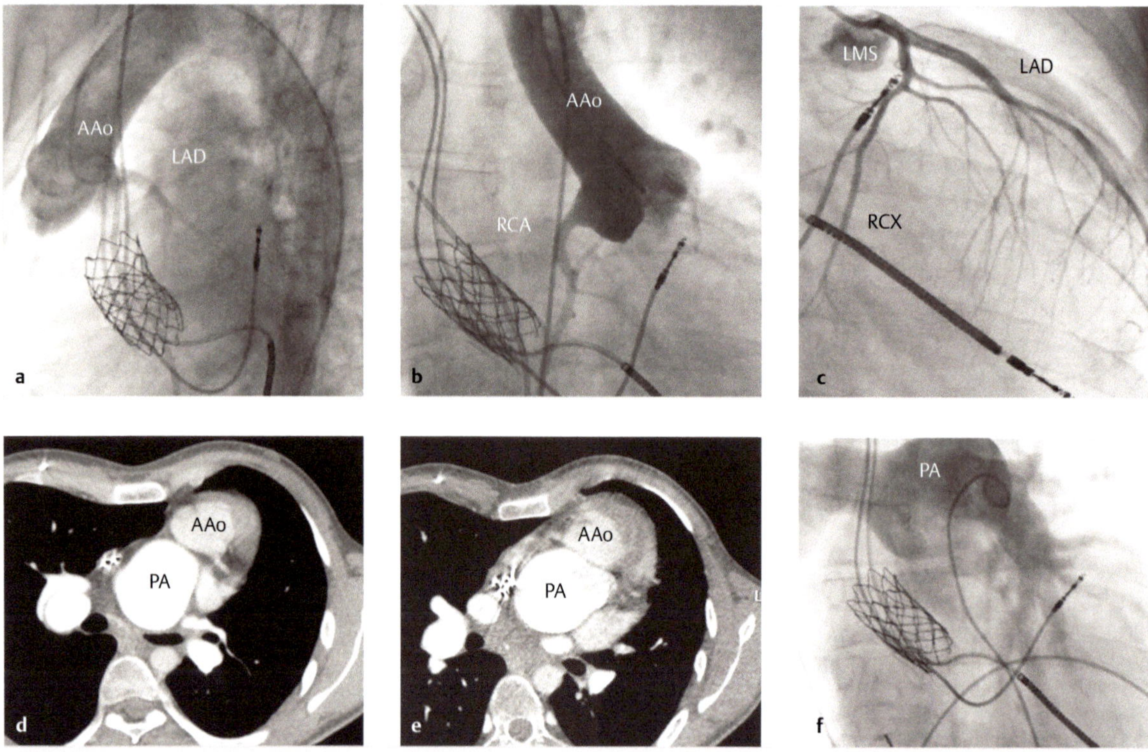

Fig. 4.84 Atrial switch operation for TGA IVS. Images of the same patients as in ▶ Fig. 4.82 and ▶ Fig. 4.83 are shown, after atrial switch operation with stent placement in the atrial tunnel.

AAo = ascending aorta
LAD = left anterior descending artery
LMS = left main stem
PA = pulmonary artery
RCA = right coronary artery
RCX = ramus circumflexus (circumflex branch)

a Invasive aortogram, lateral projection.
b b Invasive aortogram, p.-a. projection.
c Selective coronary angiogram of the left coronary tree.
d CT, transverse orientation. The dilated pulmonary artery is clearly visible (see **e**).
e CT, transverse orientation (more caudal slice).
f Pulmonary angiogram with dilated main pulmonary artery.

After Atrial Switch

The atrial tunnel, particularly near the superior vena cava (▶ Fig. 4.80, ▶ Fig. 4.81, ▶ Fig. 4.83), can only be assessed on a limited basis in older patients via TTE,[106] rendering it a primary indication for using alternative imaging methods. Stenoses or leaks can be quantified via MRI flow measurement or Doppler echocardiography. The standard sectional planes are transverse slices, primarily using rapid GE sequences (▶ Fig. 4.79c,d and,e). It is easiest to depict the entire course of the atrial tunnel, from the superior to the inferior vena cava, using angulated coronal sectional planes (▶ Fig. 4.80 and ▶ Fig. 4.81b). In doing so, an additional direct in-plane flow measurement can be performed in order to measure flow acceleration in cases of stenosis.

With adequate experience, intraatrial tunnel leaks can be discovered using MRI flow measurement, either directly or indirectly, by determining flow volume in the aorta and pulmonary artery. This allows hemodynamic significance to be assessed, especially in terms of determining whether a left–right or a right–left shunt is present.[6]

Using cine MRI in cardiac standard sectional planes, right ventricular volume, muscle mass, and function can be determined reliably.[117–120] In the future, it may be possible to also prove diffuse fibrosis of the right ventricle as a cause for "right ventricular heart failure" or to deter-

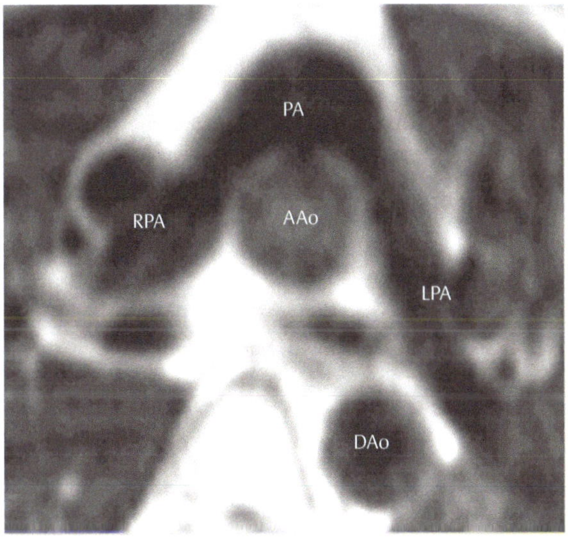

Fig. 4.85 Arterial switch operation for TGA IVS. Transverse black blood SE sequence in a patient after an arterial switch operation to treat TGA IVS using the Lecompte maneuver, with typical ventral displacement of the pulmonary artery and "embracing" of the ascending aorta by the pulmonary arterial branches.
AAo = ascending aorta
DAo = descending aorta
LPA = left pulmonary artery
PA = pulmonary artery
RPA = right pulmonary artery

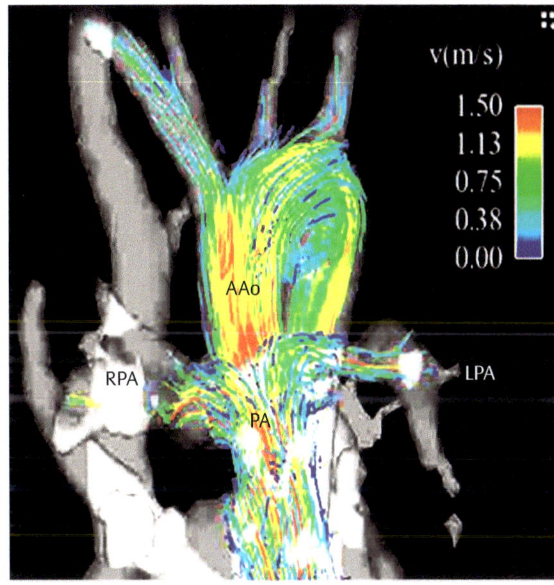

Fig. 4.86 Arterial switch operation for TGA IVS. 4-D flow visualization in a 13-year-old boy after an arterial switch operation, with minor flow acceleration in the right pulmonary artery and the ascending aorta to a maximum of 1.5 m/s during systole.
AAo = ascending aorta
LPA = left pulmonary artery
PA = pulmonary artery
PA = right pulmonary artery. (With the gracious permission of Dr. J. Geiger, Imaging Diagnostics, University Children's Hospital of Zurich.)

mine extracellular volume using the MRI technique of late contrast agent administration or parametric imaging of T1 and T2 mapping.[121] MIP or volume rendering from a contrast-enhanced MRA is well-suited to providing a spatial overview (▶ Fig. 4.81a).

After Arterial Switch

MRI can depict typical anatomy after the Lecompte maneuver is performed (▶ Fig. 4.85) using transverse SE sequences, GE sequences, or contrast-enhanced MRA in the likely event that TTE does not permit adequate visualization due to the retrosternal position of the neo-pulmonary artery and neoaorta. Cine MRI sequences in the standard sectional planes are also helpful for assessing ventricular function.[90,108,122]

Contrast-enhanced MRA should be acquired in two phases, once during the pulmonary phase, and once during the systemic phase. MRI flow measurement[90] can be used to quantify the often non-fixed, dynamic supravalvular pulmonary stenoses (▶ Fig. 4.86 and ▶ Fig. 4.87) and neoaortic valve insufficiency more accurately. In addition, flow distribution between the right and left lungs using through-plane MRI flow measurement in the left and right pulmonary arteries can be quantified accurately. In the future, this will likely be performed more frequently using 4-D flow measurement (▶ Fig. 4.86).

Since the arterial switch operation can lead to perioperative or late complications including ischemia and scar formation in the myocardium, inversion recovery GE sequences or, better yet, PSIR sequences are helpful for depicting scar tissue using late contrast agent administration (approx. 10–15 min after administering 0.1–0.2 mmol Gd-DTPA per kg body weight). This is also known as late enhancement (▶ Fig. 4.90b).[110] A stress MRI examination using adenosine or dobutamine is also suitable as an alternative to stress echocardiography or stress myocardial scintigraphy if left ventricular dysfunction is beginning to develop and myocardial ischemia is suspected.

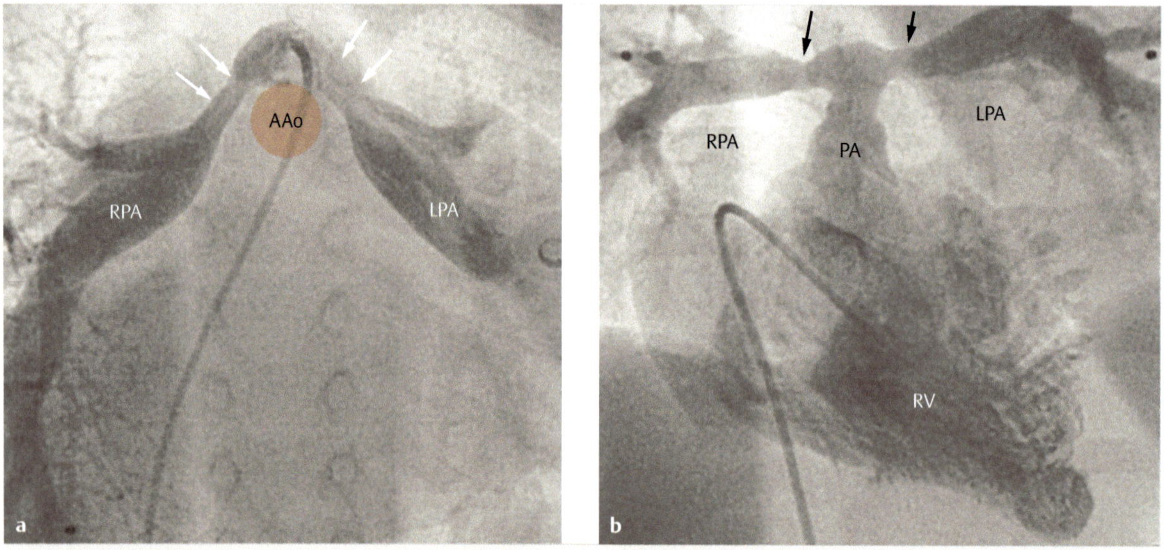

Fig. 4.87 Arterial switch operation for complete transposition of the great arteries (TGA IVS). Invasive pulmonary angiogram with bilateral pulmonary stenosis (arrows).

AAo = ascending aorta
LPA = left pulmonary artery
PA = pulmonary artery
RPA = right pulmonary artery
RV = right ventricle

a Angulated caudal projection. The red circular area indicates the ascending aorta.
b A.-p. projection.

The coronary arteries and their reinsertion into the neoaorta can be depicted directly using whole-heart sequences and the navigator technique during normal respiration, with ECG triggering.[110] This time-intensive method is a logical alternative to invasive or CT depictions in cases of normal respiration and heart rate, since stenoses generally occur proximal to the anastomosis, which can usually be depicted clearly (▶ Fig. 4.90a). View-sharing techniques and the intensive use of parallel imaging[116,123] can help shorten acquisition time.

Multi-Detector Computed Tomography (MDCT)

Native Transposition of the Great Arteries Without Prior Surgical Treatment

After MRI, multi-slice CT is the second-choice method[6,7,83,115,124–127] if it is impossible to make an adequate assessment using Doppler echocardiography or if MRI is contraindicated (e.g., after ICD implantation). In addition to clarifying morphology (▶ Fig. 4.77), particularly that of coronary anomalies (▶ Fig. 4.77e) and concurrent defects, retrospective gating can also be used to assess ventricular and valvular function.[128,129] Radiation exposure, however, remains rather high. Consequently, imaging should be performed using reduced tube currents (e.g., minDose), the step-and-shoot procedure[124,130] (also known as prospective gating), or a high-pitch mode.[126] Thus, an ECG-triggered MDCT is possible even in a single-digit mSv range, potentially even under 1 mSv in cases of low heart rate.

After Atrial Switch

Stenoses near the atrial tunnel can be depicted clearly using multi-slice CT.[129,130] Nevertheless, multi-slice CT is still the second-choice method (after MRI) for imaging atrial tunnel stenosis in this context,[6,7,83] primarily after stent placement (▶ Fig. 4.83). Multi-slice CT can use retrospective gating to quantify volume, muscle mass, and function. The use of multi-slice CT is justified, primarily before a planned reoperation, if information about the course of the coronary arteries, calcification near the planned access site, etc. is needed. In these cases, dose-sparing acquisition methods such as dose modulation (e.g., minDose), prospective gating (step-and-shoot procedure),[124,130] and flash mode (high-pitch technique) should be used.[126] Flow quantification, like with Doppler echocardiography or MRI, is not possible during multi-slice CT examinations.

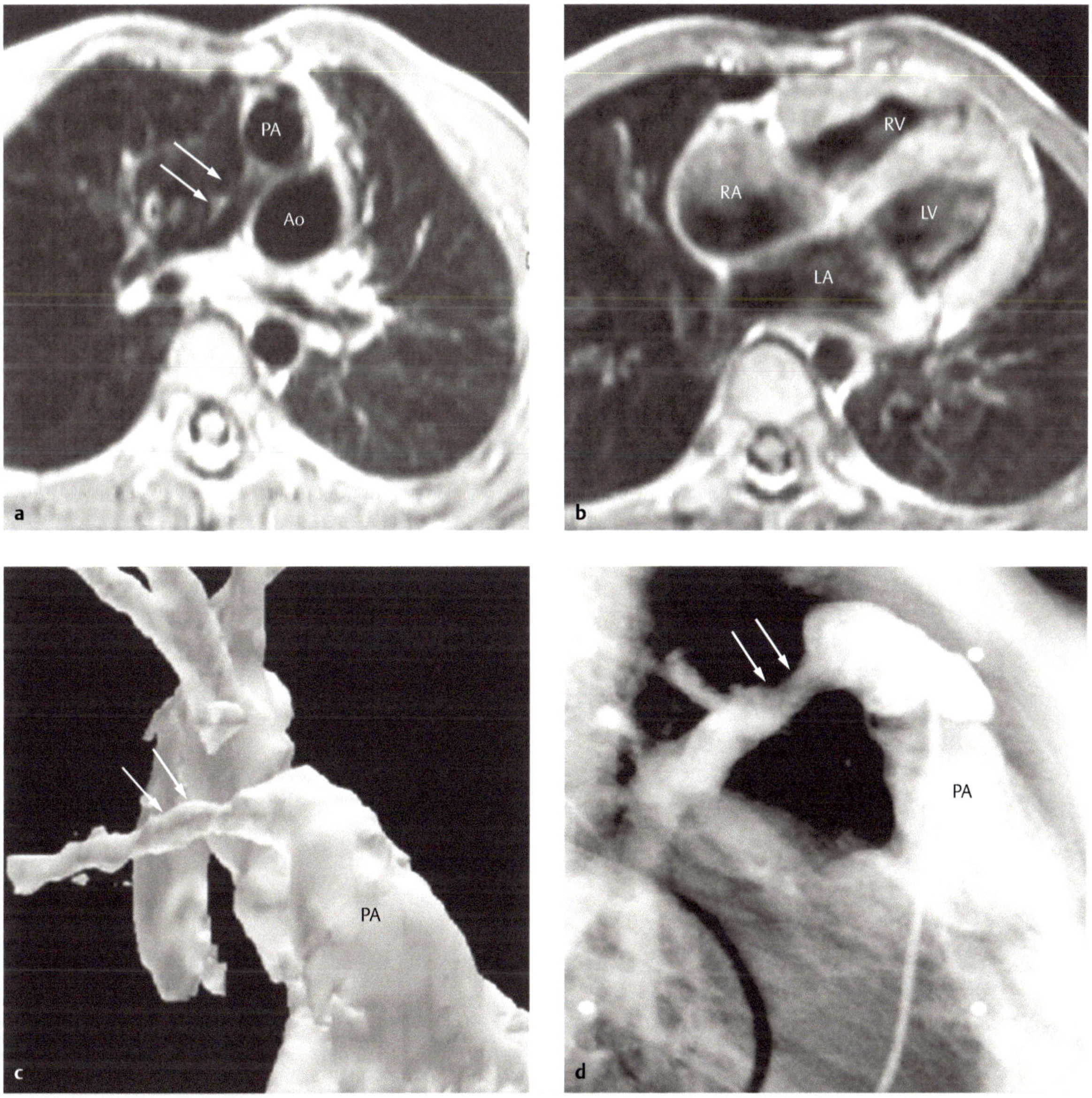

Fig. 4.88 Arterial switch operation for TGA IVS. Depiction of a higher-grade stenosis of the right pulmonary artery (**a**, **c**, **d**, arrows) in a patient after an arterial switch operation to correct TGA IVS. The left pulmonary artery is occluded.

Ao = aorta
LA = left atrium
LV = left ventricle
PA = pulmonary artery
RA = right atrium
RV = right ventricle

a Transverse MRI black blood SE sequence.
b Transverse MRI SE image. The image depicts subsequent, significant hypertrophy of the right ventricle.
c MIP reconstruction of a TOF MRA, RAO projection.
d Corresponding invasive angiogram before interventional treatment.

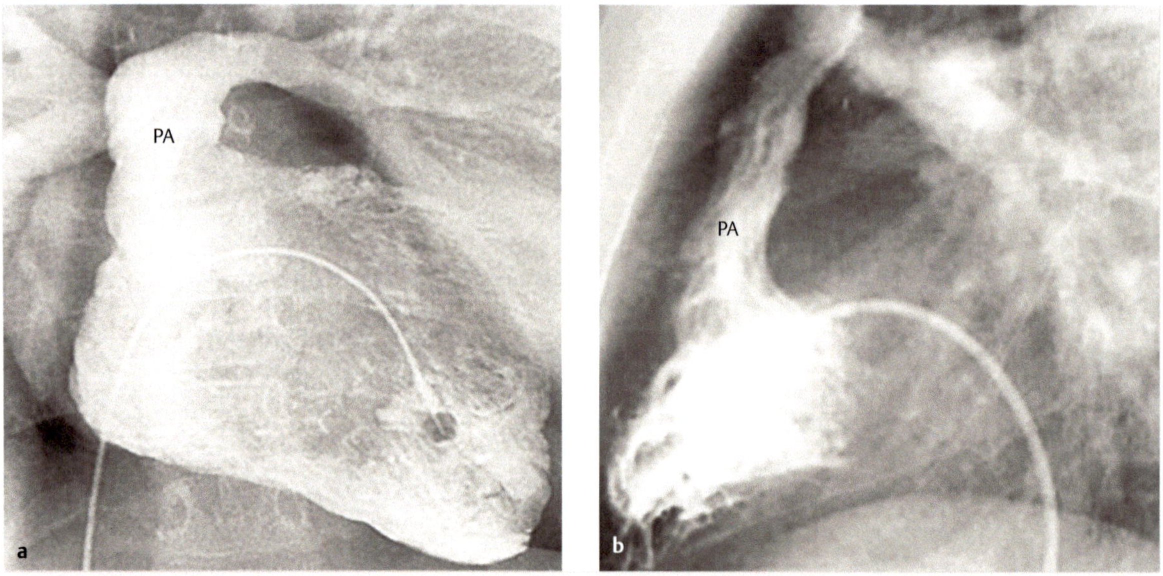

Fig. 4.89 Arterial switch operation for TGA IVS. No relevant stenoses after the operation. The invasive ventriculogram with pulmonary angiogram depicts the typical, directly retrosternal position of the pulmonary artery after performing the Lecompte maneuver.
PA = pulmonary artery
a A.-p. projection.
b Lateral projection.

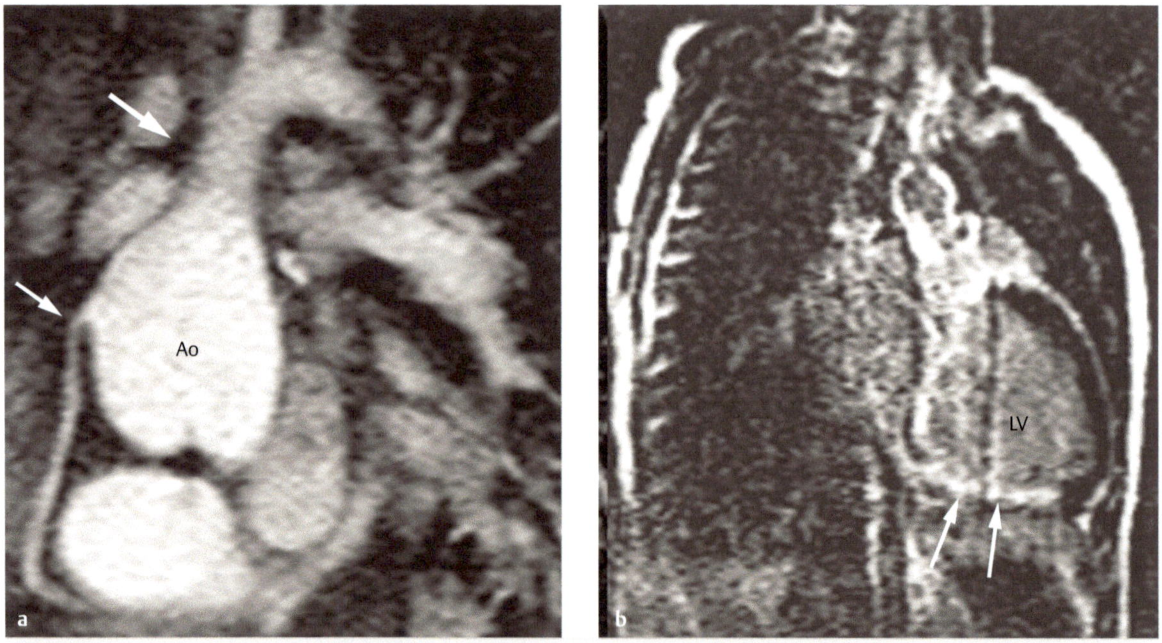

Fig. 4.90 Arterial switch operation for TGA IVS.
Ao = aorta
LV = left ventricle
a The MRI coronary angiogram of the right coronary artery of a 4-year-old girl after arterial switch operation, prepared using the navigator technique under mechanical ventilation during narcosis, depicting an origin stenosis of the right coronary artery (small arrow) and a supravalvular stenosis (large arrow) near the neoaorta.
b The corresponding late-enhancement image 15 minutes after IV administration of 0.2 mmol/kg body weight of Gd-DTPA, long axis, shows an enlarged left ventricle and a transmural scar near the posterior wall (arrow).

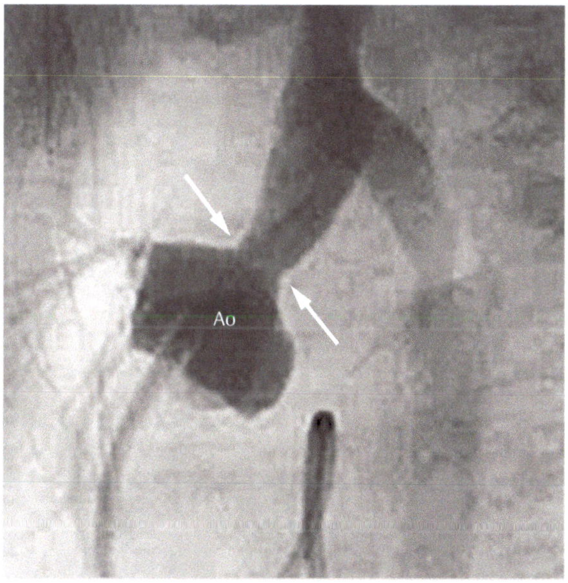

Fig. 4.91 Arterial switch operation for TGA IVS. Invasive aortogram of a patient after arterial switch operation, depicting a pronounced supravalvular aortic stenosis in the neoaorta near the pulmonary arterial branches (arrows) that were attached using the Lecompte maneuver.
Ao = Aorta

After Arterial Switch

If an inadequate acoustic window exists for TTE and MRI is contraindicated, ECG-triggered multi-slice CT is the second-choice method.[6,7,131–133] If coronary stenoses or commonly occurring supravalvular pulmonary arterial stenoses are suspected, multi-slice CT is an alternative to invasive cardiac catheter examinations, which have a higher complication rate among children and adolescents than among adults. When using dose-sparing procedures such as step-and-shoot[124,130] or flash mode,[126] comparable or even lower radiation exposure than with invasive methods can be achieved.

Radionuclide Examination

Radionuclide examinations do not play a decisive role in preoperative diagnostics for TGA, but can be used postoperatively if there is suspicion of myocardial ischemia, or to quantify shunt volume or pulmonary perfusion, provided that the latter cannot be achieved using another noninvasive methods such as echocardiography or MRI.[6]

Cardiac Catheter Exam

Diagnosing TGA IVS or ccTGA can often be done noninvasively using TTE. This means that invasive examination is only necessary if interventional measures or procedures such as a Rashkind maneuver are required, or if noninvasive diagnostics do not address all issues,[6,7] such as depicting the coronary arteries (▶ Fig. 4.84c). Invasive cardiac catheter examinations are often indispensable for hemodynamic assessment of a conduit or pulmonary artery stenosis, evaluating pulmonary hypertonia, and for treating coronary, conduit, pulmonary artery, or atrial tunnel stenoses via stent implantation, compared to surgical correction (▶ Fig. 4.82a, ▶ Fig. 4.83c,f, ▶ Fig. 4.84a,b,c,f, ▶ Fig. 4.87, ▶ Fig. 4.89, ▶ Fig. 4.91).

Summary

MRI and multi-slice CT tomographic imaging procedures only play a role for preoperative diagnostics in patients with ccTGA and no prior surgical treatment. These patients often exhibit symptoms for the first time in adulthood.

> **Note**
>
> Regular follow-up exams are recommended for patients with ccTGA to assess systemic right ventricular function and to quantify tricuspid valve insufficiency.

Doppler echocardiography and (if an intervention is needed) invasive cardiac catheter examinations are crucial for diagnosing D-TGA prior to surgery.

MRI and multi-slice CT are used primarily for postoperative follow-up examinations after atrial and arterial switch operations. Visualizing and assessing the function of the atrial tunnel and right systemic ventricle are the main indications for MRI in the case of an atrial switch operation. Multi-slice CT, in contrast, is only the first-choice method for depicting the coronary arteries noninvasively or if MRI is contraindicated. For cases of arterial switch operations, MRI is the main method for assessing supravalvular pulmonary stenoses, aortic valve insufficiency of the neoaorta, and myocardial viability, as well as for diagnosing ischemia. Multi-slice CT, however, is the first-choice method for assessing reinserted coronary arteries, and should, if possible, be performed using dose-sparing techniques such as dose modulation, prospective gating, or the high-pitch mode.

4.4.2 Common Arterial Trunk

Matthias Gutberlet, Christian Kellenberger

Definition

In this rare congenital heart defect, whereby a single ventriculo-arterial valve (trunk valve) is present, the aorta and pulmonary arteries emerge, in various spatial configurations, from a common blood vessel originating from both ventricles (truncus arteriosus) (▶ Fig. 4.92). With very few exceptions, the common arterial trunk is nearly

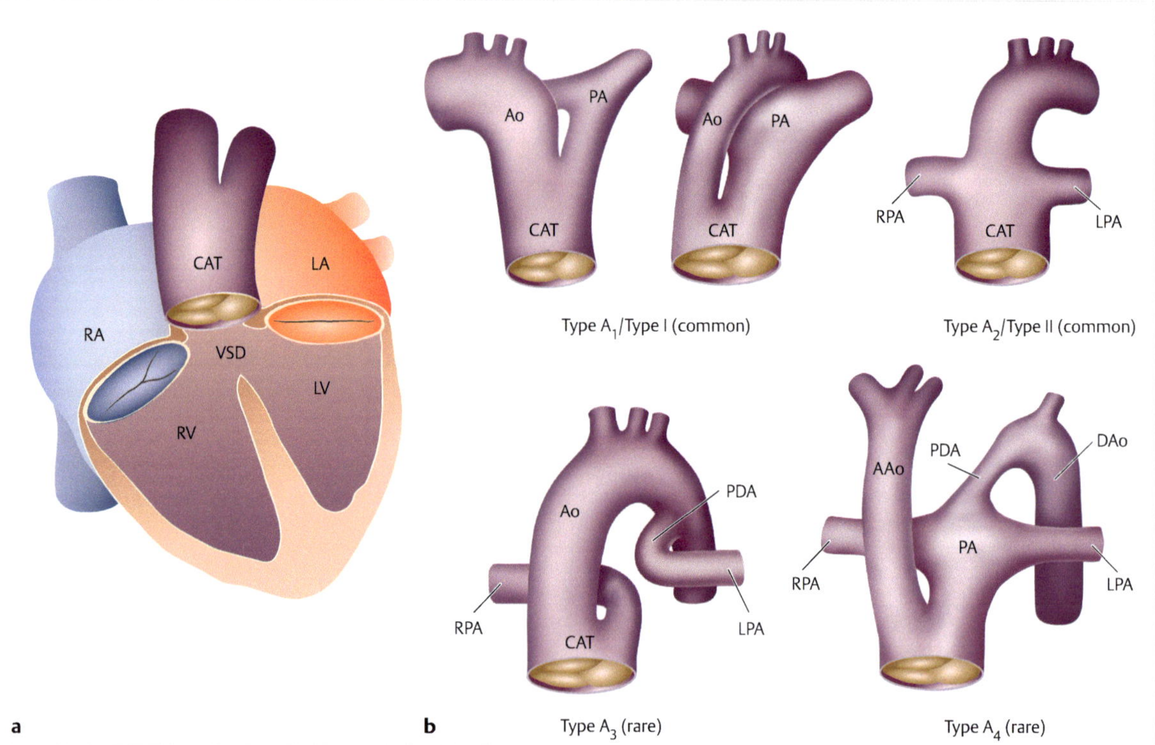

Fig. 4.92 Common arterial trunk. Schematic depiction.
AAo = ascending aorta
Ao = aorta
CAT = common arterial trunk (truncus arteriosus)
DAo = descending aorta
LPA = left pulmonary artery
PA = pulmonary artery
PDA = patent ductus arteriosus
RPA = right pulmonary artery

a Depiction of the common trunk valve for the aorta and pulmonary artery, positioned superior to the large VSD.
b Van Praagh classification of the four different forms based on the origin of the pulmonary arteries, arterial trunk, and aortic arch.[134,135] Types A_1 and A_2, which are the most common, corresponding to Collett and Edwards' types I and II.[83,134–136]

always associated with a VSD. If the central pulmonary arteries are absent, pulmonary perfusion occurs via MAPCAs.

Classification

The most common classifications are those created by Collett and Edwards[83,134–136] and Van Praagh,[134,135] which depend on the spatial position of the aorta, pulmonary arteries, and aortic arch to one another and distinguish between four different trunk forms (types I–IV or A_1–A_4; ▶ Fig. 4.92b). The two most common types, namely types A_1 and A_2 or types I and II, are identical.[83,134,137] Thus, only Van Praagh classifications will be described here.

- *Type A_1 or type I* (most common type; ▶ Fig. 4.92b): A developed trunk septum and a defect directly cranial to the trunk valve with dominant aorta or main pulmonary artery are present.
- *Type A_2 or type II* (second most common type; ▶ Fig. 4.93; also ▶ Fig. 4.92b): the trunk septum and main pulmonary artery are completely absent, and the right and left pulmonary arteries originate directly from the trunk.
- *Type A_3* (rare; ▶ Fig. 4.92b): Only one branch (right or left pulmonary artery) originates from the trunk. The second branch is supplied via the aortopulmonary collaterals or a PDA derivative. This is known as "hemitruncus."
- *Type A_4* (rare; ▶ Fig. 4.94; also ▶ Fig. 4.92b): This type corresponds to type A_1, though with a narrower or hypoplastic ascending aorta and then mostly complete aortic interruption, atresia, or aortic coarctation.

Hemodynamics and Clinical Issues

The clinical image depends on the severity of tricuspid valve insufficiency and/or stenosis, as well as pulmonary perfusion and concurrent defects. Increased pulmonary circulation leads to increased pulmonary resistance, which can eventually result in pulmonary hypertonia. The clinical picture is generally characterized by congestive heart failure.[83]

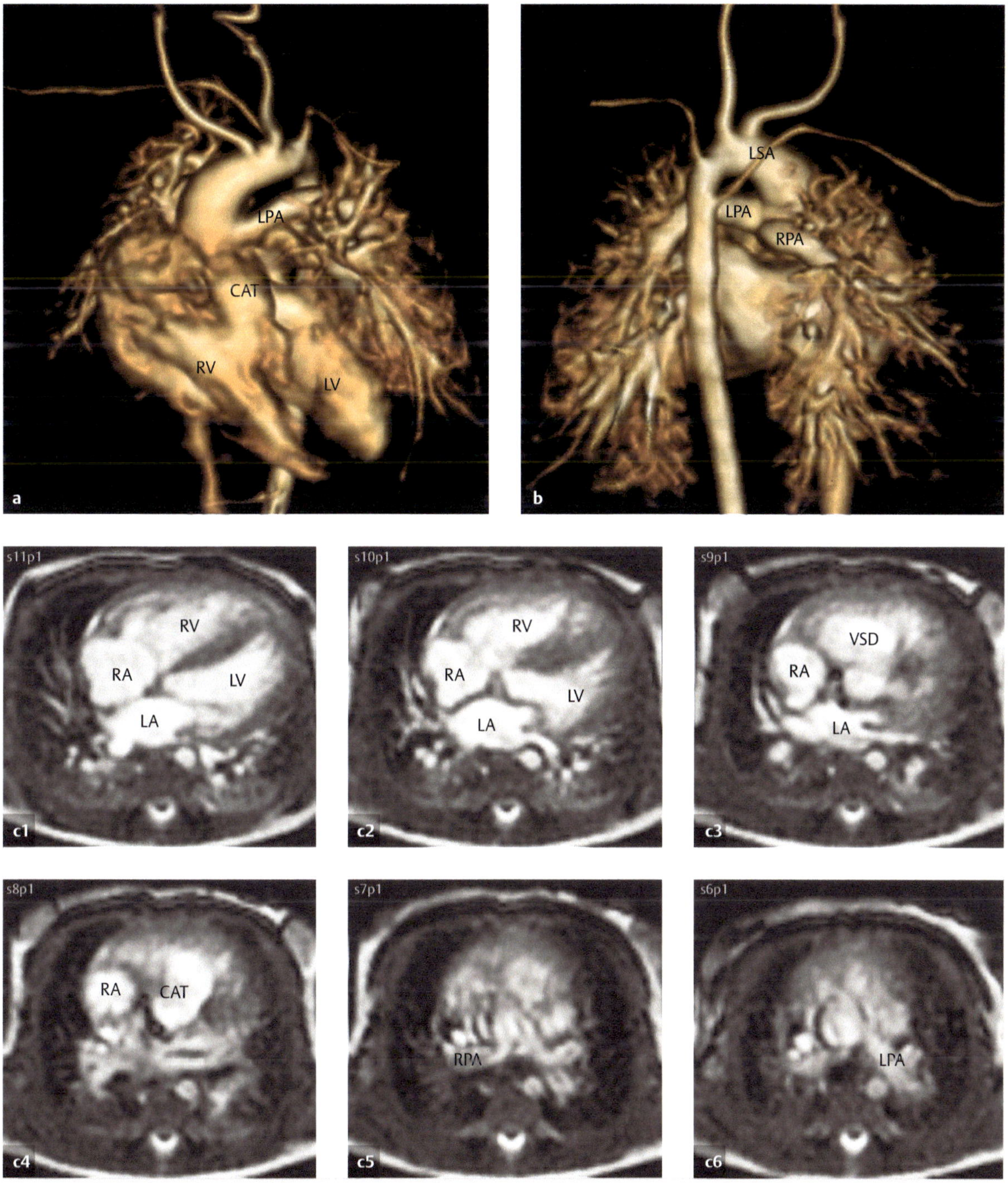

Fig. 4.93 Type A_2 common arterial trunk. MRIs of a 3-week-old girl with type A_2 (type II) common arterial trunk. The 3-D reconstructions (**a**, **b**) depict the common trunk with an origin central to the right and left ventricle. The right and left pulmonary arteries have separate origin points on the common trunk. The intact aortic arch is located on the left side with anomalous origin of the right subclavian artery (lusoria artery) as the final vessel.

CAT = common arterial trunk
LPA = left pulmonary artery
LSA = left subclavian artery
LV = left ventricle
RPA = right pulmonary artery
RV = right ventricle
VSD = ventricular septal defect

a Anterior 3-D reconstructions (volume rendering technique) of a contrast-enhanced MRA.
b Posterior 3-D reconstructions (volume rendering technique) of a contrast-enhanced MRA.
c Axial SSFP cine images, caudal to cranial, depicting the common arterial trunk cranial to a perimembranous VSD.

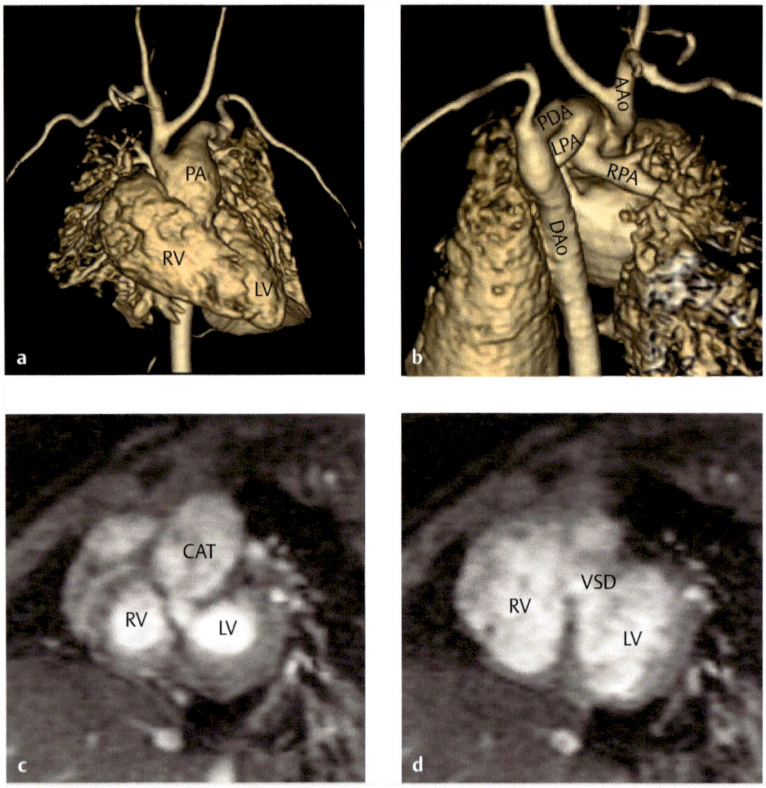

Fig. 4.94 Type A_4 common arterial trunk. MRIs of a 5-day-old boy with type A_4 (type I with type B IAA) common arterial trunk. 3-D reconstructions (**a**, **b**) depict a common trunk located centrally, superior to the right and left ventricle, with a dominant main pulmonary artery and a slightly hypoplastic ascending aorta. The aortic arch is interrupted after the origin of the left common carotid artery, and the descending aorta is supplied via the open arterial duct. SSFP cine MRIs (**c**, **d**) demonstrate the common trunk "overriding" the VSD.

AAo = ascending aorta
CAT = common arterial trunk
DAo = descending aorta
LPA = left pulmonary artery
LV = left ventricle
PA = main pulmonary artery
PDA = patent ductus arteriosus
RPA = right pulmonary artery
RV = right ventricle
VSD = ventricular septal defect

a Anterior 3-D reconstruction (volume rendering technique) of a contrast-enhanced MRA.
b Posterior 3-D reconstruction (volume rendering technique) of a contrast-enhanced MRA.
c SSFP cine MRIs, short-axis view, near the base of the heart during systole.
d SSFP cine MRIs, short-axis view, near the base of the heart during diastole.

Treatment Options and Diagnostics

Generally speaking, pulmonary artery banding is only performed in rare cases.[83] The goal is the earliest possible primary corrective surgery with patch closure of the VSD and reconstruction of the RVOT using a valve-equipped conduit between the right ventricle and pulmonary artery (▶ Fig. 4.95, ▶ Fig. 4.96, ▶ Fig. 4.97). In the event of concurrent IAA, continuity to the aorta must be restored (▶ Fig. 4.98; ▶ Fig. 4.92b). The risk of surgery depends on the type, the patient's age, the condition of the trunk valve, and the presence of coronary anomalies and concurrent defects.[83,138]

Morphological conditions can often be explained preoperatively simply by using Doppler echocardiography. Postoperatively, stenoses of the extracardiac conduit—which does not grow with the patient occur (▶ Fig. 4.97 and ▶ Fig. 4.98). Furthermore, calcifications (▶ Fig. 4.99) and valve insufficiency on the conduit or trunk valve (▶ Fig. 4.100 and ▶ Fig. 4.101) are common. For these reasons, other surgical procedures that do not use valve-equipped conduits are employed, such as those utilizing the left auricle.[138] This procedure allegedly allows the implant to better grow with the patient, though long-term results remain to be seen.

Goals and Relative Value of Diagnostic Imaging

Though *thoracic X-rays* can be used to identify global cardiac enlargement in its initial stages, as well as increased

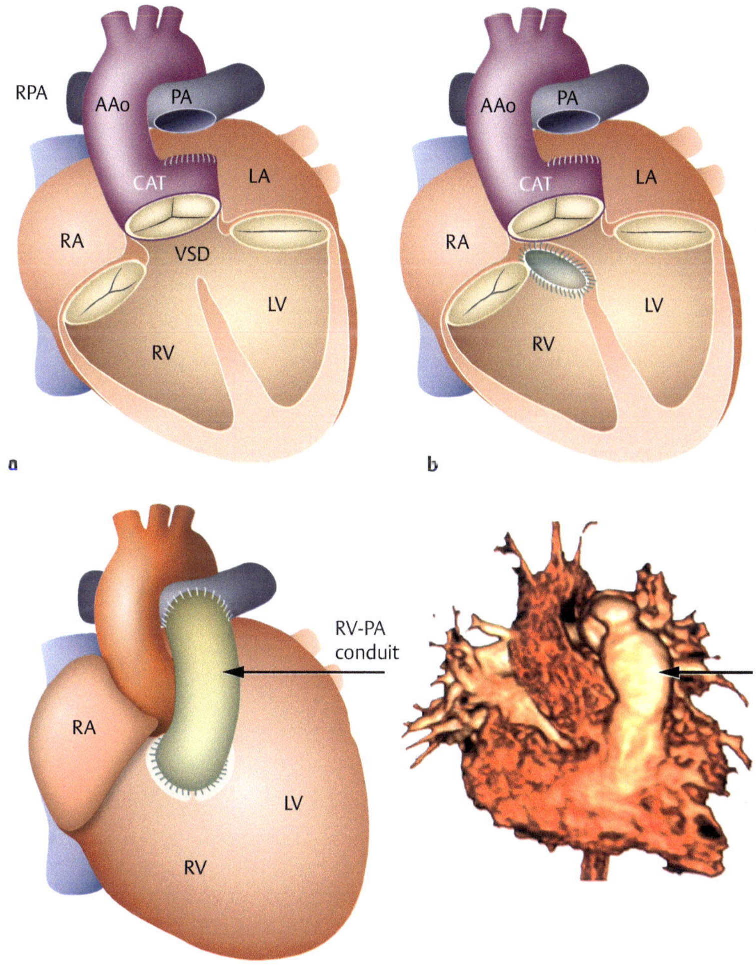

Fig. 4.95 Surgical correction of common arterial trunk. Schematic depiction of the three surgical steps (**a–c**).
CAT = common arterial trunk
LV = left ventricle
RA = right atrium
RPA = right pulmonary artery
RV = right ventricle
VSD = ventricular septal defect
a Detachment of the pulmonary artery and closure of the pulmonary stump.
b Closure of the VSD using a patch.
c Implantation of a conduit (arrow) between the right ventricle and pulmonary artery.
d 3-D reconstruction (volume rendering technique) of a contrast-enhanced MRA data set with bolus tracking near the conduit (arrow) between the right ventricle and pulmonary artery.

pulmonary volume load (▸ Fig. 4.98a) or signs of pulmonary hypertonia in later stages, there is no pathognomonic clinical picture.[83,137,139] Calcification or dilation of the conduit (▸ Fig. 4.96a) may be visible postoperatively (▸ Fig. 4.99a).

Doppler TTE is the method of choice for determining the initial diagnosis. Proving the presence of a singular semilunar valve originating from both ventricles with a malalignment VSD, and the origination of the coronary and pulmonary arteries from the arterial trunk, are decisive for diagnostic purposes. The second pulmonary artery must be identified and localized not only for classification purposes, but also for preoperative diagnostics in order to assess potential surgical connections. This can, however, present difficulties.[83] In these cases, tomographic procedures (▸ Fig. 4.93) or invasive diagnostics by means of a cardiac catheter may become necessary.

In addition to clarifying complex anatomy, especially that of the pulmonary arteries and coronaries, *invasive measurement* of pressure gradients and the calculation of vascular resistance in pulmonary and systemic circulation are crucial. Thus, tomographic procedures are generally used postoperatively. Invasive angiography is mostly used postoperatively if an intervention is also intended to be performed simultaneously (▸ Fig. 4.98b).

Fundamentally, equally clear purely anatomical depictions can be achieved using *MRI* (see ▸ Fig. 4.93, ▸ Fig. 4.94, ▸ Fig. 4.95, ▸ Fig. 4.96, ▸ Fig. 4.97, ▸ Fig. 4.98, ▸ Fig. 4.100, ▸ Fig. 4.101) or *multi-slice CT* (▸ Fig. 4.99), especially near the pulmonary arterial branches.[140–143] Noninvasive depiction of the coronary arteries, even in cases of common trunk, remains within the purview of multi-slice CT.

Pulmonary artery stenoses and valve insufficiencies, which often occur postoperatively, can be quantified both with *Doppler echocardiography* (▸ Fig. 4.101) or, in the case of limited acoustic window, via *MRI flow measurement* in order to yield absolute, precise measurements of valve insufficiency and unilateral pulmonary circulation (▸ Fig. 4.100, ▸ Fig. 4.101).

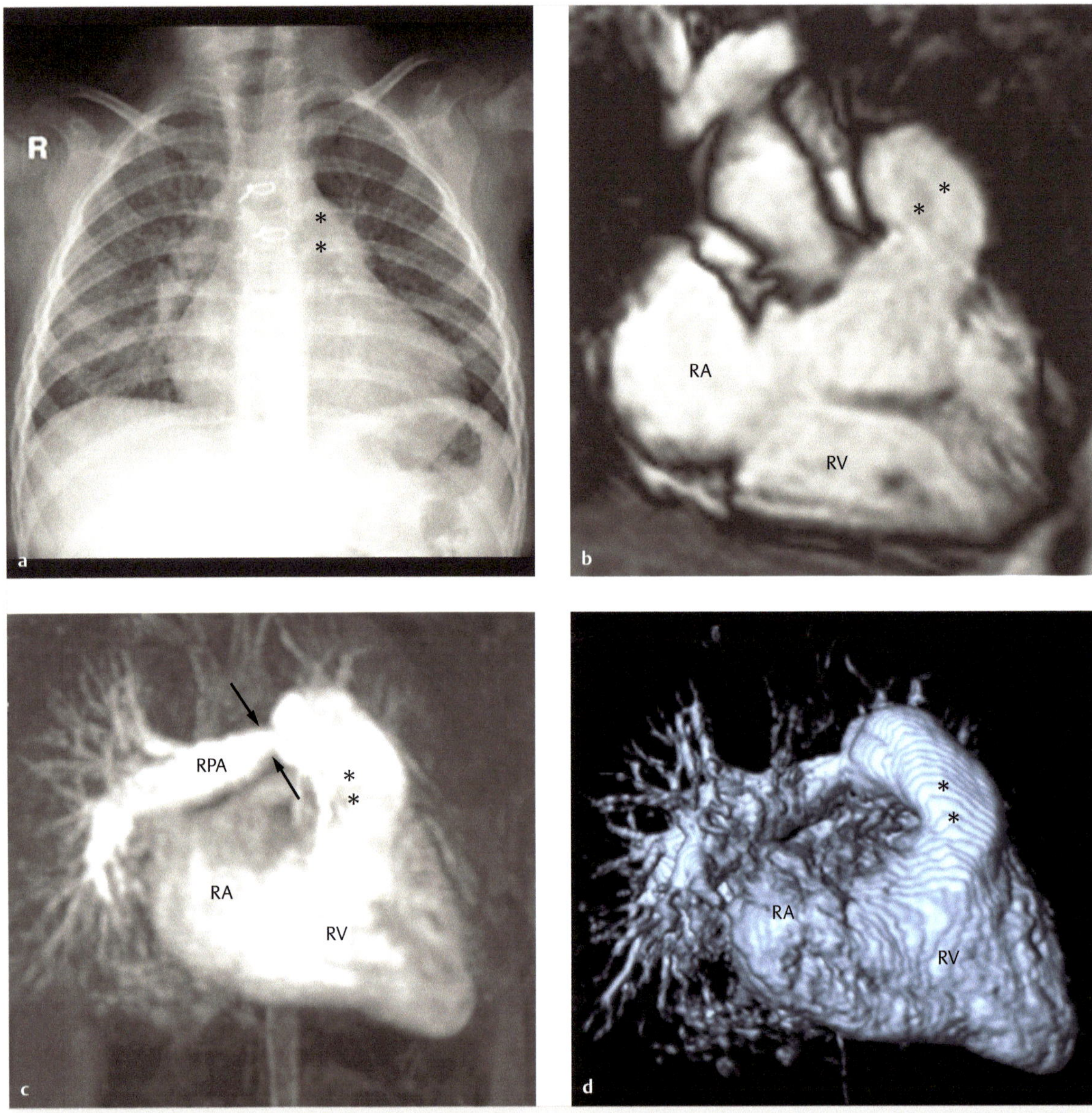

Fig. 4.96 Condition after surgical correction of type A_2 (type II) common arterial trunk. Ten-year-old girl with minor residual stenosis near the origin of the right pulmonary artery. The dilated conduit (**a–d**, two asterisks) between the right ventricle and pulmonary artery is clearly visible in MRIs (▸ Fig. 4.101 for additional patient images).

RA = right atrium
RV = right ventricle

a Thoracic X-ray, p.-a. projection.
b Coronal SSFP cine MRI.
c 3-D MIP reconstruction of a contrast-enhanced MRA data set, RAO projection, depicting the RPA origin stenosis (arrows).
d 3-D reconstruction (volume rendering technique) of a contrast-enhanced MRA data set, RAO projection.

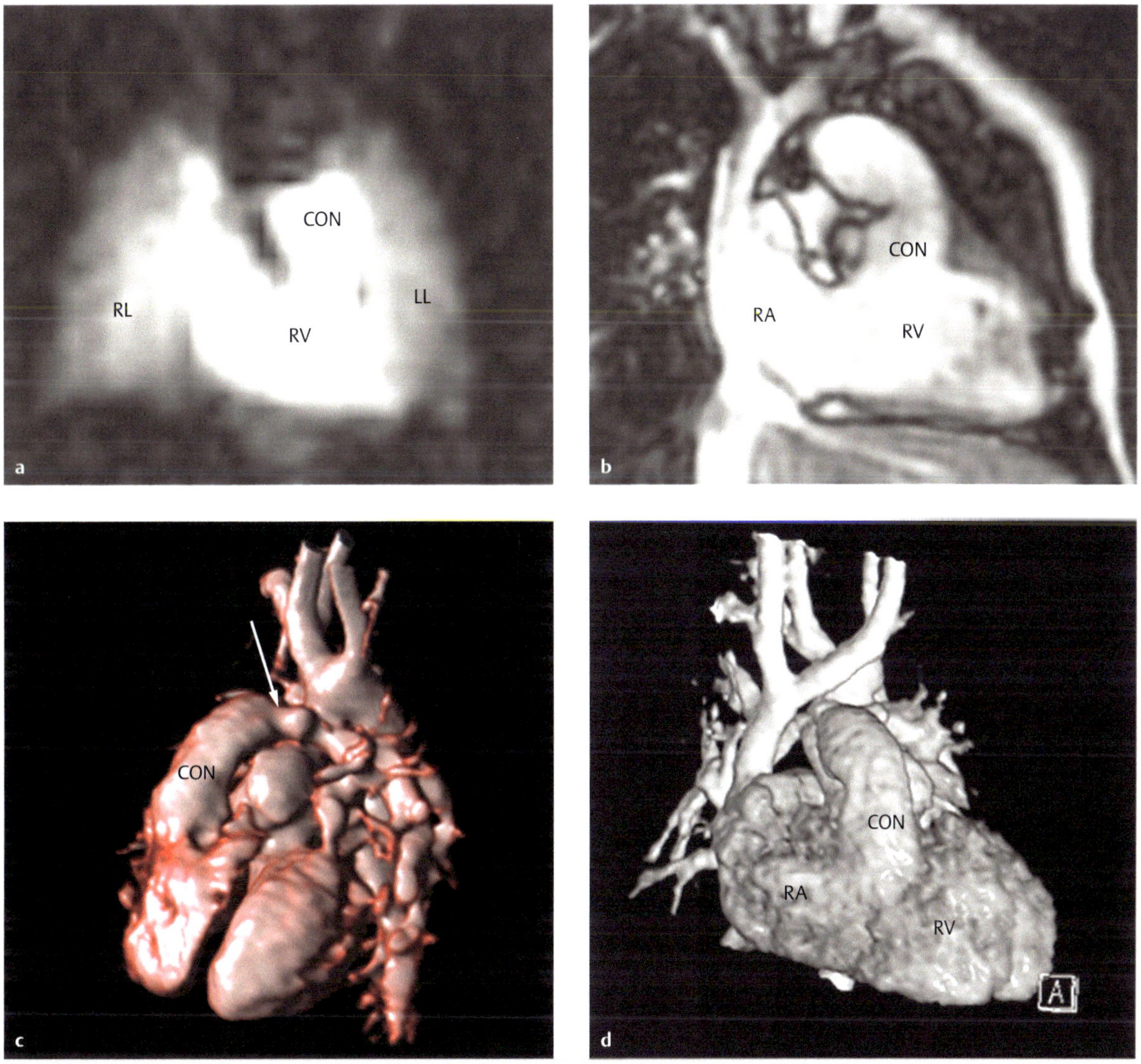

Fig. 4.97 Condition after surgical correction of type A_1 (type I) common arterial trunk. MRIs of a 4-year-old girl after surgical correction of type A_1 (type I) and IAA (type B), current stenosis of the left pulmonary artery (**c**), and relative stenosis of the ascending aorta (also ▶ Fig. 4.98).

CON = conduit
LL = left lung
RA = right atrium
RL = right lung
RV = right ventricle

a Coronal orientation of a dynamic contrast-enhanced angiogram with minor temporal delay of contrast agent inflow in the left lung and stenosis of the left pulmonary artery.

b Coronal SSFP cine MRI.

c The arrow indicates the stenosis in the left pulmonary artery.

d 3-D reconstruction (volume rendering technique) of a contrast-enhanced MRA, a.-p. projection. Depiction of a non-stenosed, valve-equipped extracardiac conduit from the right ventricle to the pulmonary artery. The pulmonary arterial bifurcation is positioned ventral to the ascending aorta after performing the Lecompte maneuver.

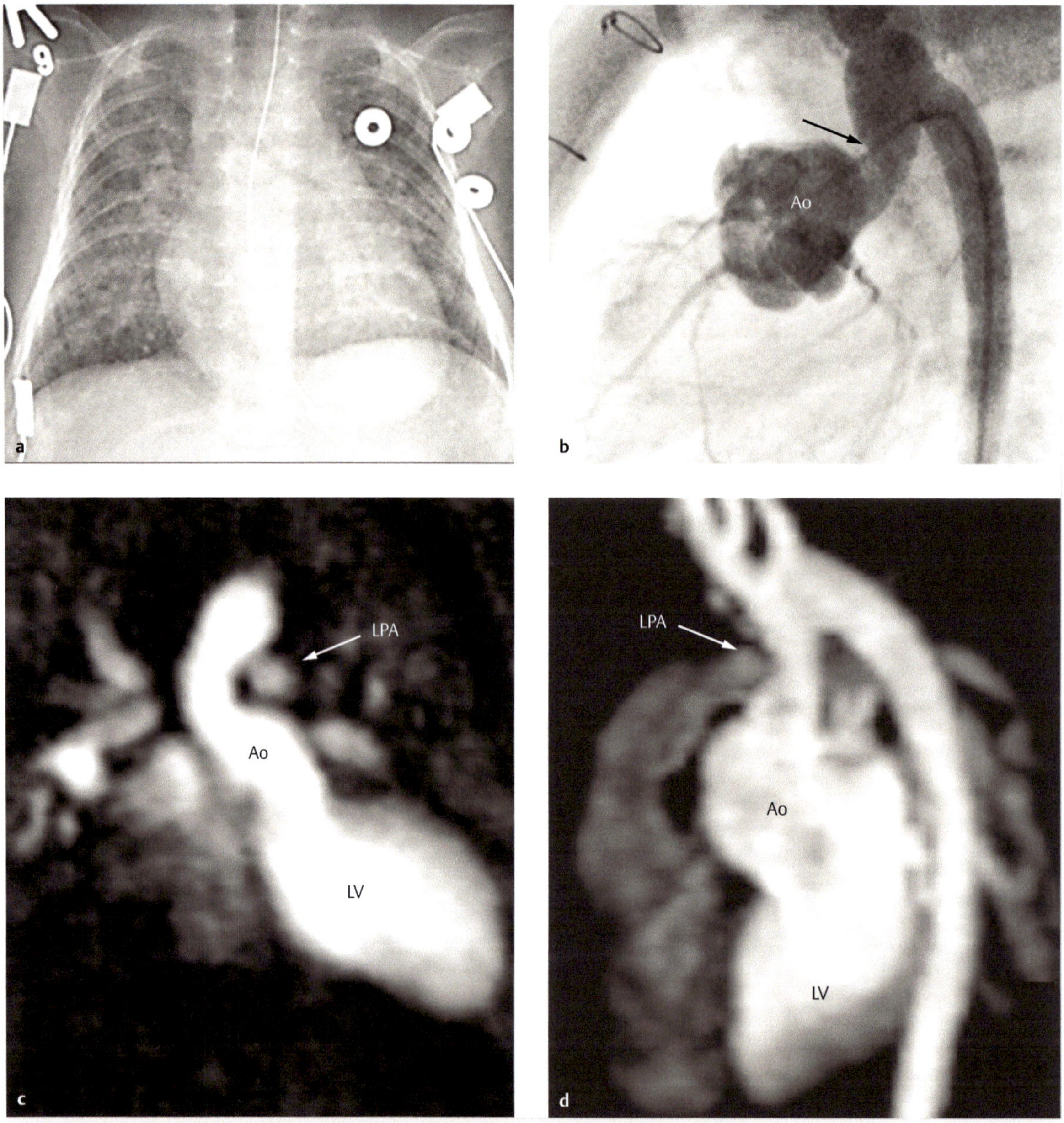

Fig. 4.98 Condition before and after surgical correction of type A_1 (type I) common arterial trunk. The thoracic X-ray (**a**) depicts an enlarged heart and volume overload in the lungs. A relative stenosis of the ascending aorta (**b**, arrow), dilated aortic root, and reconstructed aortic arch are visible via invasive angiography. The SSFP cine MRI (**c**) and 3-D MIP reconstruction (**d**) indicate the close spatial relationship between the left pulmonary artery and the relative ascending aorta stenosis after performing the Lecompte maneuver.

Ao = aorta
LPA = left pulmonary artery
LV = left ventricle

a Newborn thoracic X-ray of the 4-year-old girl from ▶ Fig. 4.97 with type A_1 (type I) common arterial trunk and IAA (type B).

b Invasive aortogram of the same patient as a 4-year-old, after surgical correction, with the detached left subclavian artery (see **d**) and Lecompte maneuver of the pulmonary arteries.

c SSFP cine MRI, coronal plane.

d 3-D MIP reconstruction of a contrast-enhanced MRI during the arterial phase, lateral projection.

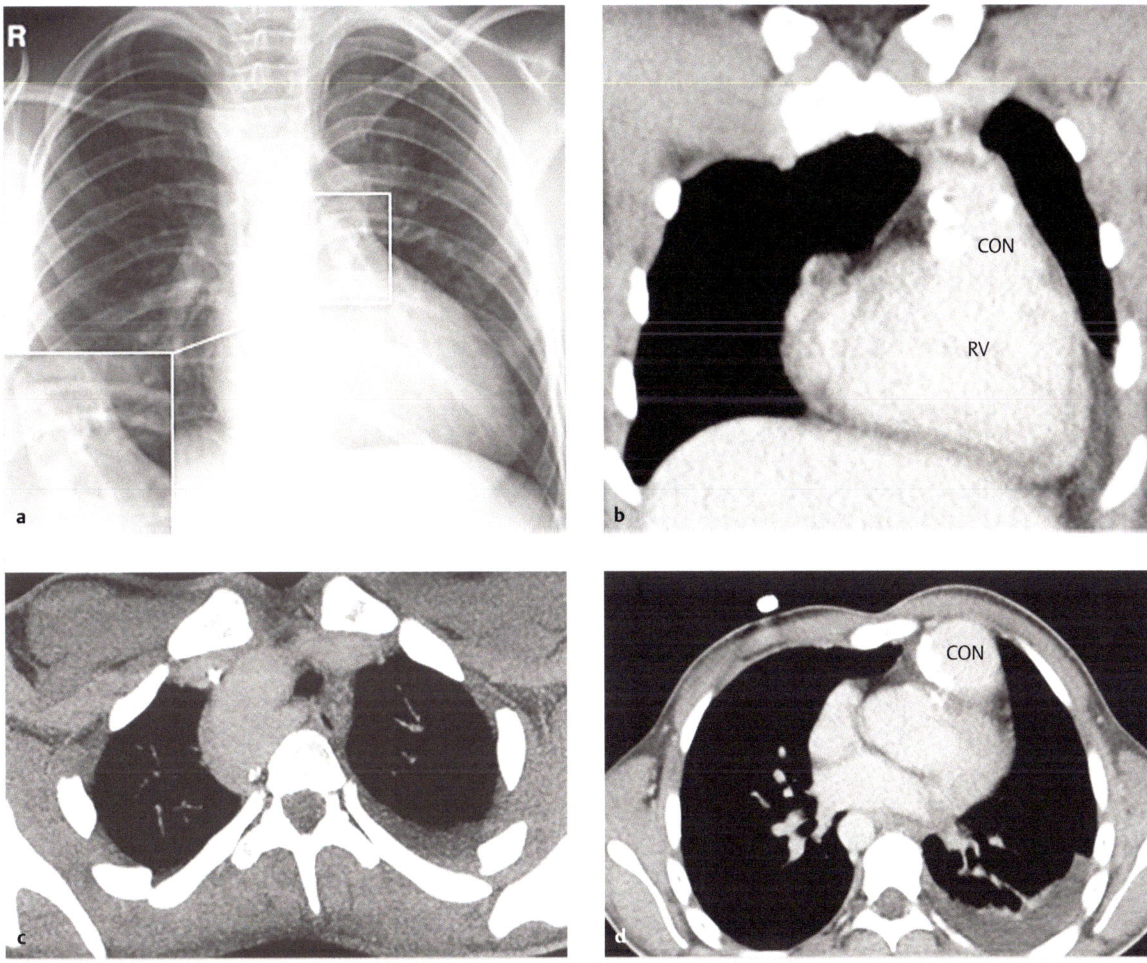

Fig. 4.99 Condition after surgical correction of common arterial trunk and two reoperations due to homograft stenosis. X-rays and CTs of a 17-year-old female patient all depict pronounced calcification near the homograft. Note the right aortic arch in **a** and **c**.
▶ Fig. 4.100 for additional depictions of this patient.

CON = conduit
RV = right ventricle

a Thoracic X-ray depicting increased conduit calcification, bottom left.
b Thoracic CT, coronal reconstruction.
c Thoracic CT, transverse reconstruction, near the “right aortic arch.”
d Thoracic CT, transverse reconstruction, near the aortic root and the ventrally located, calcified homograft.

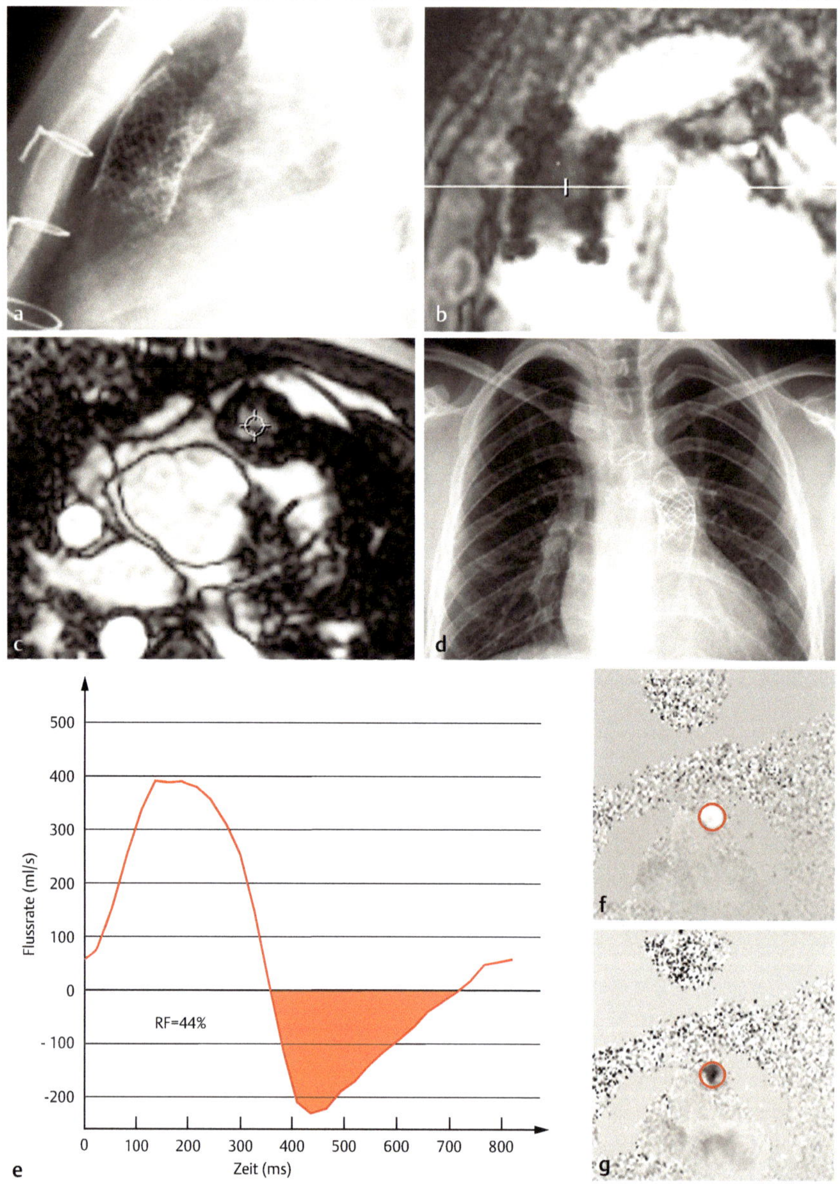

Fig. 4.100 Condition after stent implantation near a homograft stenosis, after surgical correction of common arterial trunk and multiple reoperations due to homograft stenosis. This is the same patient as in ▶ Fig. 4.99. Even in the MR SSFP cine sequence (**b**, **c**), the stent lumen is partially visible under certain circumstances (e.g., nitinol stents). The tricuspid trunk valve (neoaortic valve) is also visible in transverse slices (**c**). Depiction of flow curves (**e**) and phase images (**f**, **g**) in MRI flow measurement cranial to the implanted stent in the pulmonary arterial conduit, perpendicular to the main direction of flow (through-plane). After stent implantation in the homograft, pronounced pulmonary insufficiency (holodiastolic regurgitation) in the phase image during diastole (**g**; caudal flow depicted in black) and in the flow curve (**e**) with a measured regurgitation fraction of 44% of antegrade flow (pale red area) can be revealed.

- **a** Thoracic X-ray, lateral projection, depicting correct stent position near the RVOT and the homograft without strut breakage.
- **b** Picture detail from an SSFP cine sequence, short axis. Lateral projection like in **a** allows a view inside the nitinol stent (asterisk).
- **c** SSFP cine sequence, transverse section, corresponding to the section (white line) in **b**.
- **d** P.-a. thoracic X-ray after the final percutaneous pulmonary valve replacement using a Melody valve (Medtronic).
- **e** Depiction of flow curve via the homograft (RR interval of 822 ms). Red shaded area indicates retrograde flow and an RF of 44%.
- **f** Phase image, MRI flow measurement, cranial to the homograft during systole, with marked red region of interest for the flow curve in **e**.
- **g** Phase image, MRI flow measurement, cranial to the homograft during diastole, with marked red region of interest for the flow curve in **e**.

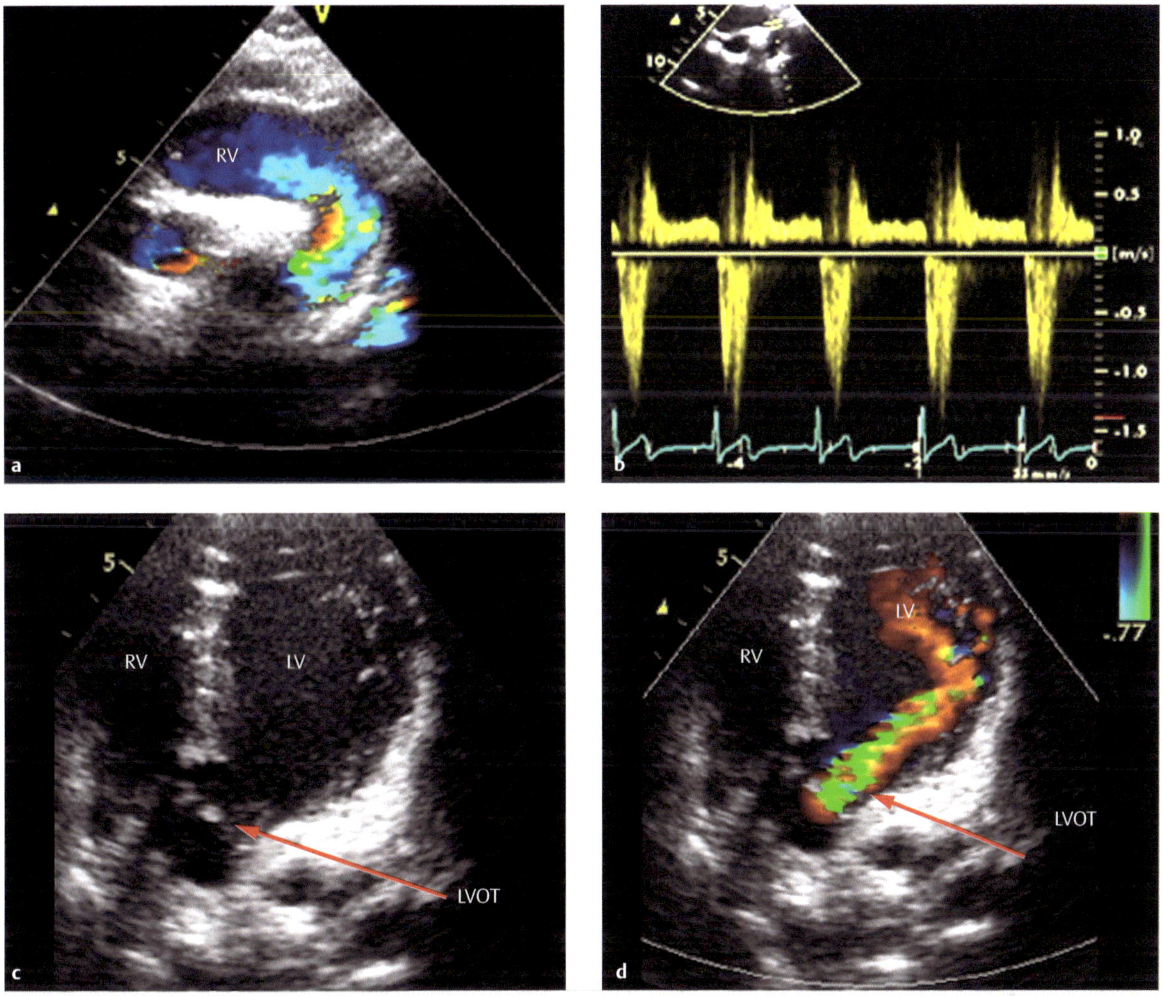

Fig. 4.101 Condition after surgical correction of type A_2 (type II) common arterial trunk. Ten-year-old female patient after surgical correction of type A_2 (type II) common arterial trunk (the same patient as in ▶ Fig. 4.96). Both color Doppler (**a**) and spectral Doppler (**b**) show holodiastolic regurgitation in the extracardiac conduit equipped with a pulmonary valve. The 5-chamber view depicts pronounced, extensive holodiastolic regurgitation (**c**, **d**, arrows) near the trunk valve in the aortic position. The dotted lines in **e** and **f** each indicate the position of the MRI through-plane flow measurement in the conduit and cranial to the trunk valve. A diastolic dephasing jet can even be seen caudal to the trunk valve using SSFP cine MRI (**f**), due to the pronounced "aortic valve insufficiency." MRI flow measurement resulted in a regurgitation fraction of 35% of antegrade flow (**h**, light blue area, pulmonary valve insufficiency). Near the conduit, the regurgitation fraction was 15% of antegrade flow (**g**, light blue area, aortic valve insufficiency).

AAo = ascending aorta
CON = conduit
LA = left atrium
LV = left ventricle
LVOT = left ventricular outflow tract
RA = right atrium
RF = regurgitation fraction
RV = right ventricle

a Color doppler echocardiography of the conduit between the right ventricle and pulmonary artery.
b Spectral doppler echocardiography of the conduit between the right ventricle and pulmonary artery.
c 2-D echocardiography of the neoaorta, 5-chamber view.
d Color echocardiography of the neoaorta, 5-chamber view.

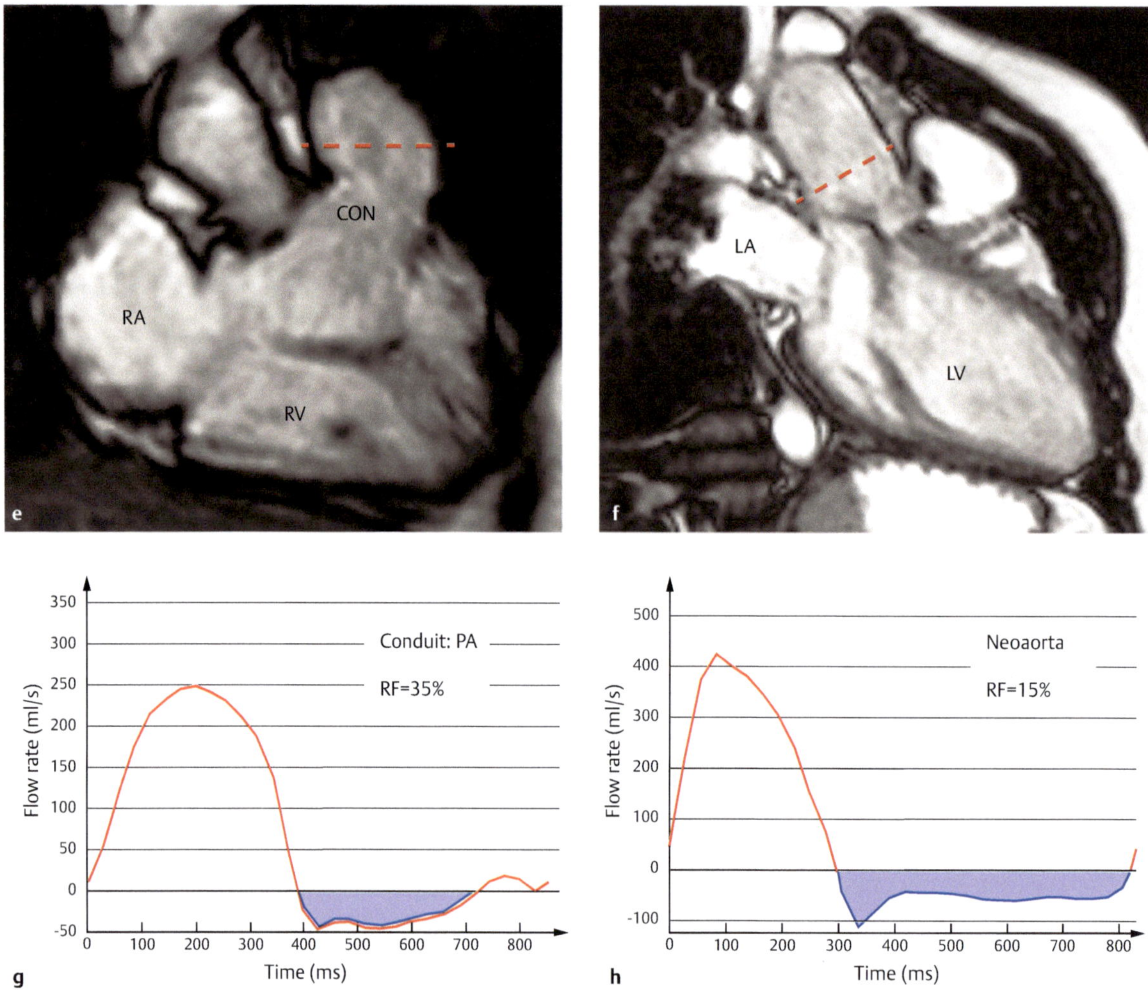

Fig. 4.101 (*Continued*) **Condition after surgical correction of type A_2 (type II) common arterial trunk.**

AAo = ascending aorta
CON = conduit
LA = left atrium
LV = left ventricle
LVOT = left ventricular outflow tract
RA = right atrium
RF = regurgitation fraction
RV = right ventricle

e SSFP cine MRI near the RVOT and conduit in the pulmonary position.
f SSFP cine MRI near the LVOT with insufficient valve in aortic position (neoaorta).
g MRI flow curve of the conduit between the right ventricle and pulmonary artery.
h MRI flow curve near the trunk valve in aortic position.

4.4.3 Hypoplastic Left Heart Syndrome (HLHS)

Ingo Dähnert, Philipp Lurz, Florentine Gräfe

Definition

HLHS is a complex congenital heart defect in which the left heart segments, though positioned correctly, are so underdeveloped or hypoplastic that the left ventricle is not able to adequately supply systemic circulation (▶ Fig. 4.102 and ▶ Fig. 4.103). Thus, pulmonary and systemic circulation must be maintained by the right ventricle, both before and after birth. *It is characterized by the ductal-dependent retrograde perfusion of the aortic arch* (▶ Fig. 4.104 and ▶ Fig. 4.105).

Classification

In typical cases, a hypoplastic left ventricle occurs in conjunction with hypoplastic mitral and aortic valves, as well as a hypoplastic ascending aorta (▶ Fig. 4.106; also ▶ Fig. 4.104 and ▶ Fig. 4.105). In addition, a distinction is made among the most common forms based on mitral valve stenosis (▶ Fig. 4.104b) or atresia (▶ Fig. 4.104a) and aortic valve stenosis or atresia, usually with an intact ventricular septum.[83]

Atypical cases occur if an unbalanced AVSD, double outlet ventricle, or another ventricular defect is present, if heterotaxia occurs, or if a PAPVR or TAPVR is concurrent with HLHS. HLHS with intact atrial septum constitutes a special case.

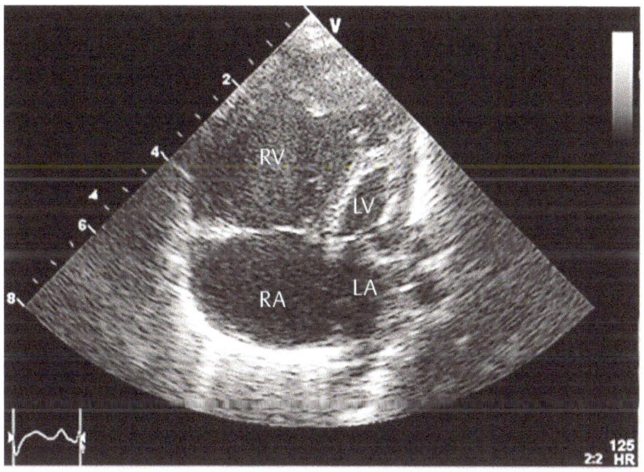

Fig. 4.102 HLHS. 2-D TTE (4-chamber view) of a newborn with HLHS. The left atrium, mitral valve, and left ventricle are hypoplastic.
LA = left atrium
LV = left ventricle
RA = right atrium
RV = right ventricle

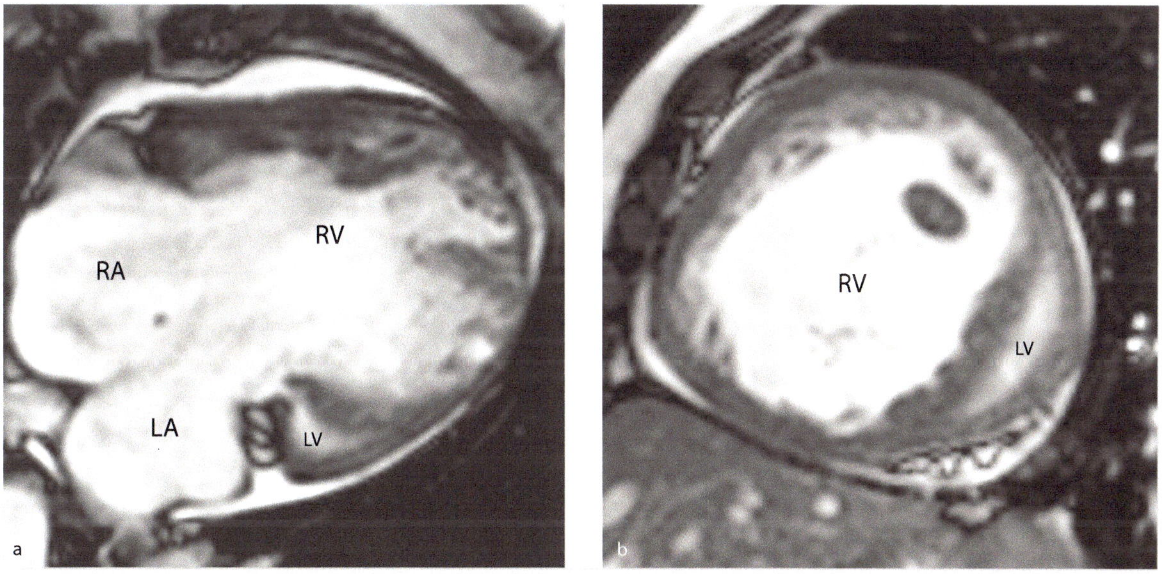

Fig. 4.103 HLHS. The SSFP cine MRI of a patient with HLHS shows a hypoplastic left ventricle with mitral valve atresia.
LA = left atrium
LV = left ventricle
RA = right atrium
RV = right ventricle
a SSFP cine MRI, 4-chamber view.
b SSFP cine MRI, short axis.

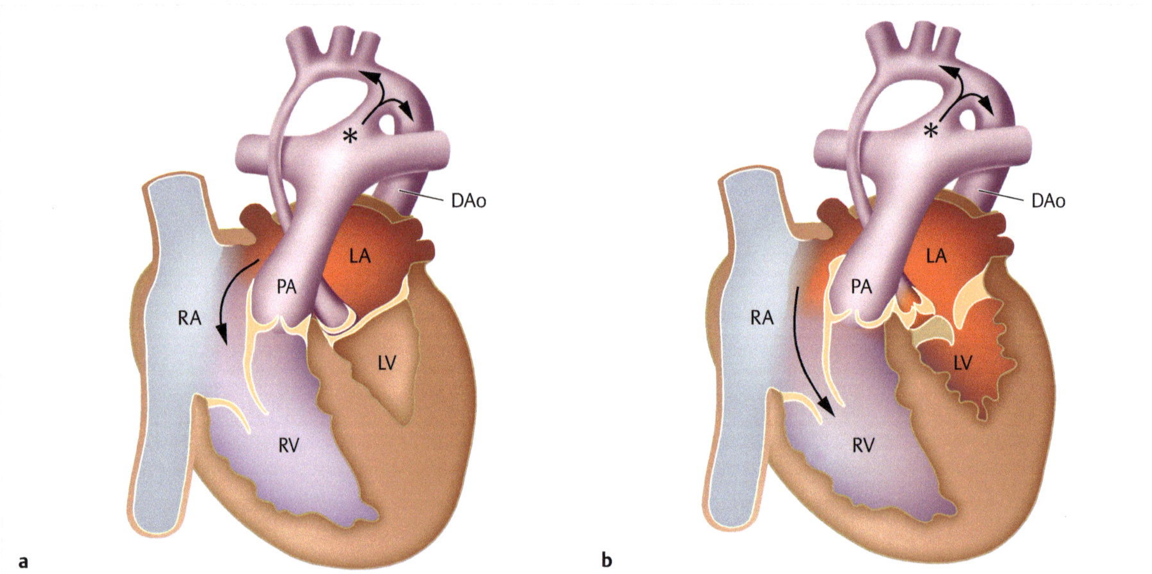

Fig. 4.104 Most common types of HLHS. Schematic depiction. The asterisk indicates the PDA.

DAo = descending aorta
LA = left atrium
LV = left ventricle
PA = pulmonary artery
RA = right atrium
RV = right ventricle.

a Mitral valve and aortic valve atresia and a rudimentary left ventricle. The arrow indicates the direction of blood flow.
b Mitral valve and aortic valve stenosis and hypoplastic ascending aorta and aortic arch, which, depending on the duct (asterisk), receives its retrograde flow (arrow) from the right ventricle via the pulmonary artery.

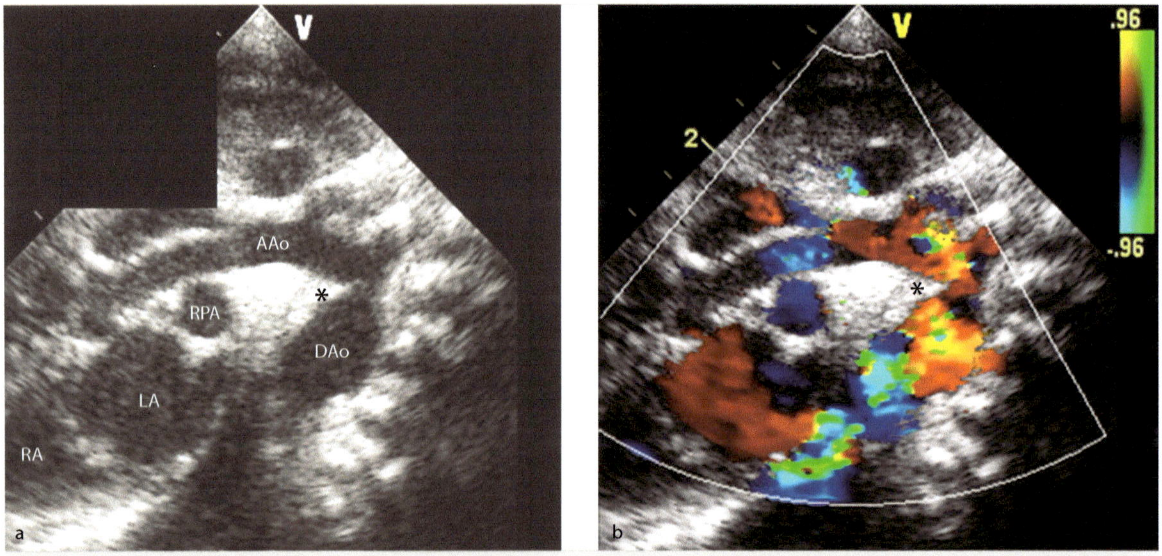

Fig. 4.105 HLHS. Newborn. Significantly enlarged descending aorta and right pulmonary artery compared to the hypoplastic ascending aorta. The color Doppler image depicts the ductal-dependent (**b**, asterisk) retrograde perfusion of the aortic arch and ascending aorta.

AAo = ascending aorta
DAo = descending aorta
LA = left atrium
RA = right atrium
RPA = right pulmonary artery

a 2-D TTE (suprasternal arch view).
b Color Doppler echocardiography (suprasternal arch view).

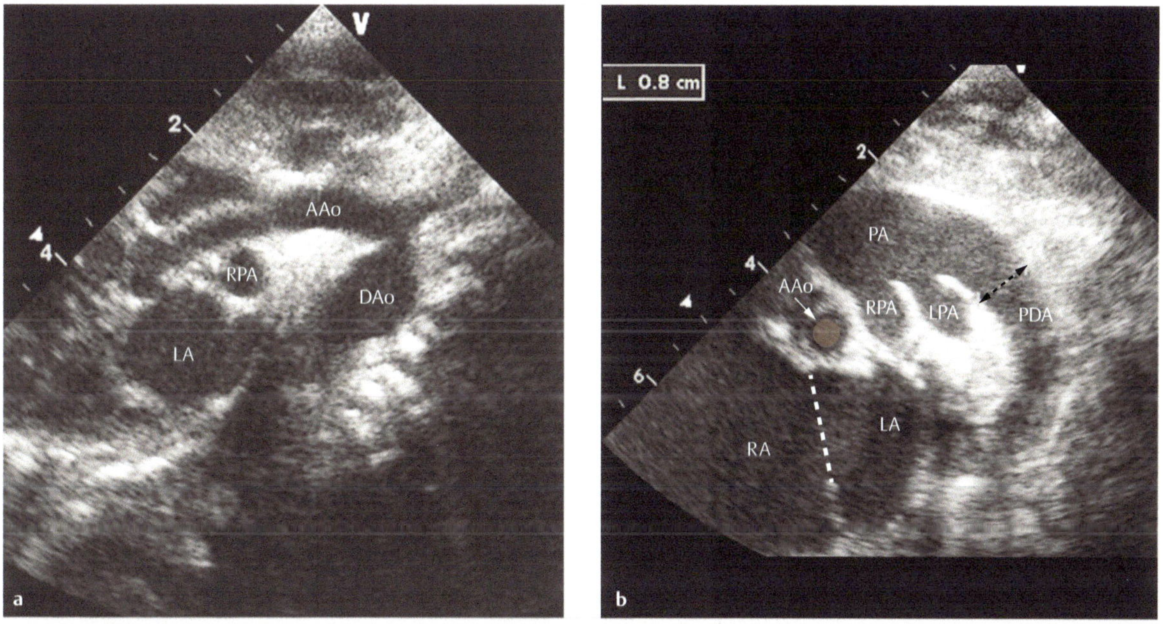

Fig. 4.106 HLHS. Two newborns.

AAo = ascending aorta
DAo = descending aorta
LA = left atrium
LPA = left pulmonary artery
PA = pulmonary artery
PDA = patent ductus arteriosus
RA = right atrium
RPA = right pulmonary artery

a 2-D TTE, suprasternal arch view, of a newborn with HLHS. The ascending aorta is significantly smaller than the descending aorta and also significantly smaller than the right pulmonary artery, as depicted in the center of the image in a orthogonal view.

b 2-D TTE (parasternal short axis) of a newborn with HLHS. The pulmonary artery dominates the image and branches into a right and a left pulmonary artery, as well as a large arterial duct (PDA) with a diameter of 8 mm (dotted double arrow). The ascending aorta (round, pale red section) is smaller than the pulmonary artery branches. The right and left atria are located posteriorly (bottom of image) and are connected to one another via a large defect (dotted line).

Hemodynamics

Typical univentricular circulation occurs with multiple abnormalities:

- Pulmonary venous retrograde flow depends on the presence and size of interatrial communication and can, for example, be hindered by a restrictive foramen ovale.
- Systemic and pulmonary venous blood mixes in the right atrium and is pumped from the right ventricle into the pulmonary arterial stem after passing through the tricuspid valve (▶ Fig. 4.104). The competence of both valves and right ventricular function are crucial to this end.
- The blood flows from the main pulmonary artery into both pulmonary arterial branches and into the aorta via the ductus arteriosus (▶ Fig. 4.104, ▶ Fig. 4.105, ▶ Fig. 4.106, ▶ Fig. 4.107). There, it provides retrograde flow into the aortic arch, arch branches, ascending aorta, and coronary arteries, and fills the descending aorta by means of antegrade flow.
- In cases of physiological duct closure, ischemia occurs throughout the body. If untreated, this leads to death. In cases of persistent duct, as well, the physiological drop in pulmonary vascular resistance causes three critical issues:
  - The right ventricle cannot increase cardiac output indefinitely, and heart failure develops.
  - Cardiac output flows increasingly into the lungs, resulting in general systemic hypoperfusion.
  - The low diastolic pressure leads to increasing ischemia, especially in the coronary arteries and the intestines.

HLHS with intact atrial septum constitutes a special case. Even prenatally, the obstruction of pulmonary venous return can cause changes to pulmonary vessels, such as arterialized veins and pulmonary parenchyma with lymphangiectasia. No perfusion is possible postnatally, and profound hypoxia develops. Only immediate surgical or catheter interventional opening of the atrial septum make it possible for the patient to survive (▶ Fig. 4.108).[144]

Clinical Issues

In typical cases, the clinical picture consists of rapid, progressive heart failure with only mild cyanosis and cardiogenic shock in cases of right ventricular failure or closure of the ductus arteriosus.

In atypical cases, the scope of cyanosis and of cardiac decompensation tendencies depends on the individual situation, though it remains ductal-dependent. If the atrial septum remains intact, the primary clinical issue is profound hypoxia immediately after birth.

Natural Progression and Indication for Treatment

The natural progression is fatal in the short-term. More than 90% of children with HLHS die within the first week of life.

The initial treatment consists of holding the ductus arteriosus open using prostaglandin infusions and, if needed, establishing or increasing interatrial communication (▶ Fig. 4.108).[145] The final treatment includes univentricular palliation in three surgical treatment steps[146] (Chapter 2.1):

- *Norwood I operation:* In the first step, the pulmonary arterial stem is connected to the neoaorta, native ascending aorta, aortic arch, and descending aorta (▶ Fig. 4.109a). Hypoplastic segments are expanded and duct tissue is removed in order to prevent the development of arch and isthmus stenoses.[147] The pulmonary artery branches are separated from the

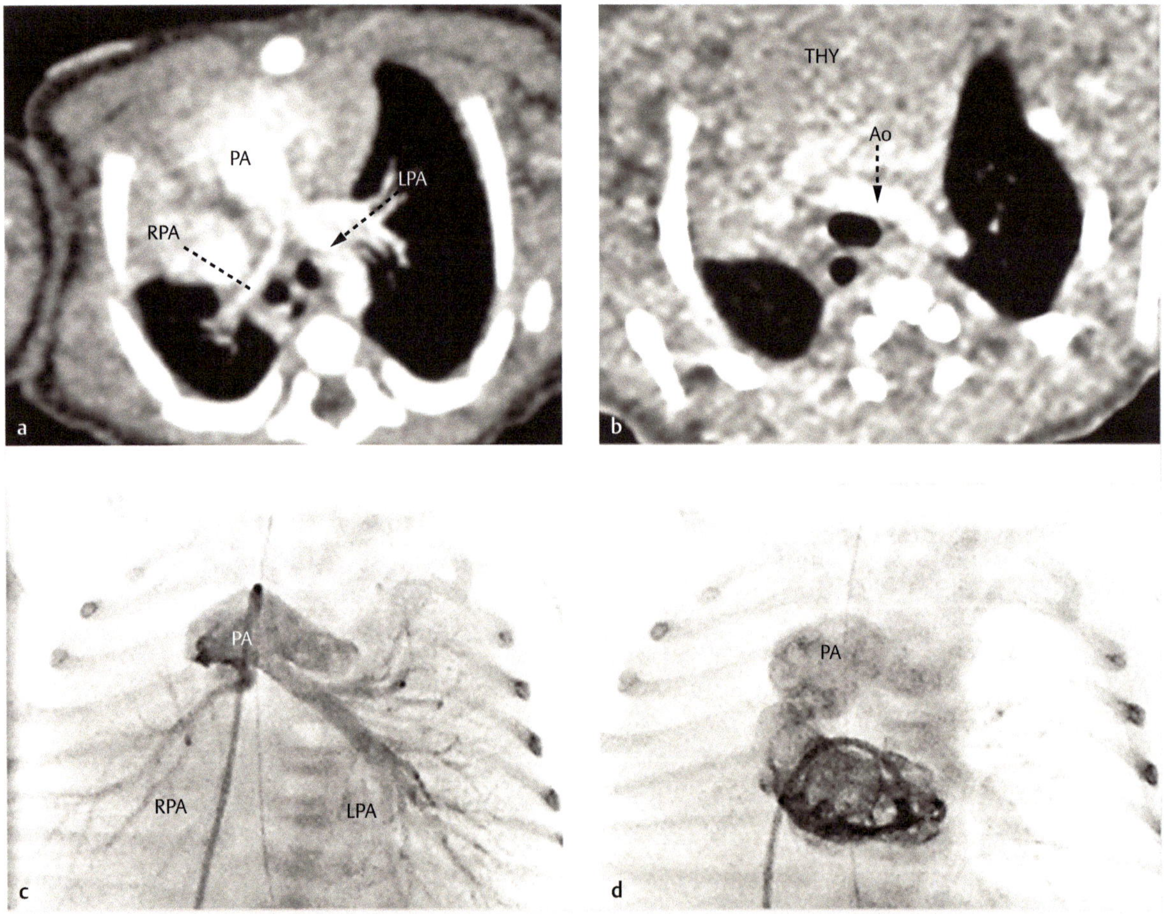

Fig. 4.107 HLHS. Newborn with HLHS, stenotic pulmonary veins with anomalous connections to the inferior vena cava (Scimitar syndrome, venolobar syndrome), pulmonary sequestration, right lung hypoplasia, hypoplastic aortic arch, dextroposition of the heart, and hypoplastic right pulmonary artery.

Ao = aorta
IVC = inferior vena cava
LPA = left pulmonary artery
PA = pulmonary artery
RPA = right pulmonary artery
THY = thymus

a The contrast-enhanced thoracic CT (80 kV, flash mode) depicts the hypoplastic right pulmonary artery in the transverse MIP reconstruction (2 mm slice).

b The contrast-enhanced thoracic CT (80 kV, flash mode) depicts the hypoplastic aortic arch (Ao) in the transverse MIP reconstruction (2 mm slice).

c Invasive pulmonary angiogram, a.-p. projection, corresponding to **a**, with hypoplastic right pulmonary artery and a catheter in the pulmonary artery.

d Corresponding pulmonary angiogram, a.-p. projection, and another catheter position (in the right ventricle).

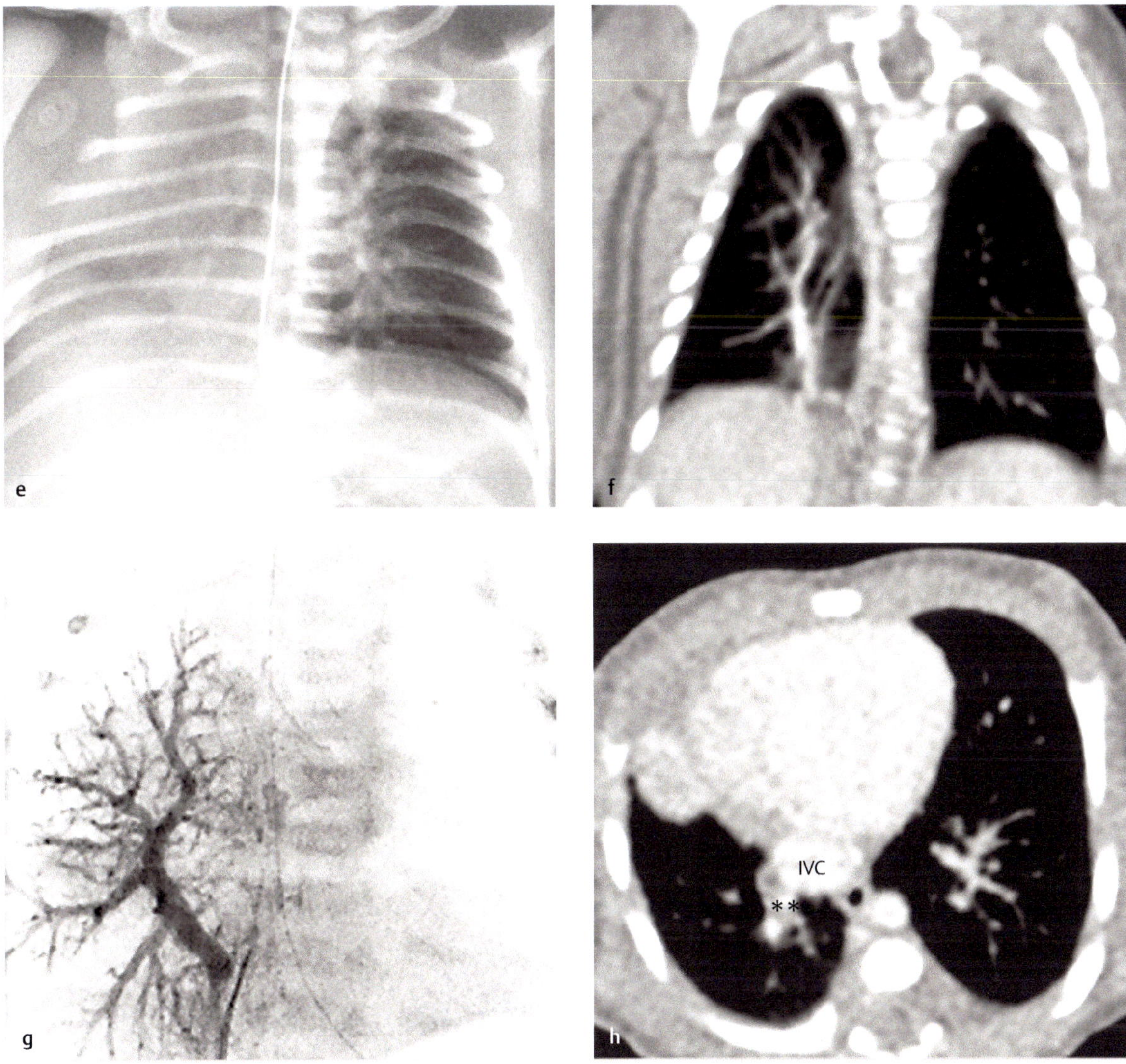

Fig 4.107 (*Continued*) **HLHS.**
Ao = aorta
IVC = inferior vena cava
LPA = left pulmonary artery
PA = pulmonary artery
RPA = right pulmonary artery
THY = thymus

e Initial p.-a. thoracic X-ray with total atelectasis of the right lung.

f The coronal CT reconstruction depicts the inferior right pulmonary veins and their anomalous connection to the inferior vena cava.

g Corresponding invasive angiogram of the inferior right pulmonary veins and their anomalous connection to the inferior vena cava.

h Transverse CT reconstruction. The inferior right pulmonary vein (double asterisk) possesses an anomalous connection to the inferior vena cava.

stem, but remain connected to one another and are perfused such that adequate oxygen saturation is achieved—yet pulmonary hyperperfusion is prevented—via a modified aortopulmonary Blalock-Taussig shunt, the original Norwood operation (▶ Fig. 4.109a and ▶ Fig. 4.110), or a right ventricular pulmonary shunt (Sano modification; ▶ Fig. 4.111).[148] If needed, interatrial communication is increased.

- *Norwood II operation:* The second palliative step involves replacing the aortopulmonary or ventricular-pulmonary connection[148] with a superior cavopulmonary anastomosis (▶ Fig. 4.109b and ▶ Fig. 4.110; bidirectional Glenn shunt).
- *Norwood III operation:* The third step involves creating a TCPC (total cavopulmonary connection, modified Fontan tunnel), comparable to the treatment for univentricular heart.

As an alternative to the Norwood operation as the first step of treatment, a hybrid procedure consisting of surgical bilateral pulmonary artery banding and catheter interventional stent implantation in the ductus arteriosus, as well as stent implantation (if needed) in the interatrial communication, has also been developed (▶ Fig. 4.108). The second step of treatment also includes the reconstructive portions of the Norwood operation (known as comprehensive Norwood).

> **Note**
>
> Heart or heart–lung transplants are another possible treatment alternative to the Norwood operation.

Numerous risk factors exist for successful treatment, which can, in part, be evaluated more closely using imaging. Cardiac risk factors include the following:

- Very small ascending aorta (diameter smaller than 2 mm)
- Atresia of the left-sided valves[148,149]
- Dysplasia and preexisting insufficiency of the tricuspid and pulmonary valves
- Caval and pulmonary venous anomalies
- Intact atrial septum

Additional risk factors include premature birth, low birth weight, surviving cardiac decompensation prior to surgery, and extracardiac defects.[150] Furthermore, potential retrograde coarctation (preductal isthmus stenosis) is a risk factor for the hybrid procedure.[151]

Preoperative Diagnostics

Preoperative diagnostics are generally performed solely using TTE (▶ Table 4.24). Ideally, diagnosis should be determined prenatally. The following parameters and structures must be depicted:

- Left cardiac segments (size of left atrium and ventricle, mitral stenosis or atresia, aortic stenosis or atresia, size of the ascending aorta and aortic arch)
- Function of the tricuspid valve, right ventricle, and pulmonary valve
- Size and, potentially, restriction of the foramen ovale (▶ Fig. 4.108) and ductus arteriosus
- All other defects

In addition to echocardiography (▶ Fig. 4.111a), regular cardiac catheter examinations (▶ Fig. 4.111, ▶ Fig. 4.112, ▶ Fig. 4.113) are often performed before the second and third steps of treatment. Cardiac MRI (▶ Fig. 4.103, ▶ Fig. 4.110) can also be helpful for quantifying right ventricular function prior to surgery.

Table 4.24 Preoperative imaging diagnostics in cases of HLHS.

Preoperative imaging methods for HLHS	Focus	Value
2-D, 3-D TTE	• Determining diagnosis • Mitral stenosis or atresia? • Aortic valve stenosis or atresia? • Size of ascending aorta • Size of ductus arteriosus • Retrograde coarctation? • Anatomy and function of the tricuspid valve and right ventricle • Type and size of interatrial communication • Ruling out pulmonary and systemic venous anomalies	+++
2-D, 3-D TEE	see TTE (only required in rare cases and only feasible under certain conditions, since most patients are newborns)	+
Cardiac MRI	• Quantifying right ventricular function • Anatomy of pulmonary and systemic veins • In borderline cases, quantifying left ventricular size and function	++ (Backup method)
MDCT	Backup method in cases of unclear echocardiography findings and contraindication against cardiac MRI; may be helpful in cases of pulmonary parenchymatic comorbidity or to prove the existence of concurrent vascular defects, such as anomalous pulmonary venous connections	+
Invasive (diagnostic) cardiac catheter tests	• Measuring pulmonary pressure and resistance, pharmacological testing • Ruling out pulmonary and systemic venous anomalies • Usually in conjunction with interventional or hybrid treatment	+ (in cases of delayed diagnosis)

HLHS, hypoplastic left heart syndrome; MDCT, multidetector computed tomography; MRI, magnetic resonance imaging; TEE, transesophageal echocardiography; TTE, transthoracic echocardiography.

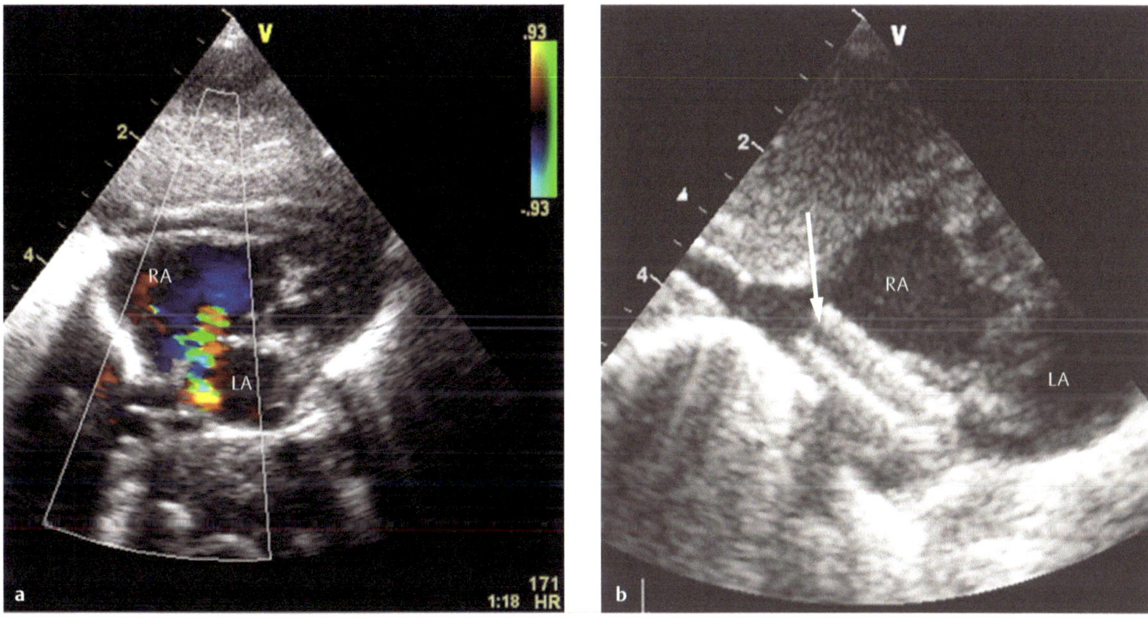

Fig. 4.108 HLHS.
LA = left atrium
RA = right atrium.

a 2-D color Doppler TTE, 4-chamber view, of a newborn with HLHS. The color flow image depicts restrictive interatrial communication.
b 2-D TTE, subcostal parasagittal axis, of a newborn with HLHS and intact atrial septum after opening the atrial septum and implanting a stent (arrow).

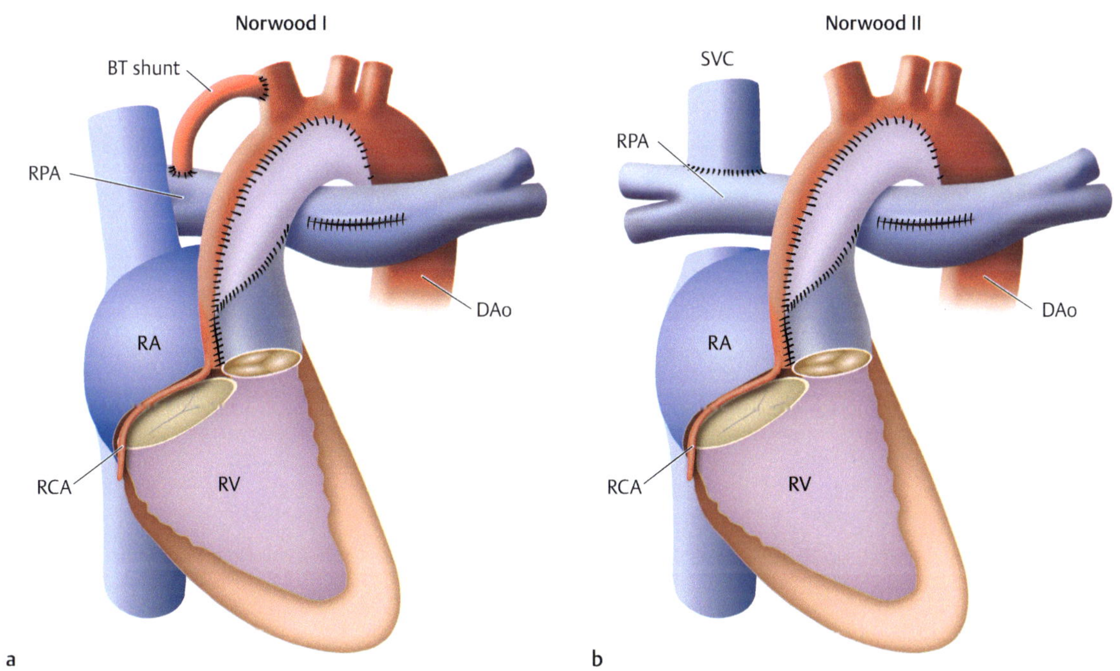

Fig. 4.109 Norwood I and II operation. Schematic depiction.
BT shunt = modified Blalock–Taussig shunt
DAo = descending aorta
RA = right atrium
RCA = right coronary artery
RPA = right pulmonary artery
RV = right ventricle
SVC = superior vena cava

a Norwood I operation with reconstruction of a neoaorta from the pulmonary artery and hypoplastic native ascending aorta, placement of a modified Blalock–Taussig shunt, and atrioseptostomy.
b Norwood II operation with placement of a bidirectional cavopulmonary anastomosis.

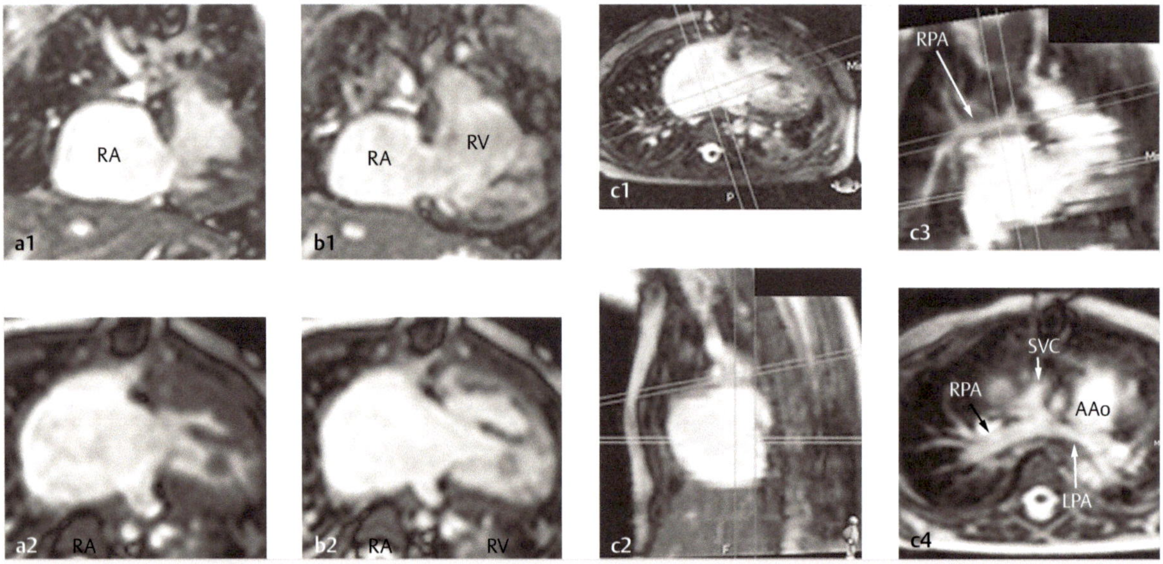

Fig. 4.110 Norwood II operation in a case of HLHS. SSFP MRI of a 10-month-old boy, 4 weeks after the Norwood II operation (▸ Fig. 4.109b) and placement of a bidirectional Glenn anastomosis of the superior vena cava in the right pulmonary artery. The cine MRIs (**a**, **b**) indicate good ventricular function. The 3-D data set was reformatted in a multiplanar fashion in order to depict the Glenn anastomosis (**c**).

AAo = ascending aorta
LPA = left pulmonary artery
RA = right atrium
RPA = right pulmonary artery
RV = right ventricle
SVC = superior vena cava.

a Cine MRI during systole in coronal (top) and transverse sections (bottom).
b Cine MRI during diastole in coronal (top) and transverse section (bottom).
c Multiplanar reformats of the 3-D data set in order to depict the Glenn anastomosis (arrows).

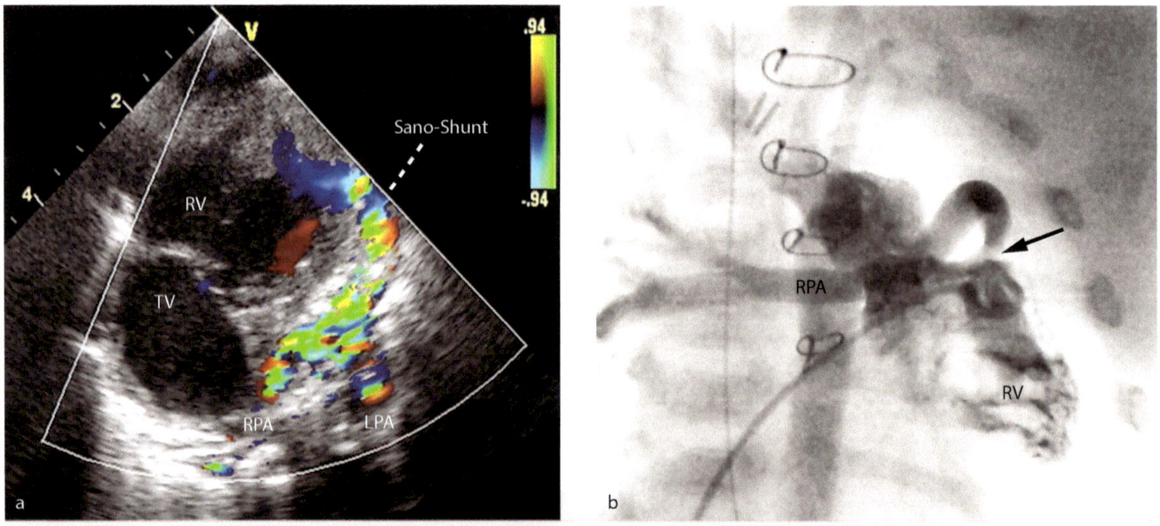

Fig. 4.111 Norwood operation in a case of HLHS. Two patients.

LPA = left pulmonary artery
RPA = right pulmonary artery
RV = right ventricle
TV = tricuspid valve

a 2-D color Doppler TTE (parasternal short axis) of an infant after the Norwood operation (Sano modification[144]) to treat HLHS. The color-coded flow indicates the right ventricular pulmonary Sano shunt and the pulmonary arterial bifurcation with the right and left pulmonary arteries.
b Ventriculogram, RAO projection, of another infant after a Norwood operation with Sano modification for HLHS. A clear stenosis (arrow) is visible on the proximal anastomosis of the Sano shunt.

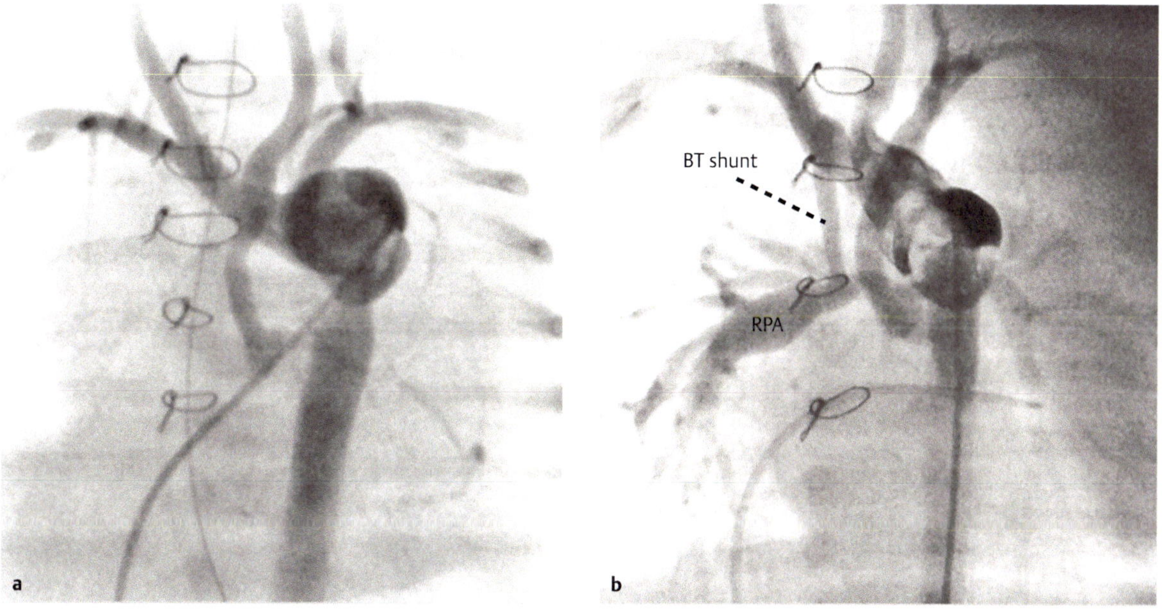

Fig. 4.112 Condition after Norwood I operation in a case of HLHS. Two patients.

BT shunt = Blalock–Taussig shunt
RPA = right pulmonary artery

a Aortogram, a.-p. projection, of an infant after Norwood I operation to treat HLHS. The pulmonary valve and pulmonary arterial stem are, as depicted schematically in ▶ Fig. 4.109a, anastomosed to the aortic arch. The retrograde perfused, hypoplastic ascending aorta is visible in the depicted arterial phase.

b Aortogram, slightly left-lateral angulated projection, of another infant after a traditional Norwood I operation to treat HLHS. The pulmonary valve and pulmonary artery are anastomosed to the aortic arch. The retrograde-perfused hypoplastic ascending aorta and modified Blalock–Taussig shunt between the brachiocephalic trunk and right pulmonary artery are clearly visible.

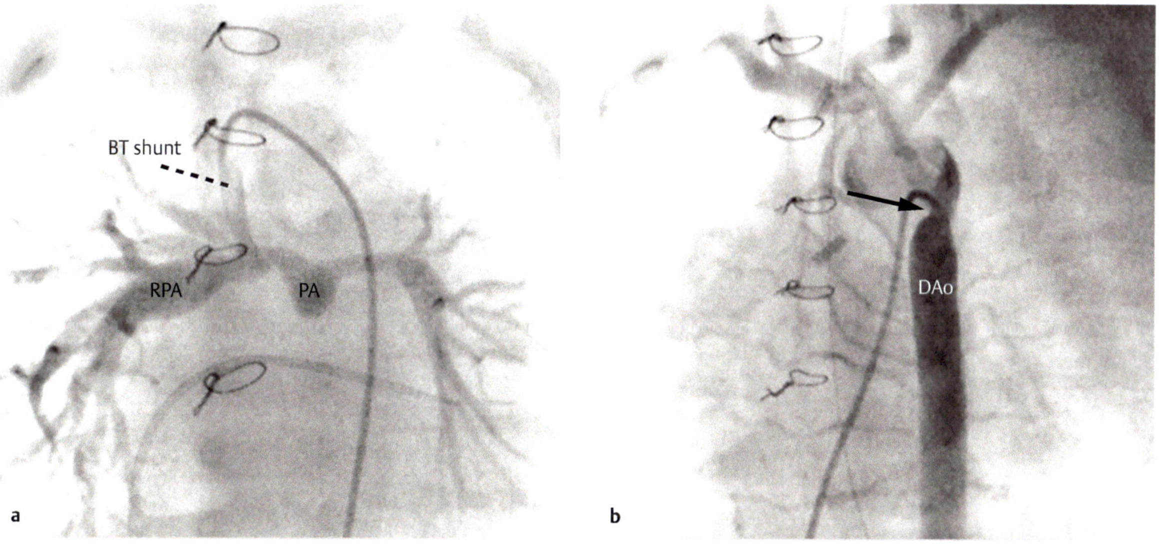

Fig. 4.113 Condition after Norwood I operation in a case of HLHS. Two patients.

BT shunt = Blalock–Taussig shunt
PA = pulmonary artery
DAo = descending aorta
RPA = right pulmonary artery

a Pulmonary angiogram, a.-p projection, of an infant after a traditional Norwood I operation to treat HLHS. The catheter crosses the aorta retrogradely before entering the modified Blalock–Taussig shunt, and depicts clear asymmetry in pulmonary arterial perfusion with relevant hypoplasia of the left main stem and its branches.

b Aortogram, a.–p. projection, of another infant after a Norwood I operation in a case of HLHS. The catheter is introduced venously into the aorta via the right ventricle and neoaortic valve. It constitutes a clear aortic coarctation (arrow).

Postoperative Issues and Imaging

Postoperatively, especially between the first and second steps of treatment (interstage interval), the hemodynamic balance between right ventricular function, pulmonary and systemic perfusion, and the extent of cyanosis constitute complex issues. Acute or chronic heart failure, tricuspid valve insufficiency, coronary ischemia, and hypoxia are possible, and require different treatment strategies. Sudden cardiac death can also occur.[152]

Obstruction of the interatrial communication, the systemic pulmonary shunt connection (▶ Fig. 4.111b), and the pulmonary arteries (▶ Fig. 4.110c and ▶ Fig. 4.113a) are possible, and can cause progressive cyanosis. Stenoses of the aortic arch and isthmus are equally critical (▶ Fig. 4.113b), since they can cause additional pressure overload for the already overloaded right ventricle. Developing aortopulmonary collaterals, like large aortopulmonary shunt connections and pulmonary valve insufficiency, also leads to low diastolic blood pressure and the risk of coronary ischemia.

Acute issues are rare after the second and third steps of treatment. Stenoses near the interatrial communication, pulmonary arteries, and aortic arch are possible. In addition to aortopulmonary collaterals, venovenous collaterals can also arise. Tricuspid valve insufficiency may develop within the scope of chronic heart failure, and arrhythmia can occur. Overall, there are no significant differences compared to other forms of univentricular heart with analogous palliative steps.[152,153]

▶ Table 4.25 provides an overview of the value of various imaging methods in postoperative diagnostics.

Table 4.25 Postoperative imaging diagnostics in cases of HLHS.

Imaging methods	Value
TTE	+++
TEE	+
Cardiac MRI	+++
MDCT	++
Invasive cardiac catheter diagnostics (before treatment steps 2 and 3 can be combined with interventional treatment)	+++

HLHS, hypoplastic left heart syndrome; MDCT, multidetector computed tomography; MRI, magnetic resonance imaging; TEE, transesophageal echocardiography; TTE, transthoracic echocardiography.

4.4.4 Univentricular Heart

Hashim Abdul-Khaliq

Definition

This rare congenital heart defect is not an isolated abnormality. Rather, it is, more precisely, a complex of defects[83,154] in which a single ventricle or univentricular heart is present from either an anatomical (▶ Fig. 4.114a and ▶ Fig. 4.115) or functional perspective (▶ Fig. 4.114b and ▶ Fig. 4.116). In the case of a functional single ventricle, two separate atria are present, though one of them only in a rudimentary form. In addition to ventricular anatomy, various forms of abnormal atrioventricular, ventriculoarterial, and venoatrial connections are often present.

Classification

The left ventricle can be hypoplastic and concurrent with various morphological entities. In cases of traditional hypoplastic left heart syndrome, the mitral valve is dysplastic or even atretic, the left atrium is hypoplastic with poor contractility, and the LVOT (including the aortic valve and ascending aorta) is hypoplastic to atretic. If, however, the right ventricle is hypoplastic, tricuspid atresia and/or pulmonary atresia is often present (▶ Fig. 4.116). Atrial situs solitus is present in most (90%) of cases of single ventricle.[83] An AVSD with unbalanced ventricles is not suited to anatomical correction. This is known as "functionally univentricular heart" and is thus treated palliatively by placing a cavopulmonary connection. If both atrioventricular valves have an inlet to the morphologic left main ventricle, this is known as "DILV" (▶ Fig. 4.117 and ▶ Fig. 4.118). If both great arteries are characterized by D-TGA and if they originate from a normal or rudimentary right ventricle, this is known as "DORV."

Hemodynamics, Natural Progression, and Indication for Treatment

Due to the "1-chamber circulation" occurring as a result of anatomical conditions, oxygen-depleted and oxygen-rich blood mix with one another, leading to central cyanosis. Balanced pulmonary and systemic circulation is an important goal of initial treatment for these young patients. Thus, pulmonary perfusion must be adequate for oxygenation and growth of the pulmonary arteries, yet cannot nullify the prerequisites for later cavopulmonary anastomosis due to increased pulmonary perfusion,

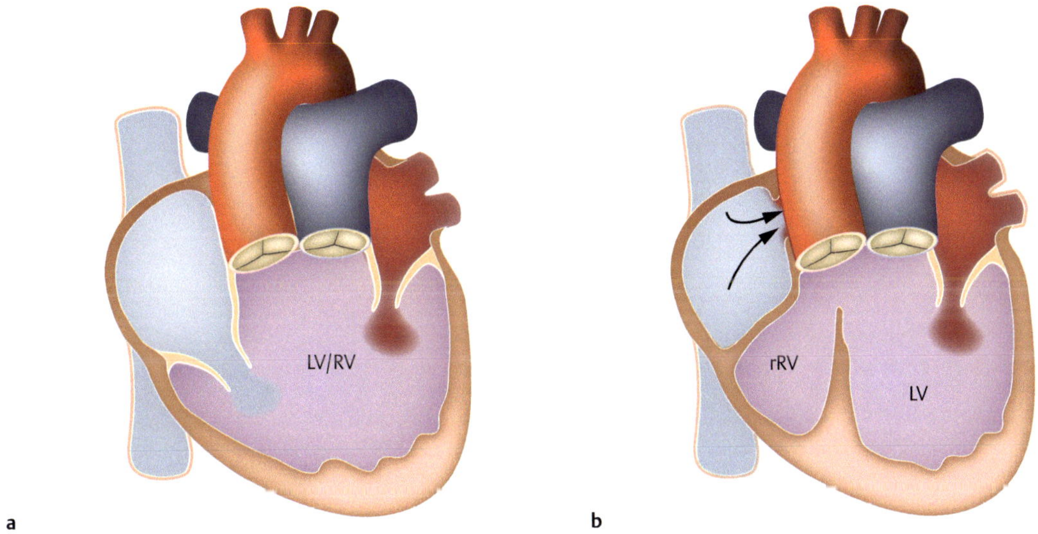

Fig. 4.114 Two forms of single ventricle or univentricular heart. Schematic depiction.
LV = left ventricle
rRV = rudimentary right ventricle
RV = right ventricle

- **a** An anatomical single ventricle with a double inlet is known as a "DILV" or "DIRV" depending on the main ventricle to which it is linked (left or right).
- **b** Common form of a functional single ventricle with rudimentary right ventricle in a case of tricuspid atresia and D-TGA.

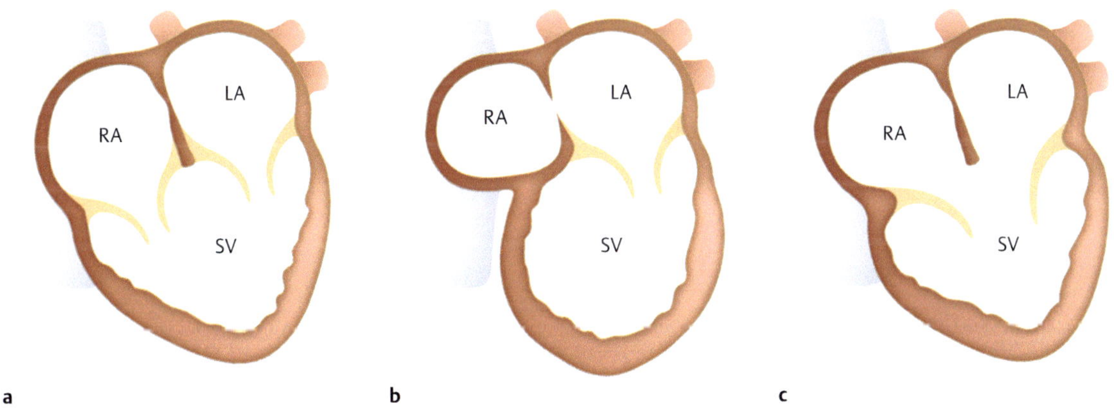

Fig. 4.115 Various potentially possible atrioventricular connections of a single ventricle. Schematic depiction.
LA = left atrium
RA = right atrium
SV = single ventricle

- **a** Double inlet.
- **b** Single inlet.
- **c** Common inlet.

which can be associated with increased pulmonary resistance and pressure. Consequently, initially elevated pulmonary circulation must be reduced via banding (pulmonary artery banding). In cases of reduced pulmonary perfusion accompanied by pulmonary atresia or stenosis, it is necessary to place an aortopulmonary anastomosis (Blalock–Taussig shunt). As a result of the overall extremely diverse anatomical and hemodynamic conditions encompassed by single ventricle, it is exceedingly difficult to draw uniform conclusions.

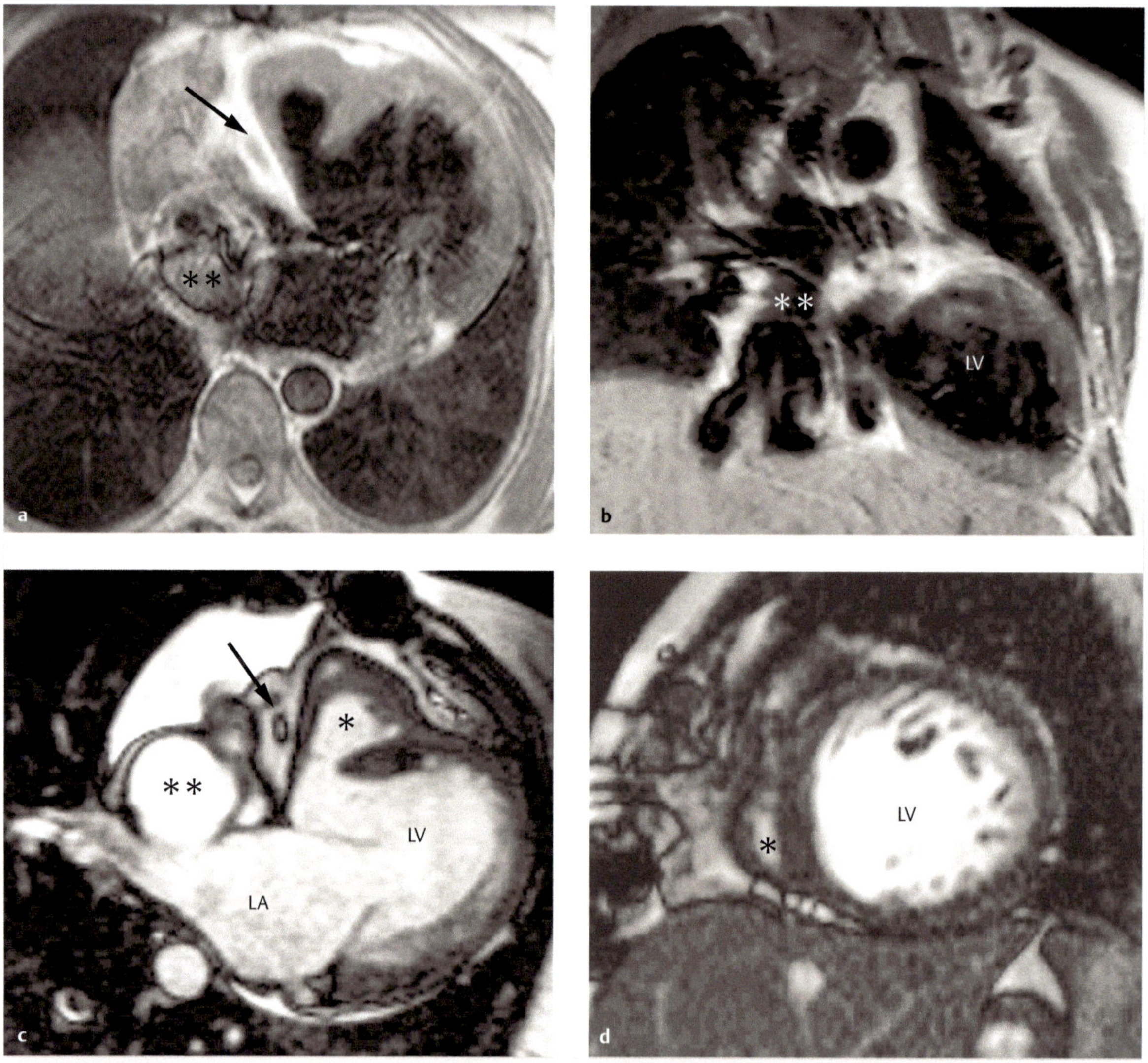

Fig. 4.116 Functional single ventricle. Thirty-four-year-old female patient with functional single ventricle, tricuspid atresia, rudimentary right ventricle (**c**, asterisk), VSD, and TCPC with an intracardiac and intraatrial Fontan tunnel (**a–c**, double asterisk), respectively. Significantly enlarged main left ventricle.

LA = left atrium

LV = left ventricle

a Transverse, ECG-triggered T1w SE image with flow artifacts caused by slow flow (double asterisk) in the Fontan tunnel. The arrow indicates the right coronary artery in the atrioventricular groove.

b Angulated coronal slice along the course of the Fontan tunnel (double asterisk) with typical anastomosis of the right and left pulmonary arteries and no evidence of stenotic anastomoses.

c SSFP cine MRI, transverse orientation. The image provides an artifact-free depiction of the Fontan tunnel (double asterisk) and rudimentary right ventricle (asterisk). The arrow indicates the position of the right coronary artery in the atrioventricular groove.

d SSFP cine MRI, short-axis, of the functional single ventricle. The rudimentary right ventricle is also visible (asterisk).

Treatment Options and Diagnostics

Because of the aforementioned cardiac and vascular anomalies, it is often impossible to attempt anatomical correction of the anatomical or functional univentricular heart. Only surgical palliative treatment in the form of gradual connection of the venous blood to the lungs (cavopulmonary anastomosis) is possible in all children with univentricular heart. The most important prerequisites for these types of surgical palliative treatments are adequately developed central and peripheral pulmonary vessels, and low pressures in pulmonary circulation. Since hypoplasia of the aortic arch is also present in cases of HLHS (Chapter 4.4.3, Hypoplastic Left Heart Syndrome (HLHS)), the arch must first be reconstructed via a Norwood I operation. Otherwise, pulmonary circulation must generally be regulated during the first step of surgical treatment, meaning it must either be improved by placing

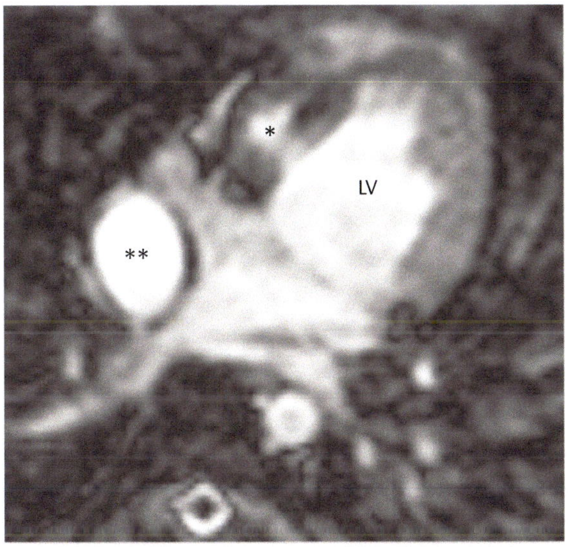

Fig. 4.117 DILV in a case of tricuspid atresia. Seven-year-old male patient with extracardiac Fontan tunnel (double asterisk) and DILV accompanied by tricuspid atresia. SSFP cine MRI, axial section. The asterisk indicates the rudimentary right ventricle. LV = left ventricle

an aortopulmonary shunt, or it must be reduced by means of pulmonary artery banding. Two steps are then generally performed in order to place a cavopulmonary anastomosis (also known as a "bidirectional Glenn shunt" or "superior cavopulmonary shunt"). The goal of these graduated surgeries is to fully divert oxygen-depleted venous blood from the superior and, later, the inferior vena cava directly into pulmonary circulation without the heart needing to pump it. This diversion was previously achieved using an atriopulmonary anastomosis or by means of a modified Fontan surgery.[83,154] In the meantime, a TCPC (*total cavopulmonary connection*) is placed, either as a lateral intraatrial or intracardiac tunnel (▸ Fig. 4.116) or, better yet, as an extraatrial or extracardiac tunnel without requiring atrial manipulation (▸ Fig. 4.117, ▸ Fig. 4.118, ▸ Fig. 4.119, ▸ Fig. 4.120).

Postoperative Issues

Initially, it was assumed that palliative treatment by means of placing an atriopulmonary anastomosis or intraatrial TCPC through the transferred atrial and ventricular contraction was more likely to generate pulsatile flow in pulmonary circulation than in the extraatrial TCPC, and thus ensure "more physiological" hemodynamics. Currently, placing an extraatrial or extracardiac TCPC is preferred, since this requires less surgical manipulation of the atria and thus reduces the risk of post-surgical rhythm disorders. Flow measurements that can be performed not just using Doppler echocardiography, but also or MRI show that pulsatile, breath-modulated flow is also present in an extracardiac TCPC (▸ Fig. 4.119m and n).[156] Nevertheless, flow is slowed, and may even be retrograde based on pulmonary pressure gradients.[157] Thus, the slowed, non-physiological flow can lead to thrombi in the Fontan tunnel (▸ Fig. 4.120c and f), stenotic anastomoses (▸ Fig. 4.118a, ▸ Fig. 4.119o and, ▸ Fig. 4.120d,e) structural changes to the pulmonary tissue caused by volume overload in cases of reduced ventricular function, or chronic hepatic congestion in cases of "failing Fontan."[158] A heart transplant is the last-resort treatment method.

Goals and Relative Value of Diagnostic Imaging

Preoperative

The strengths of imaging procedures largely correlate to those used in association with HLHS. Primary depiction of ventricular and atrial anatomy with corresponding classification of the underlying defects can usually be achieved by means of *Doppler echocardiography* (▸ Fig. 4.118c,d and ▸ Fig. 4.119b,c).

The following points should be clarified when using imaging to perform an initial evaluation of children with univentricular hearts:

- Type and size of the main atrium
- Form of atrioventricular connections (atrioventricular discordance)
- Ventriculoarterial connection (TGA, DORV)
- Type and size of the rudimentary, small ventricle
- Morphology and function of the atrioventricular valves (mitral or tricuspid atresia)
- Morphology and hemodynamics of both outflow tracts (antegrade flow via the aortic and pulmonary valves?)
- Ductal perfusion dependent upon pulmonary circulation
- Ductal perfusion dependent upon systemic circulation
- Two separate atria (PFO, ASD, restriction)
- Morphology of the atria with respect to the position of the abdominal organs (heterotaxia; right or left atrial isomerism? supracardiac, cardiac, or infracardiac PAPVR or TAPVR?)
- Connection of the systemic veins to the atrium like in cases of partial pulmonary venous anomalies (see Partial Pulmonary Venous Anomalies) or other venous anomalies (see Caval Vein Anomalies, Systemic Venous Anomalies, and Anomalous Body Venous Connections) (e.g., persistent left superior vena cava, presence of an inferior vena cava, azygos connections?)
- Concurrent defects (e.g., hypoplastic aortic arch, coarctation: ▸ Fig. 4.121)

The *cardiac catheter examination* is necessary primarily to determine pressure and resistance within pulmonary circulation and the gradients of the outflow tracts to the aorta and/or pulmonary artery, but can also be used for interventional treatments (▸ Fig. 4.121).[83]

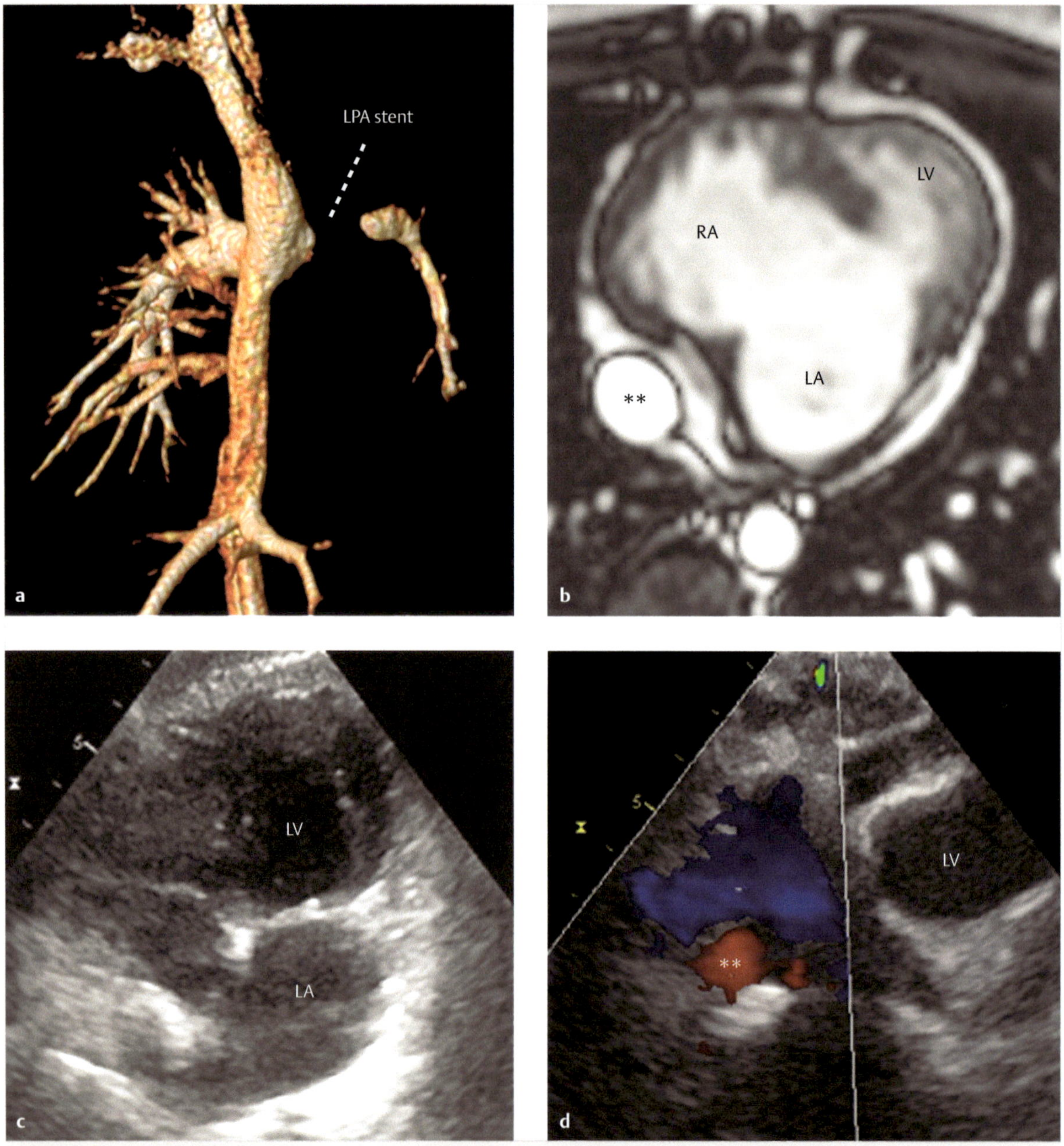

Fig. 4.118 DILV. Fourteen-year-old female patient with DILV, L-TGA, and extracardiac tunnel (**b**, **d**, double asterisk).
LA = left atrium
LPA stent = left pulmonary artery stent
LV = left ventricle
RA = right atrium

a MRI. The 3-D reconstruction using the volume rendering technique, a.-p. projection, from a contrast-enhanced MRA indicates a TCPC with signal loss near the implanted stent in the proximal left pulmonary artery.

b MRI. Depiction of the TCPC (double asterisk), unremarkable, also visible in the cross-sectional SSFP cine MRI. The enlarged atria with no atrial septum (in the sense of a DILV) is clearly visible.

c 2-D echo corresponding to the MRI from **b**.

d Color Doppler echo. Likewise unremarkable depiction of the TCPC (double asterisk).

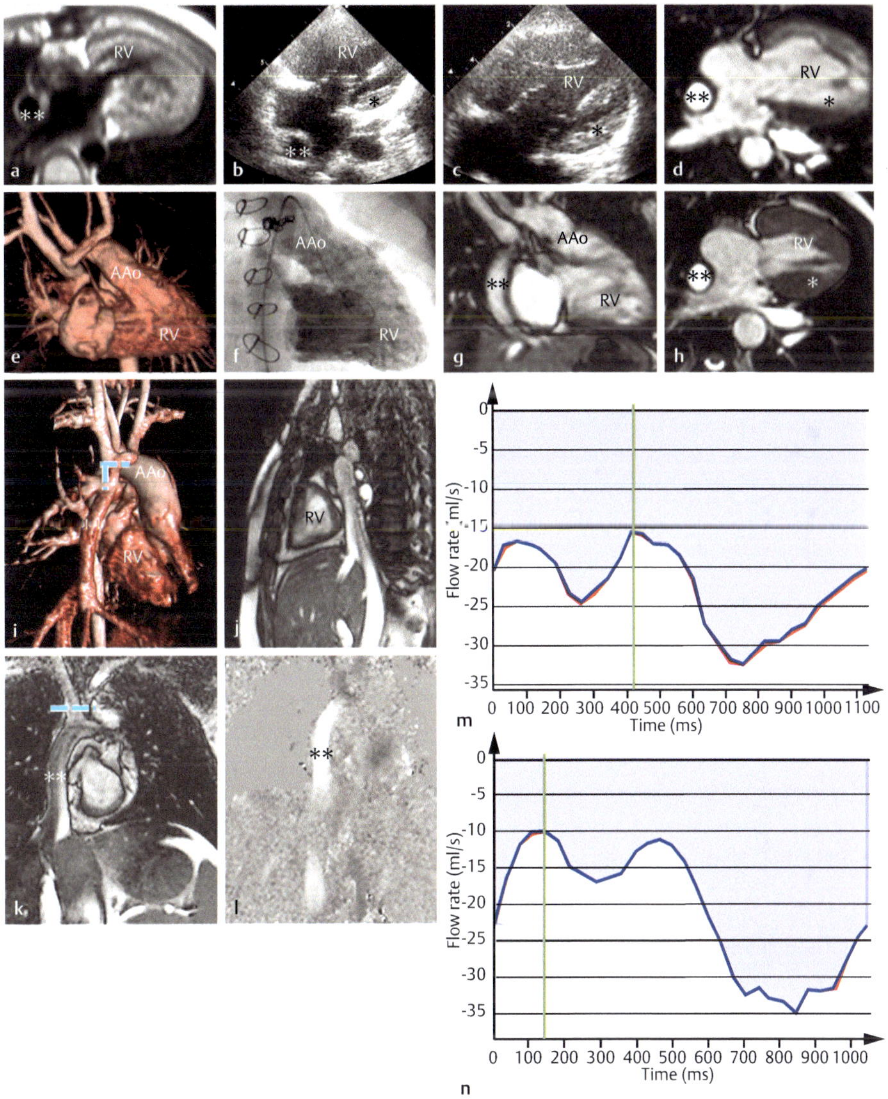

Fig. 4.119 Functional single right ventricle with DORV, extracardiac TCPC, and stent in the left pulmonary artery. The asterisk indicates the hypoplastic left ventricle (**b**, **c**, **d**, **h**), while the double asterisk indicates the extracardiac tunnel (**a**, **b**, **d**, **g–o**). Aortic coarctation is a concurrent defect (▶ Fig. 4.121).

AAo = ascending aorta
RPA = right pulmonary artery
RV = right ventricle
SVC = superior vena cava

a Transverse MR SE with flow artifacts caused by slow flow in the atrium and right ventricle.
b 2-D TTE depicting the right main ventricle, hypoplastic left ventricle (asterisk), and extracardiac tunnel (double asterisk).
c 2-D TTE, different slice. The asterisk indicates the position of the hypoplastic left ventricle.
d Transverse SSFP cine MRI during diastole. The image depicts good function of the single right ventricle during systole, in light of the partial depiction in **h**.
e Volume rendering image from a contrast-enhanced MRA depicting the DORV.
f Ventriculogram of the invasive cardiac catheter examination corresponding to **e**, depicting the aorta originating from the right ventricle.
g SSFP cine MRI, angulated coronal slice orientation, through the extracardiac TCPC (double asterisk).
h Transverse SSFP cine MRI during systole (corresponding to **d**).
i Volume rendering image from a contrast-enhanced MRA, with segmentation of the extracardiac TCPC (double asterisk; blue line for flow measurement in **m** and **n**).
j Magnitude image of a flow-sensitive GE sequence, sagittal slice orientation, through the TCPC (double asterisk).
k Magnitude image of the flow-sensitive GE sequence, coronal slice orientation, through the TCPC (blue line for flow measurement in **m** and **n**).
l Corresponding phase image of the flow-sensitive GE sequence, with regular cranial flow (pale color) in the TCPC (double asterisk).
m Biphasic caudal (negative) flow profile in the superior vena cava, no retrograde flow (no flow above the zero line).
n Biphasic (negative) flow profile to the right in the right pulmonary artery, no retrograde flow (no flow above the zero line).

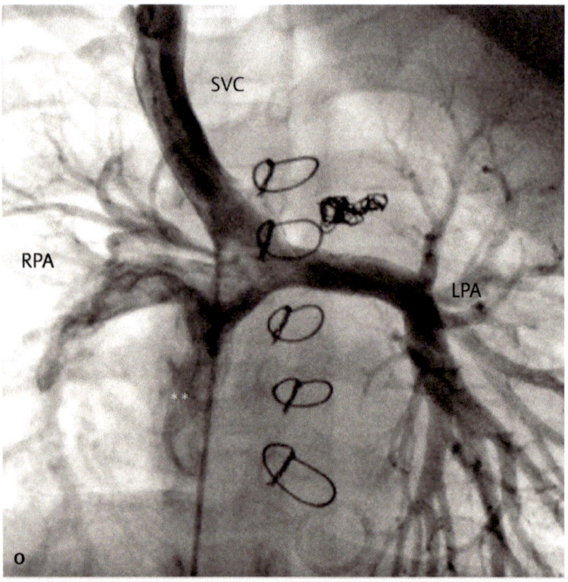

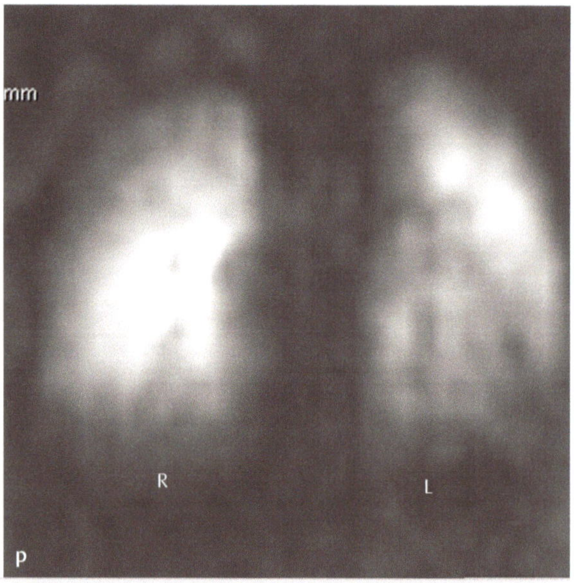

Fig 4.119 (*Continued*) **Functional single right ventricle with DORV, extracardiac TCPC, and stent in the left pulmonary artery.**
AAo = ascending aorta
RPA = right pulmonary artery
RV = right ventricle
SVC = superior vena cava

o Invasive depiction of the TCPC, with anastomoses, showing similar bilateral pulmonary perfusion.
p The dynamic MRA test bolus sequence, coronal slice orientation, also depicts similar bilateral pulmonary perfusion.

Postoperative

Tomographic procedures are used postoperatively to assess ventricular, valve, and Fontan function, as well as to prove the presence of complications such as thromboses (▶ Fig. 4.120c,f) and stenotic anastomoses (▶ Fig. 4.118a, ▶ Fig. 4.119, ▶ Fig. 4.120, and ▶ Fig. 4.121). This should be achieved primarily using Doppler echocardiography and MRI.[6,7,159,160] Especially for older patients, assessing ventricular function and the Fontan tunnel is rarely possible via Doppler echocardiography due to the limited acoustic window. The role of CT remains unclear.[6,7,157,159] It is, however, usually used as an alternative to MRI if the latter cannot be used due to contraindications or limited evaluability, such as if a stent has been implanted (▶ Fig. 4.118a and ▶ Fig. 4.120). In these cases, dose-reducing protocols, such as selecting a low kV, should be used.

Angulated coronal SSFP cine MRI sequences,[159] either axial or following the course of the Fontan tunnel (▶ Fig. 4.116c, ▶ Fig. 4.117, ▶ Fig. 4.118b, and ▶ Fig. 4.119d, g,h,j,k), are part of standard MRI examination. Depending on the underlying defects, these sequences can be used in conjunction with the short-axis slices more suitable than the axial slices for volumetric analysis of the main atrium (▶ Fig. 4.116d).

MRI remains the gold standard for volumetric and functional analysis by using SSFP sequences, particularly in cases of pathological ventricular geometry. In principle, it is also possible for morphologic assessment to only use ECG-triggered SE sequences (▶ Fig. 4.116a,b) in the same orientations. However, GE sequences are preferable because of the flow artifacts that often occur due to slowed flow (▶ Fig. 4.119a), which cannot be differentiated from thrombi, especially near the Fontan tunnel. In addition, contrast-enhanced MRA can be performed in two phases: a pulmonary arterial phase to depict the Fontan tunnel (▶ Fig. 4.118a and ▶ Fig. 4.119i) and an arterial phase (▶ Fig. 4.119 and ▶ Fig. 4.121a) with a subsequent 3-D MIP or volume rendering reconstruction. If dynamic timing of contrast agent administration is performed using a test bolus in a coronal orientation, this can be used to assess bilateral pulmonary perfusion (▶ Fig. 4.119b).

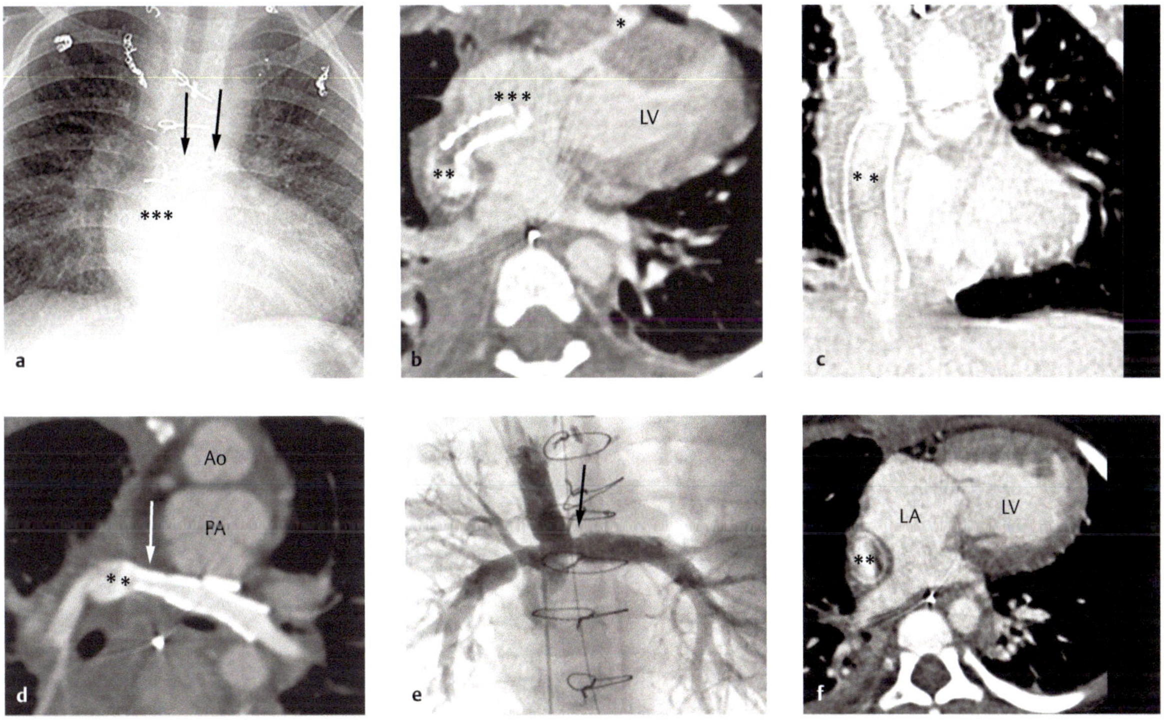

Fig. 4.120 Functionally univentricular heart. Four-year-old male patient with tricuspid atresia and functionally univentricular heart with left systemic ventricle. Condition after palliative treatment by means of extracardiac TCPC (**b**, **c**, **d**, **f**, double asterisk). The reconstructions from a contrast-enhanced CT depict parietal thrombi in the conduit of the TCPC (**b**, **c**, **f**, double asterisk), as well as flow artifacts.
Ao = aorta
LA = left atrium
LV = left ventricle
PA = pulmonary artery

- **a** Multiple coils after coil embolization of MAPCA, and well as a fenestration stent between the extracardiac conduit (TCPC) and the right atrium (triple asterisk), stents in the left pulmonary artery (arrows), an enlarged left ventricle, and pulmonary volume overload are visible in the traditional p.-a. thoracic X-ray.
- **b** Transverse reconstruction of a contrast-enhanced CT, 80 kV, using a high-pitch mode. The triple asterisk indicates the position of the right atrium.
- **c** Coronal reconstruction corresponding to **b**, depicting the parietal thrombi in the TCPC.
- **d** The transverse image depicts the anastomosis of the pulmonary artery branches with the superior vena cava (double asterisk) and multiple stents in the left pulmonary artery, with proximal stenosis (**d**, **e**, arrows). In addition, the malposition of the great arteries (MGA) with the ventrally displaced aorta and dilatated pulmonary artery, each with a tricuspid valve, are also clearly visible. The reconstruction resulted from an ECG triggered 3-D MDCT data set with isotropic voxels.
- **e** Angiogram corresponding to **d** in a.p.-projection.
- **f** Transverse reconstruction of a contrast-enhanced CT (see **b**, another slice).

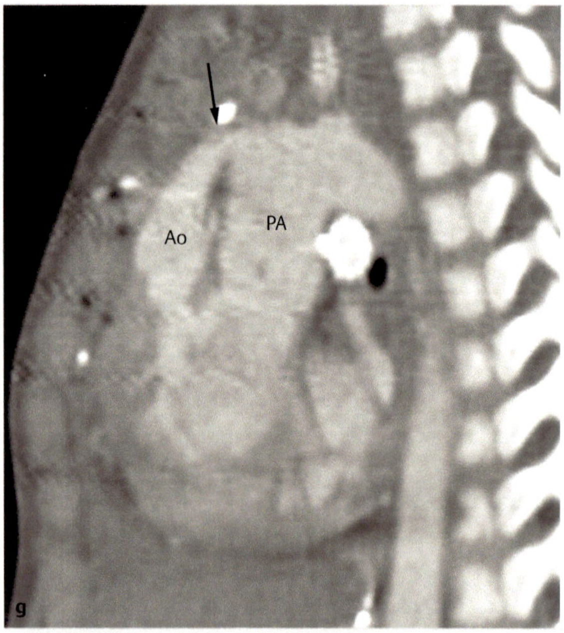

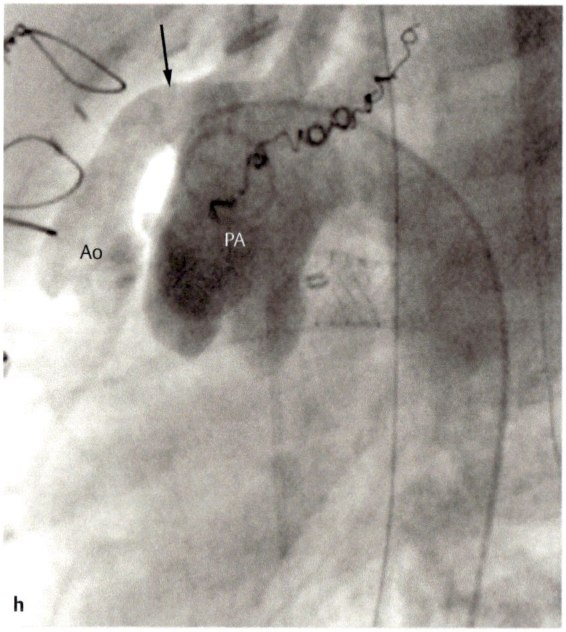

Fig 4.120 (*Continued*) **Functionally univentricular heart.**
Ao = aorta
LA = left atrium
LV = left ventricle
PA = pulmonary artery

g The sagittal reconstruction of a CT data set depicts the MGA after a Damus–Kaye–Stansel procedure[155] for achieving common systemic outflow via an end-to-end anastomosis of the main pulmonary artery branch to the aorta (**g**, **h**, arrows).
h Angiogram corresponding to **g**.

Note

In order to depict the Fontan tunnel and anastomoses of the TCPC clearly using contrast-enhanced MRA or CTA, the timing of the contrast agent bolus administration should be based on the Fontan tunnel.

Furthermore, MRI flow measurements should be performed, particularly, to assess flow ratios in the Fontan tunnel (▶ Fig. 4.119j-n) and to assess pulmonary circulation in the right and left pulmonary arteries. In the future, 4-D flow measurement will be especially helpful in this regard. The role of tissue characterization (e.g., using late enhancement or T1 mapping) during risk stratification has not yet been fully clarified.

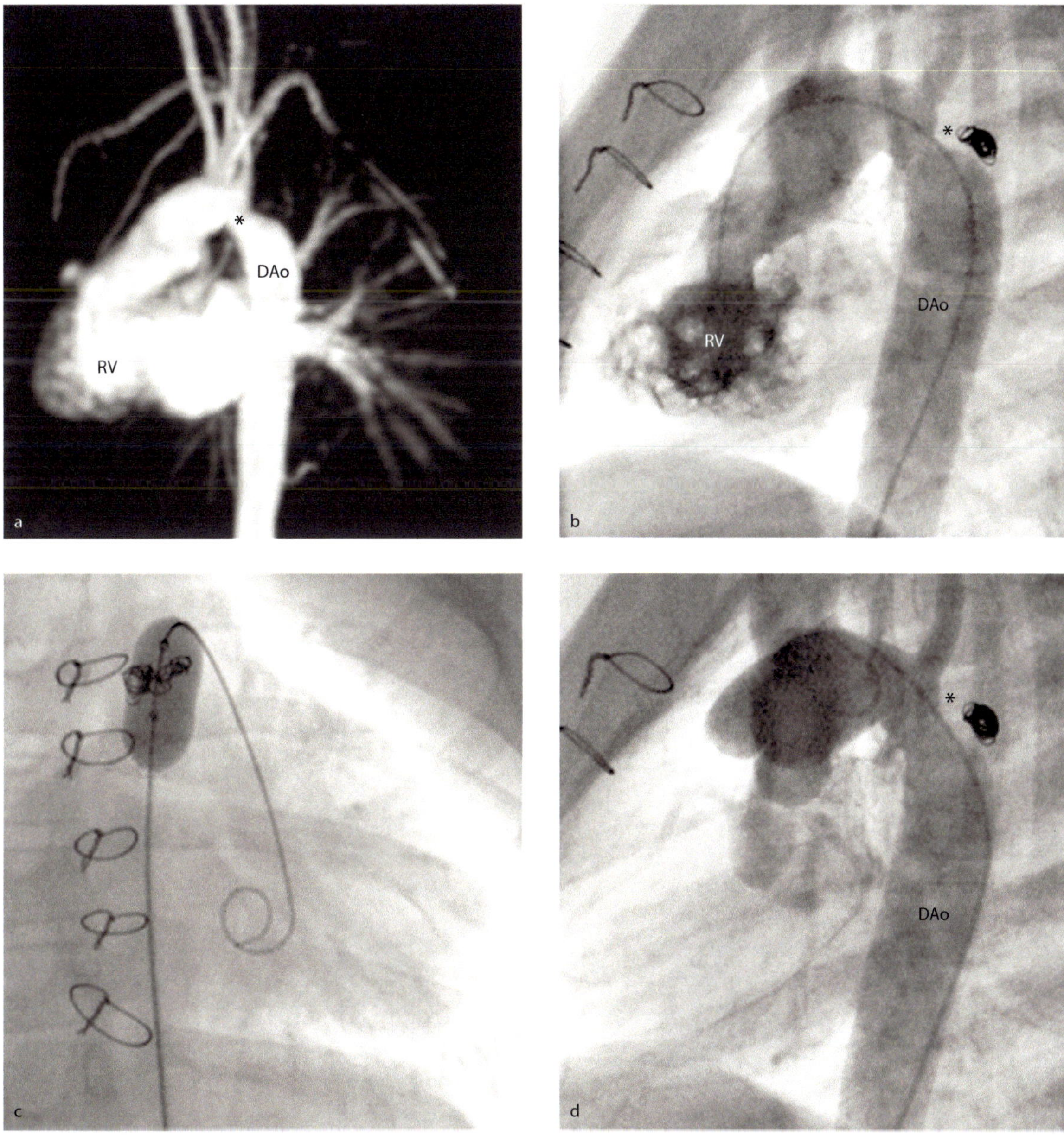

Fig. 4.121 Functional single right ventricle with DORV, extracardiac TCPC, and stent in the left pulmonary artery. Aortic coarctation as a concurrent defect. This is the same patient as in ▶ Fig. 4.119.

DAo = descending aorta

RV = right ventricle

a 3-D MIP of the arterial phase of a contrast-enhanced MRA, depicting an aortic coarctation (asterisk) as a concurrent defect in the lateral reconstruction.

b Corresponding invasive angiogram before balloon angioplasty.

c Invasive angiogram during balloon angioplasty.

d Invasive angiogram after balloon angioplasty.

4.4.5 Total Anomalous Pulmonary Venous Return

Joachim Lotz, Philipp Beerbaum, Michael Steinmetz

Definition

When this defect occurs, the pulmonary veins have no direct connection to the left atrium. Rather, all four pulmonary veins possess anomalous venous return to the caval veins, coronary sinus, or directly to the right atrium. This defect is often abbreviated as "TAPVR" or "TAPVC" ("total anomalous pulmonary venous return/connection"). This is an extremely rare illness, occurring in only 6.8 of every 100,000 live births (0.0068%).[161] The defect's distribution by gender is unclear. The Baltimore–Washington Instant Study Group has stated that the defect occurs in an 18:23 ratio between boys and girls. Literary references have also indicated that this defect is more common in male patients.

Classification

Classification is based on the site of anomalous pulmonary venous connection. A PFO (occurring in 70% of cases) or ASD II (occurring in 30% of cases) is necessary for survival. The common Craig or Gatham–Nadas classification systems[162,163] and the frequency distribution developed by Goswami et al.[164–166] will now be addressed in greater detail (▸ Fig. 4.122):

- *Supracardiac type* (45–64%; ▸ Fig. 4.123; ▸ Fig. 4.122a): The pulmonary veins merge within a collecting sinus posterior to an often very small left atrium, and then drain via an ascending vessel (vertical vein) discharging from the collecting sinus, usually into the proximal left anonymous vein—though in much rarer instances, into the superior vena cava or azygos vein. In these cases, pulmonary venous obstructions are usually, though not always, absent.
- *Cardiac or intracardiac type* (21–27%): The four pulmonary veins merge in a collecting sinus posterior to the

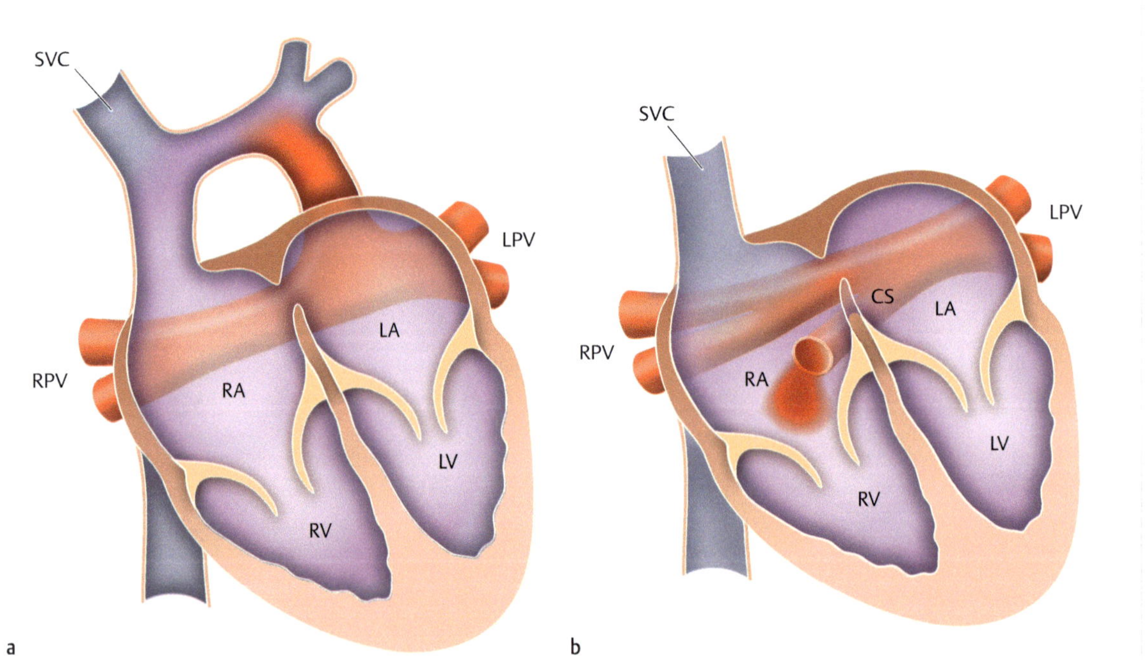

Fig. 4.122 Supracardiac and infracardiac TAPVR types. Schematic depiction.
CS = coronary sinus
LA = left atrium
LPV = left pulmonary vein
LV = left ventricle
RA = right atrium
RV = right ventricle
SVC = superior vena cava

a The most common type of supracardiac TAPVR,[167] according to Moss. The anomalous pulmonary venous connections (right and left pulmonary veins) merge dorsal to the atria and connect to a left ascending vessel that flows into a left-side, persistent superior vena cava (marked in red). The path then continues via the left anonymous vein into the right superior vena cava, and then into the right atrium.

b Intracardiac or cardiac TAPVR,[167] according to Moss. The anomalous pulmonary venous connections (right and left pulmonary veins) merge into a short vessel (marked in red) that connects to the coronary sinus. In rarer cases, the pulmonary veins can connect directly to the right atrium when this type of TAPVR is present.

heart, usually with stenosis-free drainage via the coronary sinus (approx. 18% of cases; ▶ Fig. 4.124; also ▶ Fig. 4.122b), but in rarer cases, directly into the right atrium (approx. 8% of cases; ▶ Fig. 4.125, ▶ Fig. 4.126, ▶ Fig. 4.127, ▶ Fig. 4.128).

- *Infracardiac type* (16–24%): The four pulmonary veins merge posterior to the heart (left atrium). Blood flows to the portal vein, venous duct, inferior vena cava, or (left) hepatic vein via a vessel passing through the diaphragm. This type of TAPVR is almost always associated with pulmonary venous obstructions.
- *Mixed type* (3–8%): This is a combination of various anomalous venous connections: superior vena cava and coronary sinus, anonymous vein and coronary sinus, and anonymous and infracardiac veins. This type can occur with or without pulmonary venous obstructions.

Hemodynamics

In principle, a combination of an obligate left–right shunt through a mixture of pulmonary venous and systemic venous blood with an obligate right–left shunt near the

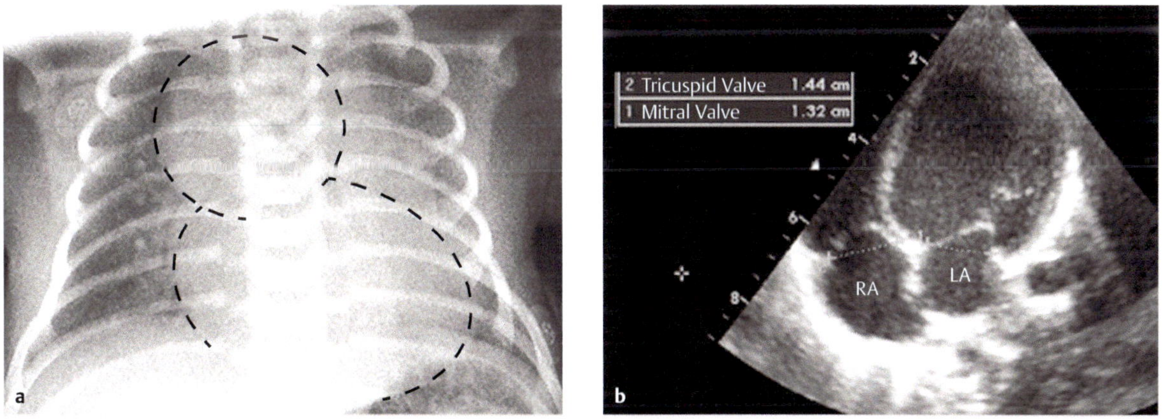

Fig. 4.123 Typical snowman or figure-eight configuration of a supracardiac TAPVR. Male newborn. Evidence of a relatively small left atrium compared to the right one.
LA = left atrium
RA = right atrium
a A.-p. "suspended" thoracic X-ray depicting the "snowman" configuration.
b Corresponding 2-D TTE image.

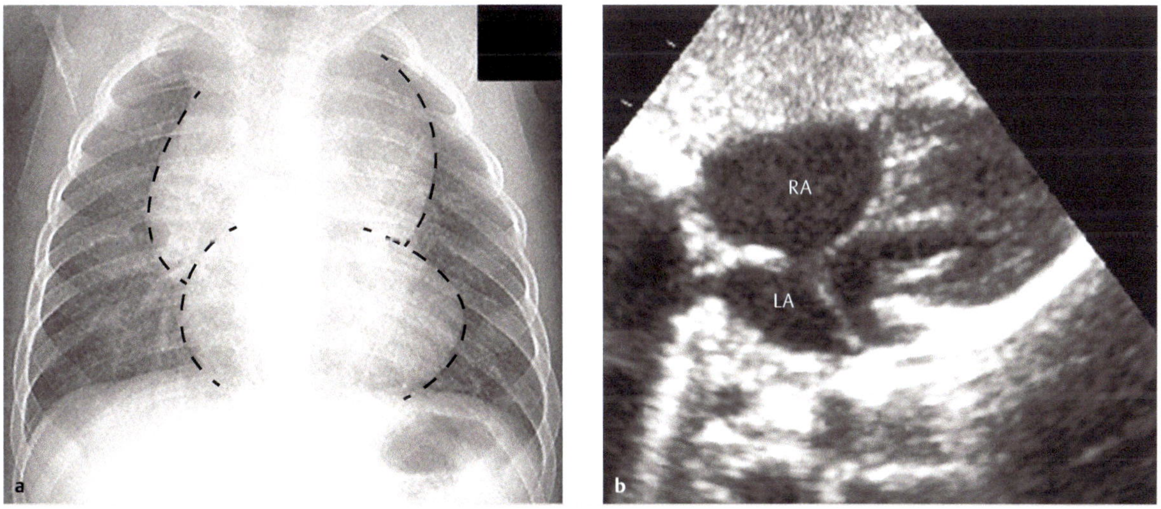

Fig. 4.124 Typical snowman or figure-eight configuration of a TAPVR with intracardiac anomalous pulmonary venous connection to the coronary sinus. Female newborn. Typical relatively small left atrium and large right atrium.
LA = left atrium
RA = right atrium
a Thoracic X-ray.
b Corresponding 2-D TTE image.

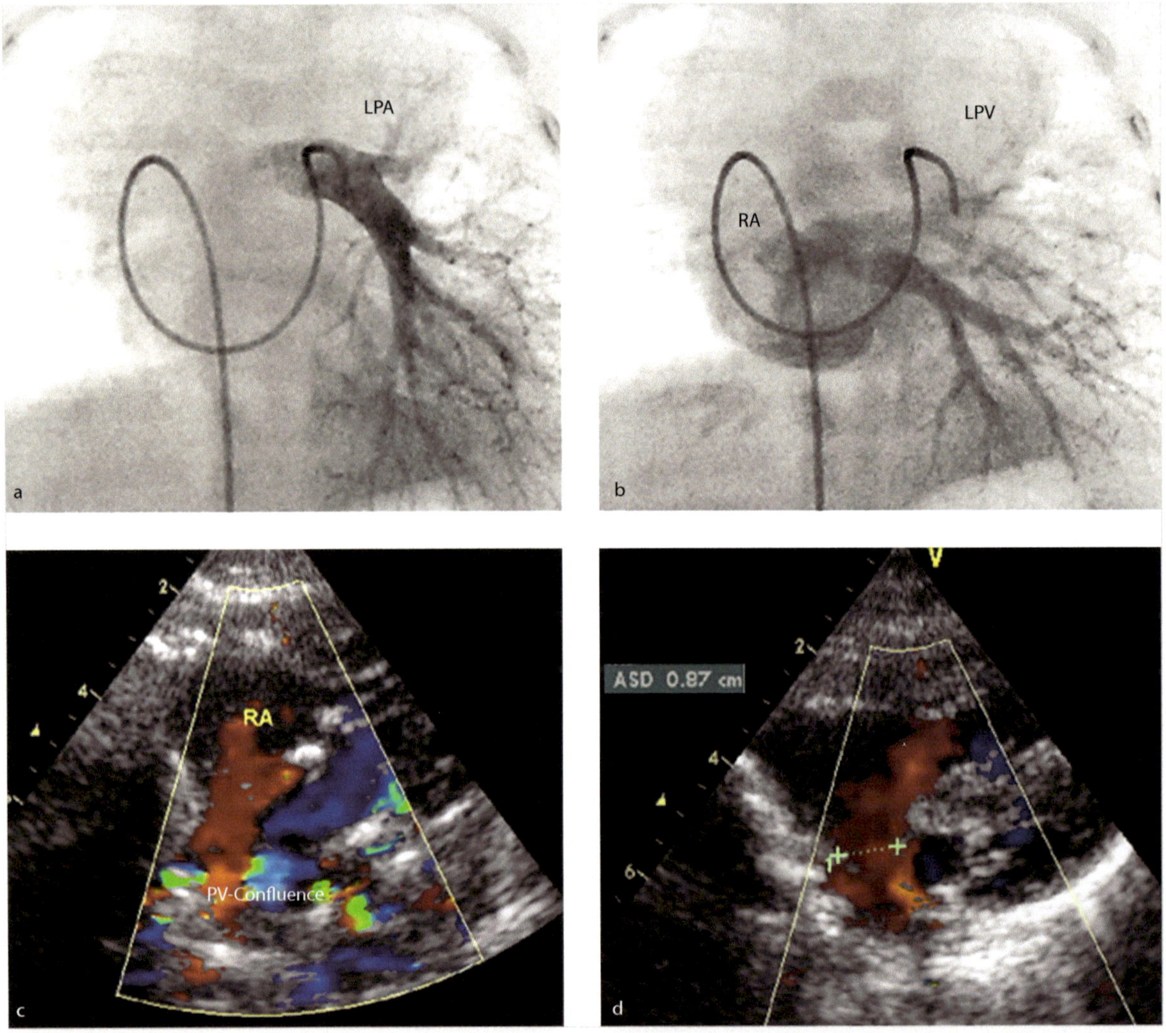

Fig. 4.125 Cardiac TAPVR with venous connection directly to the right atrium via a short pulmonary venous confluence.
LPA = left pulmonary artery
PV confluence = pulmonary vein confluence
RA = right atrium
a Invasive pulmonary angiogram depicting the pulmonary arterial phase.
b Invasive pulmonary angiogram depicting the pulmonary venous phase.
c The confluence is visible using color Doppler.
d The obligate ASD or VSD connection can be depicted and measured clearly using color Doppler.

atria occurs. This is necessary for the patient's survival, since this is the only path by which blood accesses the left side of the heart and, thus, the aorta. The size of this intraatrial communication, the degree of pulmonary venous obstruction, and the level of pulmonary arteriolar resistance determine the hemodynamic situation and clinical picture. In cases of restrictive interatrial communication, "low cardiac output" can develop. Pulmonary venous congestion accompanied by pulmonary edema, subsequent increase in pulmonary arteriolar pressure, and pulmonary hypertonia (often concurrent with progressive right ventricular heart failure) inevitably occur in cases of pulmonary venous obstruction. If no pulmonary venous obstruction is present, the left–right shunt is dominant due to the postnatal decrease in pulmonary arteriolar resistance, as well as pulmonary flooding and milder central cyanosis.

Clinical Issues

This is a cyanotic defect, since systemic and pulmonary venous return mix with one another at the latest upon reaching the right atrium, and only this mixed blood is able to reach the left side of the heart. Auscultation generally reveals a galloping rhythm and fixed heart sounds divided into two parts, with an emphasized segment of

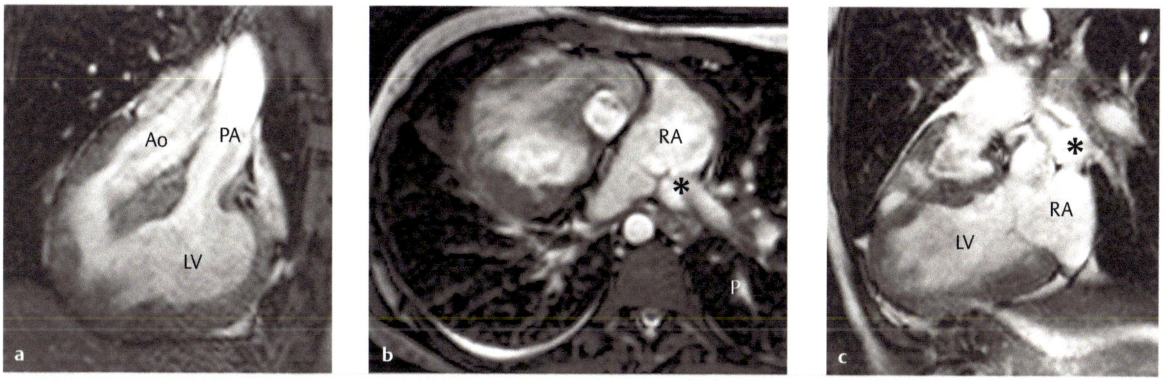

Fig. 4.126 Complete situs inversus and cardiac TAPVR with direct connection of all pulmonary veins to the right atrium. Various SSFP cine MRI of a male child.

Ao = aorta
LPV = left pulmonary vein
LV = left ventricle
PA = pulmonary artery
RA = right atrium

a Complete situs inversus, DILV, and rudimentary RVOT in an angulated sagittal cine MRI SSFP sequence.

b A cine MRI SSFP sequence in transverse orientation shows that all pulmonary veins connect to a left-displaced right atrium via a confluence (asterisk) located dorsal to the right atrium.

c Long-axis, 2-chamber view through the left ventricle depicting a stenosis between the confluence (asterisk) and atrium (see black dephasing jet) which corresponds to a hemodynamically functional pulmonary vein stenosis.

the pulmonary valve, systole as a relative pulmonary stenosis, and diastole as a relative tricuspid stenosis in cases of pronounced right heart volume overload. A distinction is made between two cases:

- *If pulmonary venous obstruction is present*, children often begin to exhibit symptoms as newborns or young infants, with progressive dyspnea caused by pulmonary edema and progressive cyanosis (decreased diffusion caused by congestion, concurrent with reduced pulmonary perfusion resulting from pulmonary hypertonia caused by the congestion). Right ventricular heart failure commonly occurs as a result of this combined pressure and volume overload.
- In contrast, if *no pulmonary venous obstruction* is present, pulmonary perfusion increases significantly. Consequently, the cyanosis may be only minor and thus remain completely undiscovered.

Natural Progression and Indication for Treatment

Children virtually always become symptomatic within the first 6 months of life, and 80% of children die if left untreated. If pulmonary venous obstructions are present, newborns exhibit significant dyspnea with progressive cyanosis, and rapid circulatory collapse can occur. Without immediate treatment, children with severe obstructions do not survive. If no pulmonary venous obstruction is present, the hemodynamic situation corresponds to that of a large ASD (pronounced volume load of the right heart and the pulmonary vessels caused by the left–right shunt of the oxygenated pulmonary venous blood to the systemic venous blood), with additional cyanosis caused by the aforementioned mixture of right atrial blood with the (obligate) right–left shunt near the atrium. Progressive heart failure accompanied by failure to thrive and tachypnea usually develops in infants. If timely surgical treatment is provided, patients usually have a normal life expectancy, provided that no pulmonary venous obstructions occur before or after surgical correction, or develop at a later date. Over the long term, however, difficult-to-treat supraventricular cardiac rhythm disorders have been documented.

Treatment Options

Surgical correction using a heart–lung machine is the only permanent treatment option. The strategy can differ and depends on the anatomy of the anomalous venous connection and of the confluence. The goal is to direct pulmonary venous blood to the left atrium, ideally by avoiding direct interventions involving the individual pulmonary veins in order to reduce the risk of postoperative pulmonary vein stenosis. In addition, the ASD must be closed.

The surgical technique depends on the anatomy of the venous return. Usually, however, an attempt is made to anastomose the confluence of the pulmonary veins posterior to the heart (known as the collecting sinus) directly to the left atrium by creating a tension-free side-to-side anastomosis and connecting it to the drainage vessel (▶ Fig. 4.129). In the event that interatrial connection is restricted, it may, in rare cases, be necessary to perform a preoperative Rashkind maneuver as a bridging procedure immediately after birth.

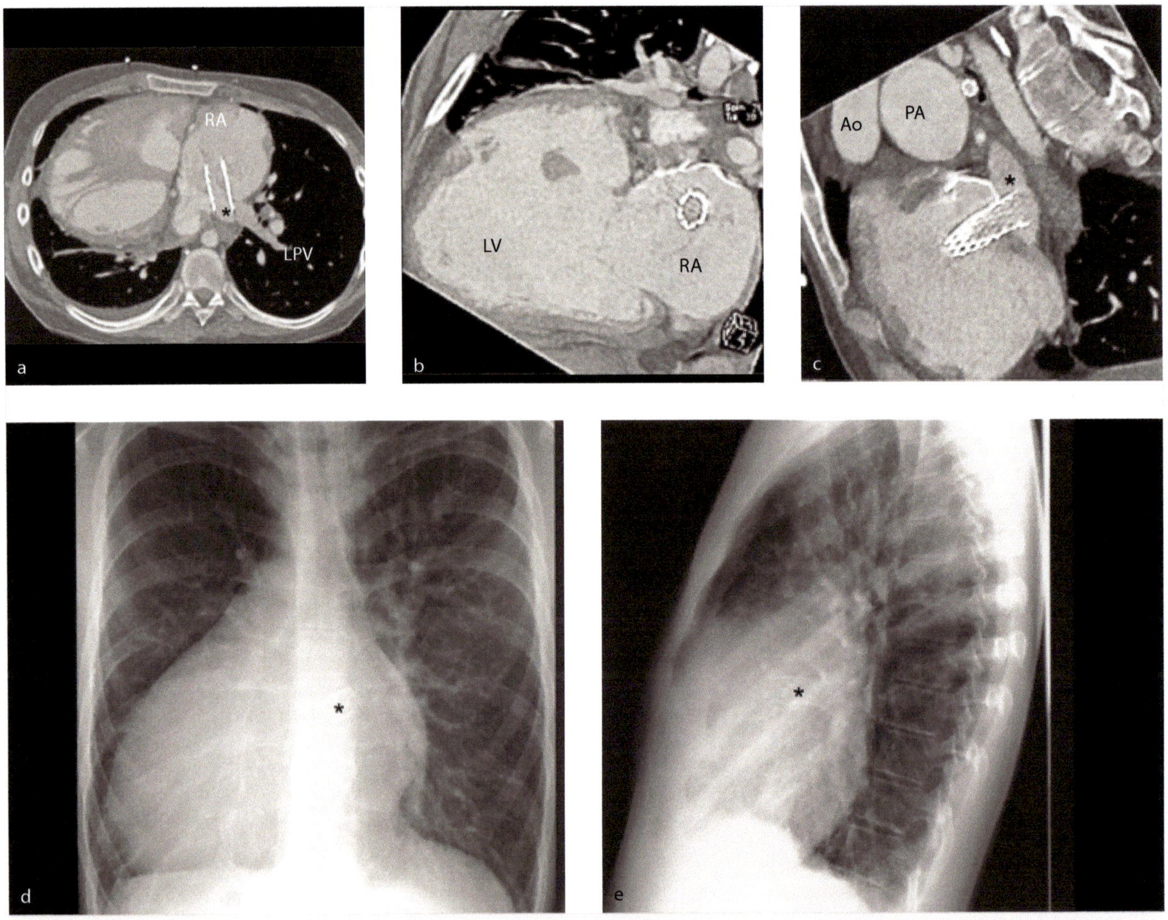

Fig. 4.127 Complete situs inversus and cardiac TAPVR with direct connection of all pulmonary veins to the right atrium. Condition after implanting a stent in the confluence. Images of the patient from ▶ Fig. 4.126 after interventional implantation of a Palmaz stent (**a**, **c–e**, asterisk) in the stenotic pulmonary venous confluence dorsal to the right atrium.

Ao = aorta
LPV = left pulmonary vein
LV = left ventricle
PA = pulmonary artery
RA = right atrium

a Transverse reconstruction of a CT data set with isotropic voxels, acquired in flash or high-pitch mode on a DSCT, with radiation exposure of less than 1 mSv.
b Coronal reconstruction.
c Sagittal reconstruction.
d Corresponding p.-a. thoracic X-ray.
e Corresponding lateral thoracic X-ray.

Note

M!

If pronounced pulmonary venous obstructions are present, this intervention is, not infrequently, performed as an emergency measure. Catheter interventional decompression of a severe pulmonary venous obstruction can, in certain cases, be useful as a temporary measure to bring the newborn into a more stable hemodynamic state before the subsequent operation. If no pulmonary venous obstruction is present, the surgery should be performed within the first 6 months of life in order to prevent pulmonary vascular disease and a failure to thrive.

Postoperative and Postinterventional Issues

The most common complication is postoperative pulmonary venous obstruction (▶ Fig. 4.126, ▶ Fig. 4.127, ▶ Fig. 4.128). Interventional or surgical treatment for restenosis is often unsatisfactory.

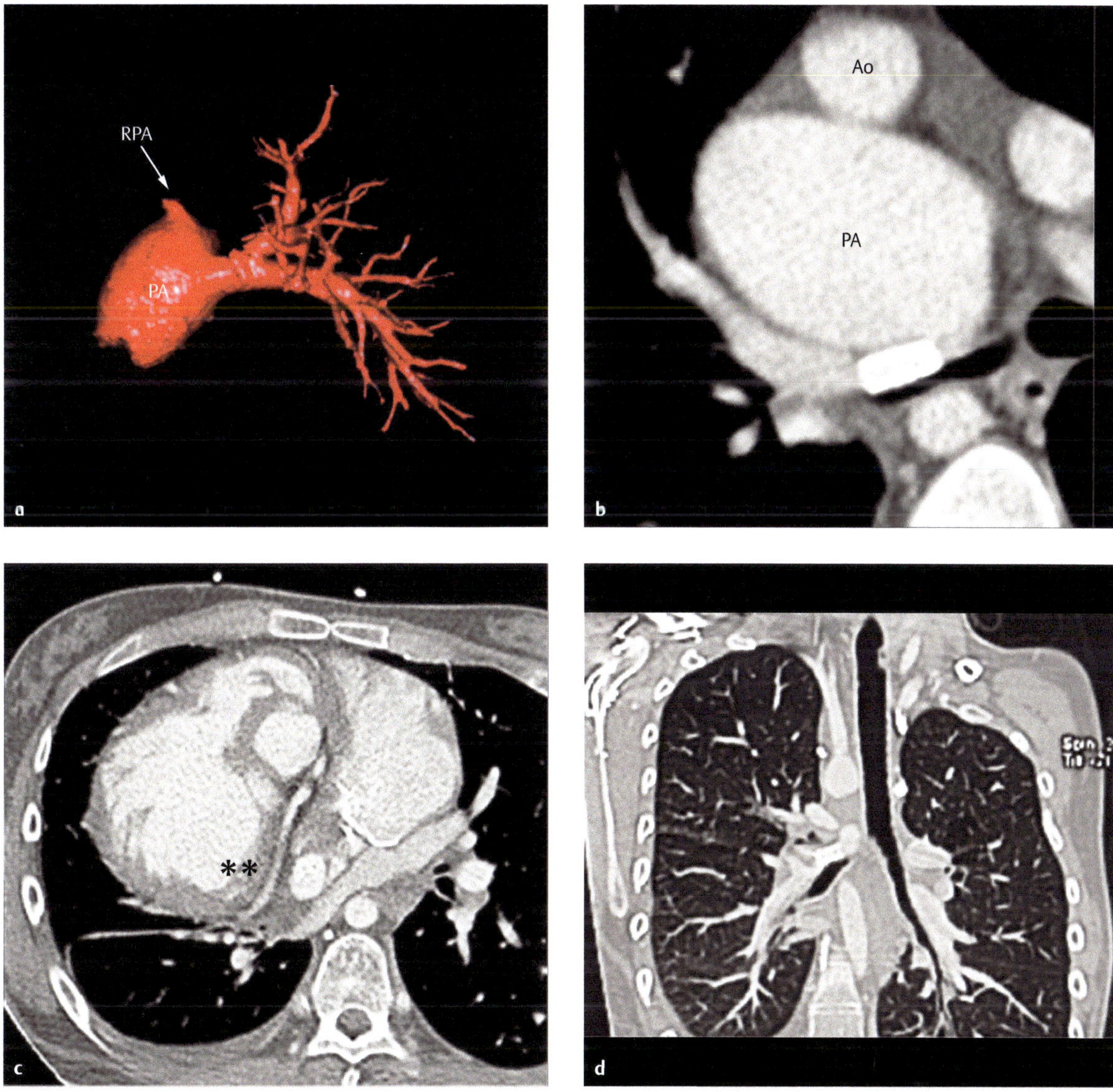

Fig. 4.128 Complete situs inversus and cardiac TAPVR with direct connection of all pulmonary veins to the right atrium. Condition after stent implantation in the right pulmonary artery. Images of the patient from ▸ Fig. 4.126 and ▸ Fig. 4.127 acquired using a CT data set.

Ao = aorta
PA = pulmonary artery
RPA = right pulmonary artery

- **a** The subtotal stenosis of the superior right pulmonary artery can be clearly seen in the 3-D reconstruction.
- **b** Transverse reconstruction of the MDCT data set after treating right pulmonary arterial stenosis by means of stent implantation.
- **c** Somewhat further caudal transverse reconstruction of the MDCT data set from **b** depicting the coronary supply (double asterisk).
- **d** Coronal reconstruction of the MDCT data set after treating right pulmonary arterial stenosis by means of stent implantation (asterisk).

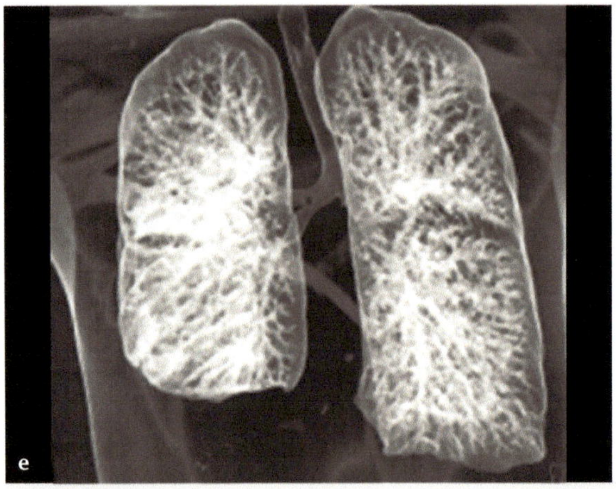

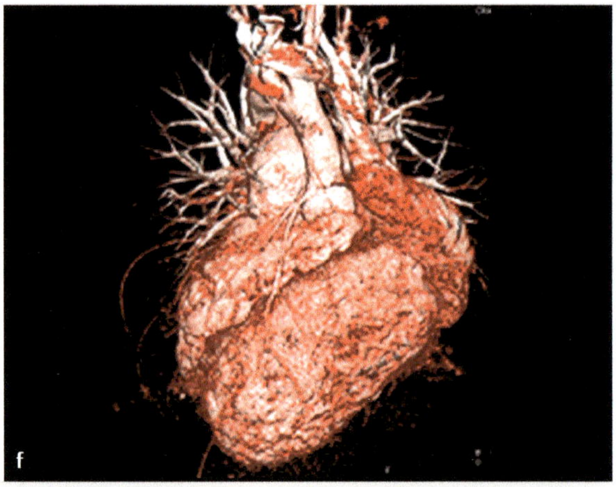

Fig 4.128 *(Continued)*
Ao = aorta
PA = pulmonary artery
RPA = right pulmonary artery

e Proof of post-interventional homogeneous pulmonary perfusion using the dual-energy technique of the used DSCT.
f Volume rendering of the 3-D data set to better depict coronary artery supply.

Goals and Relative Value of Diagnostic Imaging

Preinterventional

Preinterventional diagnostics consists almost exclusively of echocardiography (▶ Fig. 4.123, ▶ Fig. 4.124, ▶ Fig. 4.125). A preoperative MRI can be helpful in cases of complex anatomy, provided that the patient is hemodynamically stable (▶ Fig. 4.126). CTA is significantly faster and gentler for ill, artificially respirated newborns with TAPVR and pulmonary venous obstruction, and is thus the imaging method of choice (▶ Fig. 4.127 and ▶ Fig. 4.128). Cardiac catheter diagnostics are only justified in cases of very unusual anatomy with the potential for necessary interventions regarding the atrial septum or a severe pulmonary venous obstruction (stent).

The entire course of the pulmonary venous drainage should be depicted prior to the intervention, and explicit evidence of the course of all four pulmonary veins should also be shown. Imaging generally demonstrates a dilated right heart (dilatated by volume load), a small left atrium, and a narrow left ventricle (▶ Fig. 4.123b and ▶ Fig. 4.124b). A large retroatrial area can generally be seen behind the left atrium, which corresponds to the confluence of the pulmonary veins (▶ Fig. 4.125c).

Note

The typical figure-eight or snowman configuration can be seen clearly in the thoracic image of a patient without surgical correction (▶ Fig. 4.123a, ▶ Fig. 4.124a): The dilatated right heart and right atrium form the first ball of the figure-eight or snowman, while the dilated superior vena cava, innominate vein, and left vertical vein form the second ball. The two are connected via a dilated pulmonary segment.

Postinterventional

Echocardiography and MRI attempt to detect early pulmonary venous obstructions or stenosis of the surgical anastomoses.

Note

Stenotic anastomoses generally develop within the first 12 months after surgical correction. Thus, annual imaging follow-up exams are recommended during childhood.

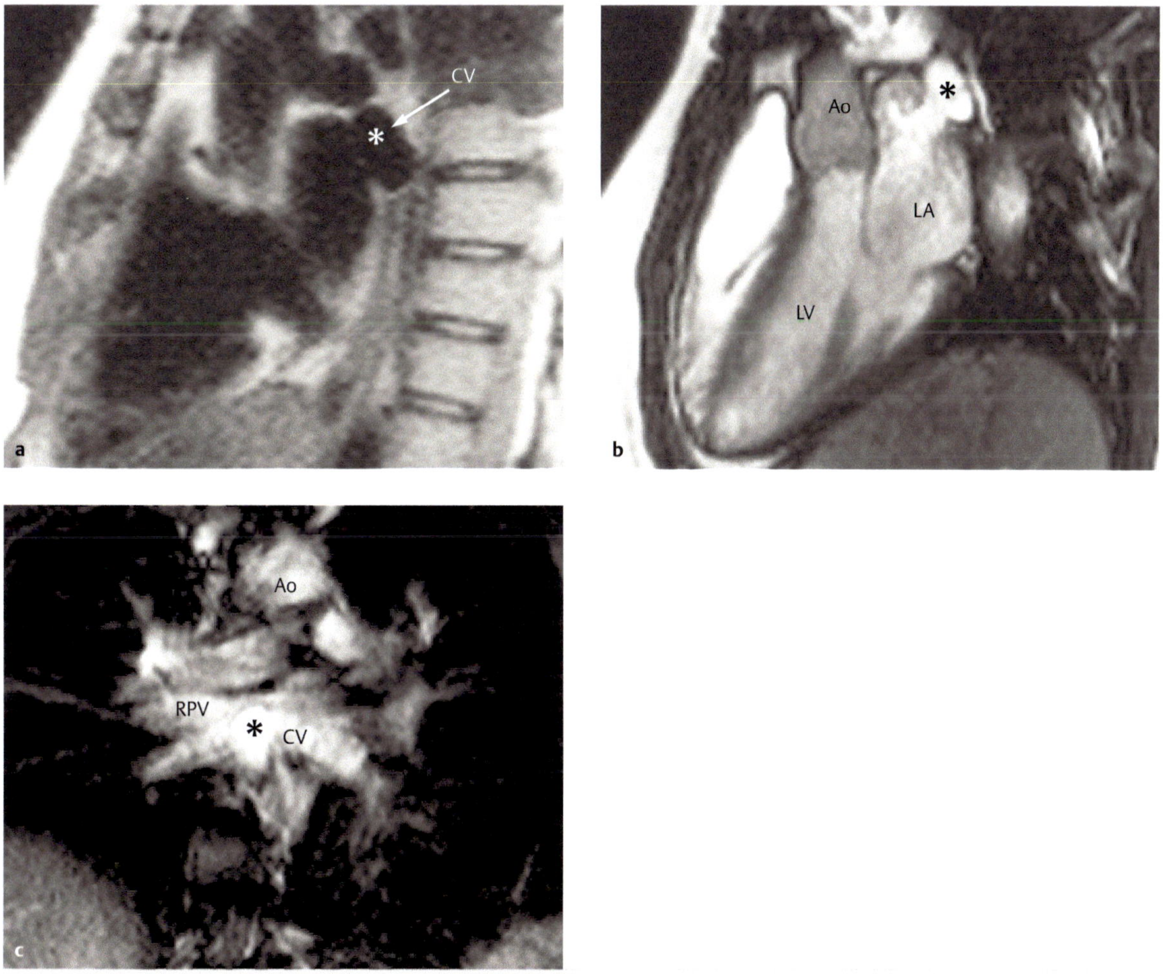

Fig. 4.129 Condition after surgical correction of TAPVR. A collecting vessel was placed dorsal to the left atrium and a window-like anastomosis (**a–c**, asterisk; diameter approx. 10 mm) of this collecting vessel to the left atrium was created.

Ao = aorta
CV = collecting vessel
LA = left atrium
RPV = right pulmonary vein

a Sagittal black blood MR SE image.
b Sagittal SSFP cine MRI.
c En face image, coronal section, clearly depicting the newly created connection to the left atrium (asterisk).

The individual pulmonary veins, surgical anastomoses, and drainage into the left atrium should be depicted. Residual shunts near the atria or ventricles should also be quantified, as well as residual changes near the former venous returns in the systemic vascular bed. If complex postoperative stenoses are present, cardiac catheter depictions are usually needed in order to be able to assess the concurrent hemodynamic situation (e.g., the presence of pulmonary hypertonia). CTA can also be very useful in this instance in order to determine further (often exceedingly difficult) invasive treatment strategies.

4.5 Vascular Anomalies

4.5.1 Partial Pulmonary Venous Anomalies

Joachim Lotz, Philipp Beerbaum, Michael Steinmetz

Definition

Compared to complete TAPVR, which occurs in 0.0068% of the population, PAPVR is relatively common, occurring in 0.3–0.5% of patients with congenital heart

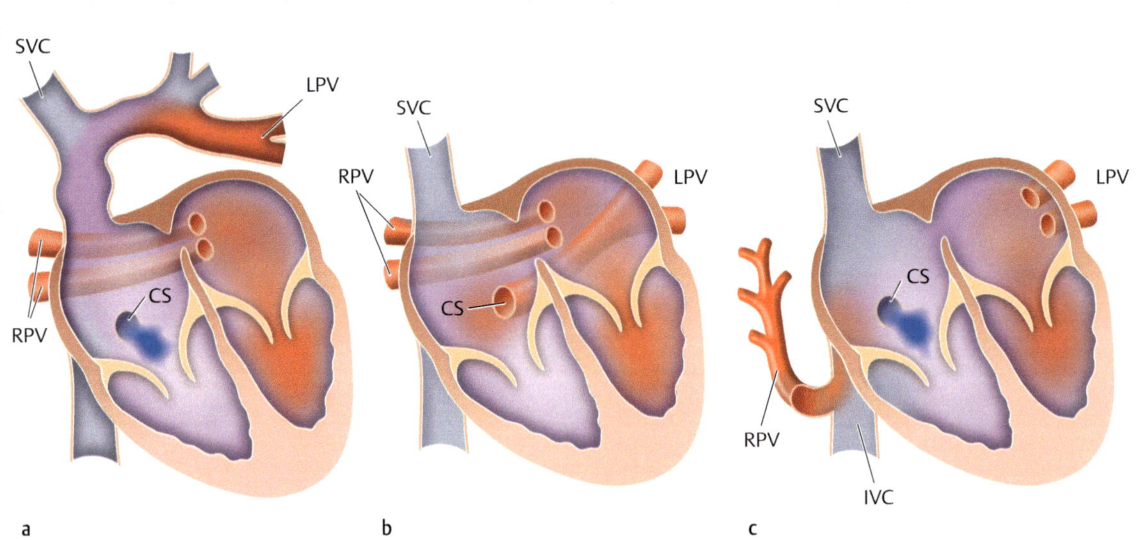

Fig. 4.130 Three typical forms of PAPVR. Schematic depiction.
CS = coronary sinus
IVC = inferior vena cava
LPV = left pulmonary vein
RPV = right pulmonary vein
SVC = superior vena cava

a Left pulmonary veins connecting to the right superior vena cava via the vertical and anonymous veins (▸ Fig. 4.135 and ▸ Fig. 4.136).
b Left pulmonary veins connecting to the coronary sinus.
c Right pulmonary veins connecting to the inferior vena cava via the scimitar vein (▸ Fig. 4.137).

defects. When this defect is present, one or more of the pulmonary veins do not connect to the left atrium.[83,167] PAPVR can occur in isolation, but more commonly occurs in conjunction with ASD, primarily sinus venosus defect (SVD).

Classification

Isolated PAPVR occurs only in rare cases, and more commonly affects the right pulmonary veins, which generally connect directly to the superior vena cava. In rarer cases, they can also connect to the inferior vena cava or directly to the right atrium. If only the left pulmonary veins are affected, they usually connect directly to the right superior vena cava via the vertical and anonymous veins[168–170] (▸ Fig. 4.130a).

In most cases, the PAPVR is associated with an ASD, primarily with a superior SVD, usually on the right side (10 times more common than on the left side). A distinction is made between the following types (▸ Fig. 4.130):

- The *right superior lobar vein(s)* connects (or connect) to the superior vena cava and/or the right atrium (▸ Fig. 4.131 to ▸ Fig. 4.134).
- The *left superior lobar vein(s)* connects (or connect) to the brachiocephalic vein via the vertical vein (33% of cases; ▸ Fig. 4.135 and ▸ Fig. 4.136). Left-side PAPVR is only associated with an SVD in 10–15% of cases.

Scimitar syndrome is a special form of PAPVR in which some or all of the right pulmonary veins (or, in rare cases, the left ones) connect to the inferior vena cava via a collecting vessel.[83,167] Venolobar pulmonary hypoplasia (also known as pulmonary venolobar syndrome) is also present. The name "scimitar" is based on the appearance of the collecting vessel adjacent to the right margin of the heart (▸ Fig. 4.137). The inferior segment, or, in some cases, all of the hypoplastic pulmonary segment veins drain into an anomalous vein. Notable components include the following:

- Scimitar vein (scimitar-shaped configuration of the vein in a p.-a. X-ray close to the right margin of the heart)
- Right pulmonary hypoplasia, with varying cardiac dextroposition
- Right pulmonary artery hypoplasia
- Anomalous arterial supply of the right inferior lobe via the aorta

The scimitar vein can have various connections:

- to the inferior vena cava, below the right hemidiaphragm (in 33% of cases),
- to the suprahepatic segment of the inferior vena cava (in 22% of cases; ▸ Fig. 4.137c),
- to the hepatic veins,
- to the portal veins (in 11% of cases),
- to the azygos vein,
- to the coronary sinus,
- to the right atrium (in 22% of cases), or
- to the left atrium (also known as *meandering pulmonary veins*).

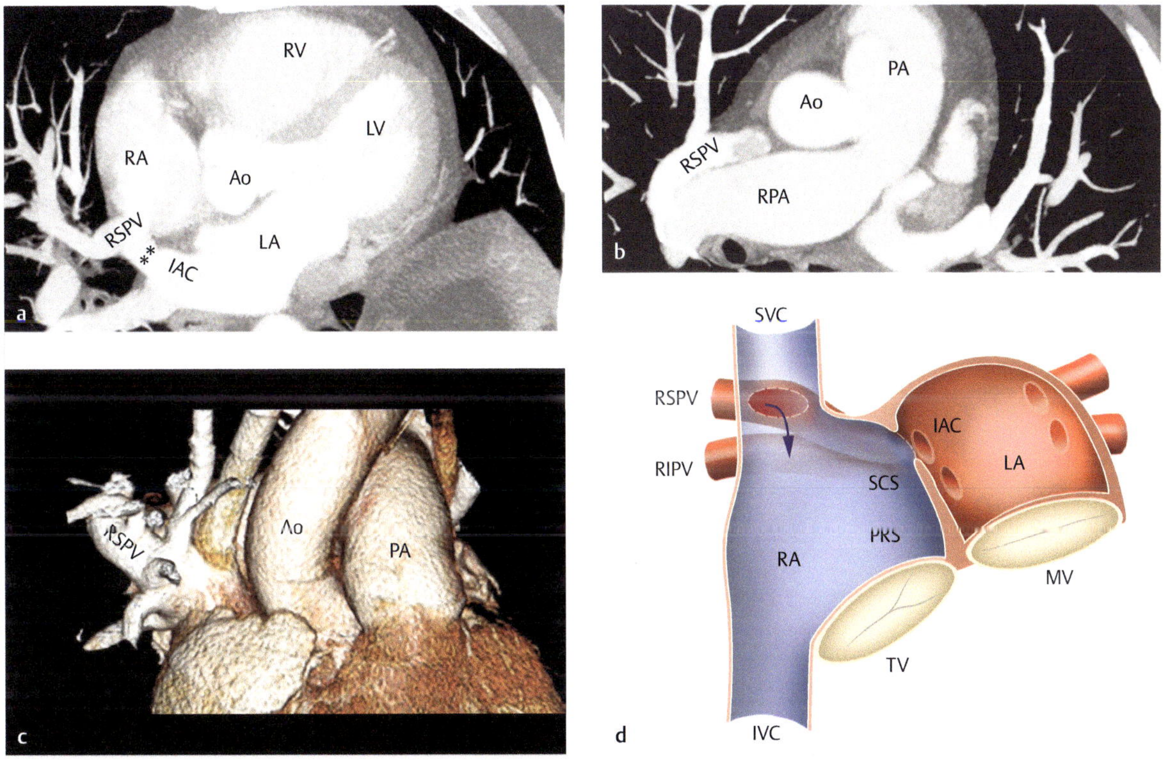

Fig. 4.131 Typical superior SVD and concurrent anomalous connection of the right superior pulmonary veins.

Ao = aorta
IAC = interatrial communication
IVC = inferior vena cava
LA = left atrium
LV = left ventricle
MV = mitral valve
PRS = primary septum
PA = pulmonary artery
RA = right atrium
RPA = right pulmonary artery
RSPV = right superior pulmonary vein
RV = right ventricle
SCS = secondary septum
SVC = superior vena cava
TV = tricuspid valve

a The MDCT reconstruction depicts the anomalous connection of the right superior pulmonary veins to the right atrium. In addition to this connection to the right atrium, interatrial communication (asterisks) is also visible.
b This axial MDCT reconstruction depicts the anomalous connection to the superior vena cava.
c The volume rendering technique used on the same patient depicts a 3-D overview of the anomalous right pulmonary venous connections.
d Most common combination in a case of PAPVR. Schematic depiction. Superior SVD with anomalous connections of the superior pulmonary veins to the superior vena cava via the lack of "roofing" (also known as unroofing) of the otherwise present common wall between the superior vena cava and the right superior pulmonary vein. According to Moss,[167] interatrial communication is not a true defect, but rather constitutes the native opening (which is generally present) of the right superior pulmonary vein into the left atrium.

Note

M!

- Approximately 90% of patients with SVD-type ASDs also have PAPVR, and 50% of patients with pulmonary venous connection, primarily on the right side, also have SVD-type ASDs. This means that all patients with an SVD-type ASD should be examined for anomalous pulmonary venous connections, particularly on the right side!
- A connection of the scimitar vein to the suprahepatic inferior vena cava (▶ Fig. 4.137) or right atrium can be an indicator of intrahepatic interruption of the inferior vena cava (see Caval Vein Anomalies, Systemic Venous Anomalies, and Anomalous Body Venous Connections).

Hemodynamics

The hemodynamic changes correspond to those of an ASD with a left–right atrial shunt. The extent of the shunt depends on the number and size of the anomalous pulmonary venous connections. Individual anomalous pulmonary venous connections usually do not lead to hemodynamically relevant shunt volumes. Unlike TAPVR, PAPVR rarely causes stenosis.

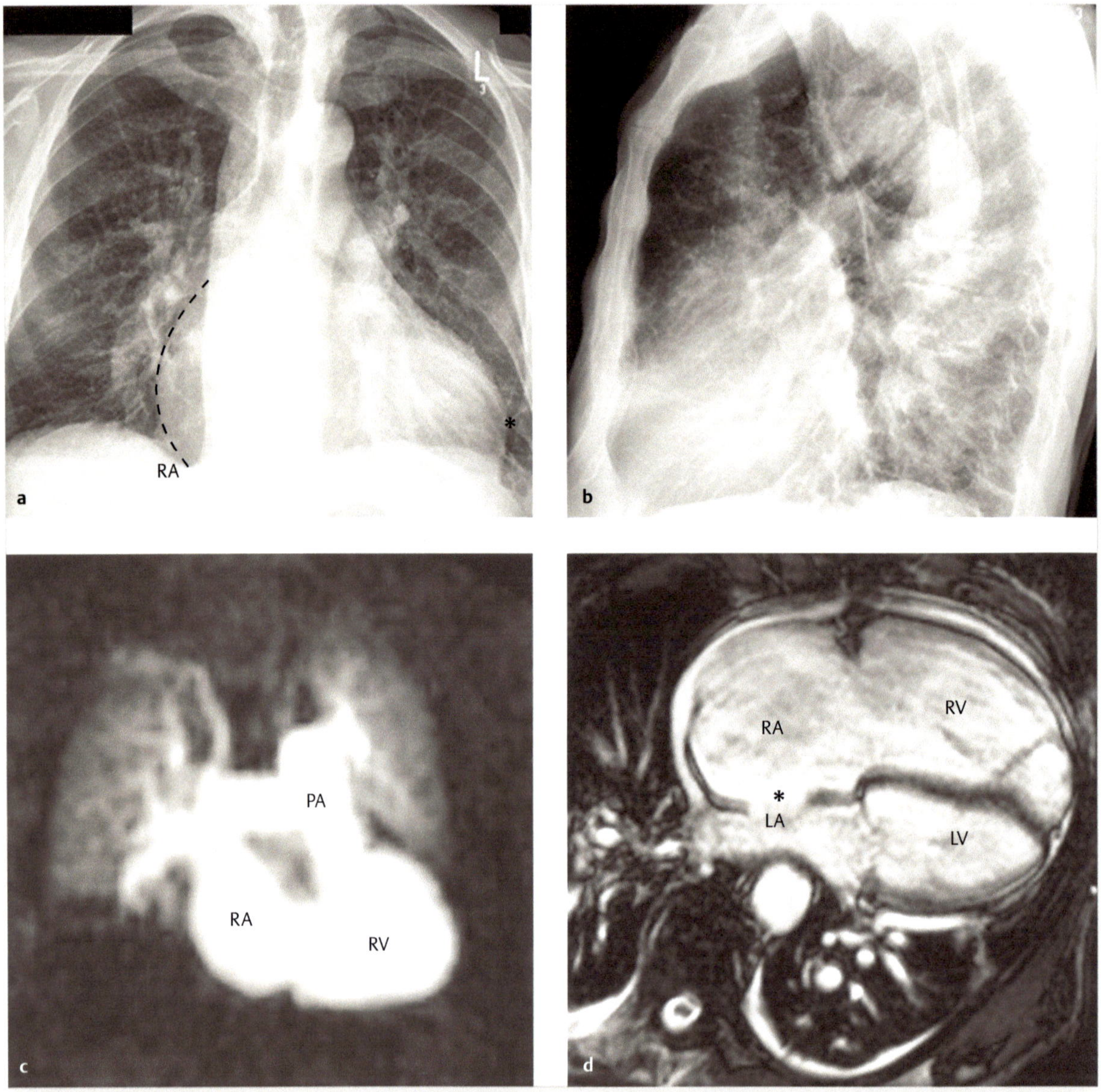

Fig. 4.132 Superior SVD and partial anomalous connection of the right pulmonary vein to the superior vena cava. Seventy-nine-year-old male patient (the same patient as in ▶ Fig. 4.133 and ▶ Fig. 4.134). The thoracic X-rays (a, b) depict a significantly enlarged, margin-forming right atrium and ventricle that displaces dorsally the left ventricle, forming the left margin, in addition to other X-ray morphological indicators of pulmonary hypertension (see MRI d). The dynamic, contrast-enhanced MRA (c) clearly depicts the dilated pulmonary arteries in the presence of known pulmonary hypertension, during the pulmonary arterial phase. The pulmonary perfusion is equal bilaterally. Both SSFP cine MRI (d) and 2-D TTE images (e–g) depict the massively enlarged right ventricle, with an internal diameter of 63 mm. MRI volumetric analysis resulted in a right ventricular EDV of 226 ml/m2 and a reduced right ventricular ejection fraction of 38%.

See Chapter 5 for the reference values. The decreased curvature of the interventricular septum can be seen as an indicator of right ventricular volume load along the parasternal short axis (f), though it cannot be fully depicted via echocardiography due to its size.

LA = left atrium
LV = left ventricle
PA = pulmonary artery
RA = right atrium
RV = right ventricle

a P.-a. standing thoracic X-ray depicting significantly elevated cardiac apex (asterisk) caused by the enlarged RV.
b Lateral standing thoracic X-ray.
c Dynamic, time-resolved contrast-enhanced MRA.
d SSFP cine MRI, 4-chamber view.

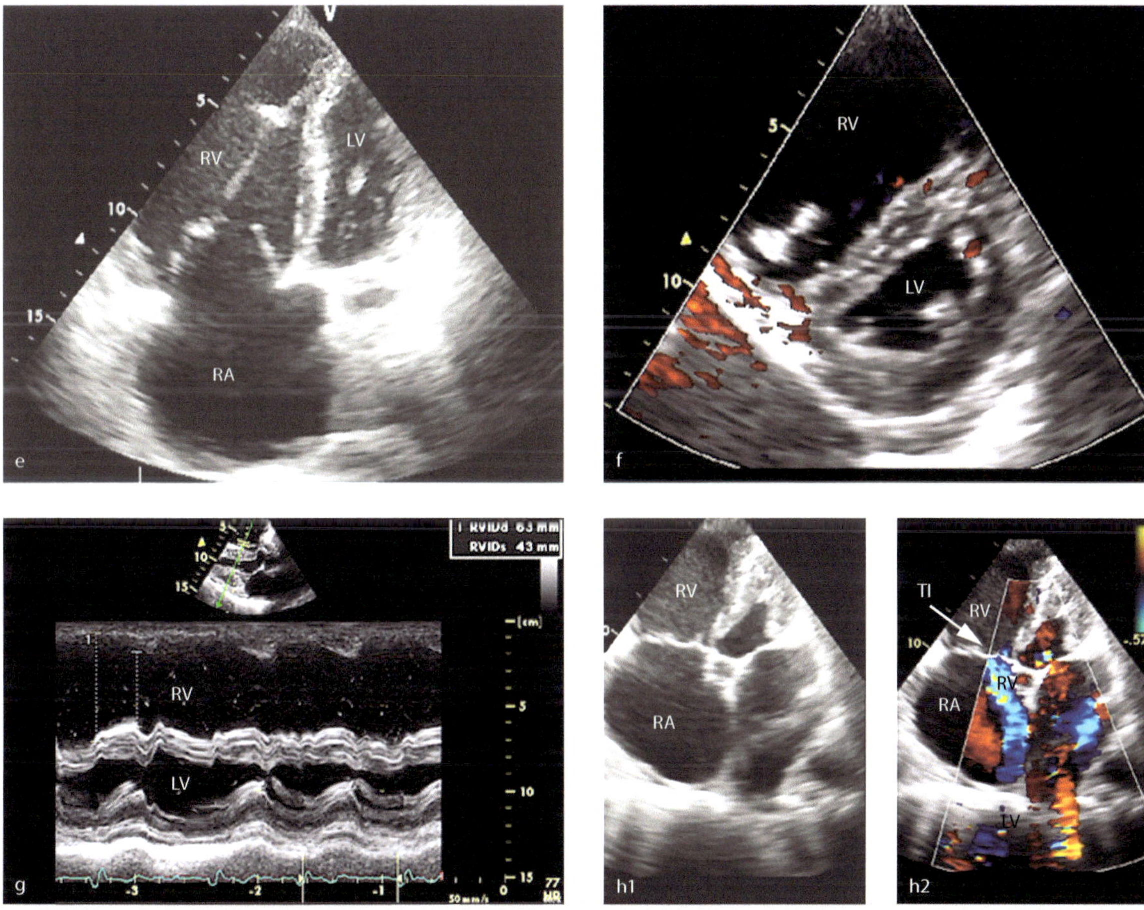

Fig 4.132 (*Continued*) **Superior SVD and partial anomalous connection of the right pulmonary vein to the superior vena cava.**

LA = left atrium
LV = left ventricle
PA = pulmonary artery
RA = right atrium
RV = right ventricle

e 2-D TTE, 4-chamber view.
f 2-D TTE, parasternal short axis. D-shaped LV due to an enlarged RV.
g 2-D TTE, M-mode.
h 2-D TTE and color Doppler echocardiography, 4-chamber view. The arrow indicates the holosystolic insufficiency jet via the tricuspid valve.

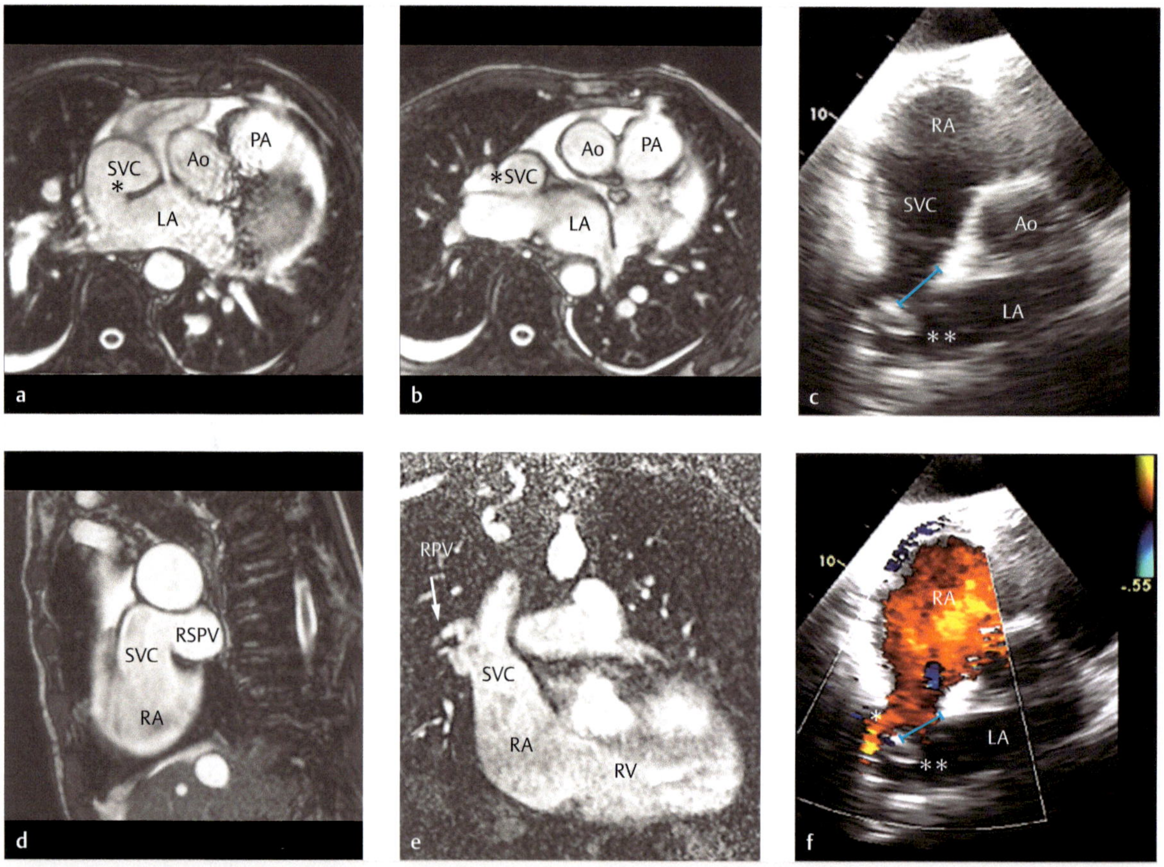

Fig. 4.133 Superior SVD with partial anomalous connection of the right pulmonary vein to the superior vena cava and right atrium. This is the same patient as in ▶ Fig. 4.132 and ▶ Fig. 4.134. 2-D echocardiography (c, f) depicts both the anomalous connection of the right pulmonary vein (asterisk) and ordinary connection of a right pulmonary vein to the left atrium (double asterisk), as well as the interatrial communication (IAC = blue line) according to Moss.167

Ao = aorta
LA = left atrium
PA = pulmonary artery
RA = right atrium
RPV = right pulmonary vein
RSPV = right superior pulmonary vein
RV = right ventricle
SVC = superior vena cava

- **a** Transverse SSFP cine MRI near the origin of the great vessels. The SVD on the posterior wall of the superior vena cava can be seen clearly (asterisk).
- **b** Transverse SSFP cine MRI near the origin of the great vessels, somewhat more cranial than in **a**. The asterisk indicates the anomalous connection of the right superior pulmonary vein to the superior vena cava.
- **c** 2-D TTE image near the right pulmonary venous connection (asterisk).
- **d** Sagittal SSFP cine MRI depicting the anomalous connection "of the right superior pulmonary vein to the superior vena cava.
- **e** Coronal reconstruction of a contrast-enhanced MRA during the pulmonary arterial phase, depicting the connection of the right pulmonary vein to the superior vena cava.
- **f** Corresponding 2-D TTE image with color Doppler (double asterisk), normal RPV.

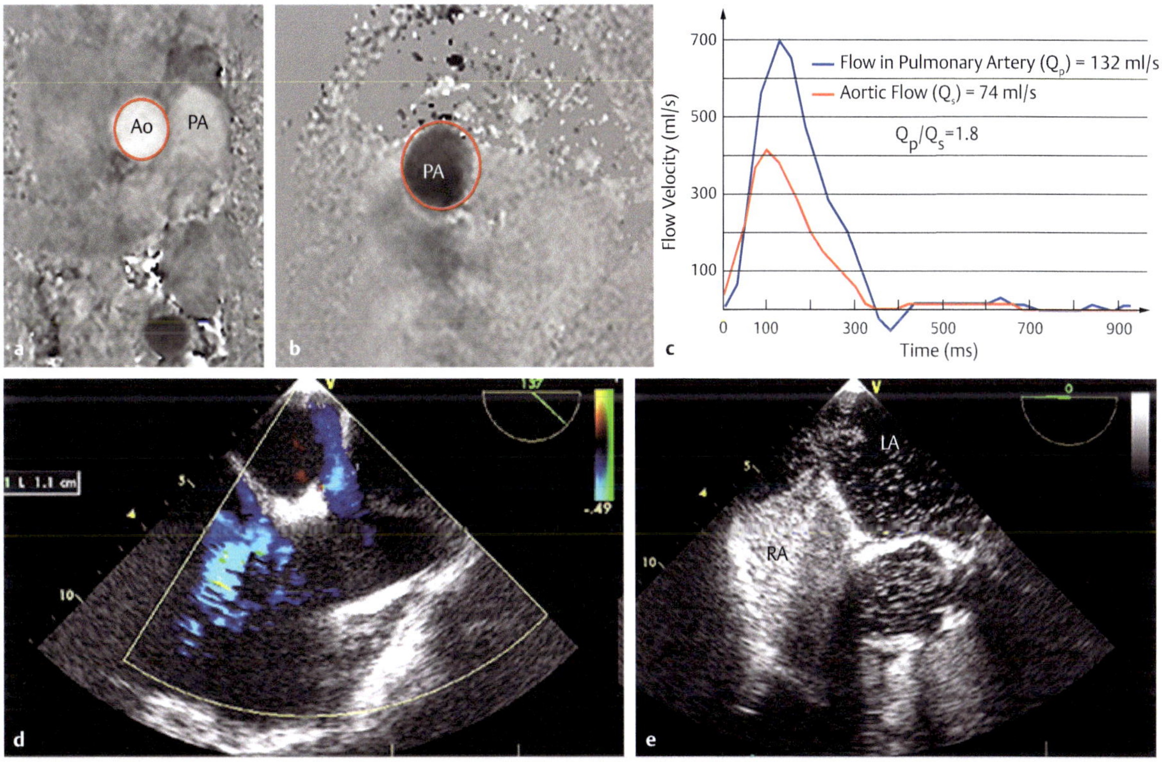

Fig. 4.134 Superior SVD with partial anomalous connection of the right pulmonary vein to the superior vena cava and right atrium. This is the same patient as in ▶ Fig. 4.132 and ▶ Fig. 4.133. The MRI flow measurements (a, b) collected in the aorta and pulmonary artery in order to determine the Qp/Qs quotient resulted in a value of 1.8 (c) and are thus relevant to treatment. Due to different angulations in the MR sectional plane for flow measurements in (a, b), the cranial flow in the aorta and pulmonary artery is light in color (a), while the cranial flow in the pulmonary artery in (b) is dark.

Ao = aorta
LA = left atrium
PA = pulmonary artery
RA = right atrium

a Through-plane 2-D MRI flow measurement in the aorta, phase contrast technique, angulated axial section perpendicular to the course of the ascending aorta. The pulmonary artery is tangentially cut, therefore flow volume in the pulmonary artery must be measured separately (**b**).

b Separate through-plane 2-D MRI flow measurement, phase contrast technique, in the pulmonary artery, angulated coronal section perpendicular to the course of the pulmonary artery.

c The resulting flow curves were superimposed upon one another. Flow volume in the pulmonary artery is significantly higher than in the aorta (Q_p/Q_s = 1.8) due to the left–right shunt.

d TEE, color Doppler, clearly depicting the superior SVD with bidirectional shunt and no superior rim.

e TEE depicting intravenous administration of an ultrasound contrast agent (Echovist, Bayer Schering), which does not enter the pulmonary vascular bed, in order to better depict the shunt near the atrium. The SVD allows contrast agent to pass from the right to the left atrium. Due to the lack of a superior rim, interventional closure of the SVD would be impossible.

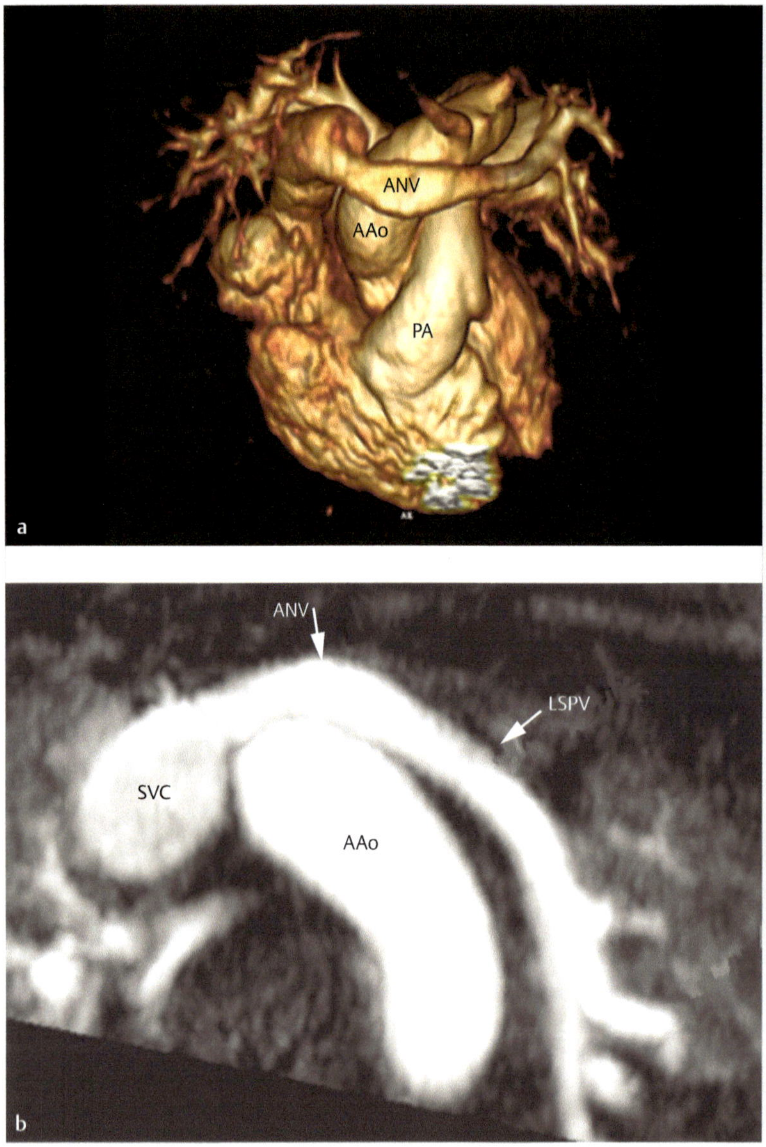

Fig. 4.135 PAPVR of the left superior vena cava via the anonymous vein to the superior vena cava as a concurrent defect to tetralogy of Fallot and Noonan syndrome. MRI of a 45-year-old male patient. The arrow in b indicates the anomalous venous connection.
AAo = ascending aorta
ANV = anonymous vein
Ao = aorta
LSPV = left superior pulmonary vein
PA = pulmonary artery
SVC = superior vena cava

a 3-D volume rendering from a contrast-enhanced MRA.

b Corresponding curved, reformatted thin-slice MIP from a contrast-enhanced MRA.

Clinical Issues

Clinical symptoms are determined by shunt volume. The number and size of anomalous pulmonary venous connection is thus significant. An unusually high shunt volume in a case of known ASD can be an indicator of concurrent PAPVR. Symptoms are generally caused by volume load of the right ventricle with subsequent right ventricular heart failure, resulting in decreased cardiac output, palpitations, and the development of arrhythmia.

Natural Progression and Indication for Treatment

Small shunts may remain asymptomatic for an entire lifetime. As a result, life expectancy is generally not affected.

If untreated, persistent PAPVR with relevant shunt volumes can lead to right ventricular dilatation (▶ Fig. 4.132 and ▶ Fig. 4.136a,b), tricuspid insufficiency (▶ Fig. 4.132h), arrhythmia, pulmonary hypertonia (▶ Fig. 4.132a,b,c), irreversible pulmonary vascular disorders, right ventricular dysfunction, and right ventricular heart failure.

Indication for surgical correction is currently analogous to that for closure of an ASD: namely, surgical treatment is provided to symptomatic patients. Asymptomatic patients receive surgery if the Q_p/Q_s exceeds 1.5 (▶ Fig. 4.134), if mild-to-moderate tricuspid valve insufficiency is present, or once the early stages of pulmonary hypertonia begin to present.

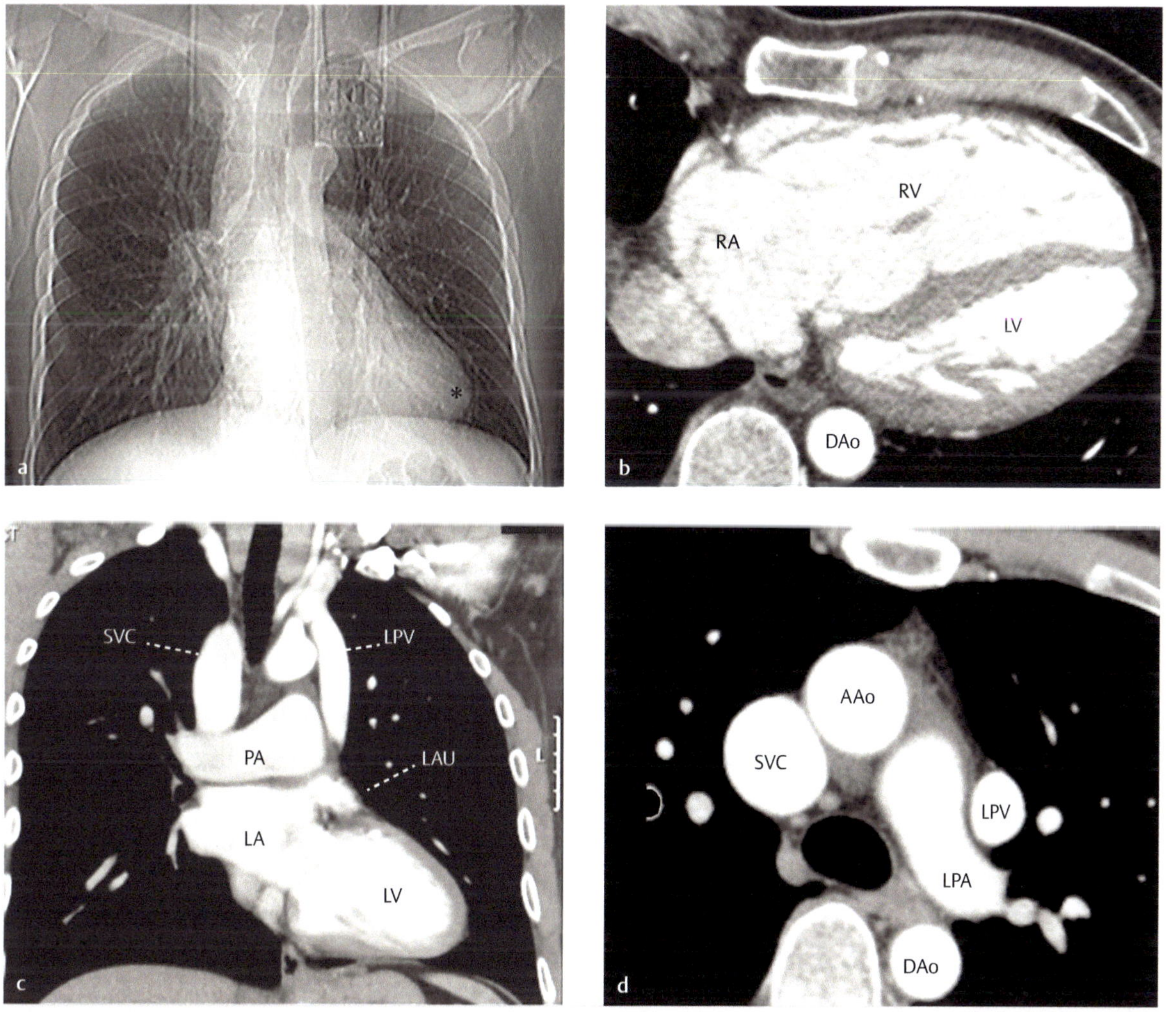

Fig. 4.136 Partial anomalous connection of the left pulmonary vein to the right superior vena cava via the vertical and anonymous veins. Prospective ECG-triggered multi-slice CTs, using the dose-sparing step-and-shoot mode, in a 53-year-old male patient. Note: The PAPVR of the left pulmonary vein and the vertical vein cannot be distinguished from a persistent left superior vena cava solely using the transverse image (d). (Courtesy: Leipzig Heart Center, Dept. of Diagnostic and Interventional Radiology, Leipzig, Germany.)

AAo = ascending aorta
DAo = descending aorta
LA = left atrium
LAU = left auricle
LPA = left pulmonary artery
LPV = left pulmonary vein
LV = left ventricle
PA = pulmonary artery
RA = right atrium
RPV = right pulmonary vein
RV = right ventricle
SVC = superior vena cava
VV = vertical vein

a The topogram depicts rounded and elevated cardiac apex (asterisk) through the large, left rim-forming right ventricle that displaces the left ventricle, as a typical sign of right ventricular enlargement.
b Significantly enlarged right ventricle with flattening of the interventricular septum indicating right ventricular volume load.
c Coronal reconstruction depicting the vertical and left pulmonary veins connecting to the anonymous vein.
d Transverse reconstruction near the great vessels depicting the significantly enlarged superior vena cava, indicating increased volume load.

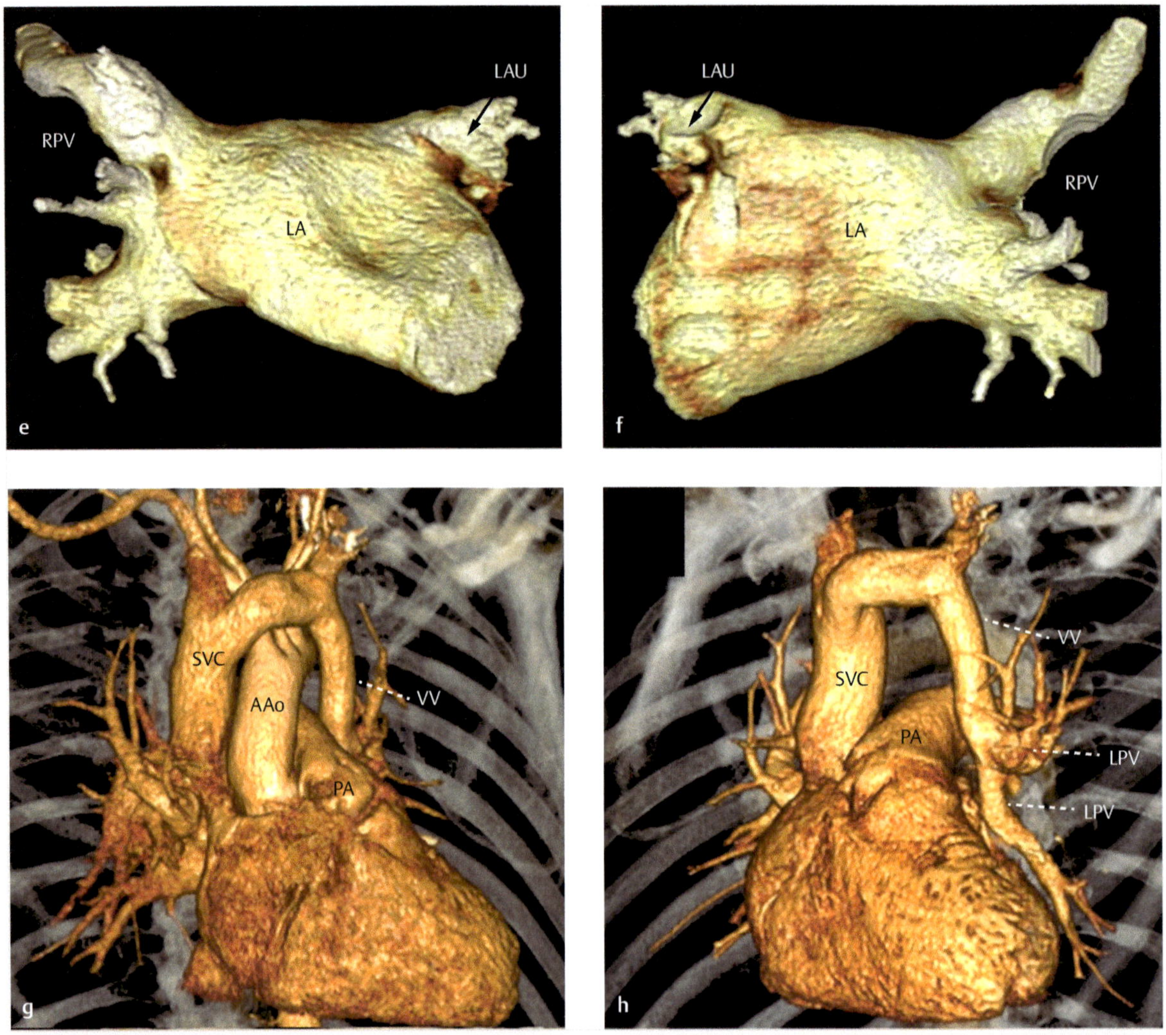

Fig 4.136 (*Continued*) **Partial anomalous connection of the left pulmonary vein to the right superior vena cava via the vertical and anonymous veins.**

AAo = ascending aorta
DAo = descending aorta
LA = left atrium
LAU = left auricle
LPA = left pulmonary artery
LPV = left pulmonary vein
LV = left ventricle
PA = pulmonary artery
RA = right atrium
RPV = right pulmonary vein
RV = right ventricle
SVC = superior vena cava
VV = vertical vein

e Volume rendering of the segmented left atrium, ventral view. Completely lack of left pulmonary veins. The left auricle can be seen clearly (**e**, **f**, arrow).

f Volume rendering of the segmented left atrium, dorsal view.

g Volume rendering depicting the great vessels, ventral view. The anomalous connection of the left pulmonary veins and vertical vein is depicted (**g**, **h**, arrows).

h Volume rendering, LAO projection, with no depiction of the aorta.

Treatment Options and Preinterventional Diagnostics

Options for surgical correction are intended to redirect the anomalous pulmonary venous connection to the left atrium. This can be achieved using direct anastomoses, tunneling through the right atrium, anastomoses to the left atrial auricle, or anastomoses to other pulmonary veins. Depicting the number and course of the anomalous pulmonary venous connections is crucial for surgical planning purposes. The number of pulmonary segments draining via the anomalous venous connections, the length of the vascular segment outside of the lungs, and the distance between the right-side venous connection and left atrium are important pieces of information. Another important criterion for deciding between surgical and conservative treatment options is the extent of shunt volume via the anomalous pulmonary venous connection.[83,167–170]

Postoperative and Postinterventional Issues

Postoperative complications include thrombosis or stenosis of the reinserted pulmonary veins and venous congestion in the upstream pulmonary segments. Pulmonary hemorrhages in cases of large pulmonary infarctions with secondary superinfections are another severe (though extremely rare) complication. Overall, surgical correction of PAPVR is considered an intervention with a low morbidity and mortality rate.[168]

Goals and Relative Value of Diagnostic Imaging

The goals of imaging are proving the existence of and characterizing anomalous pulmonary venous connections. In doing so, the diagnostic procedures performed should yield all information necessary for surgical treatment.

Echocardiography as an initial imaging modality (▶ Table 4.26) can be used to prove the existence of and to quantify an ASD (▶ Fig. 4.133e,f) or potential tricuspid insufficiency (▶ Fig. 4.132h), as well as to estimate pulmonary pressure gradients and potential right ventricular load (▶ Fig. 4.132e–h). Proving the existence of anomalous pulmonary venous connection is often only possible during childhood due to the worse imaging conditions for older patients (▶ Fig. 4.133), and can occasionally be achieved more easily using TEE (▶ Fig. 4.134d,e). Quantifying the Q_p/Q_s shunt quotients often proves the existence of a PAPVR, since the measured shunt is inconsistent with the size of the ASD.

Table 4.26 Strengths and weaknesses of various imaging procedures in cases of PAPVR.

Imaging methods	Indication	Strengths	Weaknesses
Echocardiography	I	• Initial evaluation • Shunt quantification • Right ventricular load • ASD diagnostics • Quantifying tricuspid valve insufficiency • Pulmonary hypertonia	• Localizing the PAPVR
MRI	I	• Shunt quantification • Right ventricular load • ASD diagnostics • Quantifying tricuspid valve insufficiency • Pulmonary hypertension • Localizing the PAPVR	• Diagnosing ASD and tricuspid valve insufficiency is more complicated than with echocardiography
CT	II	• PAPVR morphology	• Should be performed as an ECG-triggered cardiac CT to depict intracardiac structures (or as a pulmonary venous CT without triggering!) • Impossible to directly quantify shunt and tricuspid valve insufficiency • Radiation exposure
Cardiac catheter examination	II	• Right heart catheter: pressure charts ○ Saturation charts • Left heart catheter • Shunt quantification • Coronary anatomy • Localizing the PAPVR	• Invasive • PAPVR cannot always be depicted • Radiation exposure

ASD, atrial septal defect; CT, computed tomography; MRI, magnetic resonance imaging; PAPVR, partial anomalous pulmonary venous connection/return.

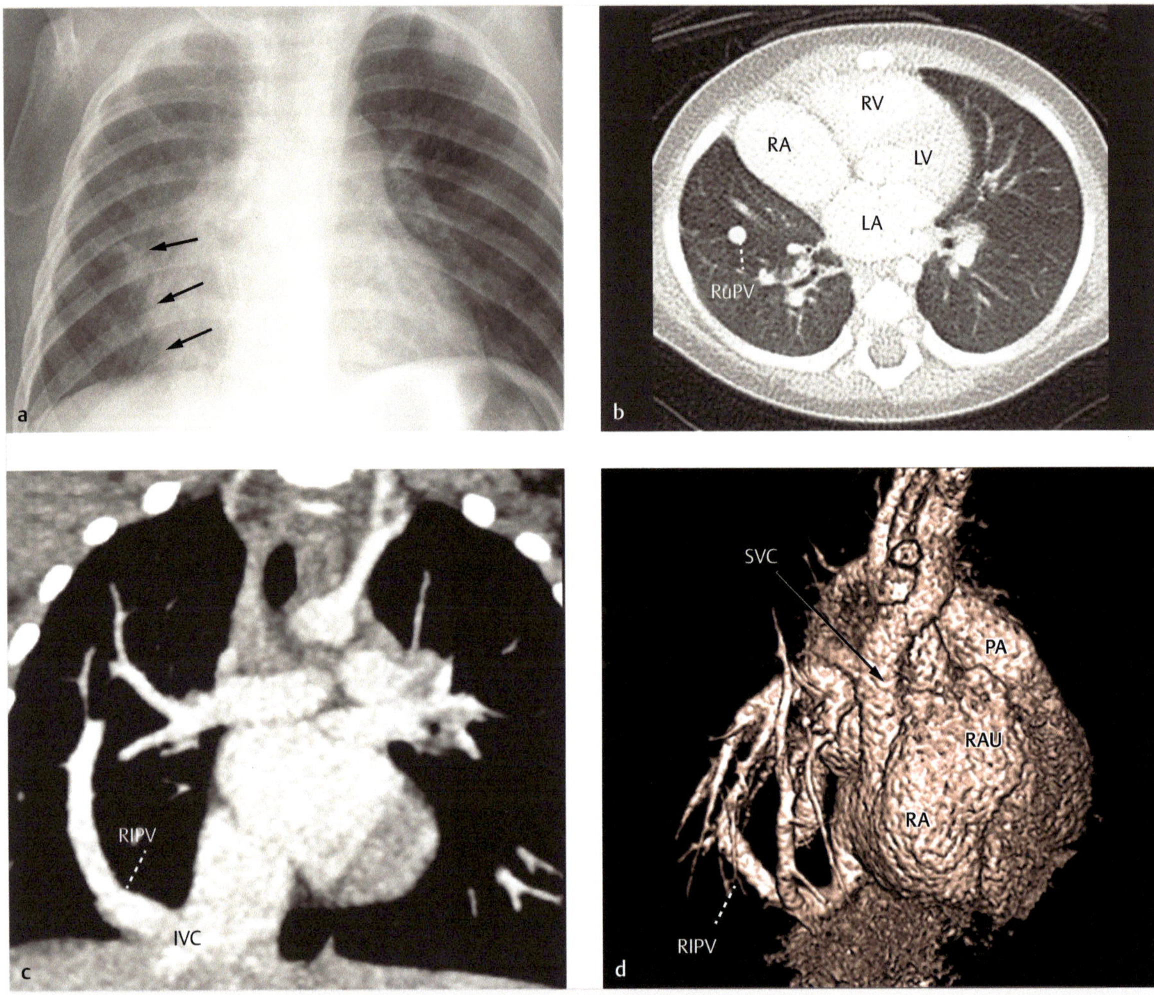

Fig. 4.137 Scimitar syndrome. Nine-month-old female infant. Both the multi-slice CT reconstruction (c) and the volume rendering technique (d) clearly depict the anomalous connection of the right inferior pulmonary vein.

IVC = inferior vena cava
LA = left atrium
LV = left ventricle
RA = right atrium
RAU = right auricle
RIPV = right inferior pulmonary vein
RSPV = right superior pulmonary vein
RV = right ventricle
SVC = superior vena cava

a P.–a. thoracic X-ray, depicting the typical scimitar-shaped anomalous connection of the inferior pulmonary veins (arrows) to the inferior vena cava above the diaphragm.

b Lung window of the multi-slice CT, transverse orientation, depicting the typical dextroposition of the heart caused by right pulmonary hypoplasia and a significantly enlarged right atrium.

c Coronal multi-slice reconstruction depicting the scimitar shape of the collecting vessel of the right inferior pulmonary vein connecting to the inferior vena cava.

d Volume rendering reconstruction from the CT data set.

MRI is the first-choice method for additional clarification beyond echocardiography.[6,7,159] In addition to global shunt quantification, it can also (under favorable circumstances) permit selective quantification of shunt volume via the individual anomalous pulmonary venous connections (▶ Fig. 4.134a-c). From a purely morphological perspective, the diameter, distance to the left atrium, and length of the free course outside of the pleura are also important results of enhanced PAPVR diagnostic procedures, in addition to the number and location of the anomalous pulmonary venous connections. For MRI sequences, SSFP cine MRI sequences should be performed in axial planes, from the liver to the origin of the supra-aortic vessels (▶ Fig. 4.132d), as well as in angulated coronal (▶ Fig. 4.133d) and sagittal planes (▶ Fig. 4.133c) in order to depict the anomalous connection.[159] The axial cine MRIs should be useful for right and left ventricular volumetric analysis from which the stroke volume can be used to estimate the Q_p/Q_s quotient. Better yet, through-plane MR flow measurement is preferable for determining shunt volume in the aorta and pulmonary arteries (▶ Fig. 4.134a-c). In the event of adequate vessel sizes, flow measurement can also be used to calculate the shunt volume of individual anomalous pulmonary venous connections. Finally, contrast-enhanced MRA or 3-D SSFP whole-heart sequences through the entire thorax can be useful for depicting the entire venous vascular system. These procedures can be used to prepare 3-D volume rendering (▶ Fig. 4.135a) and multiplanar reformatted images (▶ Fig. 4.133d and ▶ Fig. 4.135b). In the event of dynamic contrast-enhanced sequences, the procedures can also depict pulmonary perfusion (▶ Fig. 4.132c).

In addition to MRI, ECG-triggered *multi-slice CT* can also be used to depict morphology. This is especially true in young children and adolescents, provided that the corresponding dose-optimization protocols are applied (▶ Fig. 4.131, ▶ Fig. 4.136, and ▶ Fig. 4.137). Since pulmonary venous pulsation is not as pronounced, it may be possible to dispense with ECG triggering.

A *right heart catheter* is generally inserted in order to obtain objective information about pressure and oxygen saturation. An indication for a left-heart catheter may be present in cases of persistent, unclear shunt situations, additional questionable arterial vessel abnormalities, or to determine coronary status in symptomatic older patients.[159]

Plain thoracic X-rays are only helpful for diagnosing PAPVR in very rare cases. In later stages, it is possible to prove the existence of right ventricular load or pulmonary hypertonia (▶ Fig. 4.132a,b, and ▶ Fig. 4.136a). Proving the existence of saber-shaped anomalous veins on the right cardiac margin is only pathognomonic in cases of scimitar syndrome (▶ Fig. 4.137a). Postoperatively, thoracic X-rays can provide evidence of pulmonary infarction caused by pulmonary venous closure.

4.5.2 Caval Vein Anomalies, Systemic Venous Anomalies, and Anomalous Body Venous Connections

Joachim Lotz, Philipp Beerbaum, Michael Steinmetz

Definition

Inferior vena cava anomalies, systemic venous anomalies, and body vein anomalies are defects of the embryonic cardinal venous system, e.g., in the form of narrowing or even full obliteration or agenesis of the superior or inferior vena cavas, or in the form of persistent segments of the left embryonic cardinal venous system (▶ Fig. 1.5): blood flow from the body to the heart may be inhibited or can be fully asymptomatic in the event of persistent left superior vena cava (▶ Fig. 4.138). Commonly (in more than 90% of cases), systemic venous anomalies are concurrent with complex heart defects and situs ambiguus.

If the superior vena cava is obstructed, this leads to venous congestion in the head and neck. Otherwise, congestion can occur in the lower half of the body. Very full veins, a blue coloration of the skin and mucus membranes (cyanosis), and tissue swelling then become apparent.

Classification

Defects of the Superior Vena Cavas

Persistent left superior vena cava is the most common superior caval venous anomaly.[171,137] In more than 90% of cases, this vein connects to the right atrium via an expanded coronary sinus ventral to the left pulmonary artery (▶ Fig. 4.139; also ▶ Fig. 1.5). Generally, both superior vena cavas are connected, and merge with one another via an anonymous vein that may vary in terms of severity (▶ Fig. 4.138). The hemodynamic effects are dependent of the presence of a fully hypoplastic or atretic cross-linkage and right superior vena cava.

> **Note**
>
> Persistent left superior vena cava only occurs without other defects in 10% of cases.[171] Thus, imaging should also take potential concurrent defects into account, even if no symptoms are clinically manifest.

Persistent left superior vena cava can, in rare cases, be associated with defects of the coronary sinus, which may be atretic or stenotic. If this disorder is concurrent with incomplete roof formation and an ASD, this can lead to a bidirectional shunt.

Defects of the Inferior Vena Cavas

The lack of intrahepatic segment in the inferior vena cavas between the liver and renal veins with drainage via the azygos vein (also known as "azygos continuity") is one of the most common defects involving the inferior vena cavas.[137] In these cases, the hepatic veins connect almost directly to the right atrium via a small residual segment. The renal veins and the inferior vena cava connect to the azygos vein, which is dilated due to increased blood volume, and then connects to the superior vena cava. This defect usually occurs in isolation, though it is concurrent with heterotaxia syndrome in nearly all patients, primarily in conjunction with left isomerism, and can also occur in patients with polysplenia (▶ Fig. 4.139).

Direct connection of the inferior vena cava to the left atrium is an extremely rare variant which is generally concurrent with an ASD.

In rare cases, the hepatic veins that generally connect directly to the inferior vena cava can connect directly to the left or right atrium, generally within the scope of other, usually complex cardiac defects, with the corresponding

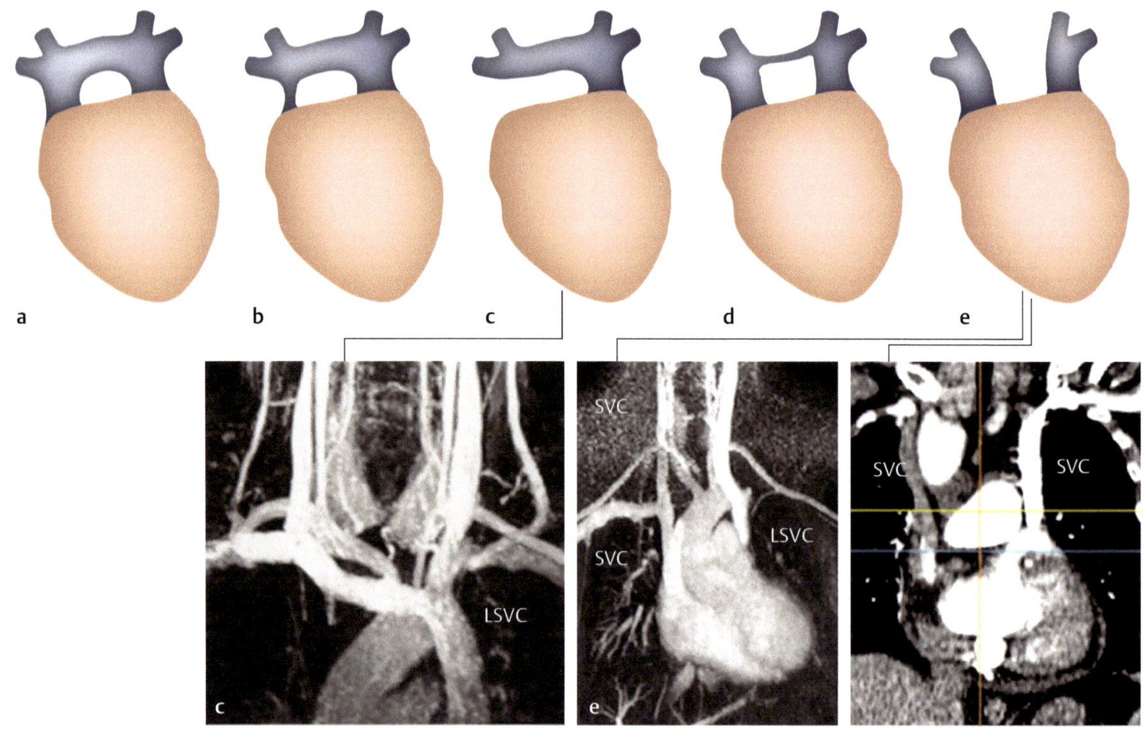

Fig. 4.138 Various possible defects of the superior vena cavas, with or without development of superior cross-linking (anonymous vein). Schematic depiction.
LSVC = (persistent) left superior vena cava
SVC = superior vena cava

- **a** Bilateral connection of the superior vena cavas with cross-linking (anonymous vein/brachiocephalic vein).
- **b** Hypoplastic right superior vena cava.
- **c** Atretic right superior vena cava. Example MRA.
- **d** Hypoplastic anonymous vein (brachiocephalic vein).
- **e** Complete lack of cross-linking. Example MRA (left) and CTA (right).

hemodynamic effects.[137] Total anomalous hepatic venous connection is often present in cases of left atrial isomerism.

Systemic venous blood is directed into the superior vena cava via the azygos and hemiazygos system in the event that the inferior cardinal venous system is obliterated. This is known as "azygos continuity syndrome."

Note

Double inferior vena cava or *persistent left inferior vena cava*—usually only within the scope of heterotaxia syndrome—are caused by the persistence of the left subcardinal and sacrocardinal venous system, and are primarily significant to urology and to visceral, cardiac, and vascular surgery prior to surgical interventions. Consequently, these defects should always be mentioned in radiological reports.

Hemodynamics and Clinical Issues

Isolated caval vein anomalies or anomalous body venous connection are asymptomatic in the majority of cases. The most common caval vein anomaly, namely persistent left superior vena cava, is asymptomatic if no concurrent defects are present and the caval vein connects to the coronary sinus. If no cross-linkage to the right superior vena cava is present, this generally leads to dilatation of the coronary sinus due to increased volume load. In the event of a hypoplastic superior vena cava, or even in its absence, this can lead to superior venous congestion. If the coronary sinus roof is absent and an ASD is present, a bidirectional shunt may develop, leading to the corresponding effects.

An absent hepatic segment of the inferior vena cava with blood drainage via the azygos vein, also known as azygos continuity, is asymptomatic when occurring in

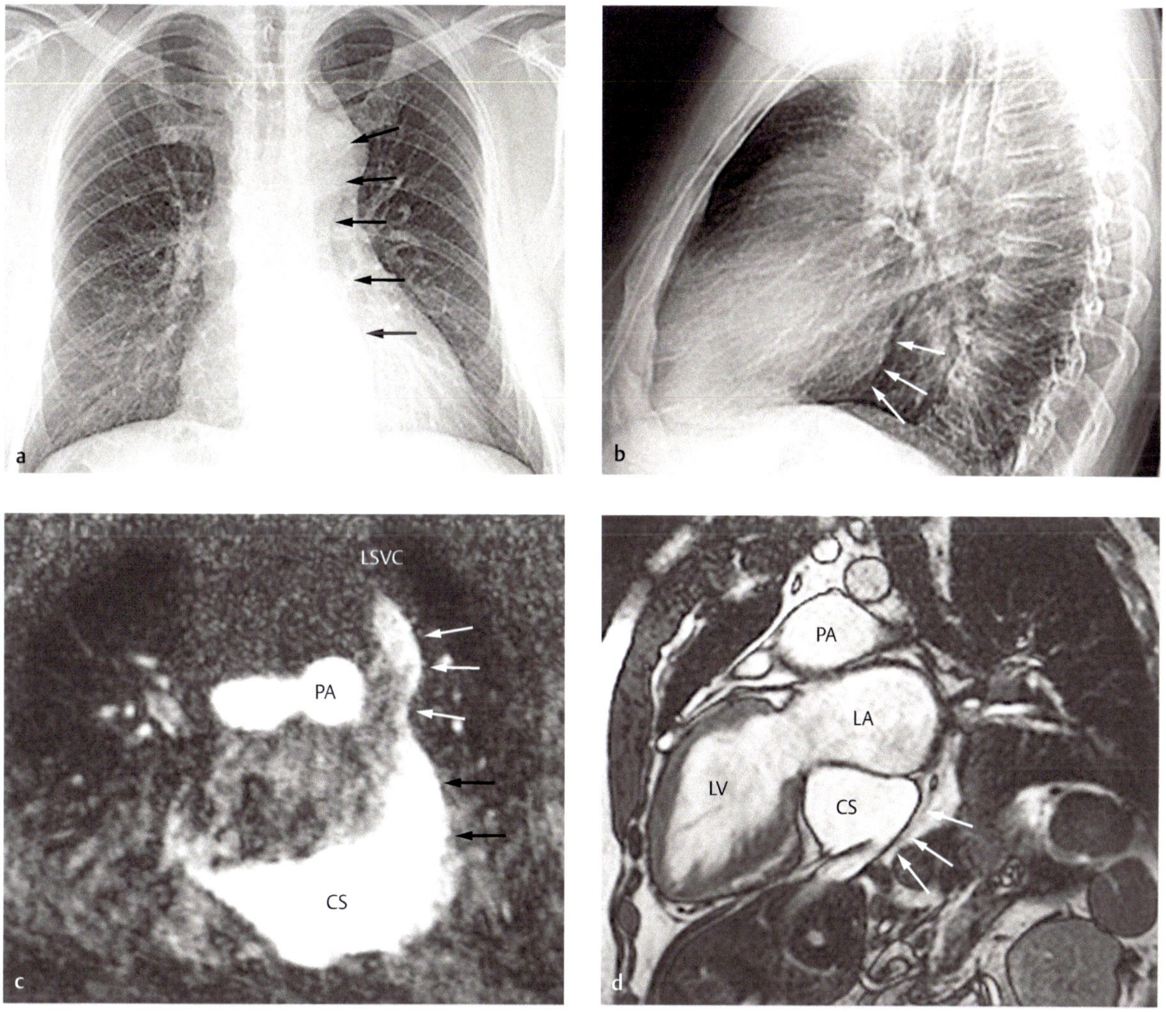

Fig. 4.139 Heterotaxia syndrome, left isomerism, polysplenia, and azygos continuity in a case of absent superior and inferior vena cavas. Fifty-two-year-old male patient. Persistent left superior vena cava with typical connection to the massively expanded coronary sinus and right atrium. Significantly enlarged hemiazygos vein connecting to the persistent left superior vena cava (j); subsequent total anomalous hepatic venous connection directly to the right atrium (i) (asterisk). The corresponding 2-D echo images, 4-chamber view (h, l), also depict the significantly dilated coronary sinus. Due to the nearly perpendicular view, no flow signal can be demonstrated in the coronary sinus using color Doppler (l). Various transverse (e–g, j), sagittal, and coronal SSFP cine MRI views depict the course of the hemiazygos vein as collateral circulation for the absent inferior vena cava, with its connection to the persistent left superior vena cava and enlarged coronary sinus. (Courtesy: Leipzig Heart Center, Dept. of Diagnostic and Interventional Radiology, Leipzig, Germany)

AAo = ascending aorta
CS = coronary sinus
DAo = descending aorta
HAV = hemiazygos vein
LA = left atrium
LSVC = (persistent) left superior vena cava
LV = left ventricle
PA = pulmonary artery
RA = right atrium
RV = right ventricle

a The contours of the persistent left superior vena cava (arrows) can be clearly seen in the p.-a. thoracic X-ray.
b The enlarged coronary sinus (arrows) can also be seen clearly on the lateral thoracic X-ray.
c Contrast-enhanced MRA, coronal slice, depicts a similar view as in **a**.
d SSFP cine MRI, angulated parasagittal slice, depicts a similar view as in **b**.

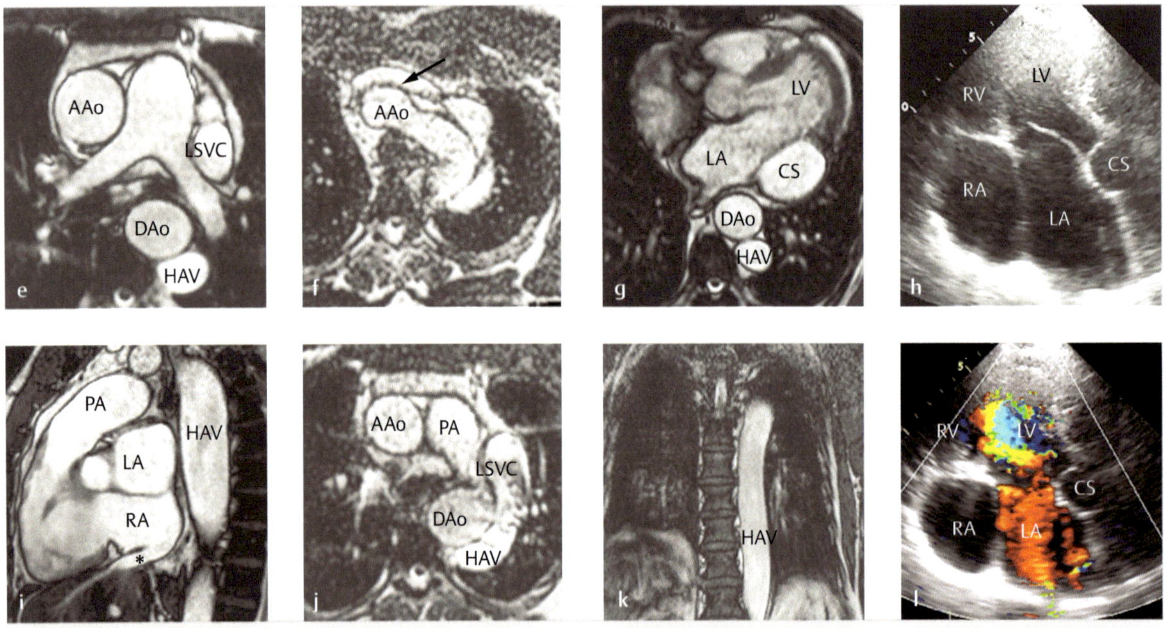

Fig 4.139 (*Continued*) **Heterotaxia syndrome, left isomerism, polysplenia, and azygos continuity in a case of absent superior and inferior vena cavas.**

AAo = ascending aorta
CS = coronary sinus
DAo = descending aorta
HAV = hemiazygos vein
LA = left atrium
LSVC = (persistent) left superior vena cava
LV = left ventricle
PA = pulmonary artery
RA = right atrium
RV = right ventricle

e Transverse SSFP cine MRI near the origin of the great vessels.
f Transverse SSFP cine MRI near the aortic arch. The arrow indicates the anonymous vein.
g Transverse SSFP cine MRI near the ventricles.
h 2-D echo image, 4-chamber view.
i Sagittal SSFP cine MRI with direct connection of the hepatic veins to the right atrium (asterisk).
j Transverse SSFP cine MRI depicting the connection of the hemiazygos vein to the persistent left superior vena cava.
k Coronal SSFP cine MRI of the dilated hemiazygos vein along its left paravertebral course.
l 2-D echo image (color Doppler), 4-chamber view. No flow signal in the coronary sinus can be depicted due to the almost perpendicular Doppler angle.

isolation and is often discovered by accident. If it occurs in conjunction with other, generally complex defects, the symptoms of the concurrent defects are predominant.

In the rare event that the inferior vena cava or hepatic veins possess an anomalous connection to the left atrium, hemodynamic effects of a right–left shunt can be determined. In addition, cyanosis may also develop. Furthermore, paradoxical embolisms may occur.[137] Persistent superior vena cava often is discovered by accident when attempting to place a venous catheter or port system: the course of the wire or catheter can be confused with an intraaortic course. This can be solved by looking at the course of the wire or catheter in the coronary sinus using a lateral X-ray or CT/phlebography.

Natural Progression and Indication for Treatment

Treatment is only required in the event of the rare hemodynamic effects of superior or inferior caval venous congestion, pronounced left–right or right–left shunt, or as a result of concurrent defects, and generally only in the form of treating the concurrent defects or addressing the shunt or venous congestion.

Goals and Relative Value of Diagnostic Imaging

Generally speaking, this diagnosis is determined as a supplementary finding before a surgery or when performing

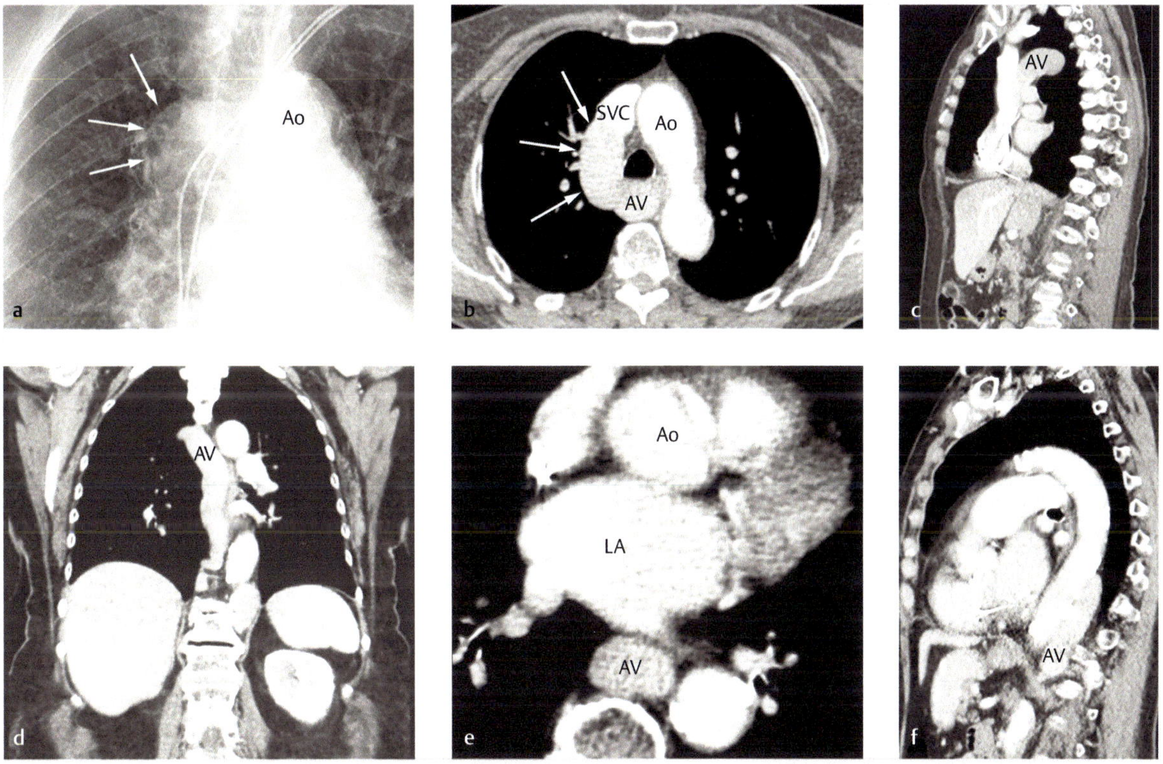

Fig. 4.140 Azygos continuity and absent inferior vena cava. Eighty-year-old female patient. The azygos continuity connects to the superior vena cava (a–c). The connection can be seen clearly both in the thoracic X-ray (a, arrows) and in CT (b, arrows).

Ao = aorta
AV = azygos vein
LA = left atrium
SVC = superior vena cava

a Extract from a p.-a. thoracic X-ray demonstrating the azygos vein (arrows) connection to the superior vena cava.
b Transverse reconstruction of a venous thoracic CT near the connection of the azygos vein (arrows) to the superior vena cava.
c Sagittal reconstruction of a venous thoracic CT near the connection of the azygos vein to the superior vena cava.
d Coronal reconstruction of a venous thoracic CT, depicting the course of the azygos continuity.
e Transverse reconstruction of a venous thoracic CT, perpendicular, through the azygos vein. The azygos vein runs ventral to the spinal column in the absence of the inferior vena cava.
f Sagittal reconstruction of a venous thoracic CT with joint depiction of the calcified aorta and azygos vein.

an imaging procedure due to another indication. In the event of defects near the inferior vena cava, this can manifest clinically in the form of deep vein thrombosis in the legs, thrombophlebitis, or venous insufficiency occurring even in young patients. Like with other vascular defects, diagnosis can often be determined at an early stage using *echocardiography* or *Doppler vascular ultrasound*.

Contrast-enhanced *MRA* (▶ Fig. 4.138) and *CTA* (▶ Fig. 4.140) are the first-choice, noninvasive methods for detecting the full scope of the defect and potential concurrent vascular anomalies. Precise quantification of shunt volume with respect to treatment relevance can still be detected using MRI, via MRI flow measurement. In principle, MRA can also be used as a time-of-flight angiogram without administering contrast agent to depict the anatomy of the caval veins. Data should be acquired during diastole, however, to ensure a better venous signal. Generally speaking, multi-phase (or, better yet, time-resolved, contrast-enhanced) MRA should be performed in order to be able to better assess the dynamics of venous flow. Two-phase acquisition is indispensable for also depicting pulmonary venous anomalies in addition to caval vein anomalies. Since the vascular system can usually be depicted with high spatial and temporal resolution using the intrinsic high contrast of SSFP MR sequences, these sequences can also be used in a transverse orientation (▶ Fig. 4.139) and, based on the results, in the following planes along the course of the vessel in order to clarify anatomical details.

Phlebography is another established, easily implemented method for depicting the superior and inferior caval venous systems. This method is, however, increasingly being replaced by MRA and CTA. An *invasive cardiac catheter examination* is only necessary for depicting anatomy in extremely rare cases, and if so, generally only to provide more information about concurrent defects.

4.5.3 Aortic Arch and Pulmonary Artery Anomalies

Gerald F. Greil, Lukas Lehmkuhl, Heiner Latus

Definition

All other anomalies of the aortic arch (▶ Fig. 4.141 and ▶ Fig. 4.142) and pulmonary arteries are generally asymptomatic embryonic defects that are based on various developmental disorders of the embryonic pharyngeal arch arteries (▶ Fig. 1.12) and occur in approximately 3% of the population (▶ Table 4.27).[137] They can, however, also lead to compression of the trachea and/or esophagus, which are adjacent to the aortic arch, at an early age (▶ Fig. 4.143).

Atypical origin of the right subclavian artery in cases of left aortic arch (also known as lusorian artery; ▶ Fig. 4.144; ▶ Fig. 4.141d), the corresponding mirrored anomaly in cases of right aortic arch (▶ Fig. 4.145; ▶ Fig. 4.141e), and double aortic arch (▶ Fig. 4.146) are among the most common anomalies, which are often discovered by accident. Rare defects include cervical aortic arch (also known as COSA syndrome; ▶ Fig. 4.147)[172] and the origin of the left pulmonary artery from the right one (also known as pulmonary sling; ▶ Fig. 4.148).

> **Note**
>
> The most common aortic arch anomaly, aortic coarctation, and the rare IAA are discussed separately with left-side defects due to their differing pathophysiology. An IAA corresponds clinically to a high-grade aortic coarctation, fully dependent on perfusion of the ductus arteriosus.

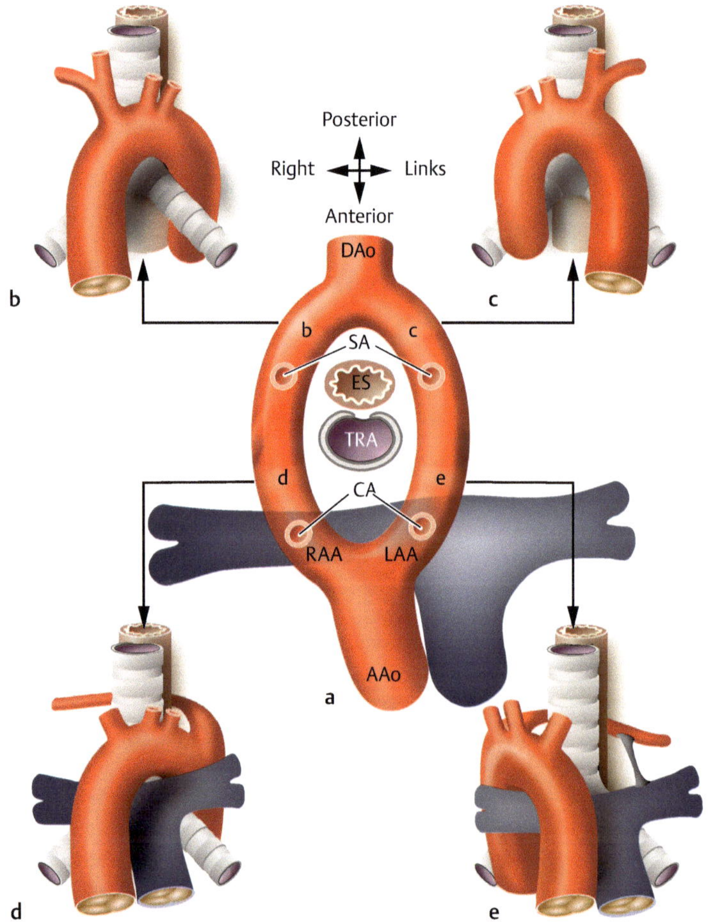

Fig. 4.141 Aortic arch anomalies. Schematic depiction.
AAo = ascending aorta
CA = carotid artery
DAo = descending aorta
ES = esophagus
LAA = left aortic arch
PA = pulmonary artery
RAA = right aortic arch
SA = subclavian artery
TRA = trachea

- **a** Primitive aortic ring.
- **b** Normal obliteration (see a, pale red, area "b") near the right aortic arch distal to the origin of the right subclavian artery, and the development of a left descending aorta.
- **c** Obliteration near the left aortic arch (see a, pale red, area "c") and development of a right aortic arch.
- **d** If the aortic arch is obliterated between the origin of the subclavian artery and the right carotid artery (see a, pale red, area "d"), this results in an aberrant right "lusoria artery."
- **e** If the aortic arch is obliterated between the origin of the subclavian artery and the left carotid artery (see a, pale red, surface "e"), this results in an aberrant left subclavian artery.

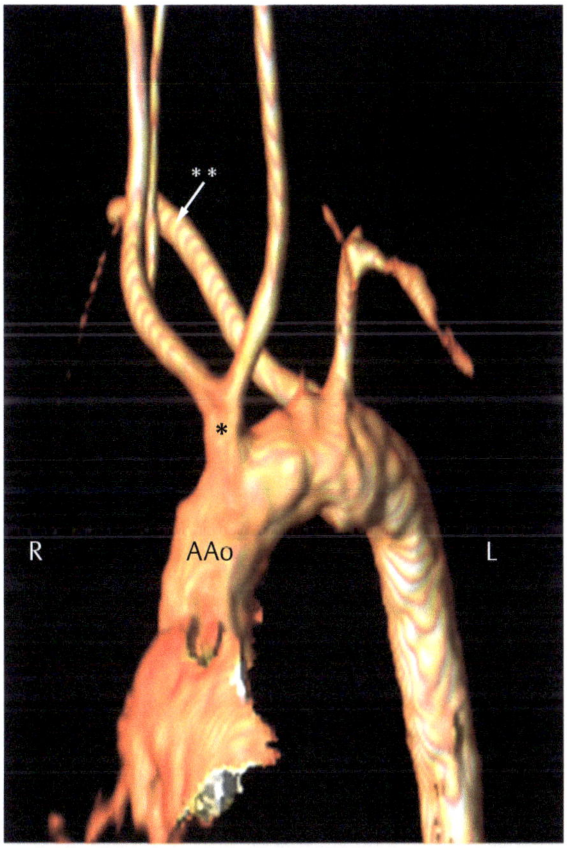

Fig. 4.142 Left-side aortic arch and lusorian artery. LAO projection of a contrast-enhanced MRA in a 20-year-old male patient with a left aortic arch, truncus bicaroticus (asterisk), and an aberrant right subclavian artery originating from the aortic arch (lusorian artery; double asterisk).
AAo = ascending aorta

Note

Remember: During embryonic development, a truncus arteriosus forms initially. Six pharyngeal arch arteries originate from this truncus and then merge to form the dorsal aortic arches. The first, second, and fifth pharyngeal arch arteries recede, and the external carotid arteries develop from the ventral aortic arches. The fourth pharyngeal arch develops from the brachiocephalic artery and the aortic arch, while the pulmonary branches develop from the sixth arch and the ductus arteriosus.

Classification

- *Vascular rings:* Defects of the fourth pharyngeal arch lead to a vascular ring around the esophagus and trachea, which may be closed, or, much more commonly—as in the case of double aortic arch—may be open, like in cases of lusorian artery:
  - Double aortic arch (▶ Fig. 4.146)
  - Aberrant subclavian artery in a case of left or right aortic arch (▶ Fig. 4.141, ▶ Fig. 4.142, ▶ Fig. 4.143, ▶ Fig. 4.144, ▶ Fig. 4.145)
  - Pulmonary sling (▶ Fig. 4.148)
- *Anomalies of the aortic arch origins* (▶ Fig. 4.147)[172]
- *Aortic coarctation,* aortic arch stenosis, and IAA

Clinical Issues

Variations in the aortic arch origins are often asymptomatic, since the vascular ring between the aorta and pulmonary artery possesses a ventral opening. Consequently, these anomalies are often described as ancillary findings within the scope of cardiovascular diagnostics (▶ Fig. 4.145). They generally first begin to exhibit symptoms

Table 4.27 Occurrence of a right aortic arch in cases of various congenital heart defects.[137]

Defect	Incidence of right aortic arch (%)
Truncus arteriosus	40–50
Tetralogy of Fallot	25–30
DORV	30
Pulmonary atresia with VSD	20
Tricuspid atresia	6–10
TGA	3–5

DORV, double outlet right ventricle; TGA, transposition of the great arteries; VSD, ventricular septal defect.

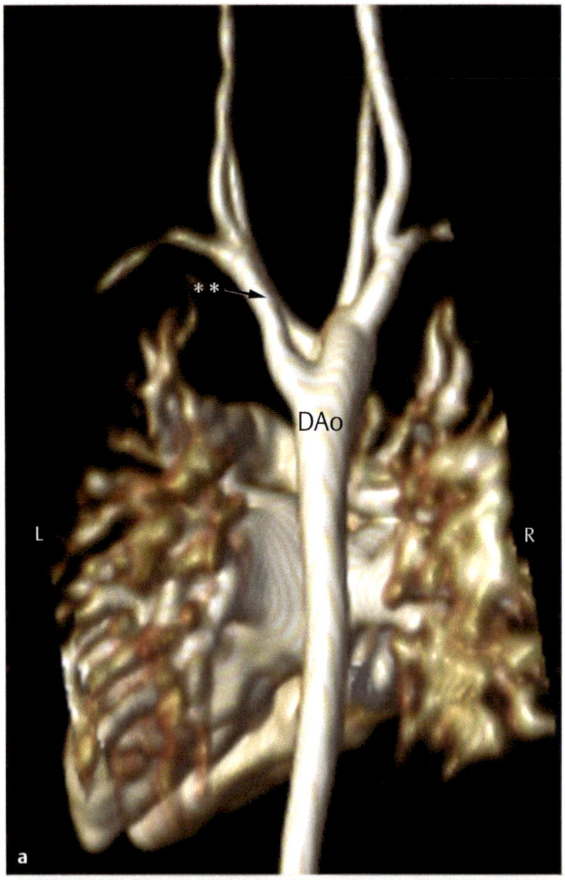

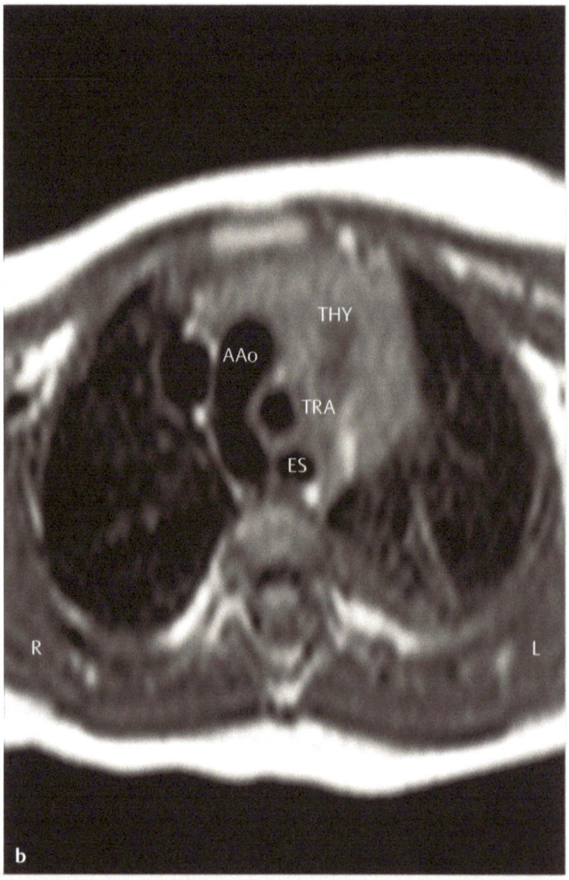

Fig. 4.143 Right-side aortic arch. Twelve-month-old infant with difficulty swallowing, a right aortic arch, and aberrant course of the left subclavian artery (double asterisk).

AAo = ascending aorta
ES = esophagus
THY = thymus
TRA = trachea

a The origin of the left subclavian artery from the descending aorta can be seen in the dorsal projection of a contrast-enhanced MRA.
b The compression of the esophagus and trachea between the left subclavian artery and the right aortic arch can be seen in the transverse black blood MRI SE sequence.

if for instance a Kommerell diverticulum is very large (▶ Fig. 4.149) or an obliterated ductus arteriosus (arterial ligament) is very short. Vascular rings (▶ Fig. 4.144) are more likely to cause complaints, particularly in "closed" or complete forms.[172] The most common complete form, double aortic arch, involves two open arches, one of which may be atretic (▶ Fig. 4.146). In addition to stridor, clinical symptoms may include increased occurrence of respiratory infections, difficulty swallowing, and even cyanosis depending on whether the esophagus or trachea are affected.

Note

"Kommerell diverticulum" is a congenital focal enlargement near the origin of an aberrant subclavian artery or lusorian artery stemming from the aortic arch or descending aorta (see ▶ Fig. 4.145 and ▶ Fig. 4.149), respectively. Its retroesophageal course can lead to dysphagia due to the diverticulum. This aortic anomaly was first described by German radiologist Kommerell in 1936,[173] and is derived from the fourth pharyngeal arch.

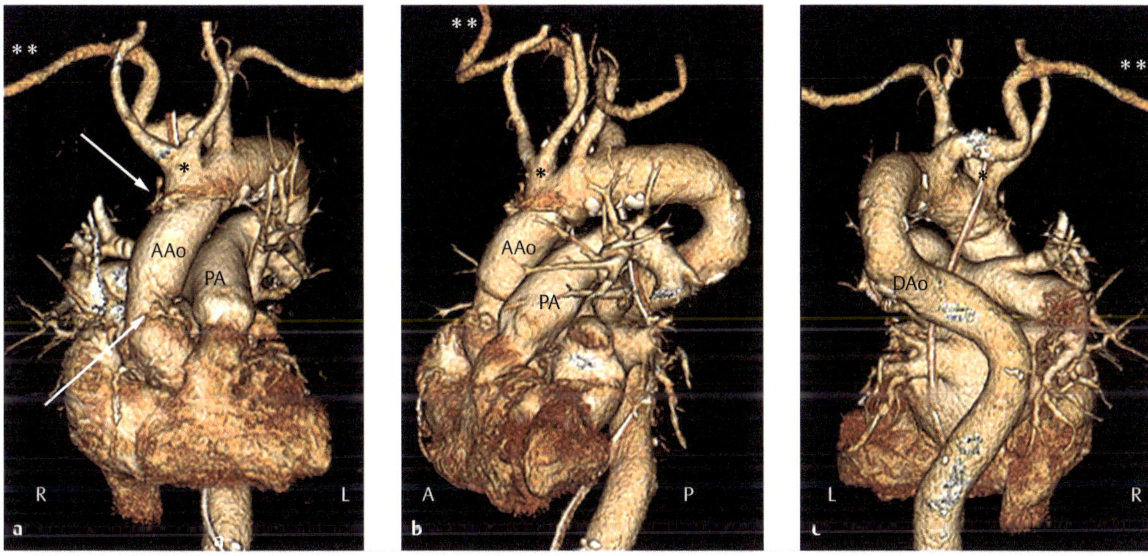

Fig. 4.144 Lusorian artery and truncus bicaroticus subclavius after replacing the ascending aorta. Seventy-seven-year-old male patient who received an aortic valve reconstruction, ascending aorta replacement, and partial arch replacement (a, arrows) due to acute type A dissection. The postoperative CT check-up reveals a truncus bicaroticus (a–c, asterisks) as an anatomical variant of the supraaortic vessels, in conjunction with a lusorian artery (a–c, double asterisk).

AAo = ascending aorta DAo = descending aorta PA = pulmonary artery

a Ventral projection of a contrast-enhanced CTA with 3-D reconstruction, volume rendering technique.

b Lateral projection of a contrast-enhanced CTA with 3-D reconstruction, volume rendering technique.

c Dorsal projection of a contrast-enhanced CTA with 3-D reconstruction, volume rendering technique.

Natural Progression, Indication for Treatment, and Treatment Options

Generally speaking, the aortic arch anomalies described here are asymptomatic and are often discovered as ancillary findings, provided that they are not concurrent with other aortic anomalies (such as coarctation or IAA). The development of symptoms, particularly compression phenomena, is facilitated by the development of aneurysms (▶ Fig. 4.149). This then constitutes an indication for surgery or interventional treatment.[174] In these cases, life-threatening conditions can be present even in infants or children. These conditions can, however, first occur later in life (▶ Fig. 4.146). The surgery addresses the life-threatening narrowing in the trachea and esophagus. Transthoracic central ligature and resection of the lusorian artery with subsequent transposition is the standard surgical procedure for treating a symptomatic lusorian artery (dysphagia) without aneurysms. This surgery has a high success rate.[174]

Isolated stenoses of the subclavian artery are now treated using a simple interventional procedure, such as percutaneous transbrachial or transfemoral angioplasty, with or without stent implantation. In cases of aneurysms (▶ Fig. 4.150; ▶ Fig. 4.149) or ruptures (▶ Fig. 4.151), hybrid endovascular interventions (if possible) are the method of choice.[174]

Goals and Relative Value of Diagnostic Imaging

If no symptoms are present, aortic and pulmonary arterial anomalies are generally first discovered later in life, as supplementary findings within the scope of a routine imaging diagnostic procedure indicated for another reason (▶ Fig. 4.145). The p.-a. *X-ray* can be used to determine a preliminary diagnosis with regard to aortic anomalies (▶ Table 4.28; ▶ Fig. 4.145 and ▶ Fig. 4.149). Thoracic X-ray imaging is not suited to dedicated diagnosis of aortic anomalies, though a barium swallow image using X-ray can be helpful for recognizing narrowing within the esophagus.

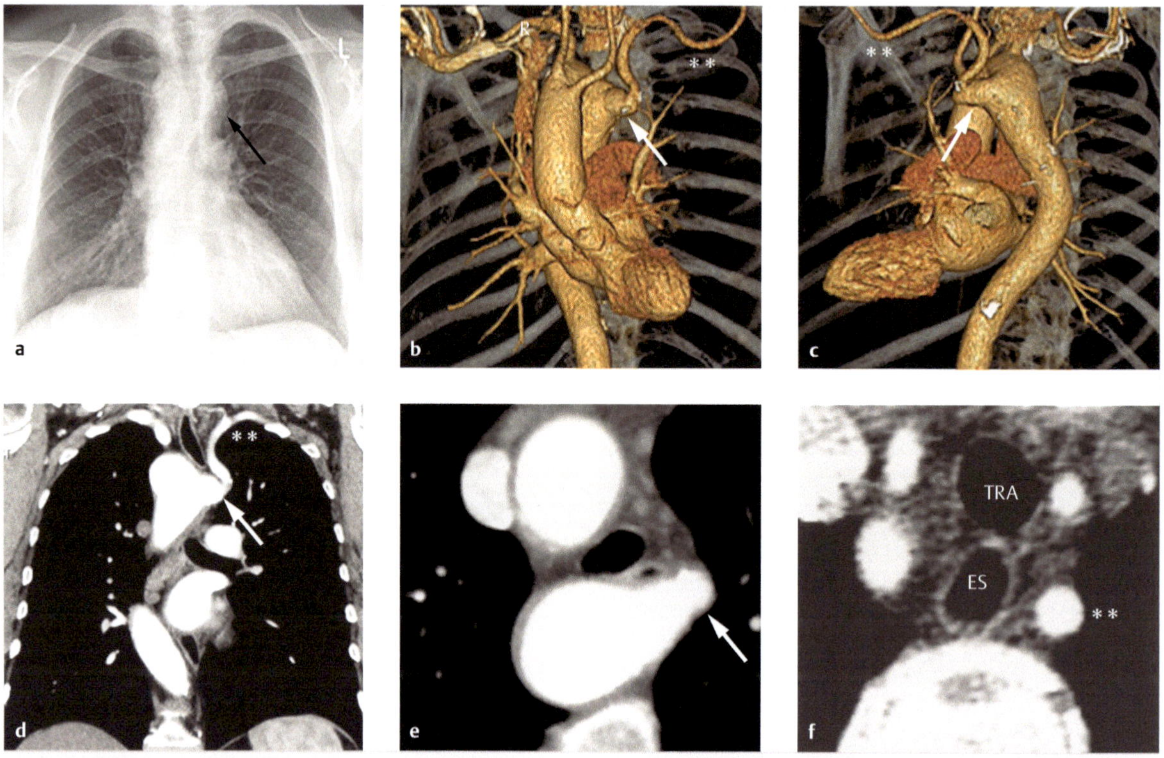

Fig. 4.145 Right aortic arch with lusorian artery. Eighty-two-year-old female patient with right aortic arch and left subclavian artery (b, c, d, f, double asterisk) originating from a Kommerell diverticulum as a lusorian artery (a–e, arrows), discovered as an ancillary finding within the scope of a CT thoracic examination to clarify ambiguous pulmonary nodules.

ES = esophagus
TRA = trachea

- **a** P.-a. thoracic X-ray with visible Kommerell diverticulum (arrow).
- **b** Ventral view of a CTA, 3-D volume rendering technique.
- **c** Dorsal view of a CTA, 3-D volume rendering technique.
- **d** Coronal reconstruction near the origin of the left subclavian artery stemming from the Kommerell diverticulum, from a contrast-enhanced thoracic CTA.
- **e** Transverse reconstruction near the origin of the left subclavian artery stemming from the Kommerell diverticulum, from a contrast-enhanced thoracic CTA.
- **f** Transverse reconstruction near the supraaortic branches of a contrast-enhanced thoracic CTA.

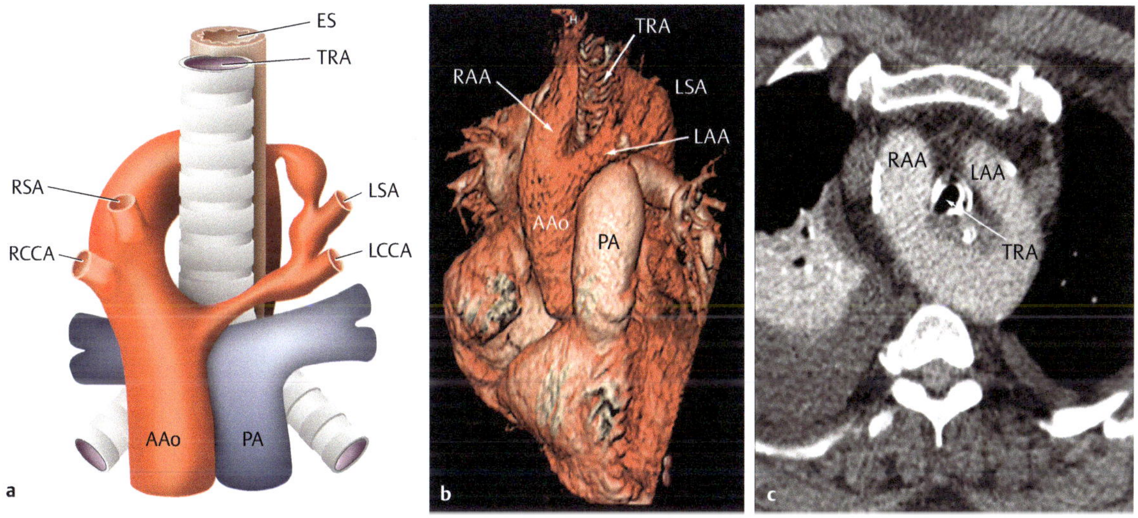

Fig. 4.146 Double aortic arch.

AAo = ascending aorta
ES = esophagus
LAA = left aortic arch
LCCA = left common carotid artery
LSA = left subclavian artery
PA = pulmonary artery
RAA = right aortic arch
RCCA = right common carotid artery
RSA = right subclavian artery
TRA = trachea

a Schematic depiction of the most common form of a closed or complete vascular ring, double aortic arch, which usually possesses an atretic segment (in this case, the left aortic arch). The right aortic arch is non-atretic, and the origins of the right common carotid artery and right subclavian artery are contained within it.

b CT reconstruction (3-D volume rendering technique), ventral view, of a 70-year-old female patient after resuscitation due to aspiration, a documented history of difficulty swallowing, detection of a double aortic arch as an ancillary finding. The double aortic arch forms a vascular sling around the esophagus and trachea. The segments of the right and left aortic arch are clearly visible.

c Axial reconstruction of a contrast-enhanced CT of the patient from **b**.

Earlier in life, particularly in infancy, certain aortic arch anomalies can be assessed fully using *echocardiography*, e.g., from a suprasternal view (▶ Fig. 4.147d). Oftentimes, it is impossible to assess the entire course of the aorta.

Consequently, contrast-enhanced *MRA*[175] and *CTA*, potentially with temporal resolution, are considered as equally useful I2 indications (that is, equal to other methods) according to the DRG, DGK, and DGPK.[7,176] For younger patients and in cases of elective diagnostics, MRI (▶ Fig. 4.142, ▶ Fig. 4.143, and ▶ Fig. 4.147b)[176] is preferred, while MDCT of the aorta is preferred for postoperative follow-up examinations (▶ Fig. 4.142), emergency diagnostics, e.g., when an aneurysm ruptures (▶ Fig. 4.149 and ▶ Fig. 4.151), or after stent implantation (▶ Fig. 4.150). In cases of stridor, or if concurrent pulmonary defects or limitations are suspected, CT has benefits that MRI does not (for example, when attempting to diagnose dysphagia caused by a defect). Summarizing the clinical symptoms and morphology for these differing anomalies results in an indication for surgical or interventional treatment.

Invasive diagnostics are generally only necessary if an intervention such as stent implantation is also planned for the same session.

▶ **Acknowledgment.** We would like to thank Mr. In der Mühle for his critical review of our initial draft of the manuscript and for searching for example images.

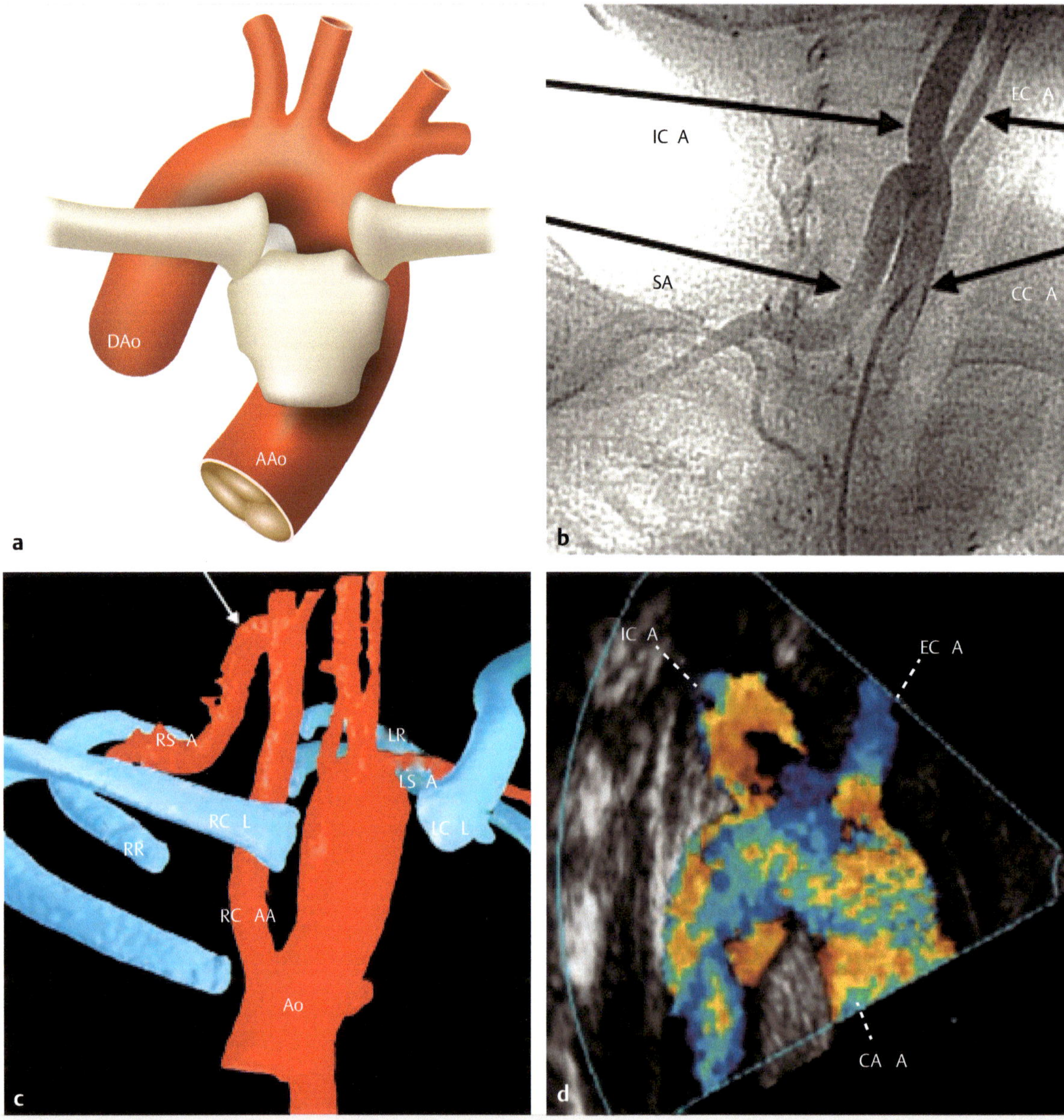

Fig. 4.147 Cervical origin of the right subclavian artery. The images depict the cervical origin of the right subclavian artery (c, arrow) near the bifurcation in the internal and external carotid arteries.

Ao = aorta
DAo = descending aorta
CCA = common carotid artery
ECA = external carotid artery
ICA = internal carotid artery
LCL = left clavicle
LR = left first rib
LSA = left subclavian artery
RCCA = right common carotid artery
RCL = right clavicle
RR = right first rib
RSA = right subclavian artery
SA = subclavian artery.

a Schematic depiction of a cervical right aortic arch with corresponding cervical origin of the subclavian artery.
b Angiographic depiction of a 4-year-old female patient with cervical origin of the RSA.
c 3-D reconstruction of the aorta and great vessels using MDCT, for the same patient as in **b**.
d Color Doppler sonogram of the patient as in **b**.

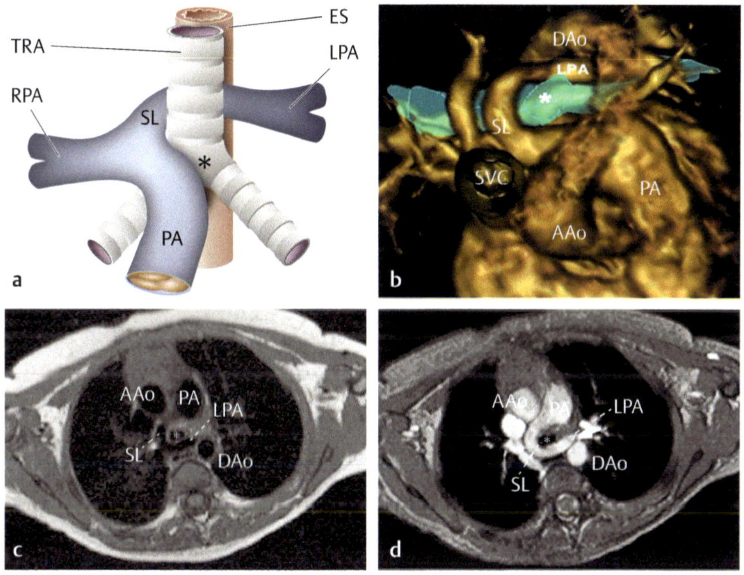

Fig. 4.148 Pulmonary sling. The trachea is marked with an asterisk.

AAo = ascending aorta
DAo = descending aorta
ES = esophagus
LPA = left pulmonary artery
PA = pulmonary artery
RPA = right pulmonary artery
SVC = superior vena cava
SL = sling

a Schematic depiction of the rare defect in which the left pulmonary artery originates from the right one (known as pulmonary sling).
b Depiction of a vascular ring using a 3-D volume rendering technique and an interleaved double-slab 3-D FISP MRA. The origin of the left pulmonary artery and sling formation around the trachea can be clearly seen in **b–d**.
c Transverse black blood MR SE sequence for the patient from **b**.
d Transverse 3-D GE sequence for the patient from **b**.

Table 4.28 Relative value of echocardiography, MRI, MDCT, and cardiac catheter examinations for comparative assessment of aortic and pulmonary arterial anomalies.

Examination parameter	Thoracic X-ray	Echocardiography		MRI	MDCT	Cardiac catheter
		TTE	TEE			
Invasiveness	Noninvasive	Noninvasive	Invasive	Noninvasive	Noninvasive	Invasive
Mobility	Yes	Yes		No	No	No
Field of view	Does not depend on acoustic window	Depends on acoustic window		Does not depend on acoustic window	Does not depend on acoustic window	Does not depend on acoustic window
Imaging options	Summation image (potentially using X-ray and esophageal barium swallow)	2-D/3-D (incl. Doppler)		2-D/3-D (4-D) (as MRA, potentially using flow measurement)	2-D/3-D (4-D) (as CTA)	2-D (3-D) (as a rotational angio intervention with fluoroscopy)
Radiation exposure	Yes	No		No	Yes	Yes
User-dependence	Relatively independent of user	Independent of user		Relatively independent of user	Relatively independent of user	Relatively independent of user
Ability to depict aortic arch morphology	Low	High	High	High	High	High
Ability to depict lungs and trachea	Low	–	–	Moderate	High	Low
Ability to depict esophageal morphology	High, if using barium swallow	Low	Low	High, if using orally administered contrast agent	High, if using orally administered contrast agent	–

CTA, computed tomographic angiography; MDCT, multidetector computed tomography; MRA, magnetic resonance angiography; MRI, magnetic resonance imaging; TEE, transesophageal echocardiography; TTE, transthoracic echocardiography.

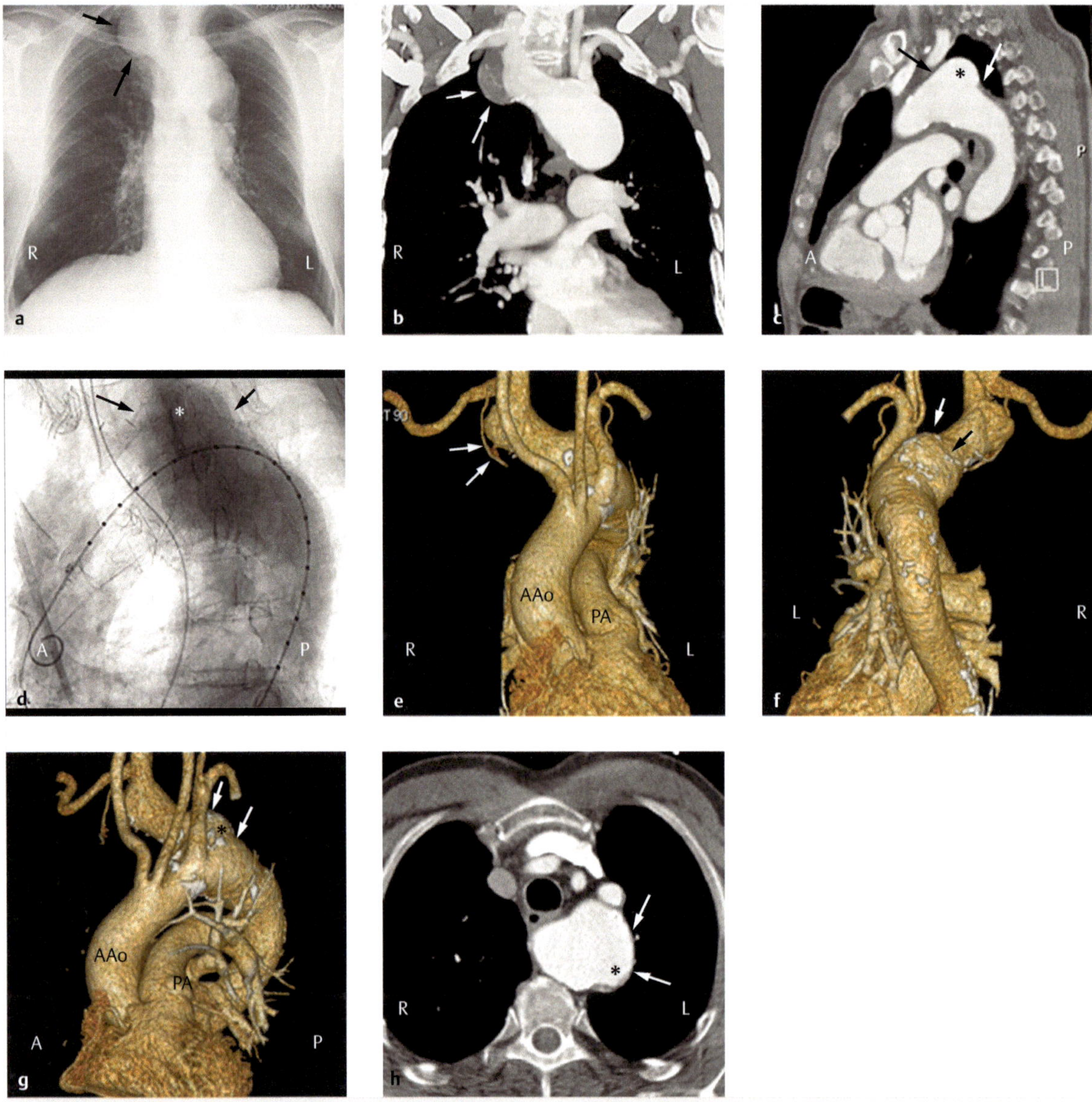

Fig. 4.149 Lusorian artery with Kommerell diverticulum. Seventy-two-year-old male patient who has complained of difficulty swallowing for a long time, and presented for treatment of Kommerell diverticulum (c, d, f–h, asterisks, and arrows). The depictions show a partially thrombosed, aneurysmatic enlargement of a lusorian artery (a, b, e, arrows) described as "Kommerell diverticulum," near the origin of the subclavian artery. The patient was treated via surgical debranching and percutaneous, endovascular stent graft implantation in the aortic arch and the proximal descending artery (▶ Fig. 4.150).

AAo = ascending aorta

PA = pulmonary artery

- **a** Traditional p.-a. thoracic X-ray.
- **b** Coronal multiplanar CT reconstruction depicting the partially thrombosed diverticulum.
- **c** Sagittal multiplanar CT reconstruction.
- **d** Interventional aortogram of the aortic arch with pigtail catheter, lateral projection.
- **e** Ventral view of a 3-D volume rendering CT reconstruction.
- **f** Dorsal view of a 3-D volume rendering CT reconstruction.
- **g** Lateral view of a 3-D volume rendering CT reconstruction.
- **h** Transverse CT reconstruction near the Kommerell diverticulum.

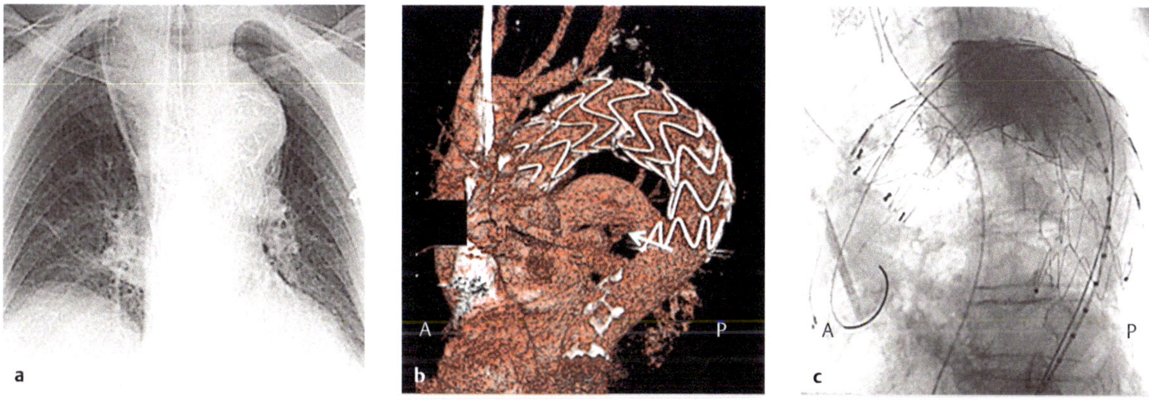

Fig. 4.150 Condition after endovascular treatment of an aneurysm in a case of lusorian artery with Kommerell diverticulum. The 72-year-old male patient from ▶ Fig. 4.149 was treated by implanting an aortic stent prosthesis in the aortic arch.

a P.-a. thoracic X-ray.

b Lateral projection of a volume rendering technique from a contrast-enhanced CTA.

c Corresponding contrast-enhanced interventional aortogram, LAO projection.

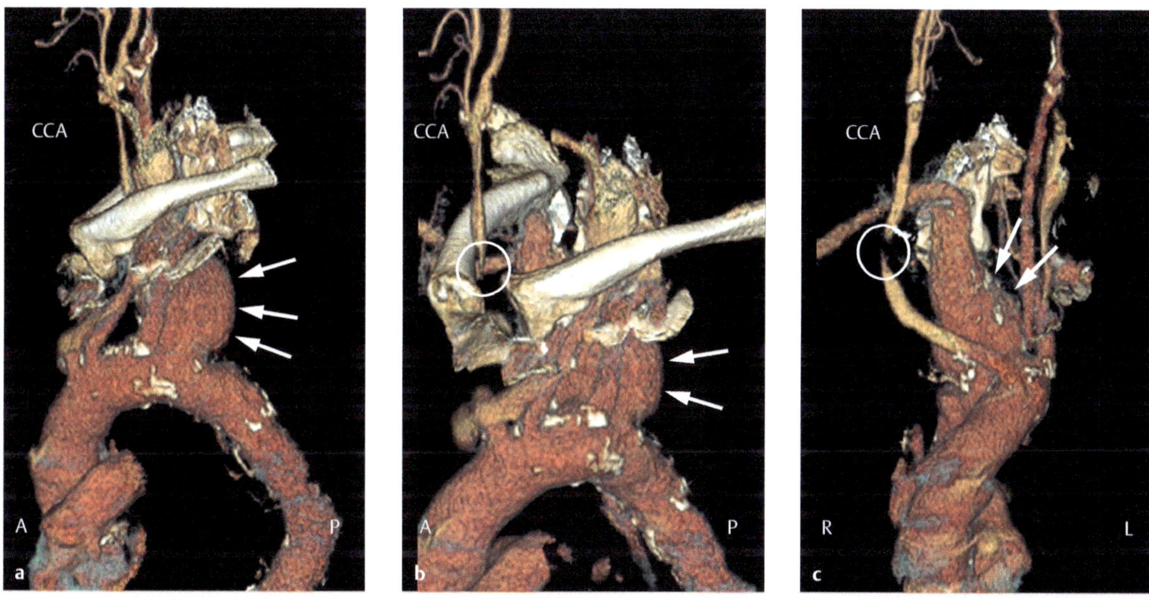

Fig. 4.151 Lusorian artery, Kommerell diverticulum, and carotid artery compression. Fifty-six-year-old female patient, presenting in the emergency room due to acute shortness of breath. The CT depicts a covered, ruptured Kommerell diverticulum (**a–c**, arrows) causing high-grade stenosis of the trachea and the right carotid artery near the clavicle (**b**, **c**, circle).

CCA = common carotid artery

a Lateral reconstruction, volume rendering technique, of a contrast-enhanced CTA depicting the bony structures.

b Fenestration with "bone removal" to depict the CCA compression.

c A.-p. projection (bones completely removed).

4.5.4 Congenital Coronary Anomalies

Marcus Makowski, Gerald F. Greil, Lukas Lehmkuhl

Definition

Congenital coronary anomalies are right or left coronary arteries originating atypically, not from the right or left coronary aortic sinuses facing the pulmonary artery, respectively (▶ Fig. 4.152, ▶ Fig. 4.153, and ▶ Fig. 4.154), with an atypical course (▶ Fig. 4.155), number, diameter, or connection (e.g., coronary arterial fistulae; ▶ Fig. 4.156).

Isolated coronary anomalies in cases of otherwise normal cardiovascular anatomy are relatively common, comprising 1–2% of anomalies.[83] Generally speaking, they are only clinically significant if they are concurrent with other congenital heart defects (▶ Fig. 4.157, ▶ Fig. 4.158, and ▶ Fig. 4.159).[177–179] Coronary fistulae may occur in arteriovenous (▶ Fig. 4.156) or arterio-systemic forms, though the right coronary artery is affected somewhat more commonly. They discharge most commonly into the right ventricle and right atrium.

Classification

For coronary anomalies, whose clinical significance can best be assessed according to the respective hemodynamic relevance of the anomaly,[180] various systems of classification exist:

- *Coronary fistulae:* Coronary fistulae are precapillary connections of the coronary arteries to the ventricles, coronary sinus (▶ Fig. 4.156), superior vena cava, or pulmonary arteries. The incidence of fistulae is approximately 1–2% in angiographic series.[181] Patients are usually asymptomatic. The patients first become clinically remarkable when the shunt volume results in relevant volume load.
- *Bland–White–Garland syndrome* (also known as anomalous left coronary artery from pulmonary artery, or "ALCAPA"): Bland–White–Garland syndrome is the second most common hemodynamically relevant anomaly, whereby the left coronary artery originates from the pulmonary artery (▶ Fig. 4.160).[182] Early diagnosis during infancy is crucial to patient survival. The postpartum reduction in pulmonary arterial resistance results in hypoperfusion of the coronary arteries effluent from the pulmonary arteries. If uncorrected, this often leads to death during infancy. The disorder can, however, first manifest in adulthood if the collaterals compensate accordingly[183] due to chronic, recurrent ischemia (▶ Fig. 4.160l).
- *Congenital coronary stenosis or atresia:* These are very rare and are only compatible with life if collateral circulation is present.[181]
- *Origin of the coronary arteries from the contralateral sinus:*
  - Origin of the left coronary artery from the contralateral sinus: either the entire left main stem (▶ Fig. 4.153) or both branches (circumflex and anterior interventricular branches) of the left coronary artery originate from the right coronary artery (▶ Fig. 4.161) or directly from the contralateral right sinus. A common ostium of all three coronaries is

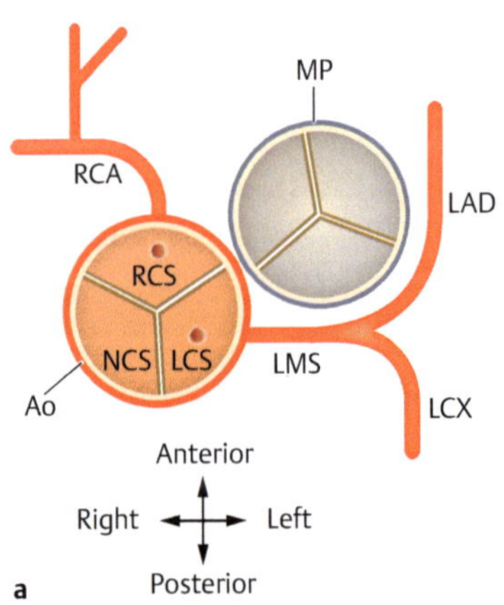

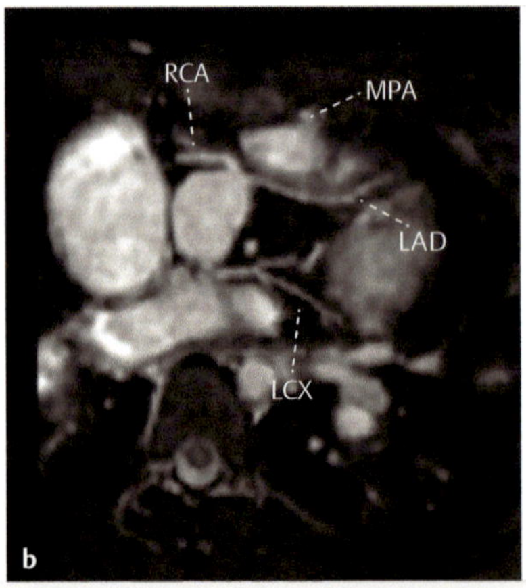

Fig. 4.152 Schematic depiction of the normal course of the coronary arteries, and atypical origin of the left anterior descending artery (LAD) from the right coronary artery.

Ao = aorta
LAD = left anterior descending artery
LCS = left coronary sinus
LCX = left circumflex artery
LMS = left main stem
MPA = main pulmonary artery (truncus pulmonalis)
NCS = non-coronary sinus (posterior or non-coronary sinus)
RCA = right coronary artery
RCS = right coronary sinus

a Schematic depiction of the normal course of the coronaries, transverse section.

b Transverse MIP reconstruction of an MRI whole heart data set, acquired using the navigator technique, in a 7-year-old male patient with isolated origin of the anterior interventricular branch from the right coronary sinus. The circumflex branch originates from the left coronary sinus.

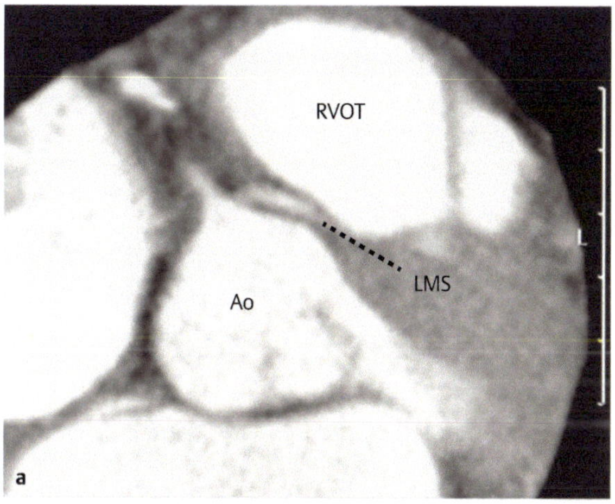

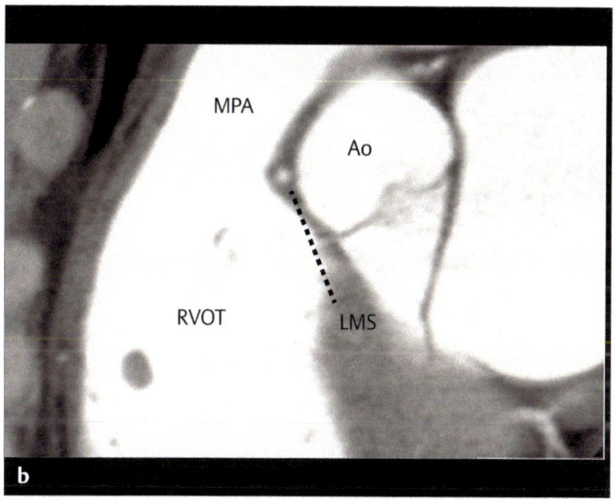

Fig. 4.153 Common origin from the right coronary artery and left main branch from the right coronary sinus. Thirty-seven-year-old woman with complaints of angina pectoris during physical exertion. The left main branch runs between the aorta and RVOT or pulmonary artery.

Ao = aorta
LMS = left main stem
MPA = main pulmonary artery
RVOT = right ventricular outflow tract

a Transverse reconstruction of a coronary CTA.
b Sagittal reconstruction of a coronary CTA.

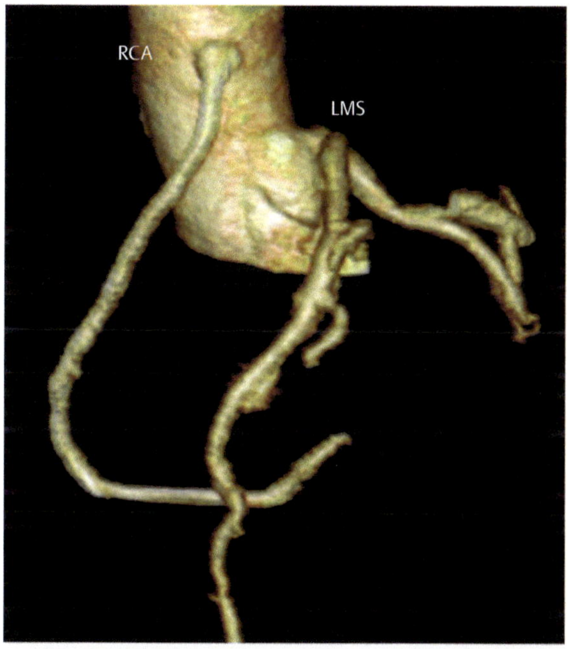

Fig. 4.154 Superior origin of the right coronary artery from the ascending aorta. Fifty-one-year-old female patient with atypical complaints of angina pectoris; coronary CTA. The coronary artery does not originate from the right coronary sinus. The left main branch originates normally from the left coronary sinus.
LMS = left main stem
RCA = right coronary artery

exceedingly rare (0.02–0.04%). Individual branches of the left coronary artery—either the anterior interventricular branch (▸ Fig. 4.152b and ▸ Fig. 4.158) or circumflex branch (▸ Fig. 4.162)—can, however, originate from the right coronary sinus or right coronary artery. The incidence of this disorder is approximately 0.7%. The circumflex branch generally runs dorsal to the aorta and non-coronary or posterior aortic sinus (▸ Fig. 4.162). Similar to the common course of the interventricular branch anterior-ventral to the pulmonary artery (▸ Fig. 4.158), this is hemodynamically irrelevant. Caution should be exercised, primarily before cardiosurgical interventions (▸ Fig. 4.161) such as surgical correction of tetralogy of Fallot or TGA in cases of an atypical course of the anterior interventricular branch ventral to the pulmonary artery (▸ Fig. 4.157 and ▸ Fig. 4.158).

  ○ Origin of the right coronary artery from the contralateral sinus of Valsalva: a right coronary artery originating from the contralateral sinus of Valsalva or left coronary artery is common. In these cases, the right coronary artery usually runs ventral to the aorta and may be located between the aorta and pulmonary artery (▸ Fig. 4.163). This can lead to stress-induced ischemia. Surgical correction should be performed in these cases.

- *Other, usually clearly hemodynamically irrelevant anomalies:* The incidence of hemodynamically irrelevant anomalies of the coronary arteries is approximately

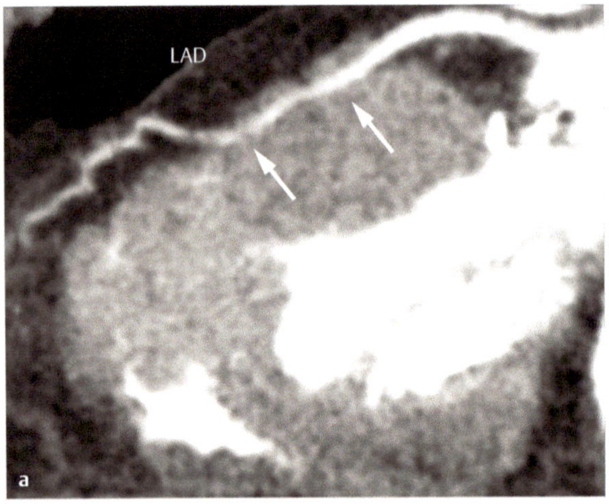

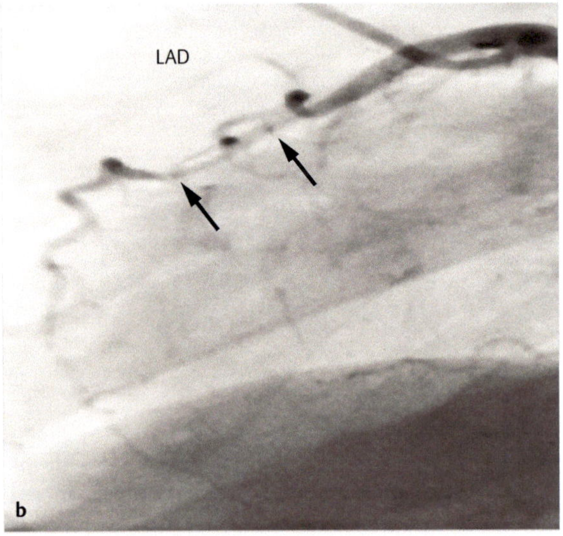

Fig. 4.155 Myocardial bridge of the anterior interventricular branch. Seventy-year-old female patient with complaints of angina pectoris before a planned aortic valve replacement. The myocardial bridge (arrows) near the midventricular anterior interventricular branch can only be depicted indirectly using a cardiac catheter, but can be depicted directly using CT.
LAD = left anterior descending artery

- **a** Curved multiplanar reformat of the anterior interventricular branch from the coronary CT data set.
- **b** Selective cardiac catheter examination of the anterior interventricular branch.

0.3–1.0%. These are generally incidental findings in asymptomatic patients that are discovered within the scope of cardiac diagnostics. It is recommended to determine diagnosis before cardiosurgical or interventional procedures for optimal surgical planning.

- *Ectopic ostium:* The ostium of the left coronary artery originates superior to the sinotubular junction in approximately 30% of cases, compared to the ostium of the right coronary artery in 8% of cases, and both ostia in 6% of cases, respectively (▶ Fig. 4.154).

Clinical Issues

The earliest possible detection of a coronary anomaly as a differential diagnosis for unclear cardiomyopathy during infancy is decisive for patient survival. Anomalies of the coronary arteries in adult patients are often diagnosed when clarifying unclear syncope, or are an incidental finding within the scope of cardiac imaging diagnostics. Coronary anomalies associated with congenital heart defects, particularly TGA or tetralogy of Fallot, are especially common (▶ Fig. 4.157, ▶ Fig. 4.158, and ▶ Fig. 4.159).[177–179]

Natural Progression and Indication for Treatment

Anomalies that could lead to myocardial hypoperfusion should be corrected surgically. Thus, early diagnosis is of vital importance to the prognosis of patients with Bland–White–Garland syndrome. In cases of decreasing pulmonary vascular resistance, this leads to hypoperfusion of the coronary artery effluent from the pulmonary artery, with corresponding damage to the myocardium (▶ Fig. 4.160k-n), heart failure, and occasionally mitral regurgitation. The course of the coronary artery between the aorta and pulmonary artery can, under stress, lead to syncope and sudden cardiac death (▶ Fig. 4.152b, ▶ Fig. 4.153, ▶ Fig. 4.161, and ▶ Fig. 4.163). It is recommended to reimplant the coronary artery ostium in the anatomically correct position.[184] Hemodynamically irrelevant coronary anomalies generally remain asymptomatic and do not require treatment.

Note

The course between the pulmonary artery and aorta (▶ Fig. 4.152b, ▶ Fig. 4.153, and ▶ Fig. 4.161d) is associated with an increased incidence of sudden cardiac death under stress conditions.[185] Surgically correcting the origin of the coronary artery is thus recommended if ischemia has already been verified.

Goals and Relative Value of Diagnostic Imaging

The value of individual imaging procedures for depicting coronary anomalies is summarized in conjunction with Kawasaki syndrome in ▶ Table 4.36. The imaging techniques currently available include echocardiography, MRI, multi-slice CT, and invasive coronary angiography using a cardiac catheter.

Coronary angiography by means of a cardiac catheter examination remains the gold standard for general depiction of the coronary arteries. As an invasive examination dependent upon radiation exposure, potentially nephrotoxic contrast agent containing iodine must be

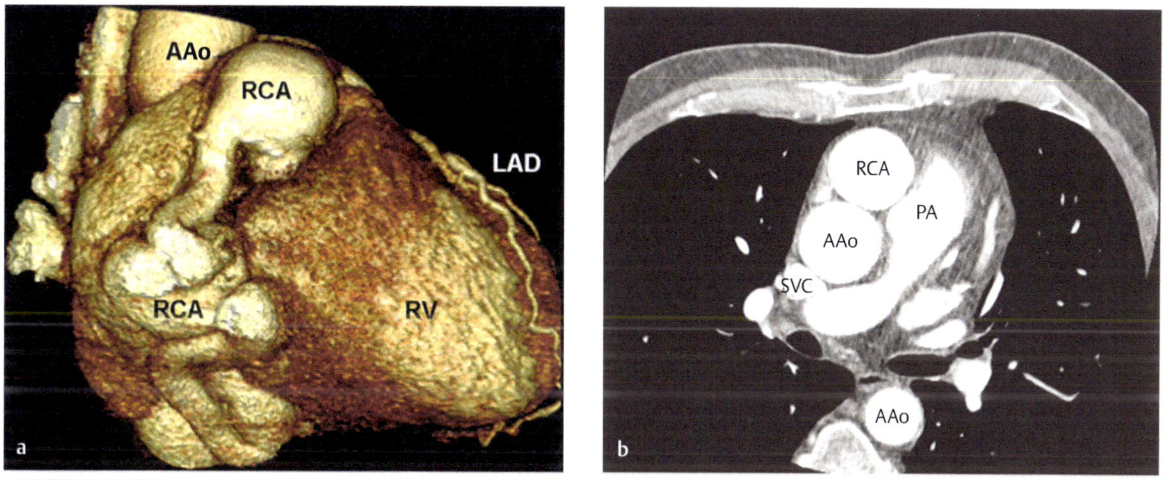

Fig. 4.156 Coronary fistula. Sixty-one-year-old male patient with a large fistula of the right coronary artery and outlet into the coronary sinus. Until a few months ago, the patient had good exercise capacity and was clinically unremarkable.

AAo = ascending aorta
LAD = left anterior descending artery
PA = pulmonary artery
RCA = right coronary artery
RV = right ventricle
SVC = superior vena cava

a 3-D surface reconstruction from an ECG-triggered CT data set.

b The cross-section of a transverse CT reconstruction depicts the right coronary artery dilated to the size of the ascending aorta.

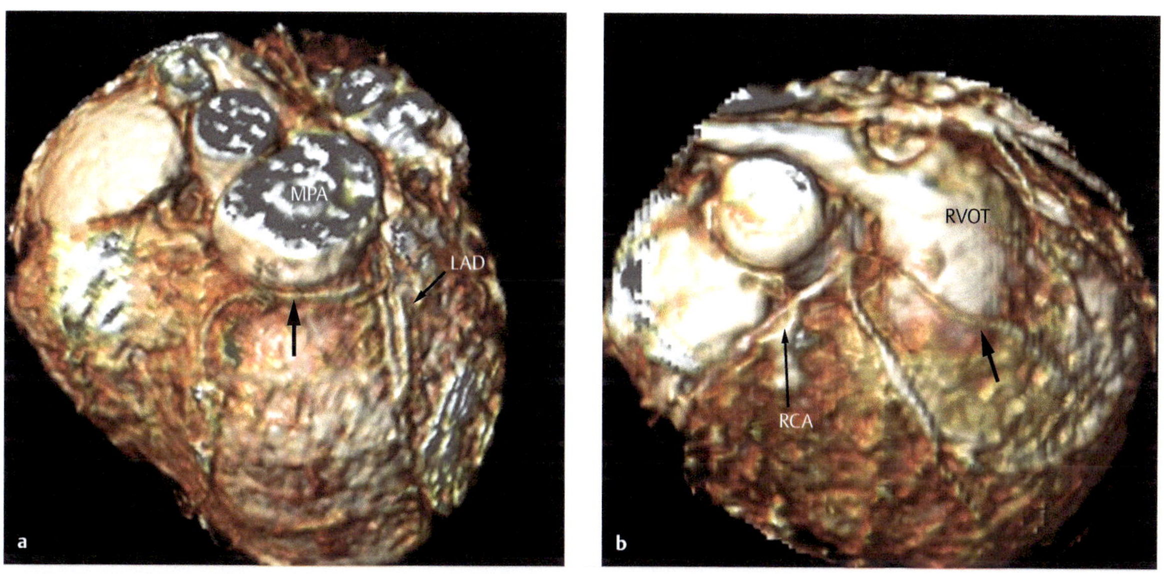

Fig. 4.157 Coronary anomalies in conjunction with tetralogy of Fallot. Two different patients.

LAD = left anterior descending artery
MPA = main pulmonary artery (truncus pulmonalis)
RCA = right coronary artery
RVOT = right ventricular outflow tract

a The volume rendering 3-D MRI data set from an SSFP sequence was recorded during normal respiration using a respiratory navigator. The 3.5-year-old male patient with surgically corrected tetralogy of Fallot received a cardiac MRI to determine right ventricular volume and function and to quantify pulmonary valve insufficiency. One side branch of the left coronary artery crosses the RVOT (arrow).

b The volume rendering 3-D MRI data set from an SSFP sequence was recorded during normal respiration using a respiratory navigator. For the 4-year-old male patient with surgically corrected tetralogy of Fallot, a side branch of the right coronary artery crosses the RVOT (arrow).

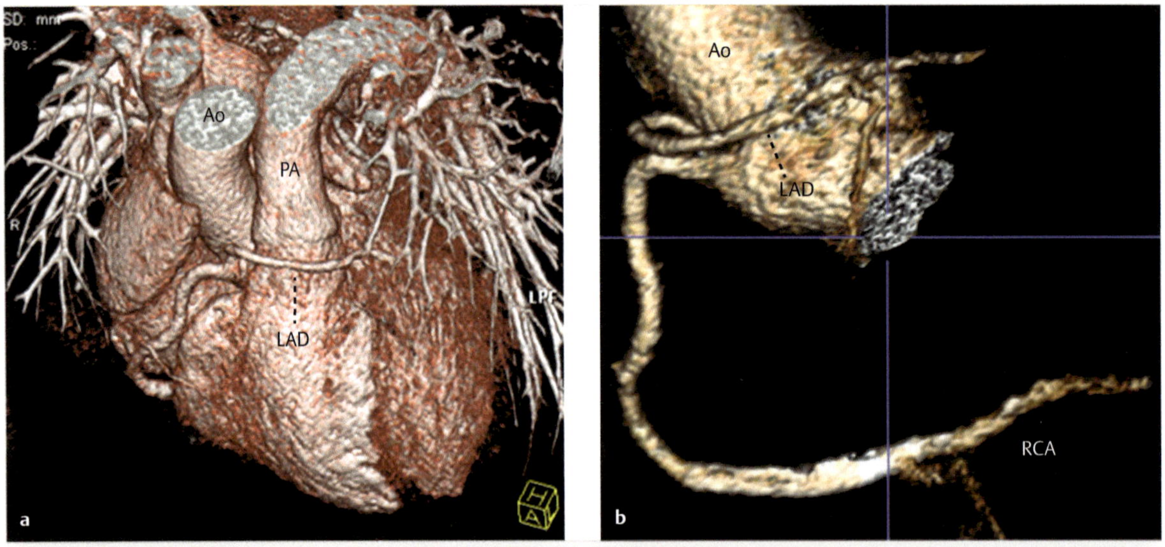

Fig. 4.158 Coronary anomalies in conjunction with coronary heart disease. Seventy-five-year-old male patient after a posterior wall infarction and stent implantation in the medial right coronary artery. The images depict an atypical origin of the left anterior descending artery from the right coronary artery with a "benign" course ventral to the pulmonary artery.

Ao = aorta
LAD = left anterior descending artery
PA = pulmonary artery
RCA = right coronary artery

a Volume rendering 3-D CT data set.
b Segmented 3-D reconstruction of the right coronary system.

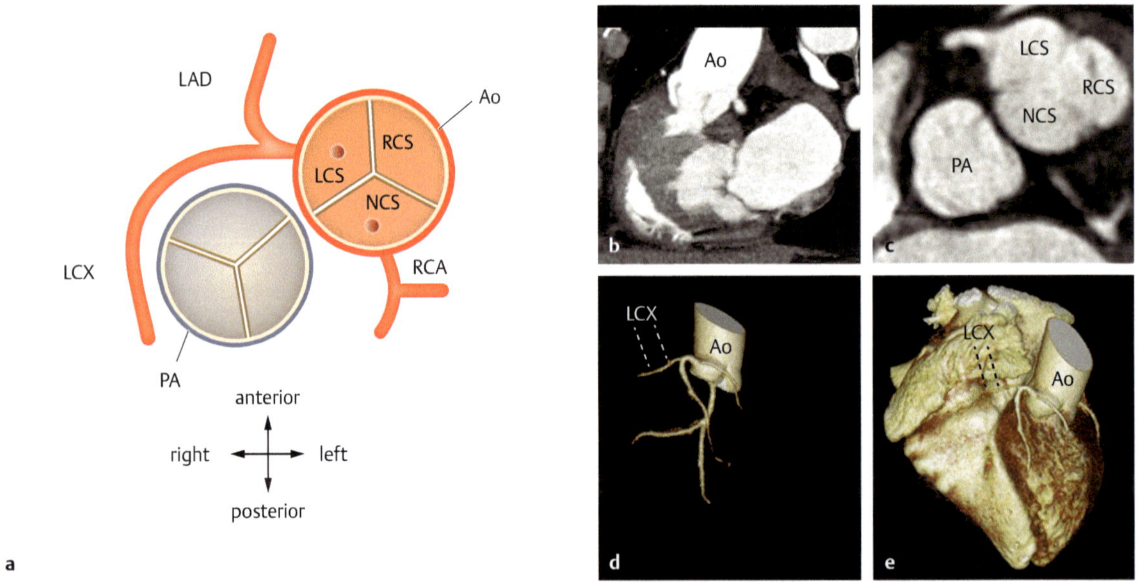

Fig. 4.159 Coronary anomalies in conjunction with ccTGA. Seventy-year-old male patient with a preoperative diagnosis of ccTGA.

Ao = aorta
LAD = left anterior descending artery
LCS = left coronary sinus
LCX = left circumflex artery
NCS = non-coronary sinus (posterior or non-coronary sinus)
PA = pulmonary artery
RCA = right coronary artery
RCS = right coronary sinus

a Schematic depiction of the coronary arterial origins of a patient with a left-localized, morphologic right ventricle. The aorta is located to the left of the pulmonary artery. The circumflex and left anterior descending artery (LAD) originate from the left coronary sinus, while the right coronary artery originates from the posterior or non-coronary sinus (as is typical).
b The angulated sagittal reconstruction of a retrospectively gated CT data set to visualize the outflow tract depicts the ventrally displaced ascending aorta with the aortic valve open during systole, and the posterior origin of the right coronary artery.
c The transverse CT reconstruction depicts the ventral origin of the left coronary artery from the left coronary sinus.
d 3-D reconstruction of the CT data set, volume rendering technique. The selective segmentation of the left coronary tree is visible.
e 3-D reconstruction of the CT data set, volume rendering technique. The anatomical course with respect to the ventricles is depicted. The circumflex branch runs through the atrioventricular groove of the right-displaced, anatomic left ventricle.

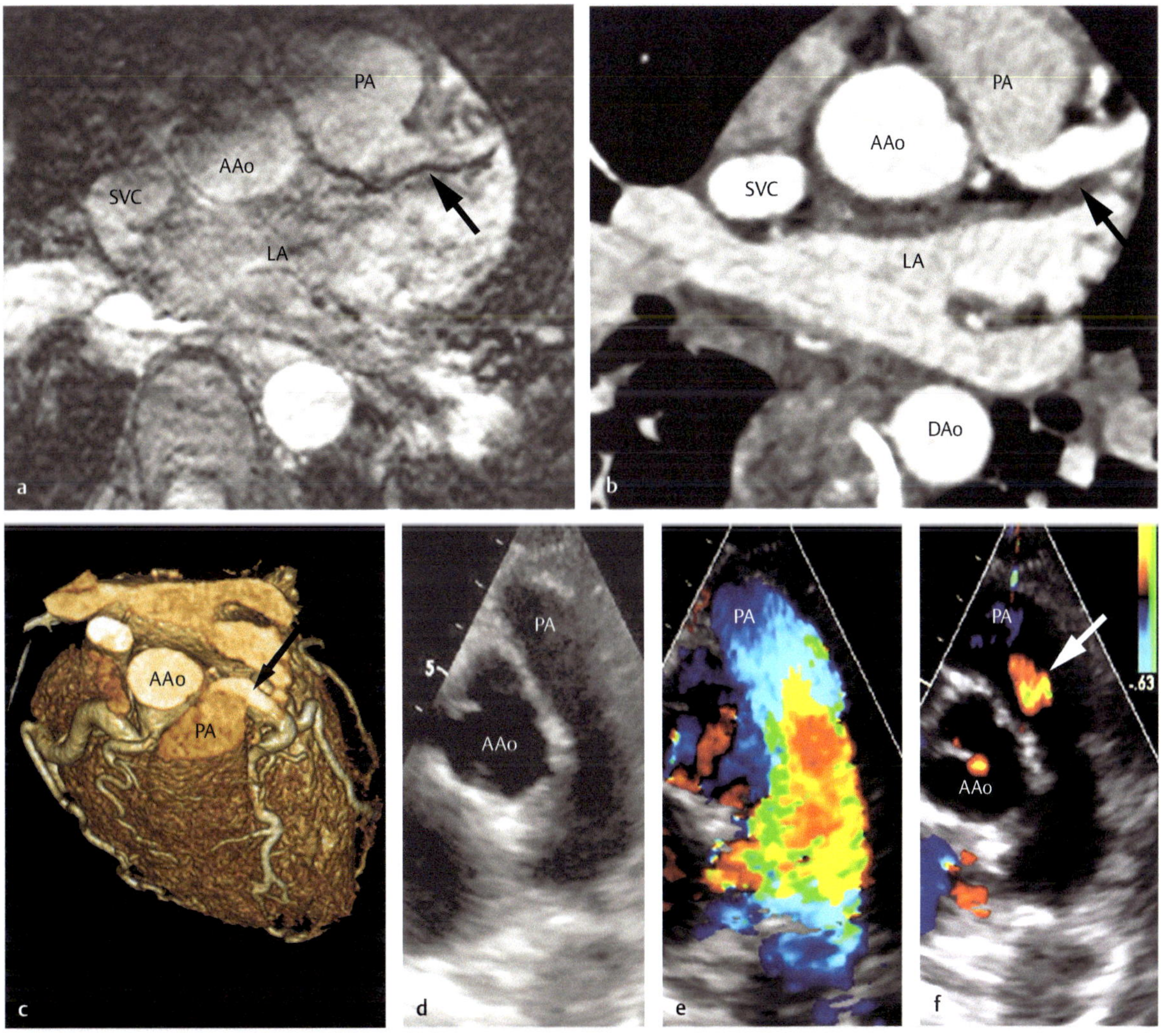

Fig. 4.160 Bland–White–Garland syndrome (ALCAPA). Thirty-year-old female patient after resuscitation due to ventricular fibrillation.

AAo = ascending aorta
AoV = aortic valve
DAo = descending aorta
LA = left atrium
LAD = left anterior descending artery
LV = left ventricle
PA = pulmonary artery
RCA = right coronary artery
SVC = superior vena cava

a Transverse reconstruction from an MRI whole heart sequence using the navigator technique, during normal respiration (acquisition time: approximately 10 minutes). The image depicts the atypical origin of the left main branch from the main pulmonary artery (arrow). The image quality, signal intensity, and contrast-to-noise ratio are, however, significantly worse than with CT (**b**) due to slow flow in the vessel and imaging without a contrast agent.

b Axial reconstruction at the same level as in **a**, of a prospectively triggered CT data set acquired in high-pitch (flash) mode (acquisition time: less than 1 second with an effective dose of less than 1 mSv), with significantly better signal-to-noise and contrast-to-noise ratio than MRI. The arrow indicates the origin of the left main coronary artery branch from the main pulmonary artery. Note the higher density in the left main coronary artery as compared to the pulmonary artery due to retrograde filling via collaterals of the enlarged RCA.

c Excerpt at the level of the origin of the left main coronary artery from the pulmonary artery, 3-D CT data set. Note the difference in density between the left main branch (arrow) and the pulmonary artery, caused by retrograde flow via collaterals of the dilated right coronary artery.

d 2-D TTE. The great vessels are visible.

e The corresponding color Doppler echocardiography image depicts systolic flow in the pulmonary artery.

f This color Doppler echocardiography image depicts the retrograde diastolic inflow into the pulmonary artery via the left main branch (arrow).

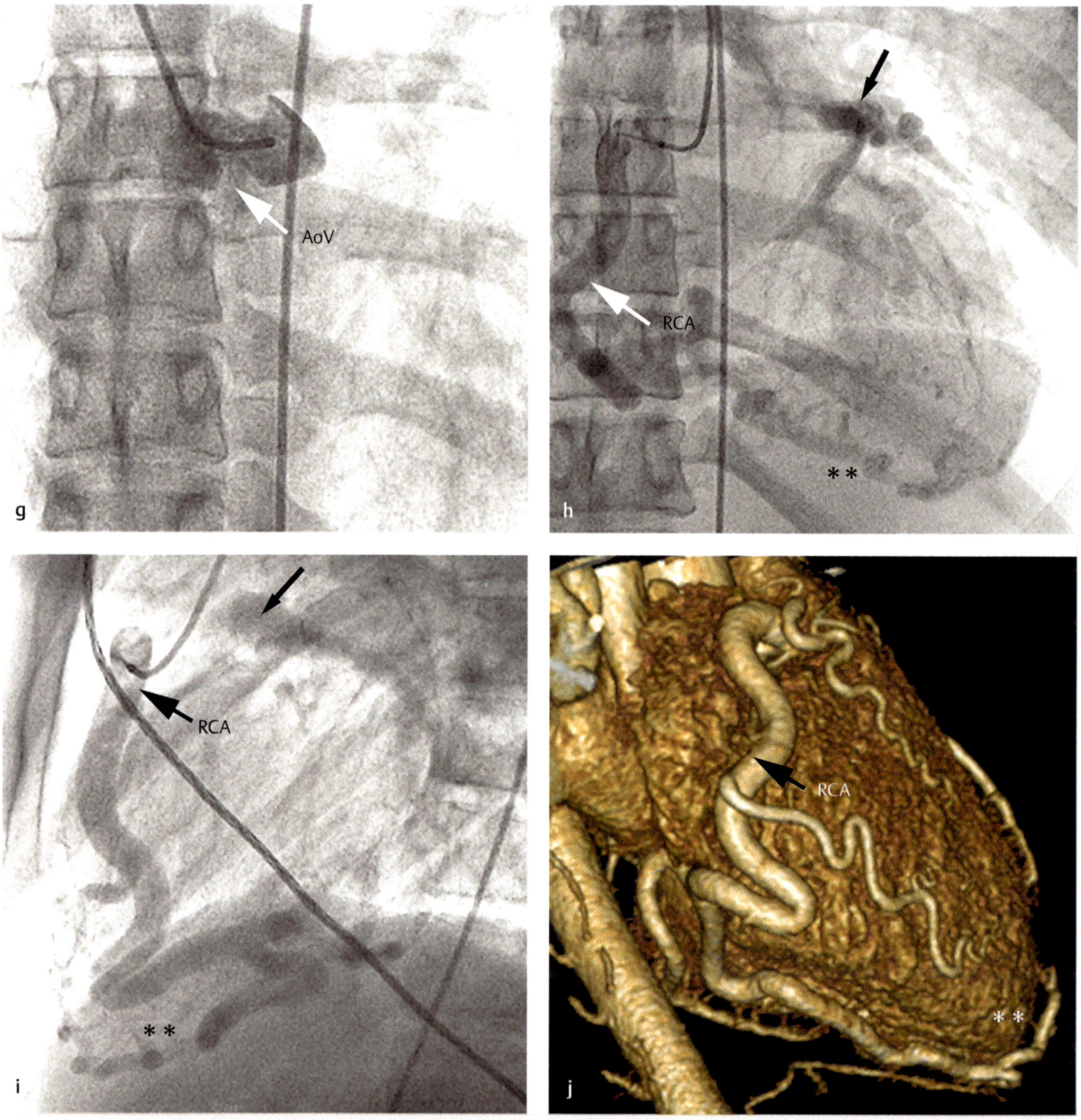

Fig 4.160 *(Continued)* **Bland–White–Garland syndrome (ALCAPA).**

AAo = ascending aorta
AoV = aortic valve
DAo = descending aorta
LA = left atrium
LAD = left anterior descending artery
LV = left ventricle
PA = pulmonary artery
RCA = right coronary artery
SVC = superior vena cava

g Selective invasive coronary angiogram. The angiogram with a pigtail catheter depicts no coronary origin near the left coronary sinus.

h Selective invasive coronary angiogram. The anomalous origin of the left main branch from the pulmonary artery is initially depicted in the selective flow coronary angiogram of the dilated right coronary artery during later stages, with retrograde filling of the left main coronary artery (**h**, **i**, arrows) via collaterals (**h**, **i**, double asterisk).

i Selective flow coronary angiogram of the RCA, later measurement point.

j In comparison, the 3-D CT reconstruction of the dilated right coronary artery, also with clear depiction of the collaterals (double asterisk) to the left coronary artery.

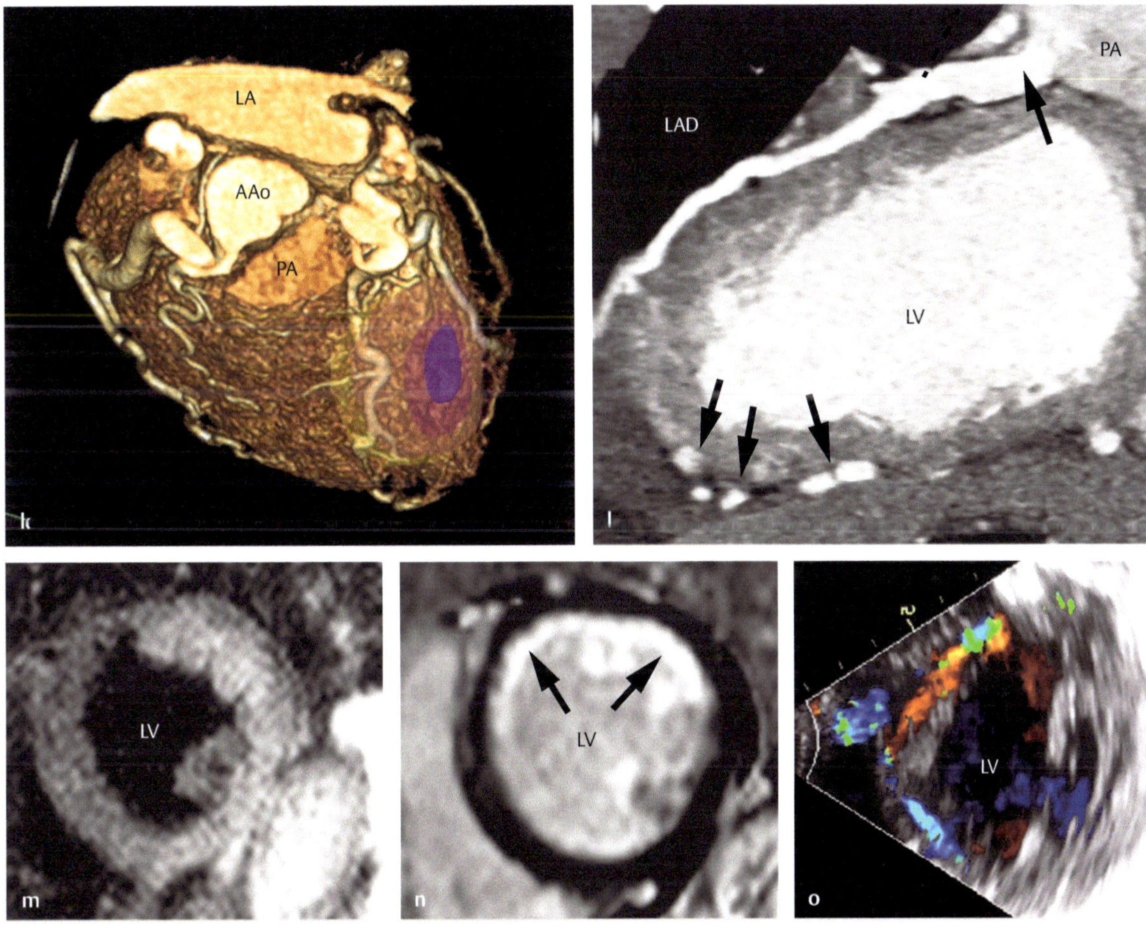

Fig 4.160 (*Continued*) **Bland–White–Garland syndrome (ALCAPA).**

AAo = ascending aorta
AoV = aortic valve
DAo = descending aorta
LA = left atrium
LAD = left anterior descending artery
LV = left ventricle
PA = pulmonary artery
RCA = right coronary artery
SVC = superior vena cava

k 3-D reconstruction from a CT data set using prospective gating in high-pitch (flash) mode near the origin of the dilated right coronary artery from the ascending aorta and the left main branch from the pulmonary artery. The region with chronic hypoperfusion is marked with color.

l Curved planar reformat of the left anterior descending artery (LAD), depicting numerous collaterals (arrows) near the posterior wall of the left ventricle. The single black arrow indicates the position of the left main branch.

m The edema-sensitive MRI sequence, short axis (T2w STIR sequence), depicting a discrete, pronounced edema as an indicator of acute anterolateral ischemia.

n The late gadolinium enhancement MRI sequence in the same orientation depicts typical ischemic subendocardial contrast agent accumulation (arrows) as an expression of subendocardial scarring within the scope of chronic ischemia caused by Bland–White–Garland syndrome, as a possible arrhythmogenic substrate for ventricular tachycardia.

o Color Doppler echocardiography depicting collaterals.

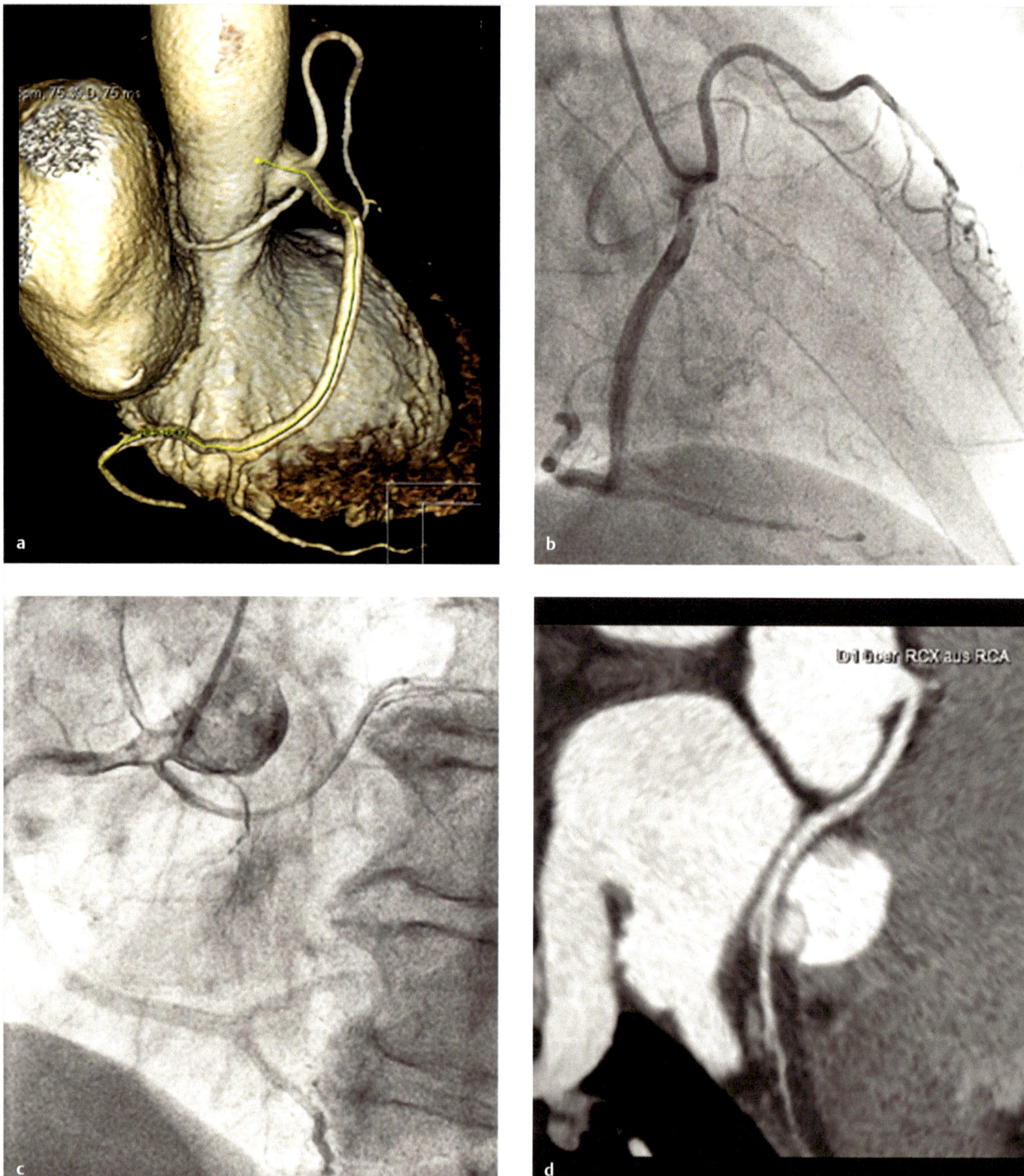

Fig. 4.161 Common origin of the circumflex branch and anterior interventricular branch from the right coronary artery, which originates from the right coronary sinus. Sixty-nine-year-old female patient. The indication for invasive diagnostics was ruling out coronary heart disease before a planned mitral valve reconstruction. The subsequent CT was performed to better diagnose the position of the course of the coronaries during a planned, minimally invasive surgical intervention.

- **a** Coronary CT with 3-D surface depiction of the heart and coronary tree. The centerline (yellow) for generating an MPR is marked in the right coronary artery.
- **b** Selective invasive depiction of the coronaries of the common origin of the circumflex and anterior interventricular branches from the right coronary artery, RAO projection.
- **c** Selective invasive depiction of the coronaries of the common origin of the circumflex and anterior interventricular branches from the right coronary artery, LAO projection.
- **d** Curved planar reformat (curved MPR) of the circumflex branch, from a 3-D CT data set.

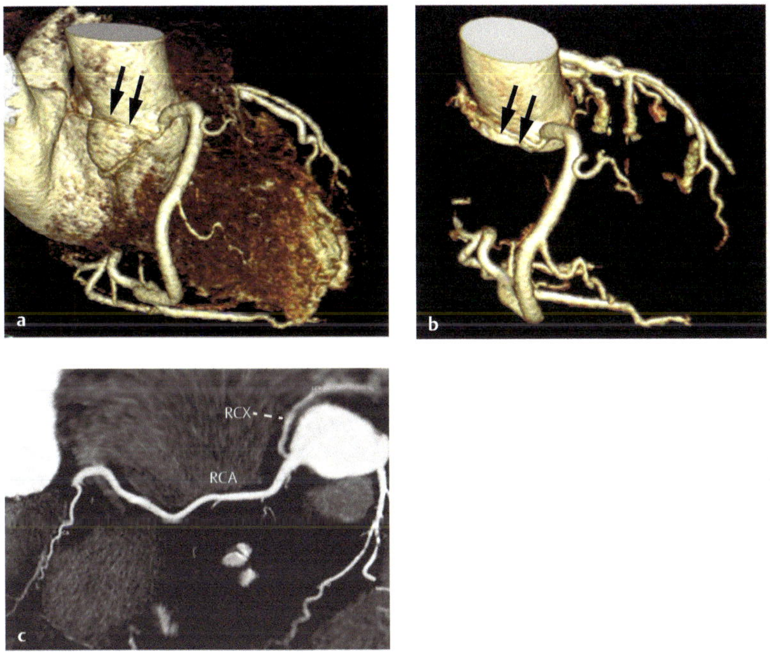

Fig. 4.162 Isolated atypical origin of the circumflex branch from the right coronary artery. Various CT reconstructions from a CT coronary angiogram in a 67-year-old male patient. The arrows in a and b indicate the origin of the circumflex branch.
RCA = right coronary artery
RCX = ramus circumflexus (circumflex branch)

a Origin of the circumflex branch (arrows).
b Origin of the circumflex branch (arrows).
c Curved reformat of the RCA and atypical origin of the Cx.

administered.[186] The spatial relationship of the coronaries to the cardiac muscle can only be depicted in a limited capacity using this method (▶ Fig. 4.155). For anomalous origins, the selective depiction of coronary arteries can last longer and be associated with higher radiation exposure than MDCT (▶ Fig. 4.160g, h, i).

In contrast, *echocardiography*, as a noninvasive and affordable procedure, is ideal for imaging in newborns and young children. The generally good acoustic window during this age usually allows the origin and course of the proximal segments of the coronaries to be depicted with precision.[187] As the patient ages, however, it becomes increasingly likely that no appropriate acoustic window for depicting the coronary arteries using echocardiography will be present.[187]

In recent years, *MRI* has been used increasingly to depict the origins and courses of the coronary arteries.[188,189] As a noninvasive method that does not expose the patient to radiation, MRI can be used to depict the origins and often the courses of the coronary arteries, particularly in adolescents and adults.[188–191]

Alternatively, coronary anatomy can also be depicted using *MDCT*, which has improved significantly in terms of spatial and temporal resolution in recent years.[192] This constitutes a logical alternative to MRI, particularly for patients who are claustrophobic or possess implants that are incompatible with MRI (e.g., cardiac pacemakers). An additional benefit of this method is better spatial resolution and better contrast-to-noise and signal-to-noise ratios (▶ Fig. 4.160a,b). This can only be achieved if contrast agent containing iodine is administered. Elevated heart rate and, in particular, arrhythmia can severely limit image quality. Due to the extremely brief acquisition times of the newest generation of CT scanners, coronary anomalies can generally still be depicted quickly, even in cases of higher heart rates, with acceptable radiation exposure compared to a cardiac catheter. This is particularly true in cases of purely morphological queries.[193] Narcosis is generally unnecessary.

> **Note**
>
> MRI (e.g., using the navigator technique) should be attempted before CT in order to depict coronary origin anomalies in compliant children and adolescents.

Nevertheless, depicting coronary anomalies is one of the few indications for cardiac CT in congenital heart disease that yields equal or better results compared to MRI and even to invasive cardiac catheterization.[7]

Other imaging techniques such as *SPECT* or *PET* now retain only secondary importance in diagnosing coronary artery anomalies in clinical routines, though they can yield valuable information for verifying the hemodynamic relevance of the anomaly (such as for stress-induced myocardial ischemia). However, in these cases, stress MRI using adenosine, regadenoson, or especially dobutamine should be rather implemented in order to prove the hemodynamic relevance of a coronary anomaly, due to the lower radiation exposure and increased spatial resolution.[194]

▶ **Acknowledgment.** The authors thank Mr. Andreas In der Mühle for his support.

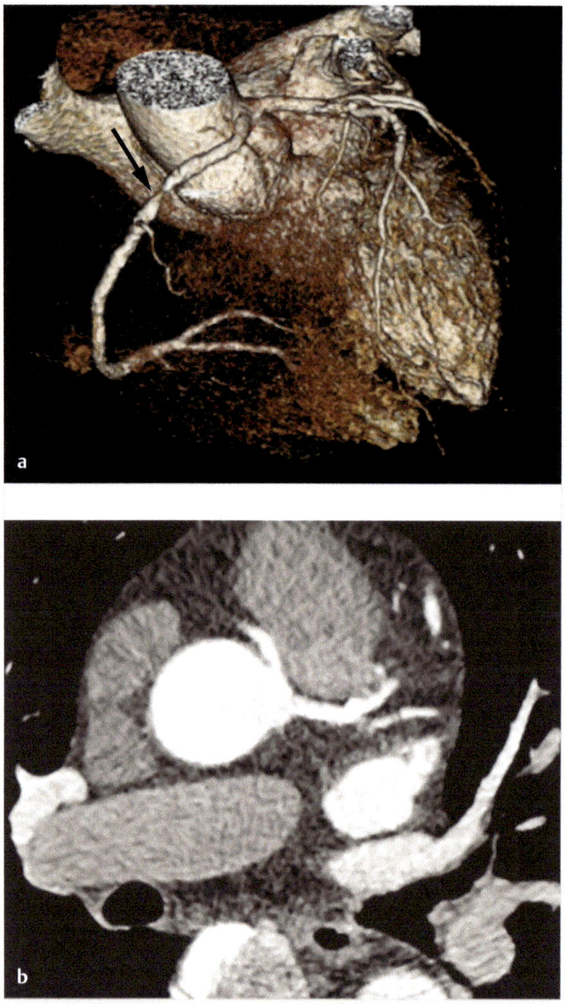

Fig. 4.163 Common origin of the right coronary artery and left main branch from the left coronary sinus, with relevant coronary stenosis in the proximal right coronary artery. CT coronary angiogram.

a The 3-D reconstruction depicts a relevant stenosis (arrow) near the proximal right coronary artery.

b The common origin of the right coronary artery and left main branch from the left coronary sinus can be seen in this transverse reconstruction.

4.5.5 Aortopulmonary Collaterals

Gerald F. Greil, Lukas Lehmkuhl, Heiner Latus

Definition

Major aortopulmonary collateral arteries (MAPCAs), collateral connections between the systemic and pulmonary vascular systems,[83] occur in conjunction with developmental issues of the central pulmonary arteries, primarily in cases of pulmonary atresia[195,196] or high-grade pulmonary stenosis (for example, concurrent with tetralogy of Fallot).

Embryology, Etiology, and Pathophysiology

Mammals form the right and left pulmonary artery from the sixth pharyngeal arch arteries during roughly the fifth week of fetal development. They then anastomose medially (proximally) with the arterial trunk and laterally (distally) with the dorsal aorta. In addition, they connect to the pulmonary vascular plexus of the primitive pulmonary buds. This plexus is also connected to the dorsal aorta by means of *intersegmental arteries*, which are already present before the development of the sixth pharyngeal arch arteries. Once these disappear, the bronchial arteries develop roughly during week 9 of fetal development. In cases of left aortic arch, the connection of the central pulmonary arteries to the left dorsal aorta is maintained by the distal segment of the sixth pharyngeal arch artery, which forms the ductus arteriosus. The distal segment of the right sixth pharyngeal arch artery and the dorsal aorta distal to the right subclavian artery disappears around week 7. In cases of a right aortic arch, the involution process is mirrored.

It is assumed that MAPCAs involve persistent intersegmental arteries,[83] which normally recede before week 5 of embryonic development, and are also not histologically identical to "bronchial arteries." Secondarily, enlarged bronchial arteries can also contribute to pulmonary perfusion via bronchopulmonary anastomoses of the arterial pulmonary vessels. Their significance to pulmonary perfusion remains minor, however, especially for patients with pulmonary atresia. A persistent fifth pharyngeal arch artery, aortopulmonary septal defect (APSD), or fistulae of the coronary arteries with pulmonary vessels can also contribute to collateral pulmonary perfusion.[83] Compared to a normally developing fetus, the pulmonary blood flow changes in the fetus for patients with pulmonary atresia and VSD: the entire blood volume flows through the aortic arch (fourth pharyngeal arch artery) into the aorta, and from there, into the ductus arteriosus (sixth pharyngeal arch artery) to the central pulmonary arteries or peripheral regions of the body. Blood flow from the right ventricle via the pulmonary outflow tract ceases, and the direction of flow in the ductus arteriosus (sixth pharyngeal arch artery) is reversed. In accordance with the aforementioned embryological development, MAPCAs often occur in conjunction with certain heart defects (▶ Table 4.29).

Note

Approximately 75% of all MAPCAs originate from the descending aorta, cranial to the passage of the diaphragm (▶ Fig. 4.164, ▶ Fig. 4.165, and ▶ Fig. 4.166). They can, however, also originate from the aortic arch (▶ Fig. 4.166e), subclavian artery, or the mammarian or intercostal arteries.

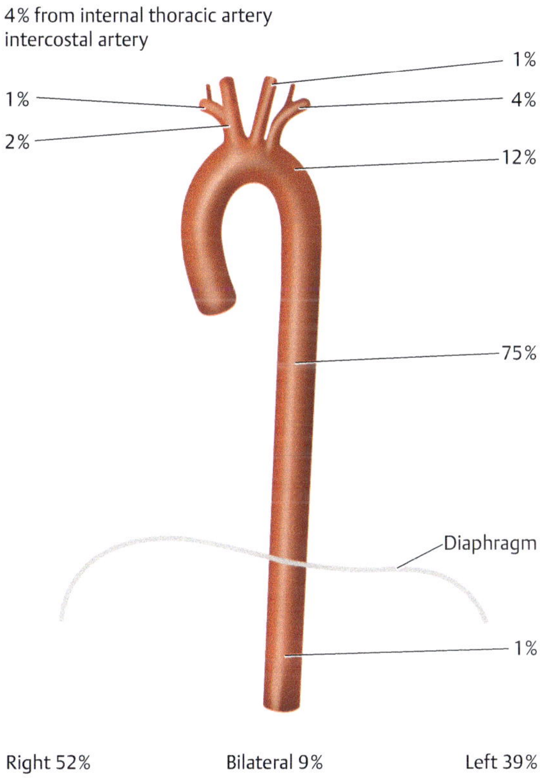

Fig. 4.164 Frequency distribution of origins of the collateral arteries. Schematic depiction. The majority of MAPCAs originate cranial to the diaphragm, more commonly on the right side than the left, though they can also occur bilaterally (▶ Fig. 4.165). Most commonly, the origin is from the descending aorta, though in rarer cases, it may be from the aortic arch, the subclavian artery, or the mammarian and intercostal arteries.

Histology

The histology of larger collaterals is described proximal as an elastic artery similar to the aorta with a distal transition to a muscular systemic artery.[197] In addition, a ductus arteriosus and stenosing MAPCA possess some structural similarities. The tendency of MAPCA toward stenosis—particularly the large MAPCA already present before birth (see ▶ Fig. 4.165)—may be caused by the embryologic development of persistent intersegmental arteries. Haworth[197] thus interpreted this as delayed closure that should have taken place during the embryonic stage.

Clinical Issues, Natural Progression, and Indication for Treatment

Due to the collaterals and often underdeveloped pulmonary arteries, corrective surgeries are rarely performed on young children. Development of the pulmonary vascular system early in childhood is decisive for prognosis. Increased pressure and flow ratios in the pulmonary vascular bed lead to pulmonary vascular obstructive diseases. If these parameters establish an equilibrium, patients may survive for a remarkably long time (see ▶ Fig. 4.165 and ▶ Fig. 4.166). Long-term observations do, however, indicate a decidedly poor prognosis for patients who do not receive surgical treatment: Marelli[198] reported on 11 MAPCA patients who were not surgically treated. The median survival time was less than 30 years. All patients exhibited symptoms classified as NYHA grade II or worse. In this group, nearly 50% (5 patients) died during the observation period.

Treatment Options

Surgical treatment for tetralogy of Fallot accompanied by pulmonary atresia was first performed by Klinner et al.,[199] using a valve-equipped conduit from the right ventricle to the central pulmonary arteries. This occurred approximately 9 years after the first open-heart surgery to correct tetralogy of Fallot, performed by Lillehei et al.[200] Previously, this disorder was treated using aortopulmonary shunts, such as Blalock–Taussig, Potts, and Waterston shunts. Wallace et al.[201] were the first to describe a successful corrective surgery on a patient with pulmonary atresia, VSD, and bilateral absence of pulmonary arteries. In this instance, a large collateral vessel supplied large segments of the left and right lungs (see ▶ Fig. 4.165). Both vessels were able to be connected using an aortic homograft. Hessel et al.[202] were the first to report a successful end-to-end anastomosis of a MAPCA originating from the descending aorta to the ipsilateral pulmonary artery. After a corrective surgery to treat pulmonary atresia or tetralogy of Fallot, the collaterals close spontaneously based on the pressure and volume ratios, or can be closed with vascular coils in the cardiac catheterization laboratory. In the event that surgical correction of the underlying heart defect is impossible, it may still be possible to treat the MAPCA stenoses that are limiting pulmonary arterial supply (▶ Fig. 4.165c) in the cardiac catheterization laboratory.

Goals and Relative Value of Diagnostic Imaging

The goal of imaging diagnostics is to depict intracardiac anatomy, particularly the pulmonary vascular supply. Classifying pulmonary vascular supply into groups I–IV (see below) can be helpful in this endeavor. In addition to depicting the origins of the collateral arteries, the goal is also to depict the intrapulmonary connections for surgical planning purposes. In accordance with embryology, patients are assigned to the following groups:

- **Group I:** Both pulmonary lobes are perfused *exclusively* by a PDA via the central pulmonary arteries (unifocal pulmonary perfusion).

- **Group II:** Both pulmonary lobes are perfused *primarily* by a PDA via the central pulmonary arteries. MAPCAs are also present (unifocal and multifocal pulmonary perfusion).
- **Group III:** The central pulmonary arteries are perfused via the MAPCA. No PDA is present. Individual pulmonary segments are perfused exclusively via the MAPCA (unifocal and multifocal pulmonary perfusion).
- **Group IV:** The pulmonary vascular bed is perfused exclusively via systemic-to-pulmonary collateral arteries that are independent of one another (multifocal pulmonary perfusion).

Intracardiac structures in newborns and children are imagined with *echocardiography* (▶ Table 4.30; ▶ Fig. 4.165h,j,k).

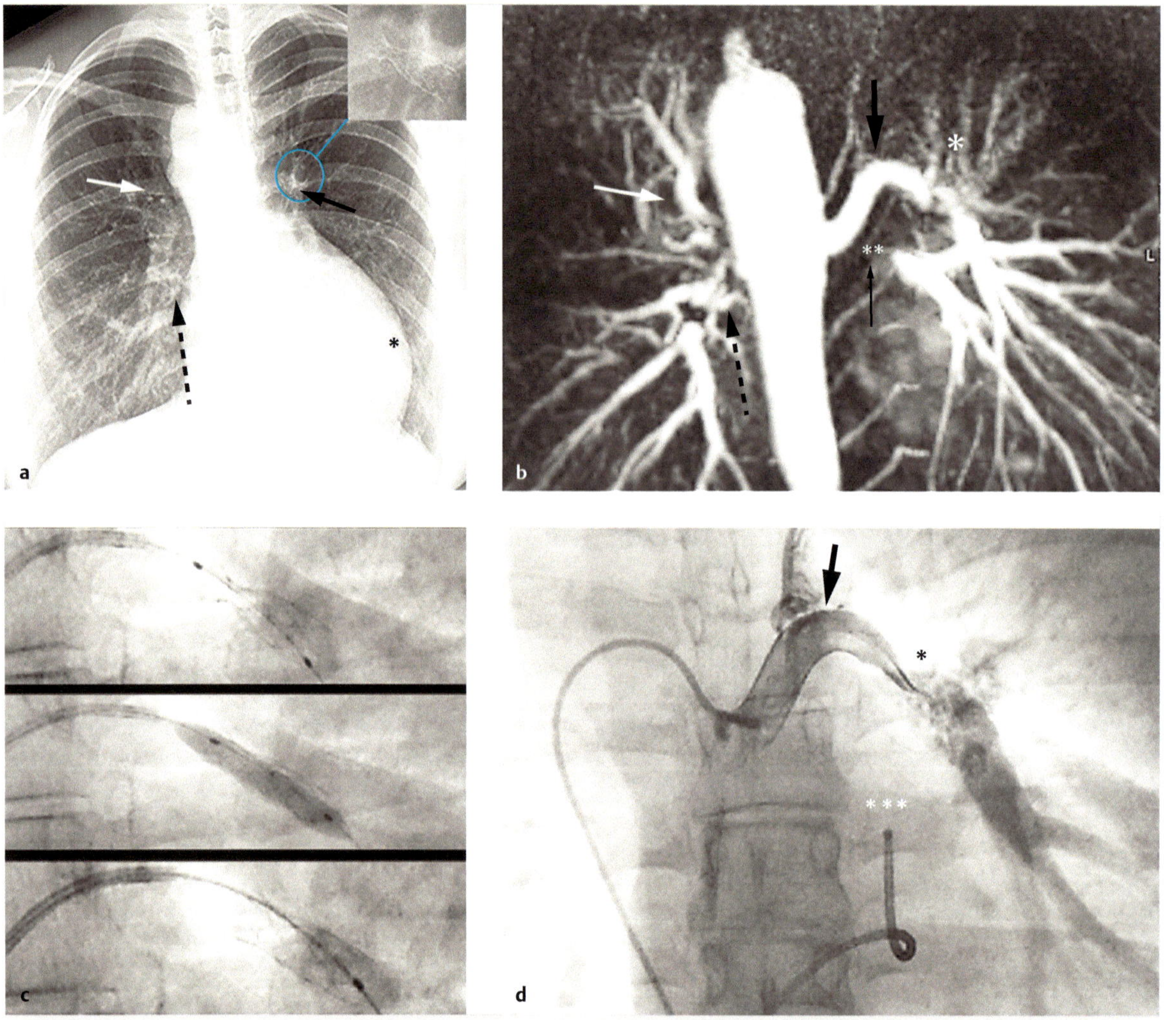

Fig. 4.165 MAPCA. Twenty-year-old cyanotic female patient with uncorrected pulmonary atresia, unbalanced AVSD in a case of large ASD-I, "straddling" atrioventricular valve, and right aortic arch rendering a 2-chamber correction impossible. This is a case of univentricular heart with right systemic ventricle, malposition of the great arteries (MGA), and hypoplastic left ventricle (g, h).

LV = left ventricle
RV = right ventricle

a The p.-a. thoracic X-ray of the patient with pulmonary atresia clearly depicts the MAPCAs (arrows) in a case of absent main pulmonary artery branch, right aortic arch, and stenosed stent in the MAPCA on the left side (blue circle and enlarged image). Also note the enlarged "single" ventricle with an elevated cardiac apex due to a hypertrophied and enlarged right systemic ventricle.

b 3-D MIP reconstruction from contrast-enhanced MRA clearly depicts the four, partially stenosed origins of the MAPCAs (arrows) from the descending aorta, with no evidence of PDA. The asterisk indicates a high-grade stenosis of the left superior MAPCA accompanied by signal voids from a metallic stent in the left inferior MAPCA (thin black arrow).

c The stent is dilated successfully.

d Selective invasive depiction of the stenosed (asterisk) superior left MAPCA (arrow; see **b**, thick black arrow) from the descending aorta with an additional catheter in the RVOT in a case of pulmonary atresia (triple asterisk).

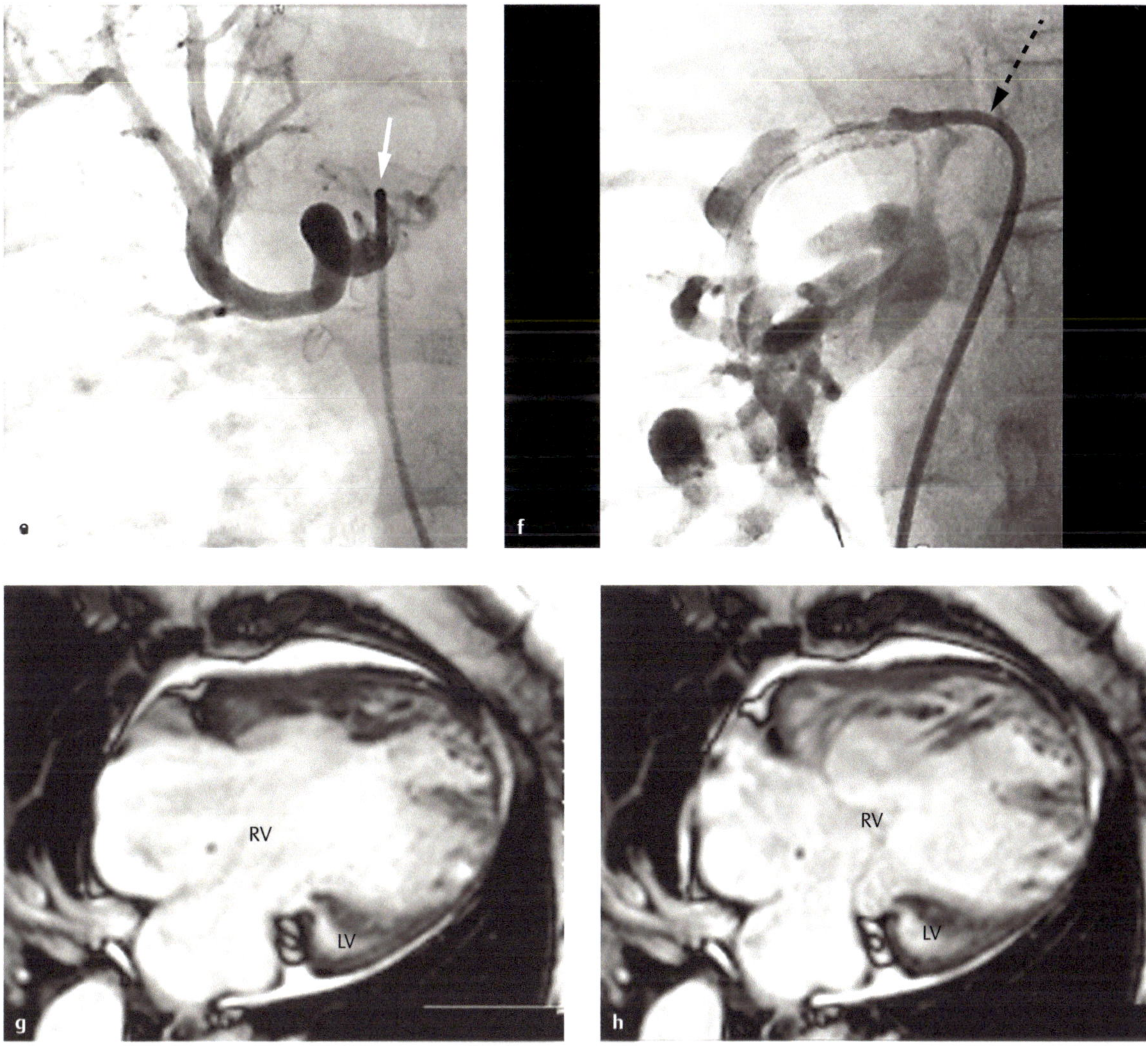

Fig 4.165 (*Continued*) **MAPCA.**

LV = left ventricle RV = right ventricle

e Selective catheterization and visualization of the first MAPCA on the right side (arrow; see **b**, white arrow).

f Selective catheterization and visualization of the second MAPCA on the right side (arrow; see **b**, dotted black arrow).

g Cine SSFP MRI, 4-chamber view, atrioventricular valve opened during diastole.

h Cine SSFP MRI, 4-chamber view, with “straddling” atrioventricular valve closed during diastole.

Table 4.29 Congenital heart defects often associated with MAPCAs, primarily in conjunction with pulmonary atresia.[83]

Congenital heart defect	Incidence (%)
VSD/ASD	79
PFO	40
Right aortic arch	26–50
Persistent left superior vena cava	24

ASD, atrial septal defect; PFO, patent foramen ovale; VSD, ventricular septal defect.

Depicting pulmonary vascular perfusion itself, however, usually requires an imaging technique that is independent of acoustic window. For these applications, ***invasive angiocardiography*** remains the gold standard. This method can selectively depict the individual collaterals once contrast agent is administered, and pressure can be measured in the individual pulmonary segments (▶ Fig. 4.165c,f and ▶ Fig. 4.166c,d). This method is invasive and requires multiple injections of contrast agent and sometimes significant volume load. The examiner’s experience is also of vital importance for successfully depicting the pulmonary vascular bed. Furthermore, invasive angiography is also associated with radiation exposure.

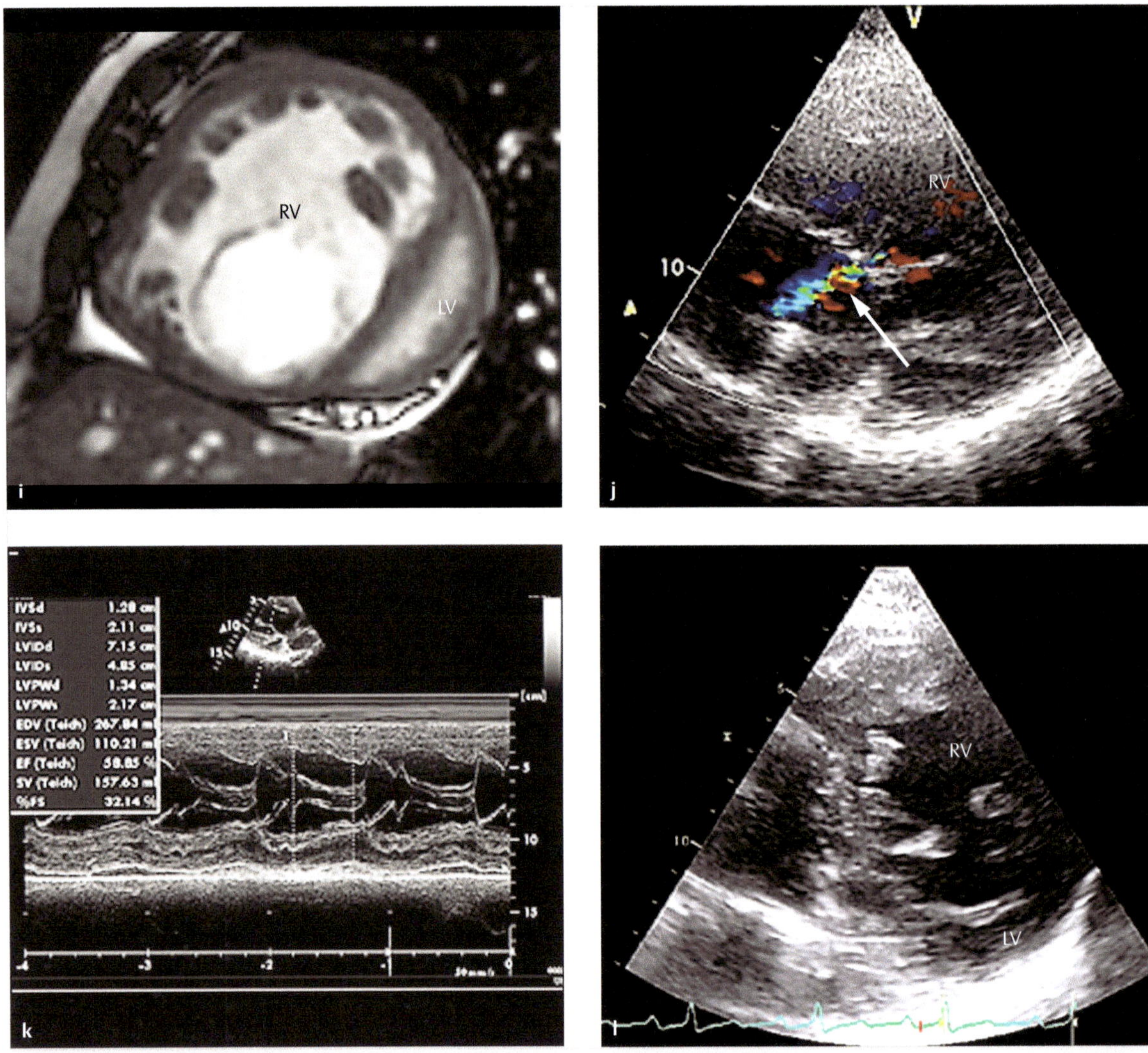

Fig 4.165 (*Continued*) **MAPCA.**
LV = left ventricle
RV = right ventricle
- **i** Cine SSFP MRI, short axis. Top view of the atrioventricular valve opened during diastole, and of the rudimentary, hypoplastic left ventricle.
- **j** 2-D TTE in color Doppler, 4-chamber view, also clearly depicting the atrioventricular valve insufficiency (arrow).
- **k** M-mode along the parasternal long axis depicting the right systemic ventricle, significantly enlarged during diastole, and a left ventricular diameter of 7.15 cm.
- **l** The short-axis slice of the 2-D TTE also depicts the opened atrioventricular valve and rudimentary, hypoplastic left ventricle.

For these reasons, contrast-enhanced *MRA* and, increasingly, *CTA* are good alternatives for depicting MAPCAs noninvasively for planning potential surgical or interventional treatment measures. The option to post-process 3-D and even 4-D data sets allows simultaneous depiction of vessels, which is often not possible during invasive cardiac catheterization. MIP reconstructions with thick slice reconstruction are particularly helpful (▶ Fig. 4.165b and ▶ Fig. 4.166b). "Flow control" using MAPCA closure (coiling) or stenosis treatment (▶ Fig. 4.165c), can currently only be performed via fluoroscopy. It does, however, benefit from good planning using noninvasive pretreatment imaging via MRA or CTA.

▶ **Acknowledgment.** We would like to thank Mr. Valverde for his critical review of the first draft of the manuscript, and for searching image examples.

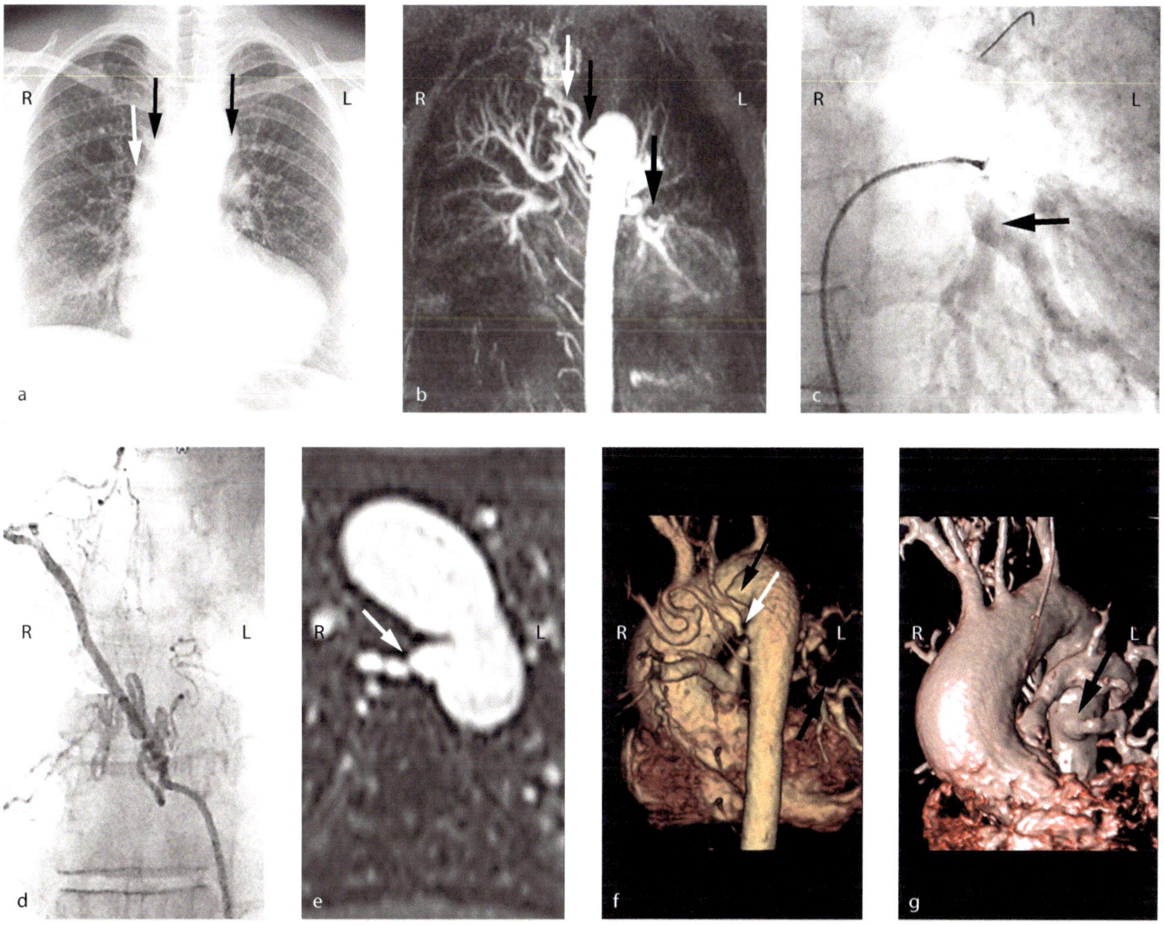

Fig. 4.166 MAPCA. Thirty-five-year-old female patient with valvular and supravalvular pulmonary atresia and a VSD. Multiple aortopulmonary collateral arteries (MAPCAs; arrows).

- **a** Multiple pulmonary collateral arteries (arrows) are faintly visible on the p.-a. chest radiograph (compare with (b)).
- **b** The MAPCAs (arrows) are definitely depicted in the 3-D MIP reconstruction of a contrast-enhanced MRA.
- **c** Selective, invasive catheter depiction of one of the MAPCAs (arrow; see **a**, **b**, thick black arrows).
- **d** Selective, invasive catheter depiction of another MAPCA (arrow; see **a**, **b**, white arrows).
- **e** The transverse reconstruction of the 3-D data from the MRA depicts an origin stenosis of the MAPCA from **d** (arrow; see **a**, **b**, white arrows) from the descending aorta to the right (dorsal view).
- **f** The 3-D reconstruction using volume rendering technique also depicts the origin stenosis of the MAPCA from **d** (white arrow; see **a**, **b**, white arrows). The thin black arrow indicates the MAPCA that is also marked in **a** and **b** using thin black arrows. The thick black arrow indicates the MAPCA that is also marked in **a** and **b** with thick black arrows.
- **g** The caudal left MAPCA from the selective depiction in **c** can be clearly seen from a ventral view (arrow; see **a**, **b**, thick black arrows).

Table 4.30 Utility of different imaging modalities for assessing major aortopulmonary collateral arteries (MAPCAs).

Parameter of interest	Echocardiography	Cardiac catheterization	MRI/MDCT
Pressure measurements	Not possible	Pressures can be measured invasively	Not possible
Interventional treatment options	None	Endovascular coiling	None
Mobility	Can be used at bedside	Stationary	Stationary
Coverage	Depends on acoustic window	Window not required	Window not required
Imaging options	2-D/3-D	2-D/3-D	2-D/3-D
User-dependence	User-dependent	Relatively standardized	Relatively standardized

MAPCAs, major aortopulmonary collateral arteries; MDCT, multidetector computed tomography; MRI, magnetic resonance imaging.

4.6 Other Disorders of the Heart and Great Vessels

4.6.1 Cardiomyopathies

Achim A. Schmaltz, Jens Bremerich, Matthias Gutberlet

There are currently two different classification systems for cardiomyopathies:

- the American classification, based primarily on etiology,[203] and
- the following classification created by the working group on myocardial and pericardial diseases of the European Society of Cardiology (ESC), based primarily on morphology.[204]

M!

Note

According to the ESC classification,[204] cardiomyopathies are disorders in which the cardiac muscle has undergone structural or functional changes in the absence of coronary heart disease, hypertonia, or valvular or congenital heart defects. They are classified as follows:

- *HCM:* hypertrophic cardiomyopathy
- *DCM:* dilated cardiomyopathy
- *ARVC:* arrhythmogenic right ventricular cardiomyopathy
- *RCM:* restrictive cardiomyopathy
- *Non-classified forms*

The distinction between primary and secondary (or other specific) forms is dropped in favor of a distinction between familial (genetic) and nonfamilial (nongenetic).

Hereinafter, the focus lies on cardiomyopathies that occur during childhood (also known as congenital), such as HCM, DCM, and a few other rare forms.

Hypertrophic Cardiomyopathy

Definition

HCM is a primary disorder of the cardiac sarcomere that causes left ventricular hypertrophy (which may differ in terms of severity and localization) for which no other cause is apparent.

Classification

In the traditional form, hypertrophy is especially pronounced in the ventricular septum (asymmetrical septal hypertrophy). This can lead to reduction of the left ventricular cavum (▶ Fig. 4.167, ▶ Fig. 4.168, and ▶ Fig. 4.169) or to obstruction of the LVOT and is then also referred to as "HOCM" (hypertrophic obstructive cardiomyopathy). Symmetrical, apical, and defined, tumorlike forms may also occur. Thickening of the endocardium near the septum may occur subaortically, and the mitral valve is often distorted and insufficient. From a histological perspective, HCM is characterized by nonparallel arrangement of the myofibrils (known as myofibrillar disarray) and fibrosis of varying severity.[205]

Etiology

With an incidence of 1:500 individuals, 55% of cases of HCM occur in patients with a familial, autosomal dominant genetic inheritance but differing penetration, while 45% of cases occur sporadically. Only 10 sarcomeric genes were known in 1989, as of now, more than 400 varying mutations have been described. Of these, the myosin heavy chain beta (MHC-ß), comprising 70–90% of cases, cardiac myosin-binding protein C, and cardiac troponin T are most commonly affected. In recent years, Z-disc, calcium transporter, and mitochondrial and lysosomal protein genes have been added. The same mutation has been identified both in HCM and DCM in individual cases.[206]

Clinical Issues

HCM most commonly manifests during adulthood, though the peak of the main complication—namely, sudden cardiac death—is during the second decade of life, and may even occur during infancy according to certain case reports. Children very rarely exhibit symptoms and only become clinically remarkable due to systolic murmur (▶ Fig. 4.167, ▶ Fig. 4.168, and ▶ Fig. 4.169). In adulthood, dyspnea and general limited physical exercise capacity are the main symptoms, though angina, palpitations, and (pre)syncope necessitate cardiological diagnostics.[203] This should draw particular attention to the potential risk factors for sudden cardiac death, which are summarized in ▶ Table 4.31.[204]

Indication for Treatment and Treatment Options

The goal of treatment is to eliminate symptoms and reduce risk factors for sudden cardiac death. Pharmacological treatment consists of administering beta blockers, calcium antagonists, or Disopyramide, though this has not yet been substantiated by prospective long-term studies. Amiodarone has been recommended to prevent ventricular tachycardia, but, like Disopyramide, has the drawback of lengthening the QT interval.

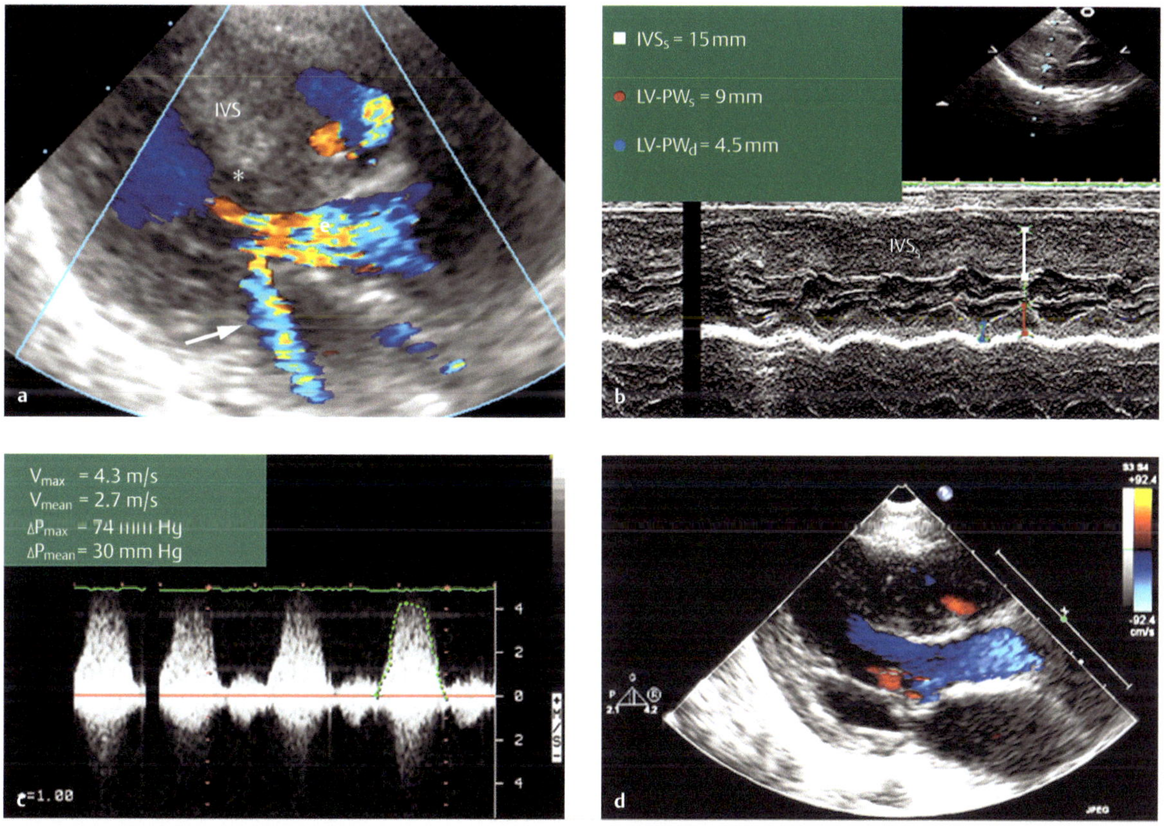

Fig. 4.167 HOCM. Three-month-old infant.
IVS = interventricular septum
IVSs = interventricular septum thickness during systole
LV-PWd = posterior left ventricular wall thickness during diastole
LV-PWs = posterior left ventricular wall thickness during systole
Δpmax = maximum pressure gradient
Δpmean = mean pressure gradient
Vmax = maximum flow velocity
Vmean = mean flow velocity

a Parasternal echocardiographic image, long axis, using color Doppler. The turbulence in the LVOT and pronounced mitral valve insufficiency can be seen clearly. The asterisk indicates the asymmetrical septal hypertrophy, while the arrow indicates the holosystolic insufficiency jet at the mitral valve in the direction of the left atrium.

b The severely thickened septum (IVS$_S$ = 15 mm) is clearly visible in M-mode.

c CW Doppler measured in the LVOT reveals a maximum flow velocity of more than 4 m/s, corresponding to a maximum instantaneous peak gradient of more than 74 mmHg.

d After a successful surgical myectomy at the age of 15 months, the LVOT is no longer narrowed, no relevant flow acceleration is depicted on Doppler images, and flow is laminal. No evidence of mitral insufficiency remains after surgery.

Table 4.31 Risk factors for sudden cardiac death in HCM patients.[204]

Traditional risk factors	Potential individual risk factors
• Young age	• LVOT obstruction
• Previous cardiac arrest	• Pronounced late gadolinium accumulation
• Unexplained syncope	• Myocardial ischemia
• Family history of sudden cardiac death	• Troponin T and troponin I mutations
• Ventricular wall thickness > 30 mm	• Atrial flutter
• Abnormal blood pressure response when under stress	• E/E_a quotient
• Intermittent ventricular tachycardia	

E/E_a, quotient calculated using the maximum early diastolic transmitral flow velocity and tissue Doppler parameters (longitudinal velocity in the lateral mitral ring); HCM, hypertrophic cardiomyopathy; LVOT, left ventricular outflow tract.

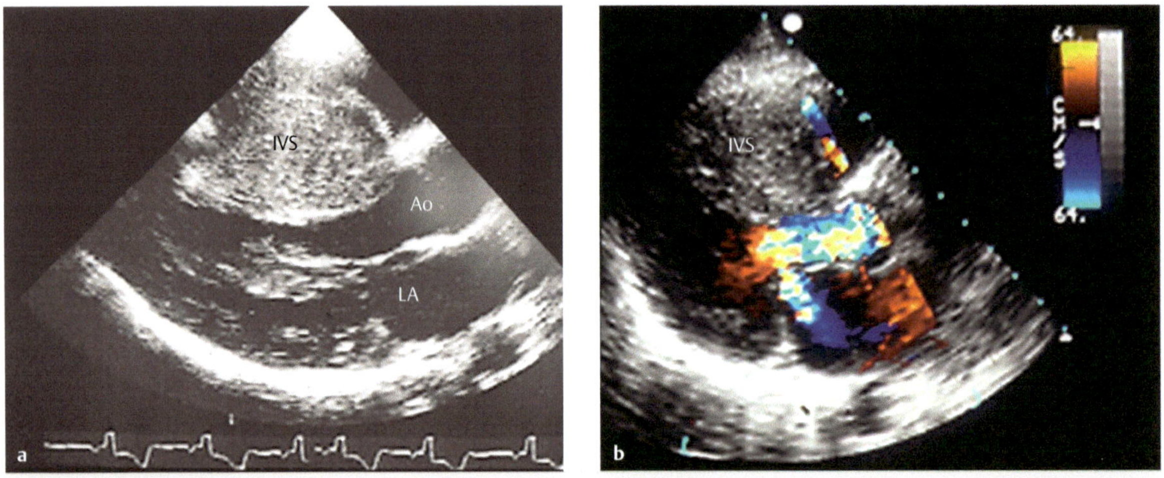

Fig. 4.168 Pompe disease.
Ao = aorta
IVS = interventricular septum
LA = left atrium
a 2-D TTE of an infant before beginning treatment, depicting a massively hypertrophied interventricular septum and obstruction of the LVOT.
b 2-D TTE, color Doppler, of the infant after 48 weeks of enzyme replacement therapy. The pronounced left ventricular hypertrophy has regressed significantly compared to **a**: the septum's thickness has decreased from 8.6 to 5.8 mm, and the thickness of the posterior wall from 11.0 to 5.4 mm, respectively.

Approximately 5% of patients reach a final stage resulting in a need for treatment for heart failure.[204] An additional 5–30% of all HCM patients possess an indication for invasive or surgical treatments under the following prerequisites:

- Gradient in the LVOT of more than 50 mmHg (▸ Fig. 4.167c,d)
- Symptoms that are limiting and resistant to pharmaceutical treatment
- NYHA class III or IV occurring in adulthood

Transaortic myectomy (▸ Fig. 4.170), according to Morrow,[207] has become the surgical treatment method of choice for children and adults. In experienced centers, this procedure has a surgical mortality rate of less than 1%, a recurrence rate of less than 2%, and a mortality rate of 0.5% each year.[208]

Alcohol-induced septal ablation is an alternative[209] method in which absolute (dehydrated) alcohol (see ▸ Fig. 4.170) is injected, causing circumscribed infarction, regression of the septal muscular bulge, and obstruction of the LVOT. This procedure appears to have a low mortality rate and a high success rate, though is associated with a high rate of atrioventricular blockage and pacemaker implantation.[209]

Dual-chamber pacing is another treatment option, though it has limited effectiveness.

Goals and Relative Value of Diagnostic Imaging

The goal of diagnostics is to verify the presence of the disorder and to determine and localize myocardial thickening and left (or in rarer cases, right) ventricular gradients, as well as to reveal cardiac rhythm disorders and rule out specific types.

ECG is preferable for depicting signs of left ventricular hypertrophy with negative T waves, but other findings (such as giant T waves) are depicted in the apical form. Long-term ECG reveals sustained or intermittent ventricular tachycardia, atrial fibrillation, or other rhythm disorders.

Echocardiography is the decisive, noninvasive imaging method of choice. The traditional criteria for M-mode (▸ Fig. 4.177b) and 2-D echocardiography of the HCM,[210] which can theoretically also be applied to other imaging modalities, are summarized as follows (see ▸ Fig. 4.167):

- Asymmetrical septal hypertrophy (septum/posterior wall ratio larger than 1.3)
- Hypodynamic septum
- Systolic anterior motion (SAM) of the mitral valve
- Anterior position of the mitral valve apparatus
- Increased diastolic apposition time of the mitral cusp to the septum
- Early systolic aortic valve closure
- Narrow left ventricle or narrow left ventricular cavum
- Flow acceleration in the LVOT
- Mitral valve insufficiency

In these cases, a precise perpendicular view or section using MRI or CT is decisive for determining the reliability of the measurement of wall thickness (▸ Fig. 4.167a,b). If HOCM is present, subvalvular stenoses and mitral valve insufficiency can be clearly depicted using color Doppler (▸ Fig. 4.167a).

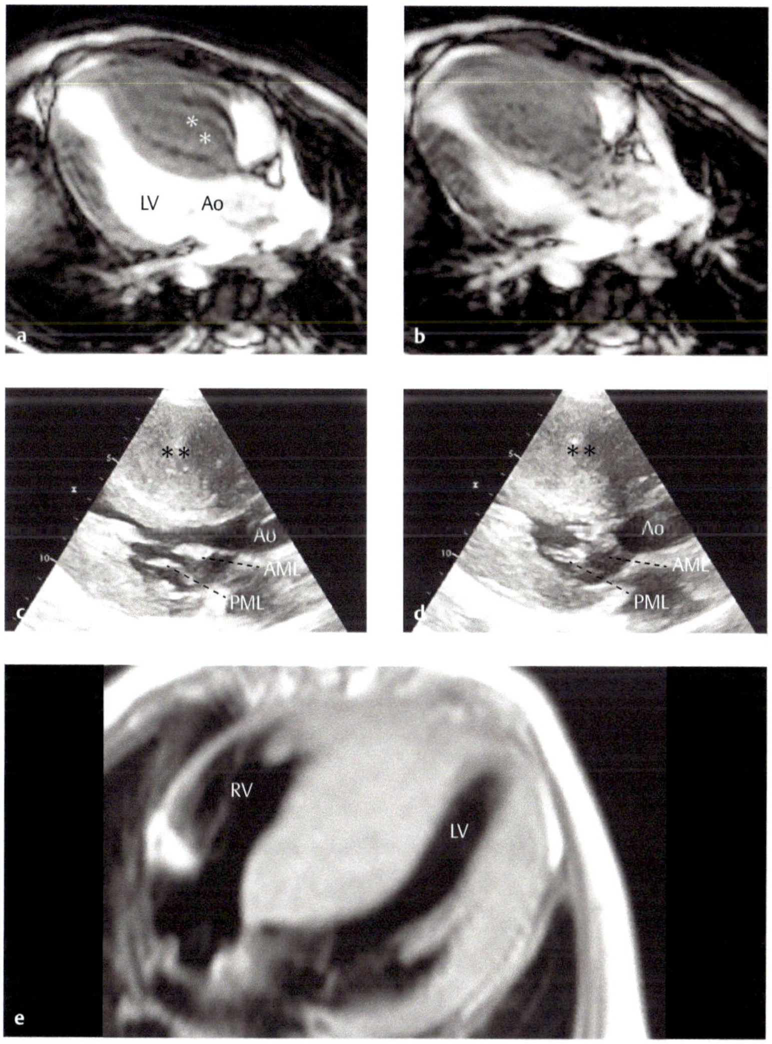

Fig. 4.169 Familial HOCM. Six-year-old boy, whose father is also affected by the disorder. Both the SSFP cine MRIs through the LVOT (a, b) and the 2-D echocardiographic images along the parasternal long axis (c, d) depict the pronounced, asymmetrical thickening, particularly of the interventricular septum (a–d, double asterisks), with a maximum end diastolic thickness of 36 mm. During systole (b), a typical systolic anterior motion phenomenon of the anterior mitral leaflet within the LVOT is clearly depicted, both in MRIs (b) (due to dephasing) and in 2-D echocardiography (d). Due to the nearly complete filling of the left ventricular cavum (b, d), a typical "hypernormal" left ventricular ejection fraction of 85% was determined. Left ventricular muscle mass was measured at 184 g/m2 using MRI (standard: 59–106 g/m2).
AML = anterior mitral leaflet
Ao = aorta
LV = left ventricle
PML = posterior mitral leaflet
RV = right ventricle

- **a** SSFP cine MRI through the LVOT during diastole.
- **b** SSFP cine MRI through the LVOT during systole.
- **c** 2-D TTE depiction, parasternal long axis, during diastole.
- **d** d 2-D echocardiographic image, parasternal long axis, during systole.
- **e** Transverse black blood SE sequence.

> **Note**
>
> Obstructions of the LVOT are only present in 25% of patients when at rest, and are even rarer in children. Consequently, performing a physiological stress test (e.g., using a bicycle ergometer) is all the more important for determining diagnosis. These tests reveal a gradient in 75% of patients.[211]

Tissue Doppler and the derived parameters—namely deformation (strain) and deformation rate (strain rate)—offer new options.[212] Systolic and early diastolic longitudinal maximum velocities in the basal wall segments of the left ventricle are reduced. This allows the quotient, calculated using the maximum early diastolic transmitral flow velocity E and tissue Doppler parameter E_a (longitudinal velocity in the lateral mitral ring), to estimate end diastolic pressure in the left ventricle. Ho et al.[213] were able to determine a positive genotype within the scope of an extensive familial examination using genotyping, with a specificity of 86% and a sensitivity of 75%, using an E_a velocity of less than 13.5 m/s, even in cases where no clinical symptoms had become manifest. On the other end of the disorder spectrum, a high E/E_a quotient (above 20.74) can be seen as a predictor of mortality, ventricular tachycardia, or syncope.[214]

When using an ECG-triggered SSFP cine sequence, *MRI* allows precise measurement of the left ventricular mass and wall thickness in all cardiac segments (▶ Fig. 4.169a,b, ▶ Fig. 4.176b,c) after manually outlining endocardial and epicardial borders. Left ventricular mass above the standard of 46–83 g/m^2 in men or 37–67 g/m^2 in women is considered hypertrophic.[215] As a result, determining physiological hypertrophy thresholds for athletes can be decidedly difficult in certain cases. In these cases, the quotient of diastolic wall strength and diastolic left ventricular volume—which should not exceed 0.15 (mm × m^2)/ml (specificity of 99%) in athletes—can also be helpful.[216] In contrast, left

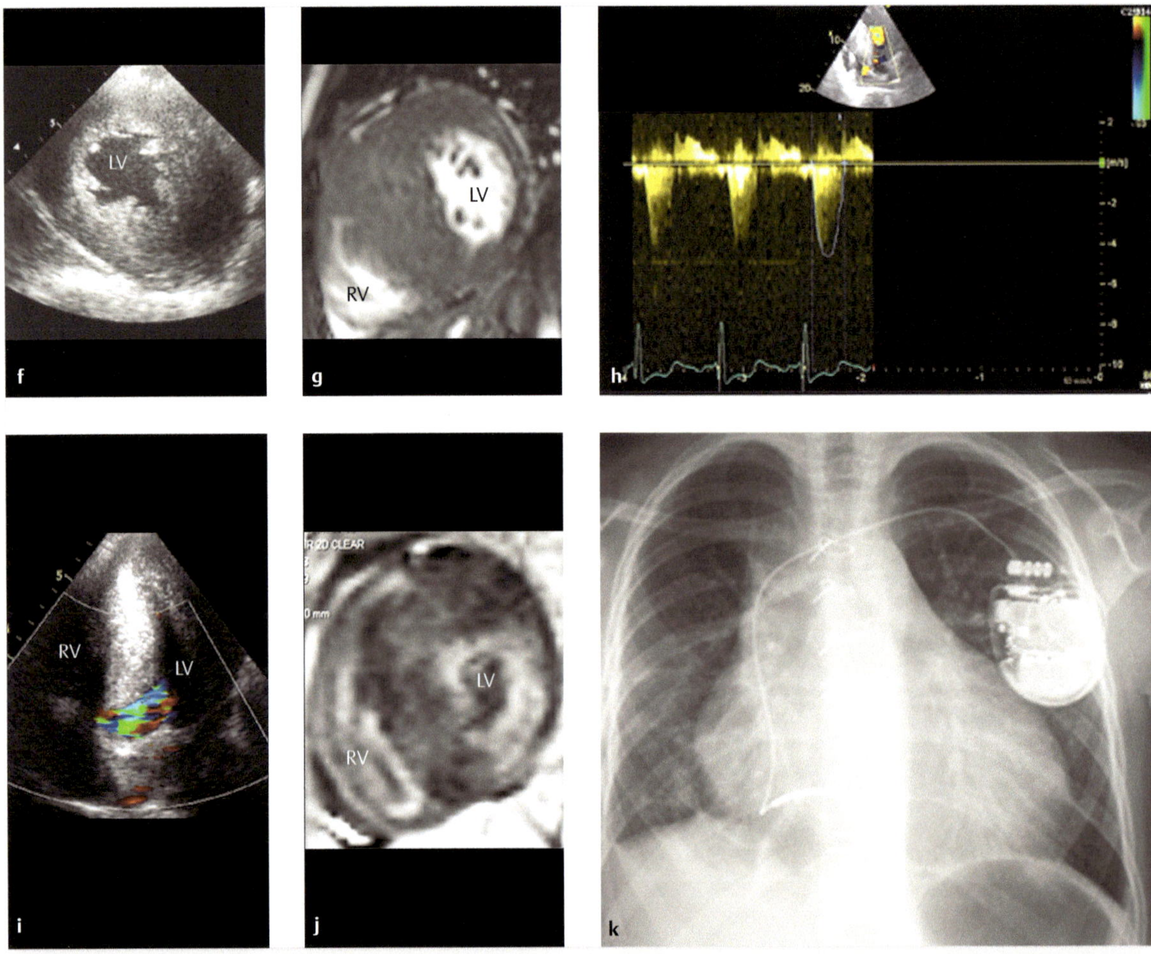

Fig 4.169 *(Continued)* **Familial HOCM.**

AML = anterior mitral leaflet
Ao = aorta
LV = left ventricle
PML = posterior mitral leaflet
RV = right ventricle

- **f** 2-D TTE, short axis, during end diastole.
- **g** Corresponding SSFP cine MRI, short axis, during end diastole.
- **h** CW Doppler near the LVOT. This yielded a maximum measured flow velocity of 4.6 m/s in line with an estimated maximum instantaneous pressure gradient of 84 mmHg.
- **i** Color Doppler near the LVOT, depicting systolic turbulence due to increased flow velocity.
- **j** Inversion recovery GE image, short axis, for late enhancement depiction with diffuse fibrosis formation.
- **k** Thoracic X-ray, of the same patient at the age of 10, after implantation of an ICD.

ventricular mass remains within the normal range in 20% of HOCM patients.[217] One significant advantage of MRI compared to echocardiography is the opportunity to perform absolutely perpendicular cross-sectional imaging through the left ventricular wall. This allowed Rickers et al.[218] to discover 10% more HOCM patients that were not diagnosed accurately using echocardiographic images. This is especially true in anatomical variants of the apical or midventricular HCM (▶ Fig. 4.169b). MRI also clearly depicts abnormalities of the mitral valve apparatus, including systolic anterior motion (SAM) of the anterior mitral leaflet and the subsequent mitral valve insufficiency (▶ Fig. 4.169b). The latter is believed, based on current knowledge, to result more from the impetus of the blood on the elongated chordae than from the Venturi effect.[208] In these cases, analyzing late gadolinium accumulation or late enhancement based on its pattern of occurrence and distribution in differential diagnosis of secondary forms is helpful. In these instances, late enhancement can be traced back to the rupturing of necrotic cell membranes and the subsequent increased distribution volume, as well as fibrotic rearrangement.[219] ▶ Table 4.32 summarizes the most important secondary forms of HCM, as well as their characteristics in MRI[220,221]; ▶ Fig. 4.171 and ▶ Fig. 4.172 depict two examples. Successful

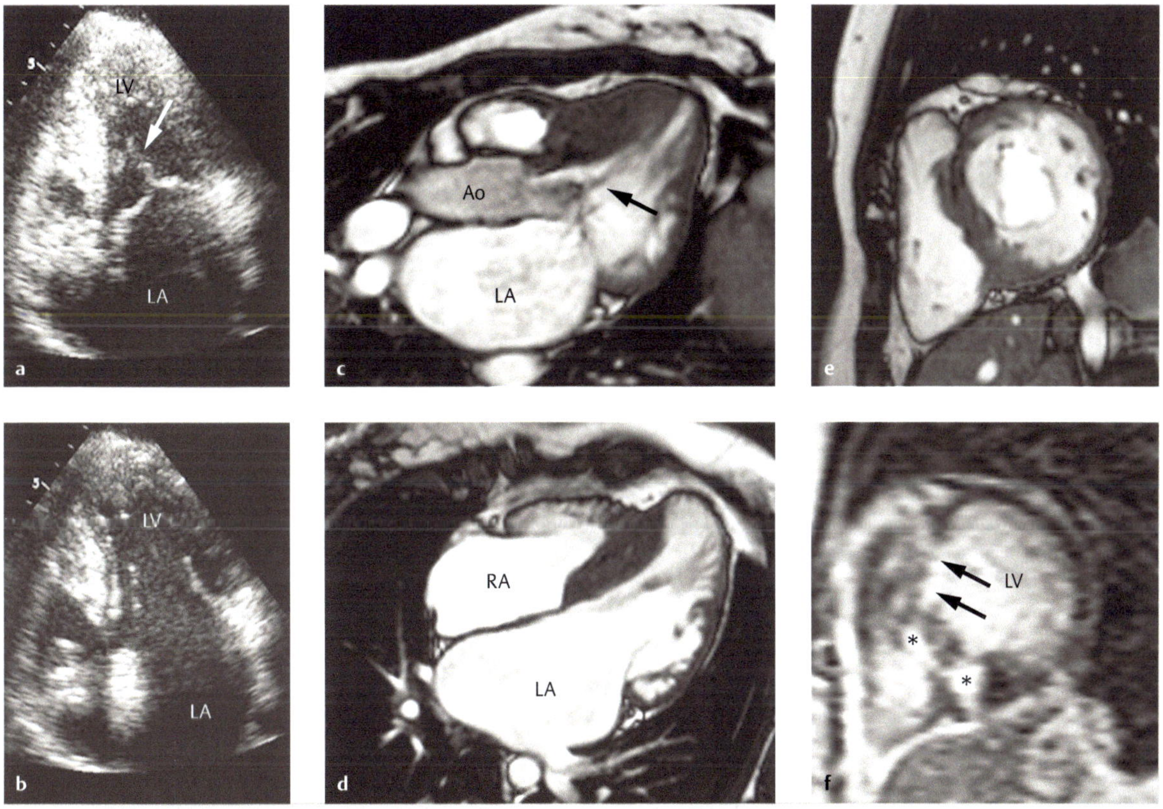

Fig. 4.170 Condition after two myectomies and transcoronary ablation of septal hypertrophy in a case of HOCM. Twenty-three-year-old woman with HOCM. Both the echocardiography (a, b) and MRIs of the LVOT (c) and MRI, 4-chamber view (d) depict a massively enlarged left atrium due to the formerly pronounced mitral valve insufficiency. The maximum flow velocity in the LVOT was measured at Vmax = 2.1 m/s using the MR phase contrast technique and CW Doppler, suggesting a small residual gradient. The anterior septal segments of the late enhancement (f) are caused by the therapeutically intended scar formation due to myectomy and septal ablation (arrows). The other patchwork-like, diffuse septal fibrosis (asterisk) is a part of the typical late enhancement pattern of HCM.

Ao = aorta
LA = left atrium
LV = left ventricle
RA = right atrium

- **a** Residual systolic anterior motion (SAM) phenomenon in the LVOT (arrow) in the 2-D TTE, 4-chamber view during systole.
- **b** 2-D TTE, 4-chamber view during diastole.
- **c** The residual systolic anterior motion (SAM) phenomenon in the LVOT (arrow) is also visible using the SSFP cine MRI sequence. The residual turbulence results in dephasing (black jet during systole, arrow).
- **d** SSFP cine MRI, 4-chamber view during diastole.
- **e** e SSFP cine MRI, short-axis view, with normal mitral valve opening during diastole.
- **f** Typical patchwork-like, pronounced late enhancement (asterisks) near the insertion point of the right ventricle using an inversion recovery GE MRI sequence, caused in part by myectomy and septal ablation (arrows).

septal thinning can be documented after surgical myectomy or alcohol ablation by means of MRI (▶ Fig. 4.170). In the future, it may be possible to use late enhancement and potentially also parametric imaging (such as T1 and T2 mapping) to stratify patient risk, especially in children.[222–224]

MDCT only plays a role in certain cases, such as after placement of an ICD (▶ Fig. 4.173).

If the noninvasive findings are unambiguous and there is a family history of the disorder, cardiac catheterization does not offer any new information (with the exception of coronary diagnostics in older patients). On the other hand, if the concentric form is present—especially in younger patients—*endomyocardial biopsy* may be the first method to reveal proof of a secondary form (Pompe disease, Fabry disease, amyloidosis) and cardiac involvement. ▶ Fig. 4.168 depicts an infant with Pompe disease immediately after diagnosis, and then after 48 weeks of enzyme replacement therapy, with significant regression of left ventricular hypertrophy.

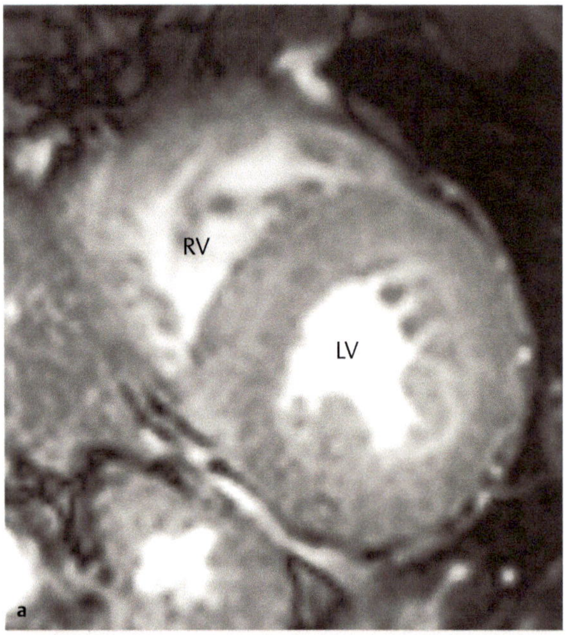

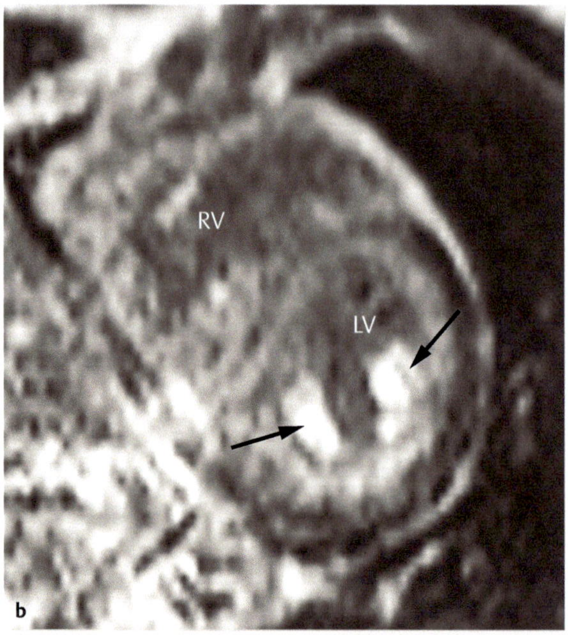

Fig. 4.171 Amyloidosis. Patient with systemic amyloidosis with cardiac involvement.
LV = left ventricle
RV = right ventricle

a The SSFP cine MRI sequence, short axis, depicts pronounced left ventricular hypertrophy.

b The phase image of the PSIR sequence depicts the typical circular, subendocardial "early" late enhancement (5 minutes after administering contrast agent) with involvement of the papillary muscles (arrow).

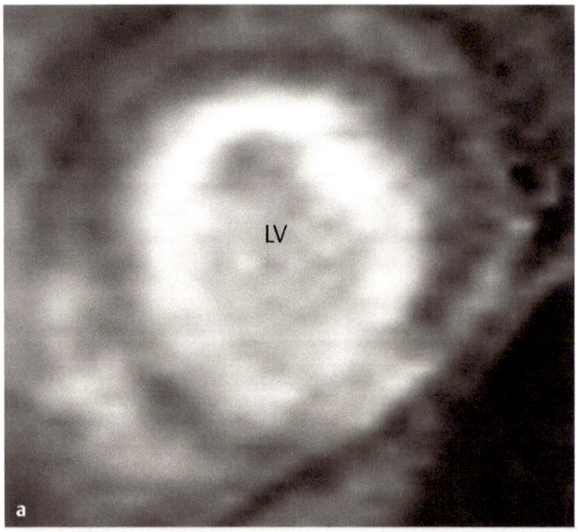

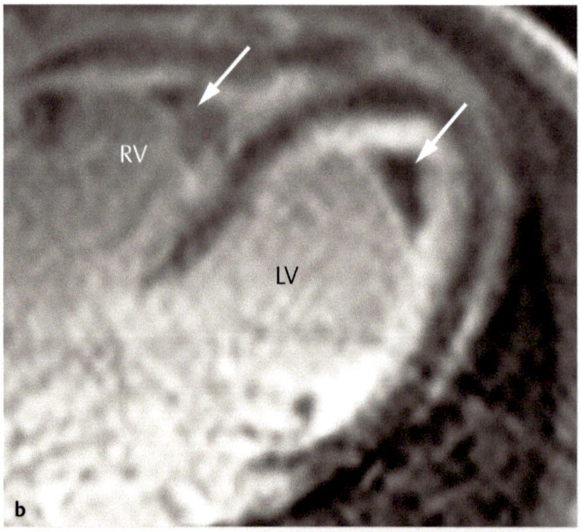

Fig. 4.172 Endomyocardial fibrosis. Seventeen-year-old male patient. Circular, subendocardial contrast agent accumulation is visible in the late enhancement sequence, as well as an apical thrombus in the left (arrow) and right ventricle (arrow).
LV = left ventricle
RV = right ventricle

a Late enhancement sequence, apical short-axis view.

b Late enhancement sequence, 4-chamber view.

Table 4.32 Differential diagnostic MRI pattern of occurrence for various secondary forms of HCM.[220,221]

Forms of HCM	MRI indications
Amyloidosis	• Late contrast enhancement in the entire myocardium (note the issue of "nullifying" the myocardium with the correct inversion pulse) • Particularly circular, subendocardial late enhancement, if measured early (less than 5–10 minutes after administering contrast agent; see ▶ Fig. 4.171; note that gadolinium is flushed from the amyloid faster than from the fibrotic focus) • Often late enhancement in papillary muscles (▶ Fig. 4.171b) • In 50% of cases pericardial and pleural effusion
Fabry disease	Late contrast enhancement, especially in the inferolateral base of the heart, but only in 50% of patients
Endomyocardial fibrosis with hypereosinophilia	• Subendocardial contrast enhancement • Thrombus formation (▶ Fig. 4.172) • Puckering of the mitral valve apparatus
Sarcoidosis	• Cardiac involvement only in 27% of cases • Contrast enhancement in all patients, often strongly pronounced in the subepicardium like in cases of myocarditis

HCM, hypertrophic cardiomyopathy; MRI, magnetic resonance imaging.

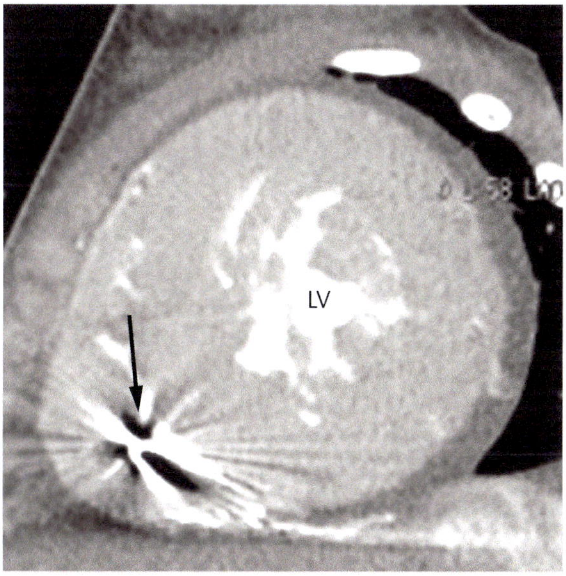

Fig. 4.173 Familial HOCM. Six-year-old boy. Short-axis MDCT reconstruction after implantation of an ICD. The arrow indicates the hardening artifact caused by the ICD lead within the likewise hypertrophic right ventricle.
LV = left ventricle

Dilated Cardiomyopathy

Definition

DCM is defined as a dilatation of one or both ventricles, for which an ischemic or post-inflammatory cause has been excluded. Its pathophysiology is based on a systolic dysfunction leading to increased diastolic pressure and wall stress that reduces the oxygen supply to the myocardium. The main histologic features of DCM are myocyte hypertrophy with increased nuclear DNA but decreased myofibrils, a variable degree of fibrosis, and an increased number of interstitial lymphocytes. Electron microscopy reveals mitochondriosis with degenerative changes and myelin figures.

Etiology and Frequency

DCM is a disorder that rarely occurs in childhood, with an incidence of only 0.34–0.86 per 100,000 children each year,[225,226] 5.5 cases of illness, and a prevalence of 36.5% per 100,000 people in the total population each year.[227] No cause can be found for two-thirds of pediatric cases (idiopathic DCM), though 16% of cases are caused by a condition after myocarditis and 9% by neuromuscular disorders, respectively. Familiar, metabolic, or syndromic disorders are rarer.[227] It is believed that familial, genetic DCM accounts for 30–50% of idiopathic forms, though this number may be even higher.[228] In recent years, numerous mutations in more than 20 genes have been identified, of which lamin A/C (LMNA) mutations may progress along a particularly malignant course.[229] This can be associated not just with DCM, but also with various forms of muscular dystrophy, lipodystrophy, neuropathy, and progeria. The proportion of post-myocarditis causes for DCM is lower, and ischemic etiology are correspondingly higher in adult patients.[230]

Clinical Issues

In pediatric patients, the disease originates during the first 2 years of life in three-fourths of cases. Often, cardiomegaly (see Myocarditis) occurs within the scope of febrile infection. Just like adults, other children may possess uncharacteristic symptoms of heart failure, such as fatigue, lack of exercise capacity, nutritional disorders, a failure to thrive, tachydyspnea, persistent cough, peripheral cyanosis, and a tendency toward edema. These also

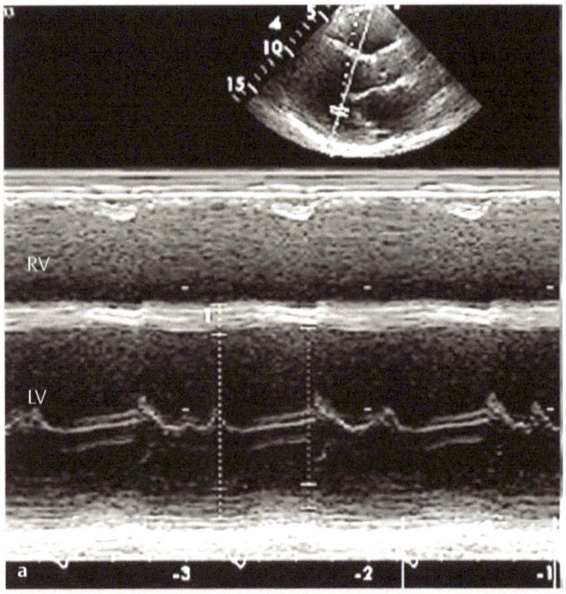

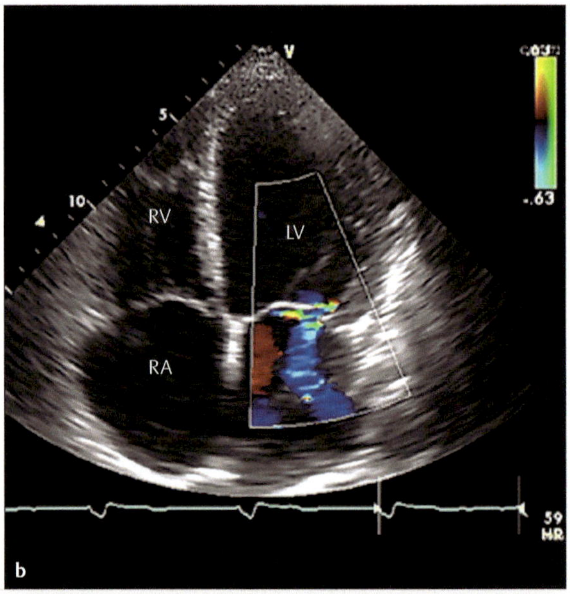

Fig. 4.174 DCM. 2-D transthoracic echocardiography in a 16-year-old boy with severe DCM (end diastolic diameter of 84 mm, end systolic diameter of 74 mm, fractional shortening of 12%) on the day before a left ventricular assist device was placed.
LV = left ventricle
RA = right atrium
RV = right ventricle
a M-Mode.
b Apical 4-chamber view, color Doppler, depicting pronounced mitral valve incompetence.

include primary complications—such as embolism, syncope, or other severe cardiac rhythm disorders—which are the initial symptoms that lead to diagnosis. The prognosis is poor: the pediatric cardiomyopathy register in the United States lists the portion of patients that did not die or require a transplant within 1 year at 69%, sinking to just 54% after 5 years.[226] Similar numbers were reported in the adult register. Felker et al. found a 10-year survival rate of less than 60%, and up to 30% of deaths were sudden.[230]

Treatment Options

Treatment for DCM is similar to that for heart failure: while the medication Digitalis only improves subjective symptoms and reduces the occurrence of hospitalization, it has no effect on survival rates. ACE inhibitors, diuretics, and slowly increased dosed beta blockers are the evidence-based treatment method for adult patients. There is little pertinent data for pediatric patients.[231] In order to prevent intracavitary and peripheral thrombi, anticoagulation treatment using coumarins is recommended during childhood, especially if a shortening fraction of less than 20% is present. Propafenones, Sotalol, or Amiodarone is recommended for anti-arrhythmia treatment, depending on the type of rhythm disorder.

Implanting an ICD can reduce the mortality rate to 30% in adult patients. If no significant contraindications (severe disorders of the central nervous system, kidneys, liver, or lungs) are present, a left ventricular assist device (▸ Fig. 4.174) or heart transplant is the last-resort treatment method.

Goals and Relative Value of Diagnostic Imaging

The goal of diagnostics is to determine the extent of left ventricular enlargement and functional impairment, reveal potential complications, and provide evidence of specific causes (particularly in cases of potential inflammatory genesis (see Myocarditis)).

ECG findings are inconsistent. Signs of left ventricular hypertrophy and a disrupted repolarization phase are usually present. It is crucial to perform a long-term ECG in order to reveal ventricular dysrhythmia and/or atrioventricular blockages and to begin anti-arrhythmic treatment.

Echocardiography clearly depicts left ventricular dilatation and reduced ventricular function. A left ventricular ejection fraction of less than 30% or a tissue Doppler velocity in the tricuspid valve ring of less than 8.5 cm/s can be predictors of urgent hospitalization, transplant, or even death in children.[232] Intracavitary thrombi are verified in a not-insubstantial number of cases.

MRI allows wall thickness and left ventricular mass, volume, and ejection fraction to be measured more precisely than echocardiography. This allowed Koikkalainen et al.[233] to use an elaborate computer program to generate a global cardiac function index (using numerous measurements of this type) in order to recognize individuals affected by familial DCM with LMNA mutations during the subclinical stage. The late gadolinium enhancement (LGE) reveals fibrosis, typically occurring in the middle of the septal left ventricular wall, as mid-wall enhancement. Fibrosis is also a predictor of death if ventricular tachycardia is also present.[234] Post-inflammatory DCM, on the other hand, typically indicates subepicardial late enhancement.[219] In addition to characterizing tissue in order to assess prognosis, MRI provides proof of the etiology by using edema-sensitive or inflammation-sensitive sequences (see Myocarditis). In the near future, MRI may also be able to use parametric imaging by means of T1 and T2 mapping to provide further explanation of the etiology of cardiomyopathies.[235]

Invasive diagnostics using cardiac catheterization and angiocardiography help rule out other structural anomalies, as well as coronary anomalies, particularly in infants. This can, however, often be detected by means of echocardiography, MRI, or even MDCT (if the corresponding dose-reduction protocols are used). Endomyocardial biopsy remains the method of choice for differentiating the disorder from endocardial fibroelastosis and chronic myocarditis.[219,235]

Rare Forms

Restrictive Cardiomyopathy

Definition and Etiology

RCM, which is particularly rare in childhood, is characterized by limited diastolic compliance in a case of normal systolic function. The atria are dilated significantly, while the ventricles often remain unremarkable. In recent years, familial forms with sarcomere gene mutations have been described.[236] Restrictive physiology also occurs in cases of amyloidosis (▶ Fig. 4.171) and endomyocardial fibrosis, whereby the former can generally be differentiated from HCM using MRI or other methods.

Clinical Issues and Natural Progression

Patients present with symptoms of severe heart failure and, if they do not receive transplants, die shortly after diagnosis.

Goals and Relative Value of Diagnostic Imaging

ECG reveals P-dextrocardia. echocardiography and MRI clearly depict the enlarged atria and the unremarkable ventricular size and systolic function. When using Doppler echocardiography, the E wave is significantly larger than the A wave when recording mitral flow, and a dip and plateau phenomenon occurs when recording pressure.

Arrhythmogenic Right Ventricular Dysplasia/Cardiomyopathy

Definition

ARVC is a genetic, autosomal-dominant inherited defect—currently with 10 known genetic variants—in which the myocardium of the right ventricle is destroyed by apoptosis and replaced by fatty and fibrotic tissue.[237,238]

Clinical Issues and Natural Progression

Due to the replacement of the right ventricular myocardium by fatty and fibrotic tissue, the right ventricular wall becomes very thin. Pulmonary circulation is sometimes maintained solely by the contraction of the right atrium. The illness can also affect the left ventricle as the patient ages. Patients generally begin to exhibit symptoms during their second decade of life or even later (▶ Fig. 4.175, ▶ Fig. 4.176, and ▶ Fig. 4.177). As a result, very few cases occurring during childhood have been reported. Prevalence is between 1 in 1,000 and 1 in 5,000 during adulthood.[237] Ventricular arrhythmia (especially under stress), persistent tachycardia with left bundle branch block in three-fourths of cases, and signs of heart failure in the remaining cases are clinically prominent.

Treatment Options

Treatment consists of avoiding physical exertion, beta blockers, and implanting an ICD (▶ Fig. 4.176a).

Goals and Relative Value of Diagnostic Imaging

Numerous major and minor diagnostic criteria have been developed, which are summarized in ▶ Table 4.33 in light of imaging procedures, an updated version compared to the original McKenna criteria.[238]

From a diagnostic perspective, *ECG* (negative T in V 1–3/4; epsilon wave) and long-term ECG are the first-choice methods.

Echocardiography reveals clearly visible, significantly enlarged right ventricular dimensions, reduced right ventricular function, and local wall motion abnormalities and small ventricular aneurysms, especially in children (▶ Fig. 4.175a, b). It is often difficult to access the right ventricle and particularly the RVOT in older children and adults.

MRI can help to assess right ventricular size and function even without limitations to the acoustic window[219] and can generally differentiate clearly between muscle, fat, and fibrotic tissue using a suitable sequence, i.e., T1w and T2w black blood SE sequences, and late enhancement sequences (▶ Fig. 4.175c,d, ▶ Fig. 4.176d-f). Though this characteristic can be considered an indicator of prognosis, it is not included in the guidelines as a fixed diagnostic marker, since assessing wall thinning and fat distribution can also lead to overdiagnosis.[239]

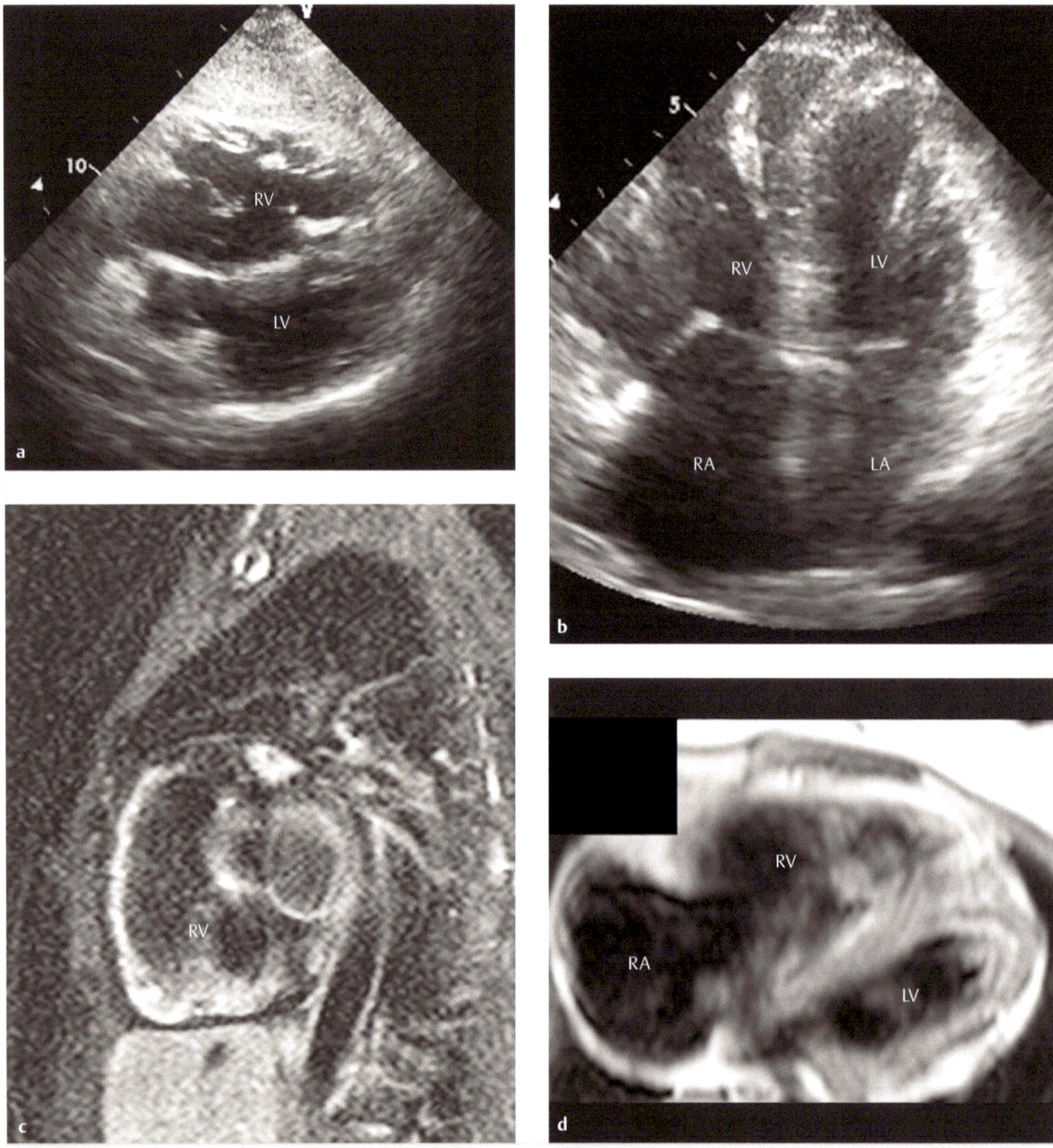

Fig. 4.175 ARVC. Fifty-year-old female patient with sustained ventricular tachycardia, electrophysiological indicators of ARVC, and significantly reduced exercise capacity. The 2-D TTE (a, b) and MRI (c–f) both depict a massively enlarged right ventricle. The maximum diameter of the RVOT along the parasternal long axis was 42 mm. Right ventricular ejection fraction was measured at 21% using MRI. Multiple small aneurysms (f, asterisks) were visible, meaning that imaging depicted the major criteria (▶ Table 4.33) for ARVC. Note that despite the pronounced late enhancement (c) in the free wall of the right ventricle, indicating fibrous tissue, this cannot be characterized as a major criterion. This is only true of histological confirmation. A fatty infiltration in the free wall of the right ventricle cannot be clearly depicted in the T1w black blood SE sequence (d), transverse slice, due to the flow artifacts caused by slow flow.

LA = left atrium
LV = left ventricle
RA = right atrium
RV = right ventricle
RVOT = right ventricular outflow tract

a 2-D TTE, substernal view.
b 2-D TTE, 4-chamber view.
c MRI late enhancement sequence, short axis, depicting a significant accumulation in the free wall of the enlarged right ventricle.
d T1w black blood SE sequence, transverse slice.

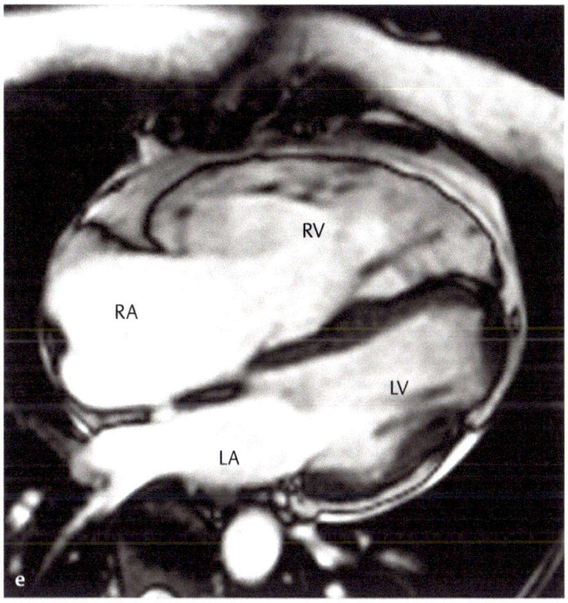

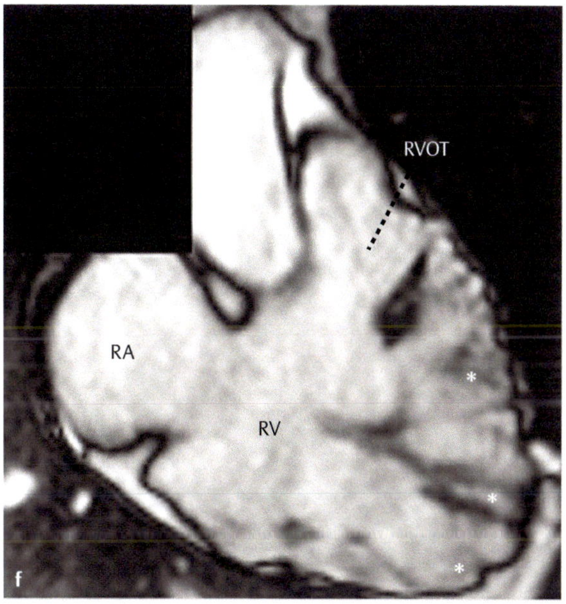

Fig 4.175 (*Continued*) **ARVC.**
LA = left atrium
LV = left ventricle
RA = right atrium
RV = right ventricle
RVOT = right ventricular outflow tract

e Corresponding SSFP cine MRI, 4-chamber view.
f SSFP cine MRI, long axis, through the right ventricle and RVOT. Multiple small aneurysms (asterisks) are visible.

> **Note**
>
> Detection of fibrosis or fat tissue by *MRI* cannot, to date, be considered a major diagnostic criterion. Diagnosis of fibro-fatty replacement is only possible using the histological results of the biopsy (▶ Table 4.33).[238]

The advantages of echocardiographic and especially MR imaging procedures are based primarily on the standard right ventricular volumetric values, which should ideally be based on the body's surface area (▶ Table 4.33).

Despite the generally good anatomical depiction of the right ventricle (▶ Fig. 4.176d,c) and the general ability to quantify the tissue-to-fat ratio, *MDCT* only plays a role if MRI is contraindicated, since the former is associated with radiation exposure. *Invasive diagnostics* are limited to electrophysiological examinations, ruling out coronary heart disease, and potentially collecting samples for biopsy.

Left Ventricular Noncompaction

Definition and Etiology

Left ventricular noncompaction cardiomyopathy (also known as "spongy myocardium") is a disorder of myocardial morphogenesis, in which compaction of the myocardial network malfunctions between the fifth and eighth weeks of embryonic development, resulting in a characteristic myocardial morphology. The compact external wall layer comprises less than one-third of the left ventricular wall, while the spongy, noncompacted trabecular network and deep recesses comprise more than two-thirds of the left ventricular wall inferior to the papillary muscles.

Noncompaction cardiomyopathy can occur in isolation, can affect both ventricles, or may be associated with other defects (▶ Fig. 4.178 and ▶ Fig. 4.179),[240,241] though it may also occur in conjunction with neuromuscular disorders, Barth syndrome, or mitochondrial disorders. In addition to rarer sporadic cases, autosomal dominant,

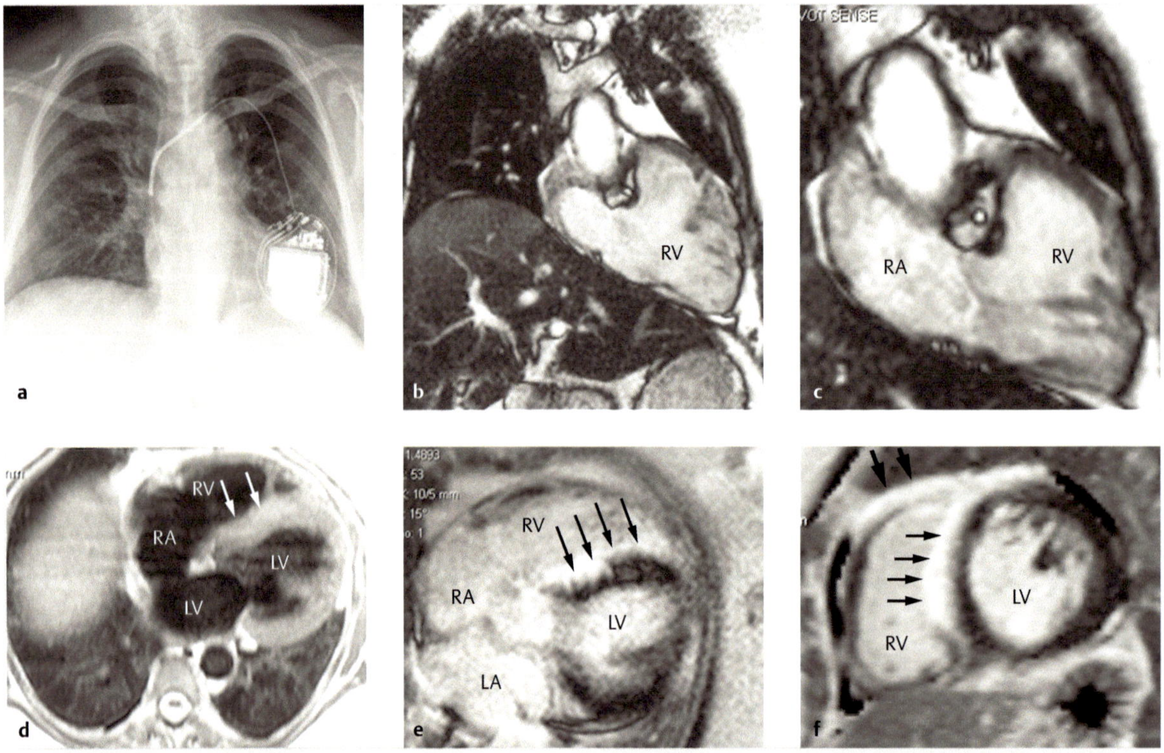

Fig. 4.176 ARVC. Fifty-five-year-old woman with sustained ventricular tachycardia and ARVC. The SSFP cine MRIs through the RVOT (b, c) depict the dilatated right ventricle with local dyskinesia, and a right ventricular EDV of 105 ml/m² (exceeding the threshold for a major criterion for women). The right ventricular ejection fraction, at 45%, was decreased only slightly, and therefore only a minor criterion for an ARVC according to the recent ESC Guidelines. Despite left ventricular involvement in late enhancement (d-f, small arrows) of the right ventricular side of the interventricular septum as an indicator for fibrosis or scar and diffuse fat deposits in the T1w SE sequences (d), the left ventricular ejection fraction, measured at 55%, remained in the normal range. Note that even the late enhancement in the anterior free wall of the right ventricle (f, large arrow) cannot be assessed as a major criterion. Only the endomyocardial biopsy is considered a major criterion.

LA = left atrium
LV = left ventricle
RA = right atrium
RV = right ventricle

- **a** P.-a. thoracic X-ray after implantation of an ICD 1 week after diagnosing ARVC.
- **b** SSFP cine MRI through the right ventricle and RVOT during diastole.
- **c** SSFP cine MRI through the right ventricle and RVOT during systole, with no significant inward wall motion. The cross-sectional lumen of the right coronary artery in the atrioventricular groove is clearly visible.
- **d** T1w SE sequence, transverse slice orientation, with fat deposits in the septum (arrows).
- **e** MRI late enhancement sequence, 4-chamber view, with significant septal and right ventricular LGE (arrows).
- **f** MRI late enhancement sequence, short axis, with significant LGE on the anterior septum (small arrows) and the free wall of the right ventricle (large arrows).

autosomal recessive, and X-chromosome inheritability has been observed in families, including mutations in various genes including G4.5, Cypher/ZASP, dystrobrevin alpha (DTNA), Lamin A/C (LMNA), and others.[242]

Clinical Issues and Treatment Options

Children and adults present with symptoms of cardiac insufficiency in up to 80% of cases. In rarer instances, ventricular tachycardia, atrial flutter, and thromboembolism complications have been observed.

Treatment is geared toward cardiac insufficiency. Information regarding prognosis varies considerably based on the classification method used.

Goals and Relative Value of Diagnostic Imaging

Echocardiography permits diagnosis as follows: at least three pronounced trabecula with deep, blood-perfused cavities are located inferior to the papillary muscles (▶ Fig. 4.178a, ▶ Fig. 4.178b, and ▶ Fig. 4.179). The end systolic ratio of noncompacted to compacted wall thickness should be more than 2, while the ratio of compacted vs. overall wall thickness should be below 0.33[241,243]

The cardiac apex sometimes cannot be depicted well by means of echocardiography in adult patients. In these cases, *MRI* should be considered for depicting noncompacted and compacted wall segments (ratio of greater than 2.3).[244] Newer studies even recommend determining absolute compacted and noncompacted muscle mass, though this can only be achieved using MRI.[240] Increased trabeculation near the cardiac apex appears less specific and less useful for differentiating between diagnoses of HCM and DCM than trabeculation near the basis of the heart and near the septum. The appearance of a typical late enhancement is a controversial discussion topic, though it does not appear to necessarily be part of the specific pathology despite histological evidence of fibroses in autopsied hearts. More likely, it is an expression of concurrent ischemia, inflammation, etc.[240]

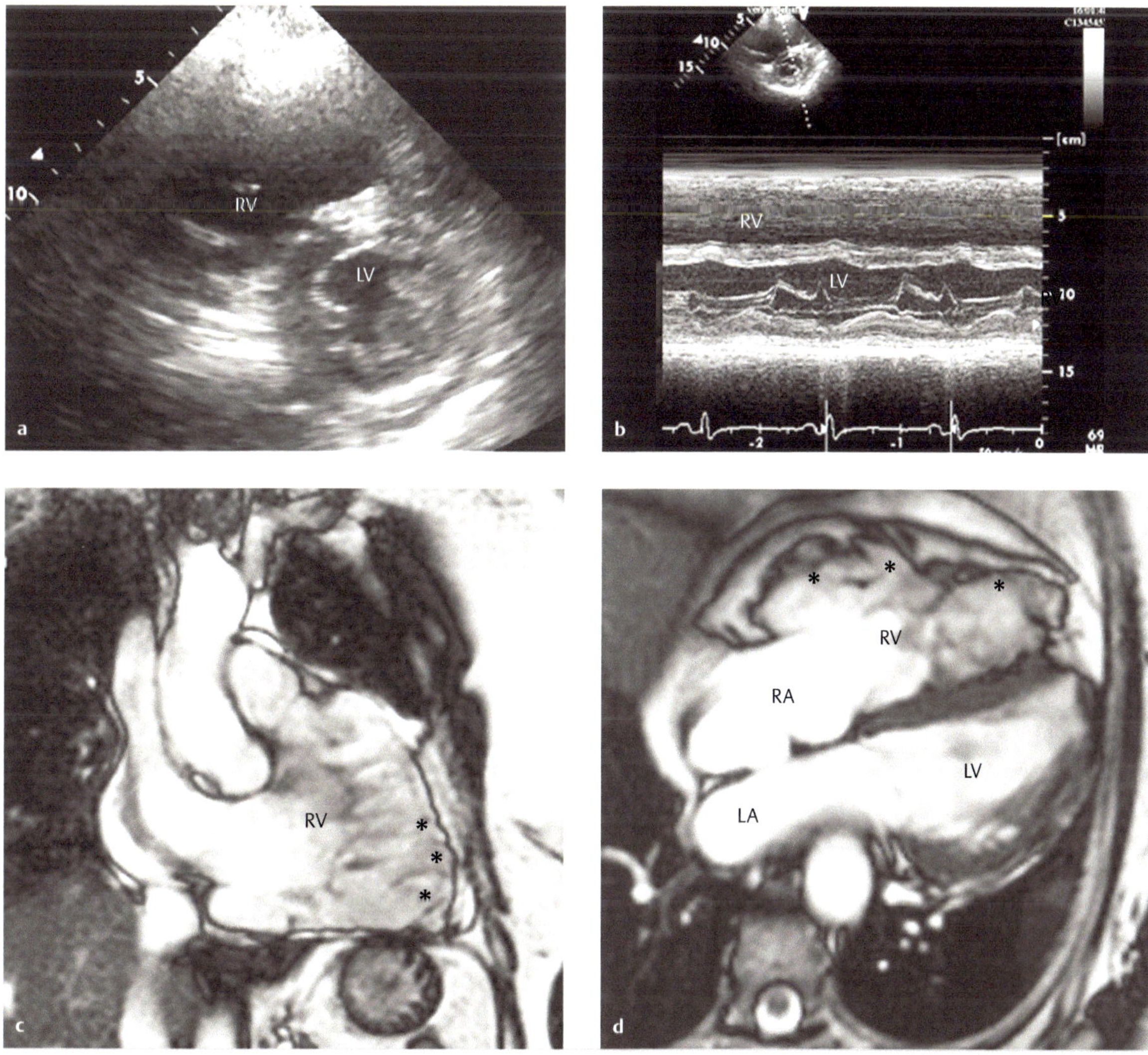

Fig. 4.177 ARVC. Sixty-six-year-old woman with major criteria of ARVC depicted in all imaging modalities. The thoracic CTs (e, f) were performed in order to rule out a pulmonary arterial embolism. Due to the low right ventricular ejection fraction of only 14% (MRI findings), a very good image quality was achieved even without ECG triggering. With the exception of TTE, the aneurysms in the right ventricle were clearly visible using all imaging modalities (c–f, asterisks).

LA = left atrium
LV = left ventricle
RA = right atrium
RV = right ventricle

a 2-D TTE, short axis, with enlarged akinetic and dyskinetic areas.
b TTE, M-mode, revealing a significantly enlarged right ventricular end diastolic diameter of more than 36 mm.
c SSFP cine MRI, long axis, from the right ventricle and RVOT. Right ventricular EDV of 194 ml/m^2 (major criterion for women: at least 100 ml/m^2; ▶ Table 4.33).
d SSFP cine MRI, 4-chamber view.

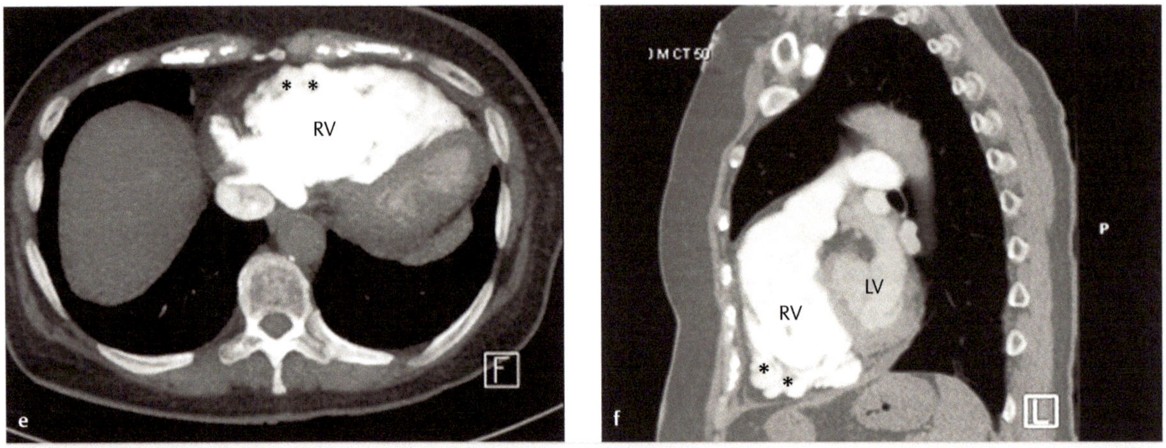

Fig 4.177 *(Continued)* **ARVC.**
LA = left atrium
LV = left ventricle
RA = right atrium
RV = right ventricle

e MDCT thoracic image, no triggering, in the pulmonary arterial phase and transverse reconstruction.
f MDCT thoracic image, no triggering, in the pulmonary arterial phase and sagittal reconstruction.

Table 4.33 Major criteria of ARVC.[238]

Criteria	Classification as major/minor criterion	2-D echocardiography	MRI	Angiography of the right ventricle
1. Structural or functional abnormalities (relevant for imaging)	Major criterion	Regional right ventricular akinesia, dyskinesia, or aneurysms *and* one of the following parameters *(during end diastole)*: a. RVOT in the parasternal long axis ≥ 32 mm (≥ 19 mm/m²) b. RVOT in the short axis ≥ 36 mm (≥ 21 mm/m²) *or* Fractional area change ≤ 33%	Right ventricular akinesia, dyskinesia, or dyssynchrony *and* one of the following parameters: c. Right ventricular EDV ≥ 110 ml/m² (men) d. Right ventricular EDV ≥ 100 ml/m² (women) *or* Right ventricular ejection fraction ≤ 40%	Regional right ventricular akinesia, dyskinesia, or aneurysms
	Minor criterion	Regional right ventricular akinesia, dyskinesia, or dyssynchrony *and* one of the following parameters *(in end diastole)*: e. RVOT in parasternal long axis 29 ≤ x < 32 mm (16 ≤ x < 19 mm/m²) f. RVOT in parasternal long axis 32 ≤ x < 36 mm (18 ≤ x < 21 mm/m²) *or* Fractional Area Change 33% < x ≤ 40%	Right ventricular akinesia, dyskinesia, or dyssynchrony *and* one of the following parameters: g. Right ventricular EDV 100 ≤ x < 110 ml/m² (men) h. Right ventricular EDV 90 ≤ x < 100 ml/m² (women) *or* Right ventricular ejection fraction 40% < x ≤ 45%	
2. Tissue characterization (currently *not* relevant for imaging; only relevant for biopsy results!)	Major criterion	Residual myocytes ≤ 60% with fatty fibrotic replacement in the wall of the right ventricle in ≥ 1 endomyocardial biopsy sample		
	Minor criterion	Residual myocytes 60% < x ≤ 75% with fatty fibrotic replacement in the wall of the right ventricle in ≥ 1 endomyocardial biopsy sample		
3. ECG changes/ arrhythmia	See references for further details[238]			
4. Family history	See references for further details[238]			

ECG, electrocardiography; MRI, magnetic resonance imaging; RVOT, right ventricular outflow tract.

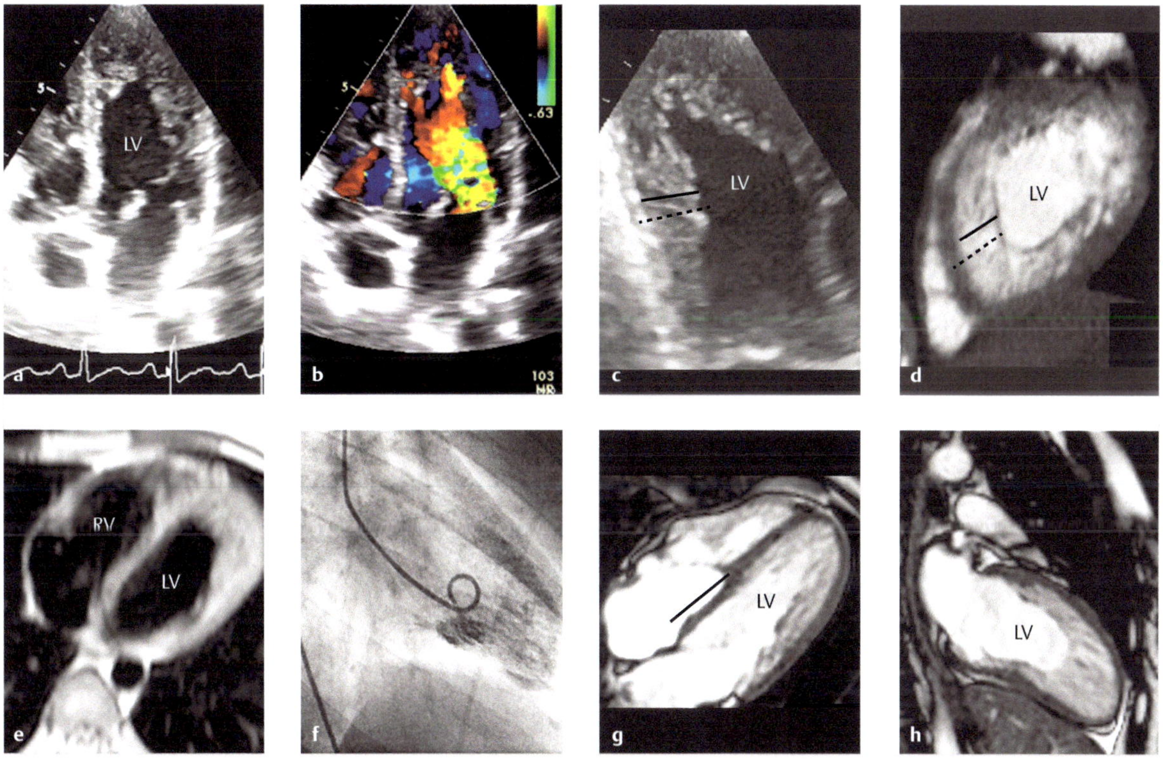

Fig. 4.178 Noncompaction cardiomyopathy. Twenty-eight-year-old woman with noncompaction cardiomyopathy of the left and right ventricle and concurrent Ebstein's anomaly. The 2-D TTE, 4-chamber view (**a**, **b**) depicts the pronounced apical and lateral trabeculation and a more than 2:1 ratio of noncompacted to compacted myocardium. This is particularly visible in the magnification image of (**c**). Echocardiographic measurement is standardized based on systole. Unlike MRI, this procedure is able to differentiate between noncompacted and compacted segments. All other imaging procedures require measurement during end diastole in order to be able to clearly distinguish the blood-filled recesses (**c**, **d**, solid line) from compacted myocardium. The dotted line in **c** and **d** indicates overall myocardial thickness (compacted + noncompacted, trabeculated myocardium). Color Doppler (**b**) can also be used. Despite measurement during diastole, slow flow in the trabecula results in only limited differentiation between noncompacted and compacted myocardium in the T1w black blood sequence (**e**). The SSFP cine MRI, 4-chamber view, depicts the septal tricuspid leaflet displaced approximately 1.8 cm apically (**g**, line) with concurrent tricuspid valve insufficiency corresponding to the concurrent Ebstein's anomaly. The left ventricular ejection fraction was already slightly limited in MRI, measured at 49%. Midventricular MRI short-axis slices (**i–l**) depict almost complete "masking" of the noncompacted myocardium in the inversion recovery GE sequence after administering contrast agent (**i**) for late enhancement due to the contrast agent in the left ventricular cavum and recesses. The "masking" of the noncompacted myocardium also occurs due to the slow flow between the trabecula in the T2w STIR black blood sequence (**j**) and due to contraction during systole (**l**). The noncompacted myocardium is clearly visible during end diastole (**k**).

LV = left ventricle
RV = right ventricle

- **a** 2-D TTE, 4-chamber view.
- **b** 2-D TTE, 4-chamber view (color Doppler).
- **c** 2-D TTE, 4-chamber view, magnification, with measurement of wall thickness of the compacted vs. noncompacted myocardium.
- **d** SSFP cine MRI, short axis, during diastole.
- **e** T1w black blood SE sequence, transverse orientation.
- **f** Invasive levocardiogram using a pigtail catheter in the left ventricle, also performed during end diastole, depicting the pronounced trabeculation of the left ventricle.
- **g** SSFP cine MRI, 4-chamber view, depicting the pathognomonic trabeculation of the basal and septal segments of the left ventricle during diastole.
- **h** SSFP cine MRI corresponding to the levocardiogram in **f**, through the long axis of the left ventricle, depicting trabeculation even more clearly during diastole.

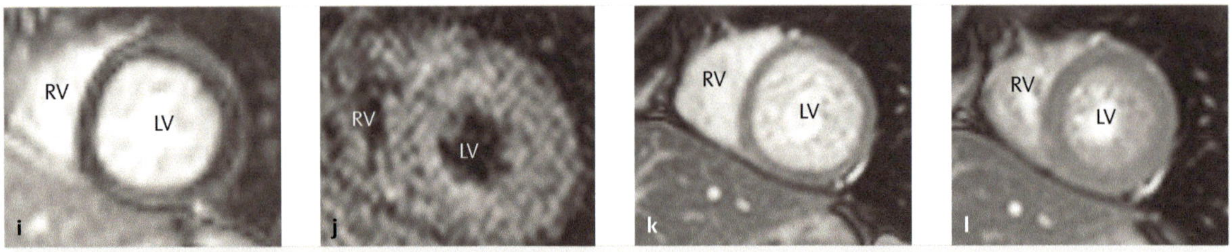

Fig 4.178 *(Continued)* **Noncompaction cardiomyopathy.**
LV = left ventricle
RV = right ventricle

- **i** Midventricular short-axis IR-GRE sequence post contrast for LGE acquired during diastole clearly depicts the "masking" of the trabeculation of the noncompacted myocardium due to the high signal intensity of the contrast enhanced "blood-pool" in between the deep recesses.
- **j** Midventricular short-axis slice, T2w STIR black blood sequence, to depict edema.
- **k** SSFP cine MRI, midventricular short-axis slice, during end diastole.
- **l** SSFP cine MRI, midventricular short-axis slice, with poor detectability of the pronounced trabeculation during systole.

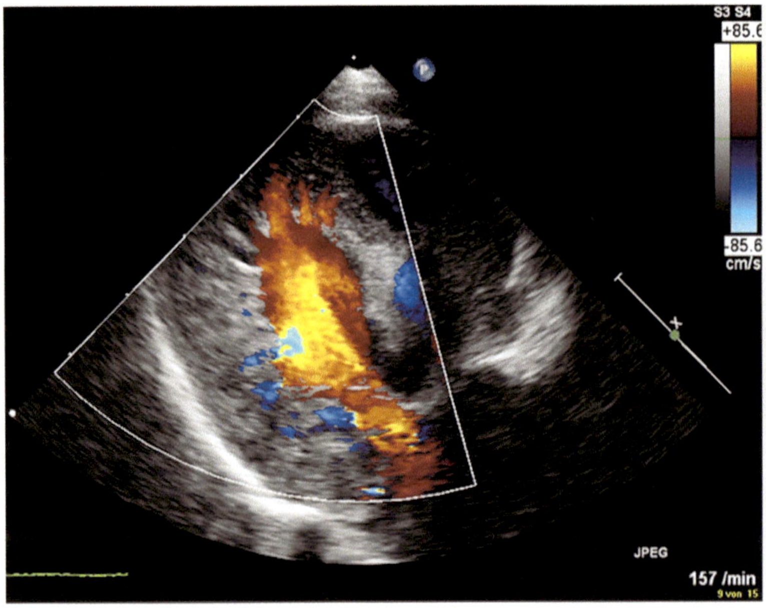

Fig. 4.179 Noncompaction cardiomyopathy. Color Doppler TTE of an infant with isolated noncompaction cardiomyopathy of the left ventricle. The deep, blood-filled recesses are clearly visible, especially at the apex.

4.6.2 Myocarditis

Achim A. Schmaltz, Jens Bremerich, Matthias Gutberlet

Definition and Classification

Myocarditis is an inflammatory disorder of the myocardium which is often not limited to a single cardiac structure, but rather can extend to the pericardium or endocardium. A distinction is made between foudroyant, acute, and chronic myocarditis based on the disorder's clinical progression.

Incidence

Inflammatory heart disorders comprise approximately 0.7% of all hospitalizations in Germany. It is believed that a larger number of cases are unreported, however, both because the inflammation process may be bland or focal. However, sudden cardiac death affects up to 17% of patients with myocarditis. Myocarditis is discovered in 1–9% of cases during routine autopsies.

Pathogenesis

From a pathohistological perspective, myocarditis can occur in either focal or diffuse forms. The type of inflammatory infiltration (either via granulocytes, giant cells, or lymphocytes) allows us to draw conclusions regarding the decidedly diverse etiology: while Chagas disease, caused by *Trypanosoma cruzi* plays a prominent role in rheumatic endomyocarditis in South America and in developing nations, Russia reports a higher mortality rate for diphtheric myocarditis. In addition, concurrent bacterial myocarditis (such as that caused by fungi, rickettsia, spirochetes, and protozoa) often occur, particularly in immunosuppressed patients.

This chapter will focus on the most significant etiology, namely *viral myocarditis*. In principle, myocarditis can be caused by any virus. The precise factors that eventually lead to the development of cardiotropic properties are unknown. Some viruses infiltrate the cells via receptors (e.g., Coxsackie adenovirus receptor), while others force their way in via the vascular endothelium (e.g., parvovirus B19) and cause organ dysfunction due to cytolysis. The Coxsackie adenovirus receptor is, however, generally not expressed on the myocytes, but rather is believed to be induced on the sarcolemma by means of cytokines. This can also cause a certain degree of genetic predisposition to inflammatory cardiomyopathy.[245] Parvovirus B19 viruses, on the other hand, find their way into the myocardium via the endothelium of the small vessels, and are verified to continue their in situ hybridization there.[246]

Viral damage to the myocardium can, on the one hand, occur directly by means of a viral protein that interferes with host cell metabolism and can, for example, cause a loss in cytoskeletal integrity by splitting the dystrophin.[247] On the other hand, viruses trigger an immune process that produces cross-reacting antibodies for active B lymphocytes solely against viral (but increasingly also against myocardial) antigens. The resultant cytokines then induce cell adhesion molecules and lead to an imbalance in metalloprotease and its inhibitors, and finally to limited contractility in the myocytes. Finally, the cytotoxic T lymphocytes cause direct cytolysis in the myofibrils. The tumor necrosis factor (TNF) alpha, interferon (IFN) gamma, and interleukin (IL)-12 produced by the macrophages exacerbate inflammation, while IL-10 has an anti-inflammatory, disease-limiting effect during autoimmune responses.

Initially, various mouse models (followed by human models) demonstrated that based on the previously unknown host factors, the virus persists in the cardiac myocytes at a low replication rate[246] and, once there, maintains chronic inflammation characterized by the evidence of T lymphocytes and inflammatory mediators such as IL-1 beta and TNF alpha. The extent of viral replication can be quantified by verifying single-strand RNA molecules with negative po larity, which are the product of the initial replication step of the normally positively charged RNA molecules. If the inflammation process has subsided, the uncharacteristic histological situation of fibrosis with hypertrophy of individual myofibrils and ultrastructural degenerative changes suggesting a case of clinically dilated, functionally limited heart (also known as DCM (see Dilated Cardiomyopathy)) persists. The corresponding, irreversible fibrotic or scar tissue changes (if large enough) can be verified using imaging procedures. ▸ Fig. 4.180 provides a schematic depiction of the pathogenesis of myocarditis and its development into DCM.

Clinical Issues

Clinical issues are, overall, rather vague, and can range from fully subjective asymptomatic states to symptoms similar to myocardial infarction, or even to sudden cardiac death. Oftentimes, clinical symptoms begin with complaints of heart failure, which can follow varying progressions: on one end of the spectrum is sudden cardiac death after a prior banal gastrointestinal or respiratory infection, which is often found to be caused by acute myocarditis in forensic examinations. Other patients experience progressive heart failure and subsequent multiorgan failure. These patients can only be kept alive using extracorporal membrane oxygenation or various mechanical life support systems.[248] On the other end of the spectrum are asymptomatic children solely with ECG repolarization disorders, in which 3 of 12 have histological verification of myocarditis.[249]

Cardiac or retrosternal pain, sustained or nonsustained ventricular tachycardia, and any other functional disorder of the heart, atrial flutter, total atrioventricular block,[250] or an ECG depicting a myocardial infarction are considered the main symptoms of myocarditis.[251] A mortality rate of 50% and a heart transplant rate of 20% are recorded in childhood,[248] and only 2% of these disorders heal. An epidemiological study from the United States[252] depicts two frequency peaks for myocarditis during childhood: one up to age 2, and another between ages 14 and 18 (▸ Fig. 4.181).

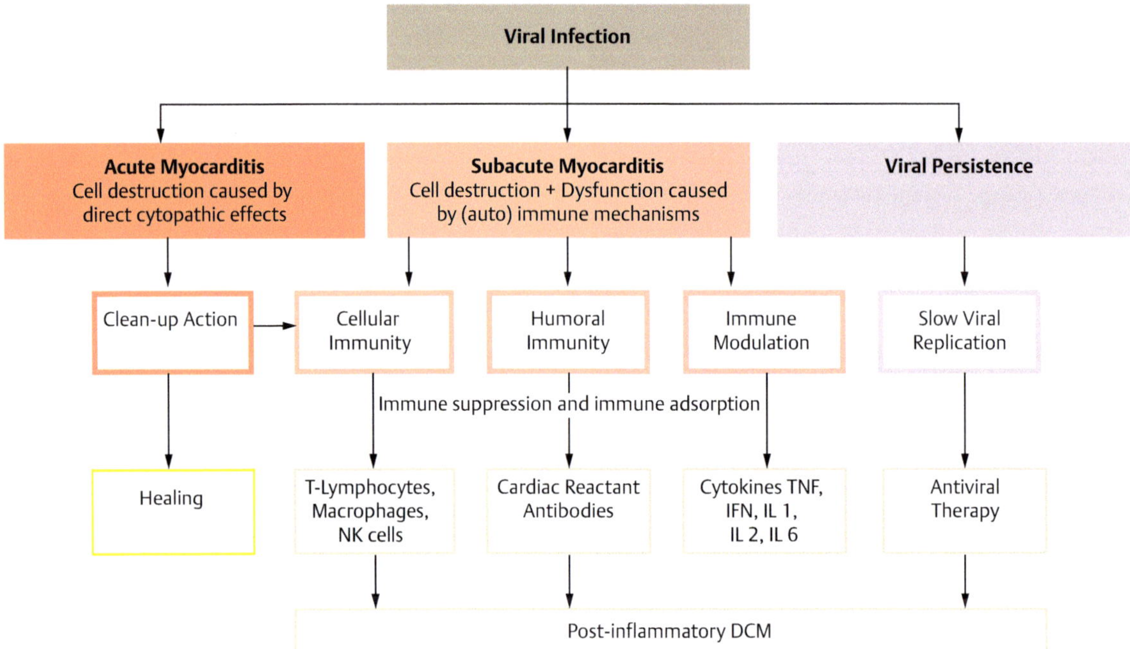

Fig. 4.180 Pathogenesis of viral myocarditis or inflammatory cardiomyopathy. Schematic depiction.
IFN = interferon
IL = interleukin
NK cells = natural killer cells
TNF = tumor necrosis factor.

Goals and Relative Value of Diagnostic Imaging

Note

The more nonspecific the clinical signs of myocarditis, the more diverse the diagnostic measures.

ECG can document new atrioventricular or bundle branch blocks[250] as well as ST changes, while long-term ECG can verify rhythm disorders. The specificity of this method is very low.

Laboratory diagnostics attempt to verify the destruction of myocytes based on the concentration of troponin I or T and CK-MB, though they are unable to distinguish between ischemic and inflammatory causes. The sensitivity and negative predictive value is indicated at 53–56%.[256] The prevalence of elevated troponin levels in a case of histologically verified myocarditis is only 35–45%.[257]

Echocardiographic findings in a case of myocarditis are also rather nonspecific[258]: left ventricular dilatation and dysfunction indicate a high degree of severity, yet may be naturally absent in a case of focal myocarditis. In the former instance, intraventricular thrombi can form (▶ Fig. 4.182) and pericardial effusion can also occur.[259] Right ventricular dysfunction was also found to be an independent predictor of death or heart transplant.[260] Mild forms of dysfunction were discovered using tissue Doppler. Changes to echogenicity are believed to rely on the extent of tissue edema and cellular infiltration. Felker et al.[258] demonstrated that in a case of fulminant myocarditis, unlike in acute forms, the left ventricle is not yet dilated, though septum thickness (edema!) is above average (▶ Fig. 4.183).

The *nuclear medicine procedures* of gallium-67 scintigraphy for chronic inflammation and monoclonal indium-111 antimyosin antibodies have become less prominent among the generally relatively young patients due to the not insignificant radiation exposure and the limited availability of nuclides. Instead, cardiac MRI is used.[254]

Despite progress in diagnostics using noninvasive imaging procedures, ***endomyocardial biopsy*** remains the gold standard for verifying myocarditis.[261] In these cases, the initially implemented Dallas criteria, defined purely based on histology, constitute the foundations that have been decisively improved by implementing immunohistochemistry and molecular biology. The use of various antibodies permits the lymphocyte infiltration cells to be characterized precisely, and the polymerase chain reaction[249] can be used to verify and identify the viral genome (▶ Fig. 4.184). Due to the so-called sampling error, biopsies provide only moderate sensitivity, but excellent specificity (▶ Table 4.34). They even permit us to distinguish between chronic myocarditis with viral persistence and virus-negative, autoimmune mediation with the corresponding treatment results,

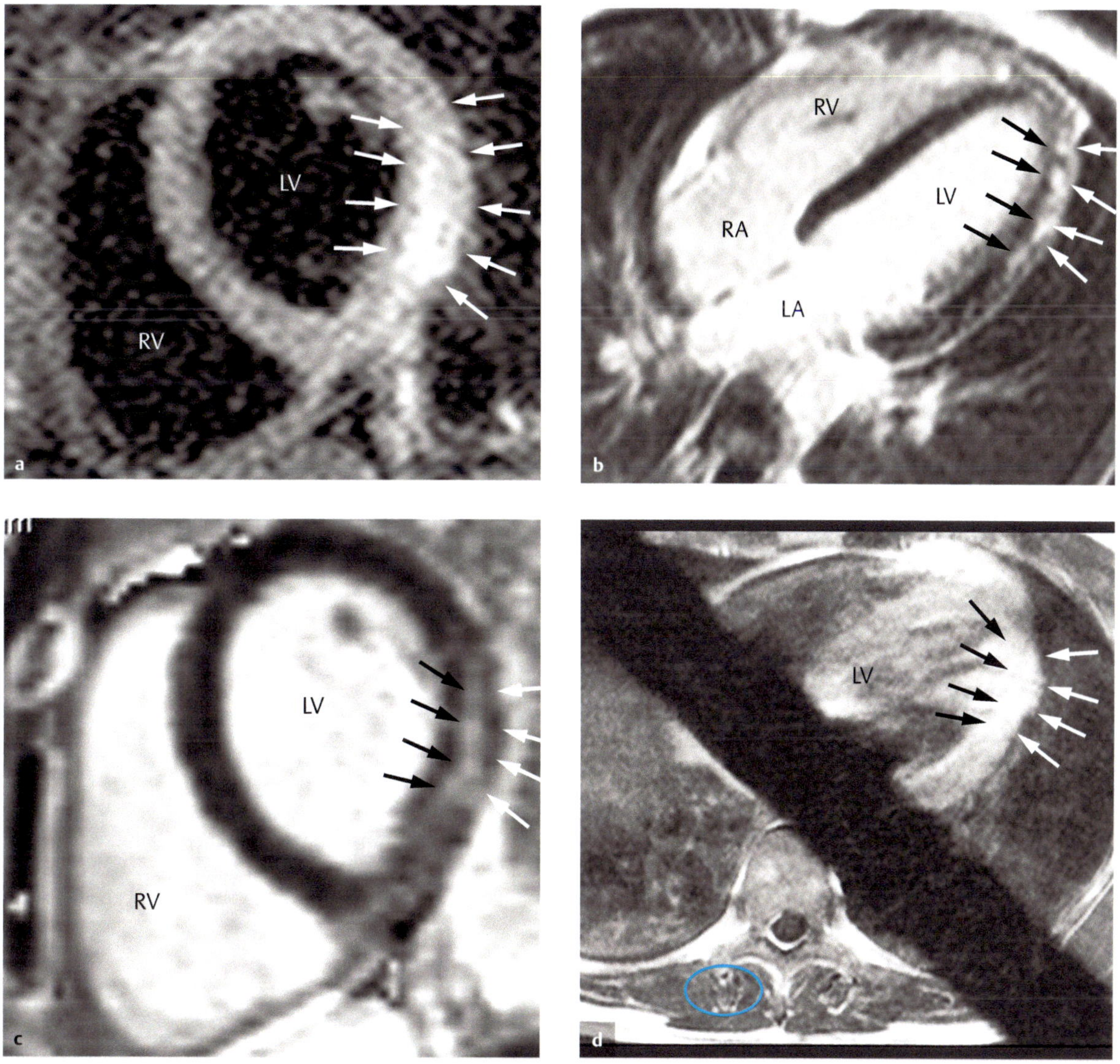

Fig. 4.181 Acute myocarditis. Cardiac MRI of a 17-year-old male patient with acute chest pain and infarct-like myocarditis 10 days after an influenza infection: typical ST elevation, elevated troponin concentration, and apparent infection. TTE verifies pericardial effusion and normal left ventricular function.

LA = left atrium
LV = left ventricle
RA = right atrium
RV = right ventricle

- **a** T2w STIR sequence, short axis, with focal, inferolateral edema (arrows). The relative water content with an edema ratio (ER) of 2.7 (standard: less than 2.0) was also significantly elevated. The left ventricular ejection fraction, measured at 57% by means of MRI, remained in the normal range. Note: Data was acquired using only the integrated body coil. The surface coil was not used.
- **b** The 2-D inversion recovery GE sequence, transverse slice, 10 minutes after i.v. administration of 0.15 mmol Gd-DTPA/kg body weight, depicts the subepicardial late enhancement typical for myocarditis (**b**, **c**, arrows).
- **c** Corresponding phase image for the 2-D PSIR sequence, short-axis slice with subepicardial LGE (arrows)
- **d** The transverse T1w SE sequence for determining global relative enhancement[253–255] in order to verify hyperemia depicts both discrete focal contrast accumulation (arrows) and an elevated global relative enhancement of 5 (standard: less than 4). Note the black saturation slice via the left atrium to reduce flow artifacts and the region of interest (blue circle) near the right erector spinae muscle in order to determine the global relative enhancement.[253–255] Data was acquired using only a body coil. The surface coil was not used.

though they are reserved for cases of left ventricular dilatation and functional limitation due to the inherent, not insignificant risk of complications.[253,261]

Thus, noninvasive diagnosis of myocarditis by means of *cardiac MRI* has become all the more significant in clinical routines, especially in recent years. Although

Gagliardi et al.[262] had already described the increased contrast in T2w SE sequences due to tissue edema in a small series of 11 children in 1991, the benefits of contrast-enhanced T1w SE sequences for verifying muscular inflammation and gadolinium enhancement in necrotic and fibrotic tissue became clear years later, beginning with the work of Friedrich et al. in 1998. In the meantime, the indication, progression, MRI protocols, and criteria have been clearly defined[253–255] and the sensitivity, specificity, and diagnostic accuracy have been evaluated in comparison to endomyocardial biopsy.[254,255,263]

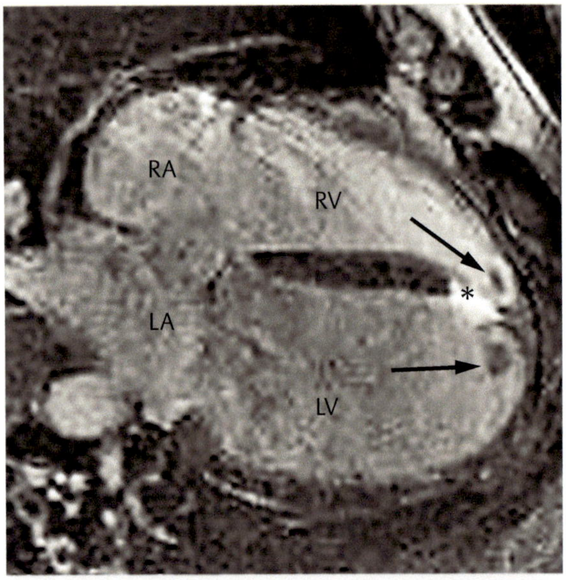

Fig. 4.182 Acute myocarditis. Young man with parvovirus B19 myocarditis and elevated troponin "similar to infarction" verified by means of biopsy. Apical septal, subendocardial scarring (asterisk) and right and left ventricular thrombi (arrows) are visible in the inversion recovery GE sequence 10 minutes after i.v. administration of 0.15 mmol Gd-DTPA/kg body weight.
LA = left atrium
LV = left ventricle
RA = right atrium
RV = right ventricle

Note

Since the individually applied MRI sequences are of varying significance, multiple sequences should always be used to verify the diagnosis.[253,254] In order to determine quantitative parameters such as global relative enhancement in T1w SE sequences before and after administering contrast agent to verify capillary leakage or relative water content (edema ratio) in T2w STIR image, note that standard values exist only for the use of the integrated body coil.

The T2w sequences (▶ Fig. 4.185 and ▶ Fig. 4.186; ▶ Fig. 4.181a and ▶ Fig. 4.183b) and early contrast agent accumulation in T1w SE sequences (▶ Fig. 4.181d) are useful for verifying active inflammation by visualizing focal changes or determining the edema ratio. In contrast, late enhancement 10–15 minutes after IV administration of Gadolinium-Diethylenetriaminepentaacetic acid (Gd-DTPA) with typical subepicardial accumulation (▶ Fig. 4.181b) is more typical of irreversible cell destruction with necrosis

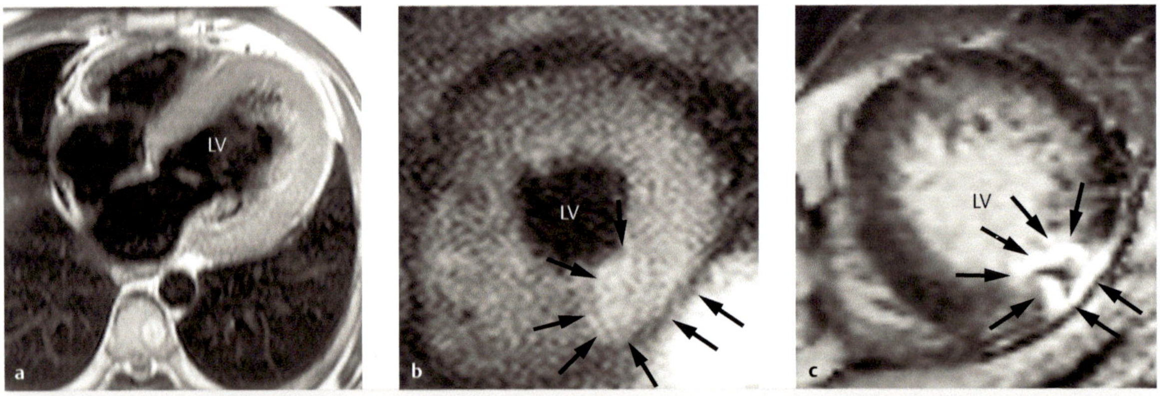

Fig. 4.183 Acute myocarditis. Thirty-five-year-old male patient.
LV = left ventricle

- **a** The transverse T1w black blood SE image depicts significant "myocardial thickening," particularly in the apex due to edema.
- **b** The short-axis slice of an edema-sensitive T2w STIR sequence depicts both myocardial thickening and focal inferior edema (arrows). Note: the body coil should be used in order to achieve the greatest possible homogeneity, even if the body coil increases image noise compared to surface coils.
- **c** The corresponding inversion recovery GE sequence for verifying late enhancement depicts necrotic or fibrotic tissue (arrow) near the focal edema (**b**).

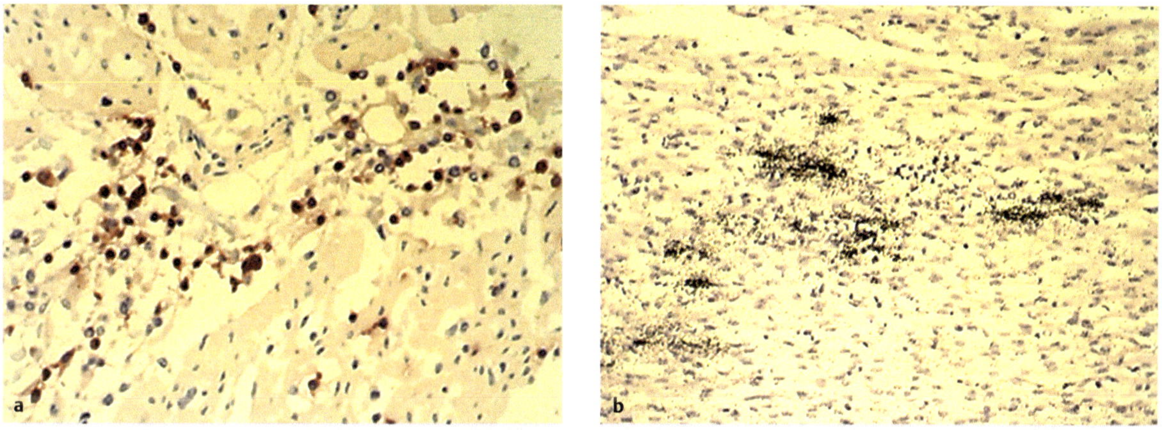

Fig. 4.184 Endomyocardial biopsy of a chronic viral myocarditis. (Courtesy: Professor Dr. R. Kandolf, Tübingen, Germany)

a Adhesion and penetration of CD3-positive T lymphocytes, particularly near the capillary endothelium, in a case of parvovirus B19 myocarditis.

b In situ hybridization of a radioactive labeled, enterovirus-specific RNA sample in a case of Coxsackievirus myocarditis.

Table 4.34 Effectiveness of various methods for diagnosing myocarditis.[235,254,257]

Diagnostic method	Sensitivity (%)	Specificity (%)
ECG changes	47	Unknown
Troponin	34	89
CK-MB	6	100
Myosin or viral antibodies	25–32	40
Indium-111 antimyosin scintigraphy	85–91	34–53
Endomyocardial biopsy		
• Dallas criteria	35–50	78–89
• Polymerase chain reaction	38	80–100
T2w MRI (edema ratio)[254]	70 (45–100)	71 (50–100)
T2w MRI[254]		
• Early enhancement	74 (49–85)	83 (33–100)
• Late gadolinium enhancement	59 (31–95)	86 (46–100)
T1 mapping[235]		
• Native	Acute: 88 (74–96) Chronic: 24 (15–41)	Acute: 67 (41–87) Chronic: 94 (21–100)
• ECV	Acute: 75 (60–88) Chronic: 69 (55–82)	Acute: 72 (47–90) Chronic: 61 (36–83)
T2 mapping[235]	Acute: 85 (71–94) Chronic: 71 (57–85)	Acute: 68 (43–87) Chronic: 72 (47–90)

CK-MB, creatine kinase-MB; ECG, electrocardiography; MRI, magnetic resonance imaging; T2w, T2-weighted.

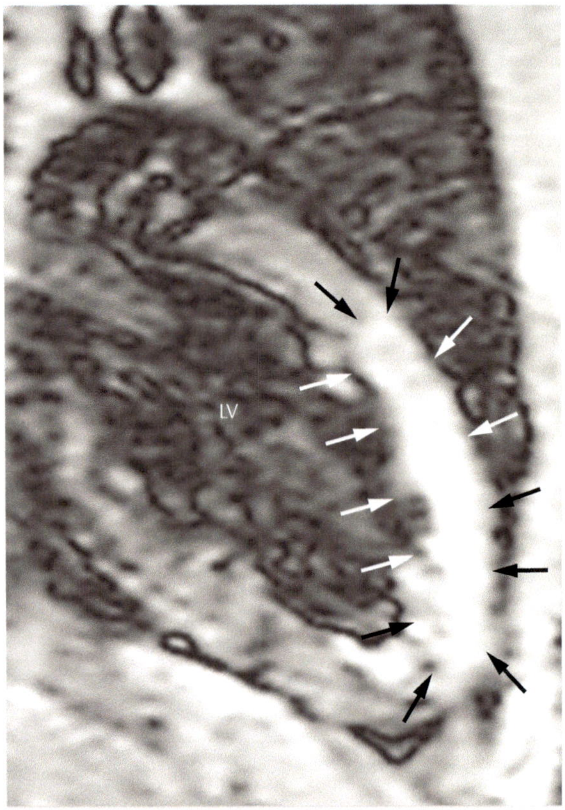

Fig. 4.185 **Acute myocarditis.** Cardiac MRI of a 16-year-old boy with acute retrosternal pain, intermittent right bundle branch block, and elevated troponin. The T2w STIR sequence clearly depicts the elevated signal intensity (arrows) at the anterior wall and apex of the LV as an expression of inflammatory edema.
LV = left ventricle

and fibrosis formation, which cannot always be verified. The lack of late enhancement does not definitively rule out active myocarditis. Late enhancement is thus verifiable especially in patients with myocarditis considered "infarct-like."

Note

Subepicardial late enhancement often occurs in cases of myocarditis (▶ Fig. 4.181b) and is pathognomonic for myocarditis. Midwall enhancement (▶ Fig. 4.186c) or even subendocardial (▶ Fig. 4.182) or transmural late contrast accumulation (▶ Fig. 4.183c) is, however, also possible in cases of myocarditis, whereas subepicardial enhancement never occurs in ischemic heart disease.

If the Lake Louise criteria for positively diagnosing active myocarditis require at least 2 of the 3 most commonly used parameters (T2w edema-sensitive sequence, early and/or late contrast enhancement), this results in a sensitivity of 67–86%, a specificity of 91–95%, and an accuracy of 78% in a pooled data analysis.[253,254] Later works depicted favorable results, primarily in diagnosing acute myocarditis and, consequently, "infarct-like" myocarditis.[263] In contrast, MRI diagnostics yielded significantly worse results in cases of chronic myocarditis (▶ Table 4.35). Liu and Yan[257] emphasized this diagnostic progress by means of cardiac MRI and compared the value of the various methods in ▶ Table 4.34. Further improvement in the reliability of these methods is expected in the future, especially for parametric imaging by means of T1 and T2 mapping.[254] Initial studies with results verified via

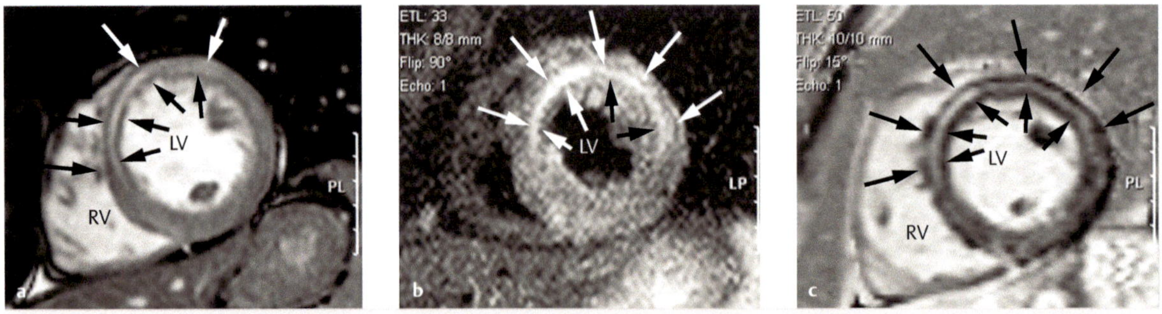

Fig. 4.186 Acute myocarditis confirmed via biopsy. Thirty-year-old male patient presents with pronounced late gadolinium midwall enhancement (a and c, arrows) near the left ventricular anterior wall, which can also occur in cases of DCM (see Dilated Cardiomyopathy). The focal midventricular edema in the T2w STIR sequence (b) also permits differentiation, and acute inflammation is assumed.
LV = left ventricle
RV = right ventricle

a A SSFP cine MRI sequence, midventricular short axis, after administering contrast agent.
b T2w STIR sequence, midventricular short axis, with significant, corresponding intramyocardial edema.
c Corresponding late enhancement MRI sequence (phase image of the 2-D PSIR), midventricular short axis.

biopsy seem to depict primarily benefits, especially for T2 mapping, in terms of verifying chronic myocarditis[235] (▶ Table 4.34).

The significant differential diagnoses of myocarditis (especially during childhood) can be best ruled out using the following methods:

- Decompensated congenital heart defects: Echocardiography, MRI
- Endocardial fibroelastosis (▶ Table 4.32, ▶ Fig. 4.172): Echocardiography, MRI, biopsy
- Paroxysmal tachycardia: Long-term ECG
- Bland–White–Garland syndrome (see Congenital Coronary Anomalies): Echocardiography, MRI, MDCT, angiography
- DCM: Biopsy, potentially MRI for differential diagnosis

Treatment Options

Acute myocarditis

Progress (albeit not entirely satisfactory) in imaging diagnostics remains in stark contrast to progress in treatment options. For cases of acute myocarditis, treatment goals after ruling out all nonviral etiologies (and thus those requiring specific treatment) consists of combating or preventing the spread of inflammation and addressing heart failure. In order to do so, antiviral treatment requires knowledge of the underlying virus.[245] Nevertheless, myocarditis treatment remains somewhat experimental in nature. Administering i.v. immunoglobin during the acute phase is not evidence-based, and is associated with significant volume load, particularly in pediatric patients.[264] Animal trials substantiate ordering bed rest in order to prevent the spread of inflammation, supplemented by administering ACE inhibitors. In foudroyant cases, addressing shock and heart failure is the main goal, which can even necessitate placing a left ventricular assist device (▶ Fig. 4.187).[248]

Chronic Myocarditis

Chronic myocarditis can require various treatment strategies depending on whether a persistent virus is present or if there are indications of autoimmune origins. Earlier, large-scale studies that did not take these differences into account used various forms of immune suppression or modulation and yielded contradictory results.[265–267]

Numerous multicenter studies[268,269]—one using pediatric patients[270]—have been performing IFN treatment based on the precise pathohistological clarification of the stage of inflammation in cases of viral persistence (or immune suppression in cases of autoreactive forms). Due to the lack of participation, however, the studies initiated with pediatric patients have been readjusted in the interim. No multicenter, randomized study has yet been conducted[271] with regard to immune absorption. Furthermore, no evidence-based treatment for chronic myocarditis is yet available.[272]

Table 4.35 Overview of the results of MRI diagnosis in patients with symptoms similar to infarction, for the various available MRI parameters.[254,263]

Myocarditis resembling infarction ($n = 37$)	Sensitivity (%)	Specificity (%)	Precision (%)	NPV (%)	PPV (%)
Edema ratio (T2w STIR)	69 (52–86)	63 (29–96)	68 (52–83)	36	87
Global relative enhancement (T1w early)	79 (65–94)	63 (29–96)	76 (62–90)	46	89
Late enhancement (T1w late)	83 (69–97)	63 (29–96)	78 (65–92)	50	76
At least 2 of 3 are positive	86 (74–99)	75 (45–100)	84 (72–96)	60	93

NPV, negative predictive value; PPV, positive predictive value; STIR, Short tau inversion recovery; T1w, T1-weighted; T2w, T2-weighted.

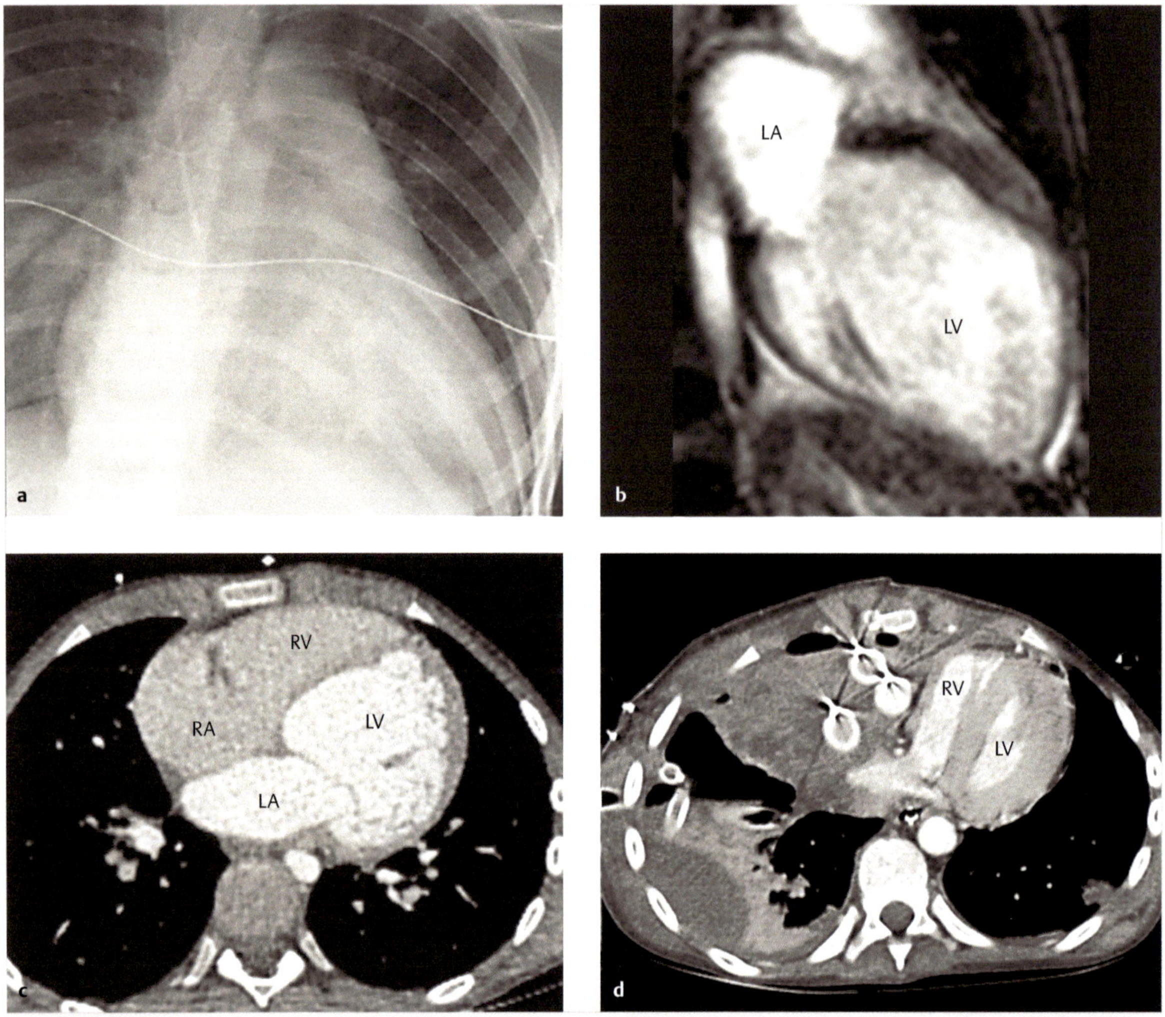

Fig. 4.187 Foudroyant acute myocarditis after influenza infection. Thirteen-year-old boy. Significantly enlarged left ventricle with significantly limited left ventricular function, MRI (left ventricular ejection fraction of 14%, left ventricular EDV of 256 ml or 208 ml/m2, global relative enhancement of 6.0 [standard: less than 4.5], edema ratio of 2.1 [standard: less than 2]). As the patient's clinical condition worsened, a left ventricular assist device (LVAD) was implanted, resulting in ventricular size reduction in the follow-up MDCT by means of pressure reduction (d).

LA = left atrium
LV = left ventricle
RA = right atrium
RV = right ventricle

- **a** P.-a. thoracic X-ray with massively enlarged left ventricle and pulmonary venous congestion.
- **b** The long axis of the SSFP cine MRI also depict the significantly enlarged left ventricle.
- **c** MDCT before implantation of a left ventricular assist device (**d**).
- **d** MDCT after implantation of a left ventricular assist device, already depicting significantly improved contractility with a corresponding reduction of LV size. The image depicts the left ventricle during systole.

4.6.3 Kawasaki Syndrome

Markcus Makowski, Gerald F. Greil

Definition

Kawasaki syndrome is a syndrome complex whose clinical picture is dominated by systemic vasculitis associated with necrotic inflammation of the vascular musculature. The vascular musculature of the small arterioles and venules is first affected, followed by the great arteries. The inflammation occurring in the coronary arteries is of particular clinical importance.

Kawasaki syndrome (also known as "mucocutaneous lymph node syndrome") has replaced acute rheumatic fever as the most common cause of acquired heart diseases in children and adolescents in highly industrialized nations.[273,274] It was first described by Japanese physician

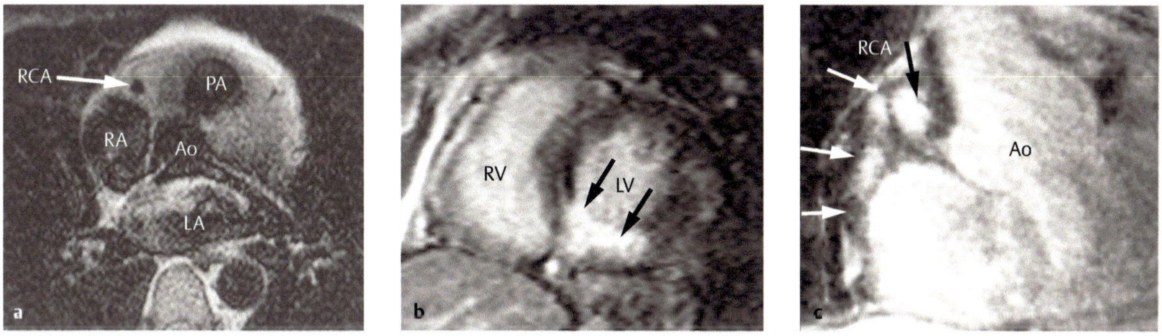

Fig. 4.188 Kawasaki syndrome. Seven-year-old male patient with Kawasaki syndrome and an aneurysmatic right coronary artery with wall thickening.

Ao = aorta
LA = left atrium
LV = left ventricle
PA = pulmonary artery
RA = right atrium
RCA = right coronary artery
RV = right ventricle.

a T1w black blood turbo SE image, transverse slice, near the origin of the great vessels. Right coronary artery, perpendicular slice.

b The inversion recovery GE sequence (late gadolinium enhancement), midventricular short-axis slice, depicts an inferior scar (arrows).

c A 2-D single-shot sequence for depicting the coronary arteries, angulated sagittal section, depicting multiple saccular aneurysms (arrows) in the right coronary artery. The image was acquired during a breath-holding command.

Kawasaki in 1967.[275,276] It is a neonatal and pediatric disease (peak of illness: ages 6 months to 5 years) which affects boys approximately 1.5 times more often than girls. A secondary illness is also possible in 2–3% of cases.[274,277]

Clinical Issues and Natural Progression

Kawasaki syndrome can be diagnosed if coronary aneurysms[278] and at least one of the following symptoms are present after 5 days of high, antibiotic-resistant fever. Alternately, in the event that coronary aneurysms are absent, diagnosis can be determined if at least four of the following symptoms are present[277,279]:

- Changes to extremities (acute: swelling and reddening of the hands and feet, convalescence: membranous desquamation of the fingertips)
- Nonspecific polymorphic exanthema of the body's trunk
- Bilateral conjunctivitis
- Changes to the lips and oral cavity (chapped lips, strawberry tongue, enanthem, rhagades)
- Generally unilateral cervical lymph node swelling (usually at least 1.5 cm)

This is particularly important to coronary imaging for these patients.[280] Coronary aneurysms varying in size and shape can develop, primarily localized in the main coronary arterial branches (▸ Fig. 4.188).[273] Inflammation in the myocardium within the scope of pancarditis or endocarditis can also occur, which can lead to decreased left ventricular function or even to valve insufficiency.[281,282] Pericardial effusion can occur within the scope of pericarditis. Coronary aneurysms occur in 15–25% of patients with untreated Kawasaki syndrome.[283] Approximately one-half of all children and adolescents who develop coronary aneurysms during the acute phase have unremarkable vessels during cardiac catheter examinations 1–2 years later. Between 50% and 75% of all coronary aneurysms heal spontaneously 1–2 years after Kawasaki syndrome develops. The size of the aneurysms determines the likelihood of subsequent damage to the coronary arteries.[274]

The following factors had a positive influence on healing:

- Patient age under 1 year when Kawasaki syndrome developed.
- Spindle-shaped vs. saccular morphology of the coronary aneurysms.
- Development of coronary aneurysms in the distal coronary arteries.

Classification and Indication for Treatment

Note

The risk of developing myocardial infarction is highest during the first year after the disease develops (▸ Fig. 4.188b). Long-term management of Kawasaki syndrome is based on the risk of developing myocardial infarction.

The amended AHA guidelines permit patient risk to be classified into five discrete classes,[273] wherein the risk of myocardial infarction is lowest in class I and highest in class V:

- *Class I:* No morphological changes to the coronary arteries

- *Class II:* Temporary changes to the coronary arteries that recede after 6–8 weeks
- *Class III:* Small or medium aneurysms in a main coronary artery
- *Class IV:* A large aneurysm or multiple large aneurysms, or multiple complicated aneurysms in the same coronary artery
- *Class V:* Stenosis of a coronary artery

Consequently, serial assessment of the size and position of the coronary aneurysms and coronary artery stenoses is necessary in order to make treatment decisions.

Treatment Options

Due to preexisting vasculitis, anti-inflammatory medications (e.g., steroids, acetyl salicylic acid, immunoglobins, etc.) were used for treatment in the past.[273] The introduction of ***immunoglobin treatment*** helped significantly reduce the incidence of coronary artery aneurysms.[284] Clinicians consistently recommend administering immunoglobin (2 g/kg body weight) as early as possible.[285]

Administering high doses of ***acetyl salicylic acid*** during the acute phase (80–100 mg/[kg body weight × day] in 4 individual doses) is also generally recommended. Steroid administration, however, remains debated. Low-dose acetyl salicylic acid treatment (3–5 mg/kg body weight) is continued for up to 8 weeks, provided that coronary status remains unremarkable. If coronary aneurysms or coronary artery stenoses are present, acetyl salicylic acid treatment is continued indefinitely. This is not just due to the latter's anti-inflammatory effects. Rather, this treatment helps prevent myocardial infarction due to thrombosis formation near the coronary aneurysms or coronary stenoses, which are particularly likely to occur in the distal segments of the coronary aneurysms.

Depending on the extent of damage to the coronary arteries, medication treatment can be supplemented using Dipyridamole. If the aneurysms are of adequate size, marcumarization may also be necessary.[277,286] In cases of acute aneurysmal thrombosis, clinicians should consider thrombolysis using streptokinase, urokinase, or tissue plasminogen activator.

Surgical attempts to treat high-grade stenosis (within the scope of a coronary bypass surgery) or complete closure of the coronary arteries have been undertaken in certain critical cases, though with limited success. Stent implantation is similarly debated for this patient group. Currently, it is not recommended during the acute phase of Kawasaki syndrome.

Goals and Relative Value of Diagnostic Imaging

Kawasaki syndrome is a challenge for clinicians, since aneurysms can often develop while remaining clinically unnoticed. Later consequences, such as myocardial infarction (▶ Fig. 4.188b) or sudden cardiac death, may not occur until years later. Repeated examinations of the entire cardiovascular system, particularly the coronary arteries, may be necessary for affected patients. Since follow-up examinations are often needed, imaging techniques with the lowest possible degree of invasiveness and radiation exposure should be implemented, particularly for pediatric or adolescent patients. The benefits and drawbacks of the currently available imaging techniques are listed in ▶ Table 4.36.

Table 4.36 Value of various imaging techniques for assessing Kawasaki syndrome.

Examination parameter	Echocardiography	MRI	MDCT	SPECT	PET	Cardiac catheter
Invasiveness	Noninvasive	Noninvasive	Noninvasive	Noninvasive	Noninvasive	Invasive
Pressure measurement	No pressure measurement	No pressure measurement	No pressure measurement	No pressure measurement	No pressure measurement	Pressure measurement possible using an intervention
Mobility	Mobile	Stationary	Stationary	Stationary	Stationary	Stationary
Field of view	Dependent upon acoustic window	Independent of acoustic window	Independent of acoustic window	Independent of acoustic window	Independent of acoustic window	Independent of acoustic window
Imaging options	2-D/3-D	2-D/3-D	2-D/3-D	2-D/3-D	2-D/3-D	2-D/3-D
Radiation exposure	None	None	Radiation exposure	Radiation exposure	Radiation exposure	Radiation exposure
User-dependence	User dependent	Relatively independent of user	Relatively independent of user	Relatively independent of user	Relatively independent of user	Relatively independent of user

MDCT, multidetector computed tomography; MRI, magnetic resonance imaging; PET, Position emissions tomogram; SPECT, Single-photon emission computed tomogram.

Echocardiography is the screening method of choice if Kawasaki syndrome is suspected.[287] The reliability of this technique is, however, extremely dependent upon the examiner's experience. 2-D TTE is normally sufficient to this end in pediatric patients, but is usually inadequate for adolescent patients due to the reduced acoustic window.[288,289] Echocardiography is not currently used in clinical routines for diagnosing coronary artery stenoses for patients with Kawasaki syndrome. Stress echocardiography is not a routine procedure for this patient group.

Cardiac catheter examination remains the gold standard if coronary aneurysms or coronary artery stenoses are suspected. Nevertheless, this method is invasive and associated with radiation exposure. The latter is associated with elevated risk, particularly in children.[186]

Consequently, *MRI* can be a promising alternative to invasive cardiac catheter examinations.[281,290] Furthermore, MRI can be implemented to assess myocardial infarction for patients with Kawasaki syndrome after i.v. administration of Gd-DTPA using late contrast agent enhancement, also known as LGE (▶ Fig. 4.188b). Both the lumen and coronary wall thickness can be depicted and measured using MRI. This allows additional potential points for precise risk stratification and direct assessment of treatment approaches.[291] The coronary aneurysm wall has been depicted successfully using MRI, and significant thickening compared to healthy test subjects has been verified.[291] MRI generally depicts the coronary lumen with a whole-heart 3-D sequence using a respiratory navigator. At this time, the acquisition time is approximately 6–9 minutes. Aneurysms and wall thickening are generally acquired using black blood SE sequences rather than rapid GE sequences (▶ Fig. 4.188a). Single-shot 2-D sequences using the breath-holding technique, which can be implemented along the course of the coronary arteries (ideally along the right one), yield adequate visualizations (▶ Fig. 4.188c). Stress MRI examinations are implemented as a promising method for verifying stress ischemia within this patient group.

Multi-slice CT is a rapid and robust alternative for everyday clinical practice, especially if MRI is contraindicated. This technique generally allows very rapid, reliable depiction of coronary aneurysms[292] and stenoses. Coronary stenoses can be depicted more clearly using this technique than with MRI due to the very high spatial resolution, which is accurate even in the sub-millimeter range.[293] In addition, this technique allows coronary calcifications to be visualized. New, optimized examination protocols enable significant reduction in patients' radiation exposure. Unlike MRI, using contrast agent with multi-slice CT is always required. Thus, i.v. access must be available. Small vascular diameter and significant radiation exposure, primarily in children with generally high heart rates that limit the use of dose-sparing protocols, are the drawbacks of this technique for pediatric and adolescent patients. New techniques offering a significant improvement in acquisition speed and further reduction in radiation exposure are anticipated.

Though *SPECT* and *PET* permit the depiction of myocardial perfusion defects,[294] these techniques are rarely used in clinical routines for patients with Kawasaki syndrome due to the high radiation exposure and limited availability.[281]

4.6.4 Marfan Syndrome

Heiner Latus, Gerald F. Greil

Definition

Marfan syndrome is characterized by a multisystemic connective tissue weakness, which targets the cardiovascular system, eyes, and skeleton. Its characteristics were first described by Frenchman Antoine Bernard-Jean Marfan in 1896, after whom the complex of symptoms was named. This syndrome occurs in approximately 1:5000 people.[295] Marfan syndrome is autosomal dominant inheritable and demonstrates complete penetration, though variable expression. Approximately one-third of cases are caused by new mutations.[296]

Etiology

In the majority of cases, this syndrome is caused by a mutation in the fibrillin 1 gene on the long arm of chromosome 15 (15q21).[297,298] This leads to changes in the glycoprotein fibrillin (hence the term "fibrillinopathy"), which, in addition to collagen and elastin, is an essential component of the extracellular connective tissue matrix. Microfibrils are responsible for the elastic properties of connective tissue and can be found in various organ systems. This explains the broad spectrum of clinical manifestation, histological changes to the blood vessels accompanied by degradation of the extracellular matrix, the loss of elastic fibers, hypertrophic smooth muscle cells, and cystic medial necrosis.[299,300] These structural changes to the vascular wall lead to increased sensitivity to shear force, which can result in dilatation and dissection of the vascular wall over the long term (▶ Fig. 4.189, ▶ Fig. 4.190, ▶ Fig. 4.191, ▶ Fig. 4.192).

Clinical Issues

Due to the varying severity of symptoms, international clinical criteria have been defined (Ghent Nosology[302]). In the meantime, aortic root aneurysms and aortic root dissection with lens dislocation are the primary clinical signs, and suffice for diagnosis.[303] Mutations in the fibrillin 1 gene can be verified using molecular genetic analysis. Diagnostics are complicated by the overlap with other connective tissue disorders and phenotypes similar to Marfan syndrome, such as Loeys–Dietz syndrome, Shprintzen–Goldberg syndrome, or MASS syndrome, which also affect the mitral valves, aorta, skeleton, and skin.

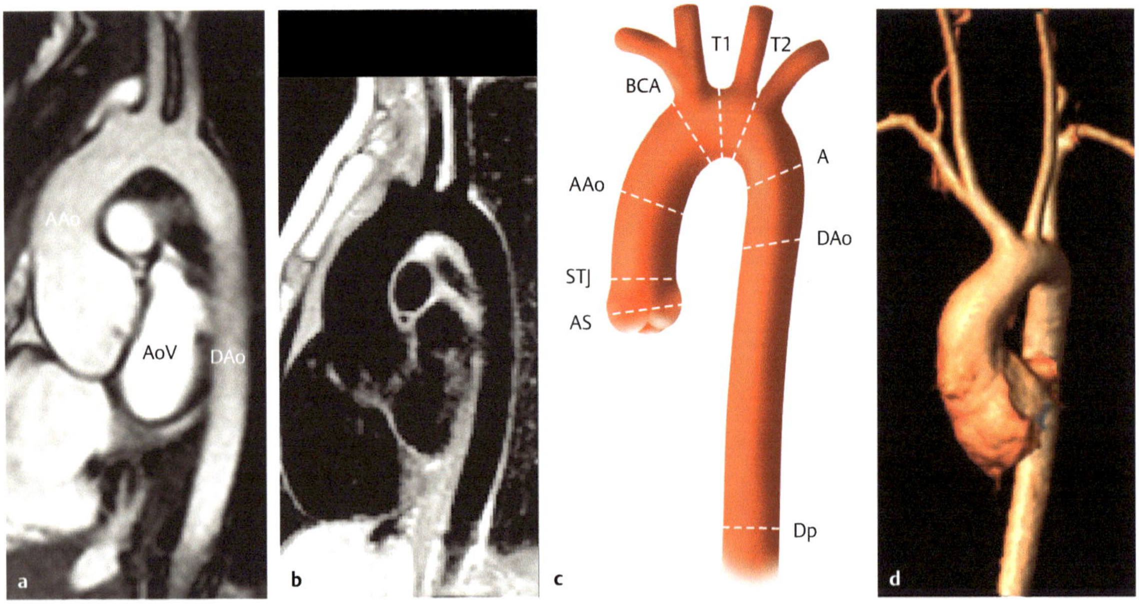

Fig. 4.189 Aortic root dilatation in a case of Marfan syndrome. Seven-year-old male patient. Note that an SSFP sequence (a) during systole and two perpendicular slices must be used to determine the diameter. This patient's Z-scores (Chapter 5) for the sinus (5.7), sinotubular junction (7.2), and ascending aorta (5.7) are significantly higher than the published standard values.[301]

AAo = ascending aorta
AoV = aortic valve
AS = aortic sinus
BCA = brachiocephalic artery
DAo = descending aorta
DP = diaphragmatic passage
IA = isthmus area
STJ = sinotubular junction
T1 = first transverse diameter
T2 = second transverse diameter

a SSFP cine sequence, angulated parasagittal plane, through the entire thoracic aorta during systole.
b Black blood SE sequence, angulated parasagittal plane, through the entire thoracic aorta during diastole.
c Schematic depiction of the diameters to be measured.
d The pronounced dilatation of the aortic root is clearly visible in the 3-D reconstruction from a contrast-enhanced MRA using the volume rendering technique.

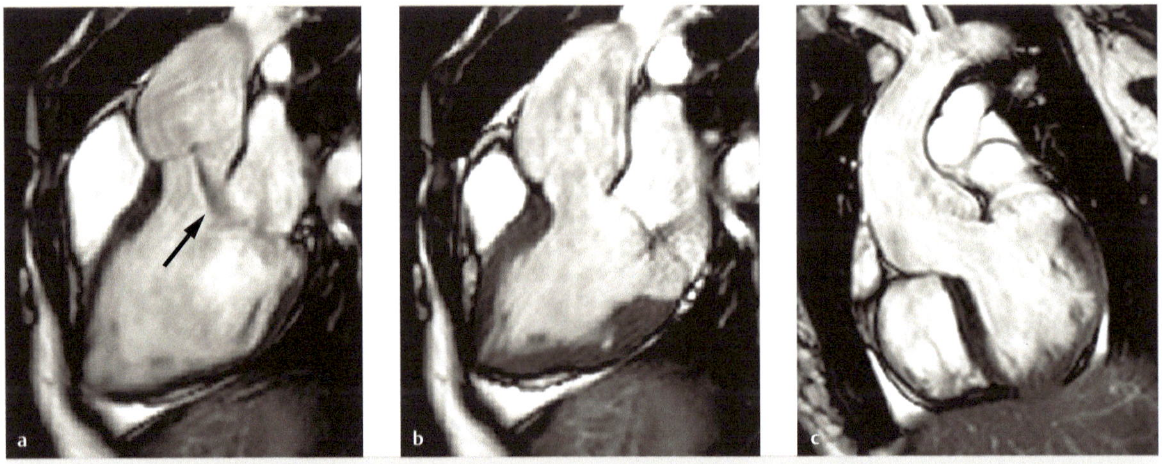

Fig. 4.190 Significantly dilated aortic root in a case of Marfan syndrome. SSFP cine MRIs. Note the significant change in diameter between diastole (a) and systole (b) in the aortic root. A clear insufficiency jet (a, arrow) caused by dephasing is visible during diastole, inferior to the aortic valve.

a Section through the LVOT and aortic root during diastole.
b Section through the LVOT and aortic root during systole.
c Sagittal section through the aortic root, ascending aorta, and aortic arch during systole.

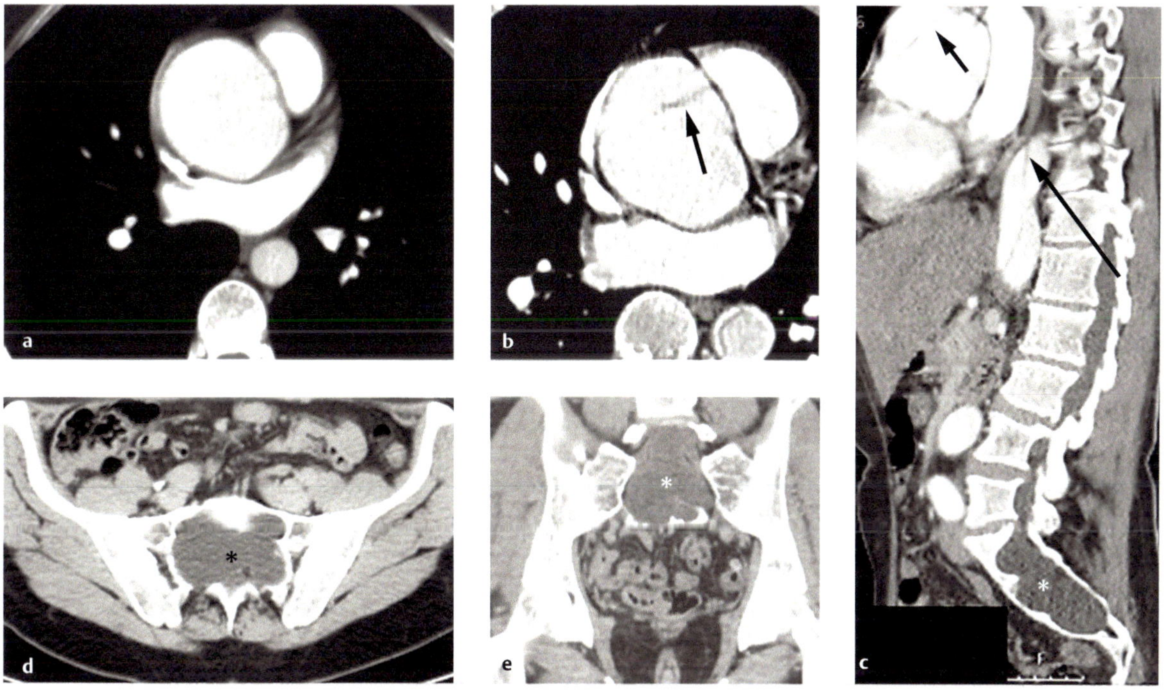

Fig. 4.191 Aortic dissection in a case of Marfan syndrome. A 43-year-old male patient with Marfan syndrome, demonstrating dilatation in the aorta to a maximum of 5.8 cm (a) during the initial examination. Acute type A dissection (b, arrow, and c, short arrow) 3 months later, extending to the descending aorta (c, long arrow). The reconstructions near the os sacrum depict the pronounced dural sac ectasia (c–e, asterisks) typical for Marfan syndrome. The patient then underwent aortic valve, ascending aorta, and partial aortic arch replacement.

a Initial examination using ECG-triggered MDCT.
b ECG-triggered, emergency MDCT examination 3 months later due to suspicion of acute type A dissection.
c Sagittal reconstruction.
d Transverse reconstruction near the os sacrum.
e Coronal reconstruction near the os sacrum.

Cardiovascular System

Within the cardiovascular system, the *aorta*, myocardium, and cardiac valves are affected. The pathological vascular changes can lead to thinning in the vascular walls and reduced flexibility, which can allow aneurysms to form, particularly in the aortic root.[304] Aortic root aneurysms can be verified in approximately 60% of patients with Marfan syndrome by age 35 (see ▶ Fig. 4.190). By age 60, 96% are affected. Men are at an increased risk for this disorder.[305] Aneurysms seldom form in more distal sites (ascending aorta: 19%, aortic arch: 16%, descending aorta: 15%). Dissection or rupture of the vascular wall generally constitute acute, life-threatening complications. The proximal aorta is most commonly affected in these cases.

> **Note**
>
> According to the Stanford classification, type A dissection constitutes an immediate indication for surgery (▶ Fig. 4.191b,c). CT examination in the intensive care unit is the method of choice, and should, if possible, always be ECG-triggered.

The *mitral valve* is most commonly affected, corresponding to mitral valve prolapse. Generally speaking, the leaflets do not suffer from myxomatous degeneration, but rather are thinner and longer than normal. The posterior leaflet prolapses most commonly. Two-thirds of Marfan syndrome patients suffer from mitral valve disorders even at a young age (▶ Fig. 4.192e), and these disorders are progressive in approximately one-fourth of patients. Both sexes are equally affected.[305] From a treatment perspective, mitral valve reconstruction or mitral valve replacement should be considered.[306]

Prolapse of the *tricuspid valve* usually occurs in conjunction with mitral valve prolapse. Due to the aortic root dilatation and stretching of the annulus, reduced coaptation occurs in the aortic semilunar valve, with subsequent aortic valve insufficiency (▶ Fig. 4.190a, ▶ Fig. 4.192l).[307]

Cardiomyopathy was first recorded in a patient with Marfan syndrome in 1985.[308] Further studies verified the *dilatation and functional impairment of the right and left ventricles*.[309–311] The study performed by Yetman et al. associated this dilatation with an elevated risk for the occurrence of life-threatening arrhythmias. Alpendurada et al. discovered a reduced ejection fraction of 25% among Marfan syndrome patients with no relevant valve disease.[312] Pectus excavatum, which often occurs in Marfan syndrome patients, can limit the function of the right and left ventricles (▶ Fig. 4.192k).[313]

Extracardiac Manifestations

Typically, approximately 80% of Marfan syndrome patients also possess lens subluxation (ectopia lentis). The typical skeletal characteristics are long, narrow extremities (dolichostenomelia), arachnodactyly, hyperextendable joints, and pectus excavatum and carinatum. Lumbosacral dural ectasia (▶ Fig. 4.191c,d,e), skin striations, and a tendency toward recurrent pneumothorax can also occur.

Indication for Treatment and Treatment Options

In order to avoid progressive aortic dilatation and dissection, *medication treatment* should begin immediately after diagnosis. Treatment with propranolol has been demonstrated to have positive effects on the progression of aortic dilatation.[314] Dose should be based on resting heart rate, which should be below 60 per minute for adults.[315] Based on newer knowledge, angiotensin II blockers[316] and ACE inhibitors such as Perindopril[317] appear to be effective.

Due to increased mortality within the scope of emergency aortic root replacement (generally due to dissection),[318]

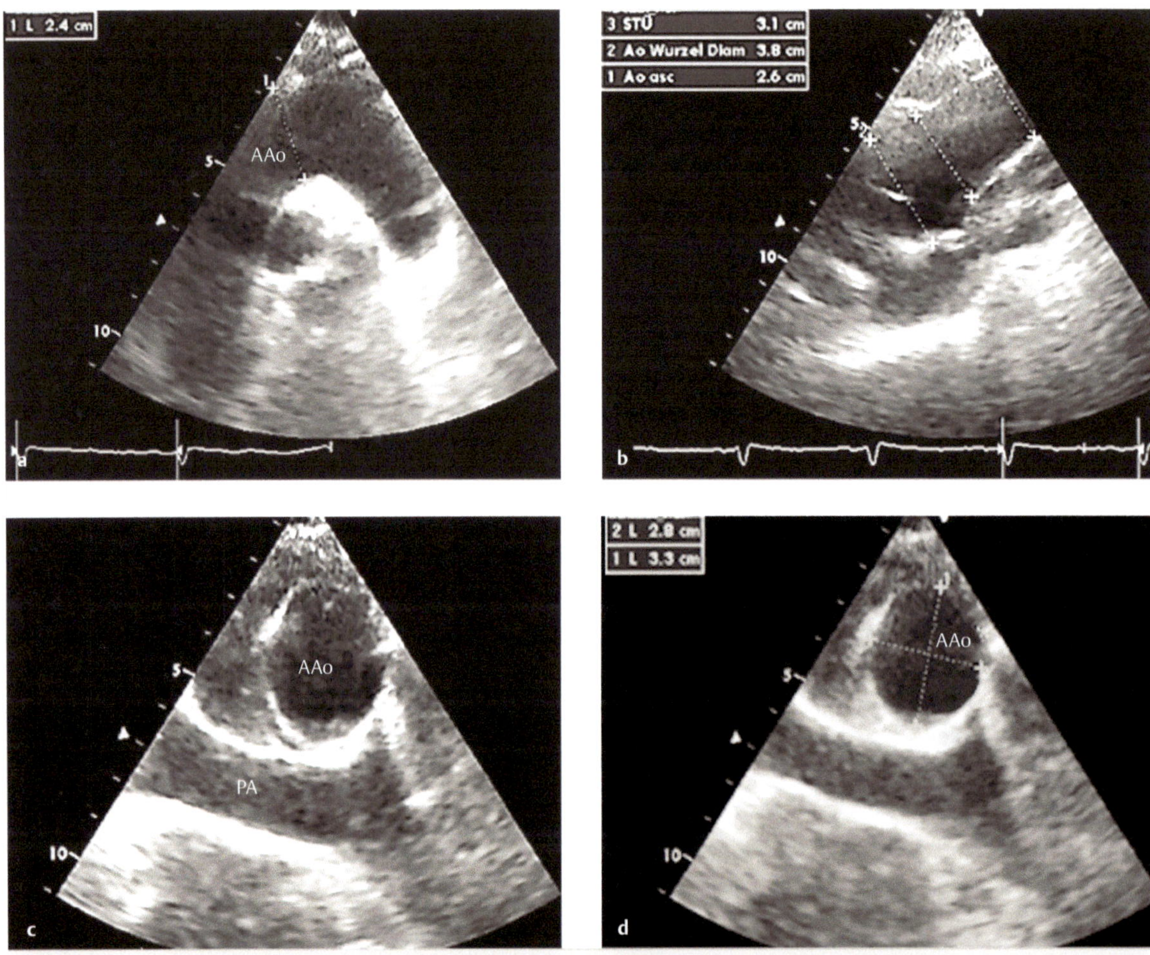

Fig. 4.192 Dilated aortic root in a case of Marfan syndrome. Thirty-two-year-old female patient with Marfan syndrome and a family history (father died from aortic rupture due to acute type A dissection). The aortic root is enlarged to a maximum of 3.8 cm (b). Color Doppler depicts moderate mitral valve insufficiency (e). The topogram (g) of the corresponding MDCT depicts the osteosynthesis material near the spinal column, condition after scoliosis surgery and pectus excavatum. The aortic root, dilated to a maximum of 4 cm, is depicted in h–j. The MDCT pulmonary window (k) depicts clear pectus excavatum with ventricular narrowing. MRI flow measurements revealed a minor regurgitation fraction of 5% (l, light blue area), only.

AAo = ascending aorta
PA = pulmonary artery
a 2-D TTE, suprasternal view.
b 2-D TTE, parasternal long axis.
c 2-D TTE, transverse slice.
d 2-D TTE, transverse slice, with diameter values acquired during systole.

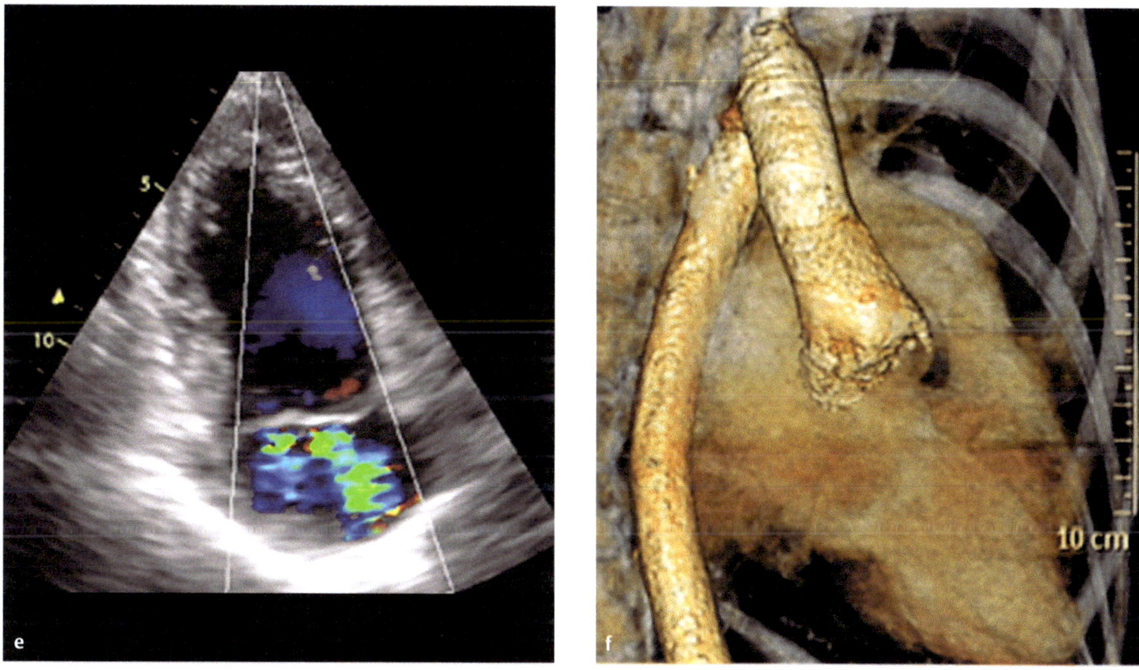

Fig 4.192 *(Continued)* **Dilated aortic root in a case of Marfan syndrome.**
AAo = ascending aorta
PA = pulmonary artery

e 2-D TTE, 4-chamber view (color Doppler), during systole.
f 3-D reconstruction from a CTA using volume rendering technique.

both American and European guidelines[6] recommend an elective *aortic root replacement* starting at a vessel diameter of more than 5 cm (▸ Fig. 4.191a). Additional criteria include severe aortic and mitral valve insufficiency, a family history of dissection (▸ Fig. 4.192), rapid increase in dilatation, and planned pregnancy. Complete replacement of the aortic root and ascending aorta by means of a valve-equipped, premade conduit (composite prosthesis) can be performed independently of aortic valve function (Bentall procedure[319–321]). Alternatively, only the ascending aorta can be replaced if the aortic valve leaflets appear unremarkable under macroscopic examination. The valve-preserving surgeries can be performed using the Yacoub (remodeling technique) or David (reimplantation technique) methods. For the former, the wall of the aortic root is replaced by a prosthesis, and the valve is stitched to the prosthesis (Yacoub method). For the David procedure, the aortic valve is reconstructed, and the coronary arteries are reimplanted near the prosthesis. The David procedure is preferred for patients with Marfan syndrome nowadays, since this procedure offers the opportunity to tighten and thereby stabilize the annulus, while in the Yacoub technique the aortic root can further dilate.[322,323] The valve-preserving technique requires fewer reinterventions compared to total aortic root replacement. Nevertheless, the latter yields significantly fewer thromboembolic complications.[322]

> **Note**
>
> If the leaflets are anatomically intact, the guidelines promote the use of valve-preserving aortic root replacement procedures.

Improvements in medication and surgical treatment have increased the life expectancy of Marfan syndrome patients from an average of 32 years[324] to 40 years.[325] In these cases, a family history of severe cardiovascular events is associated with lower life expectancy.[326]

Goals and Relative Value of Diagnostic Imaging

Based on the described changes to the cardiovascular system, adequate imaging (both within the scope of primary diagnostics and in postinterventional follow-up examinations) is of crucial clinical importance.

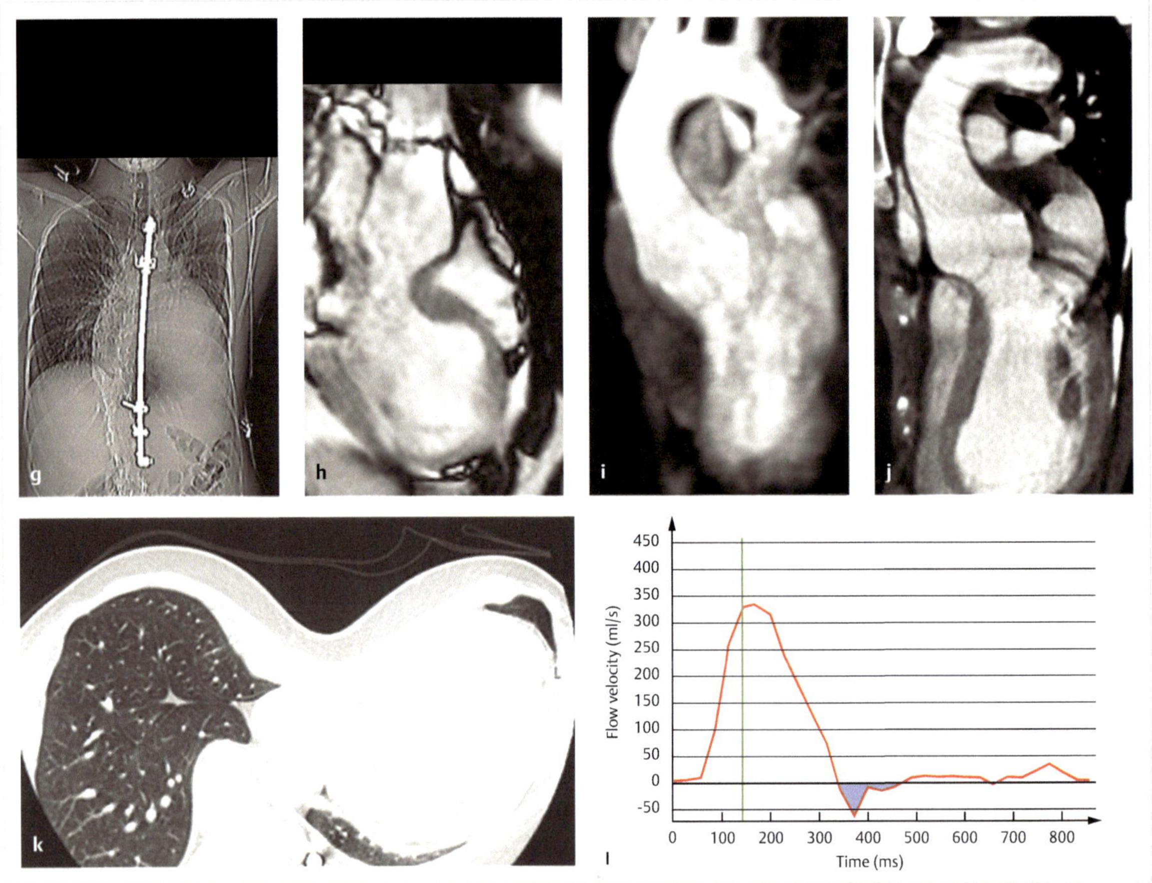

Fig 4.192 (*Continued*) **Dilated aortic root in a case of Marfan syndrome..**
AAo = ascending aorta
PA = pulmonary artery
g Topogram of the MDCT.
h SSFP cine MRI through the LVOT.
i 3-D MIP reconstruction of a contrast-enhanced MRA.
j LVOT reconstruction of a CTA.
k Pulmonary window of an MDCT.
l Results of MR flow measurements via the aortic valve, using the phase contrast technique.

Within the scope of initial diagnostics, the European guidelines[6] recommend a *TTE* (▶ Fig. 4.192a-d) and measurement of aortic diameter in defined locations (▶ Fig. 4.189c), including the aortic annulus, aortic sinus, sinotubular junction, and distal descending aorta. Biventricular function and the heart valves should also be assessed. Furthermore, the entire aorta should be depicted using either CT or MRI. Follow-up examinations should be performed promptly, based on the initial size of the aorta and its increase in size.

If acute aortic dissection is suspected, TEE or *MDCT* (▶ Fig. 4.191a,b) are the imaging methods of choice, based on availability.[327]

> **Note**
>
> A CT coronary angiogram should be performed before a planned surgery. The coronaries should not be depicted invasively due to the risk of dissection.

MRI permits radiation-free, noninvasive depiction of all important structures, including the entire aorta, and detection of aneurysms, dissections (entry and re-entry of intimal tears and dissection membrane),[328] and ruptures. In the event of asymmetrical dilatation, tomographic procedures by means of MRI and MDCT are superior to echocardiography.[329] In order to achieve this precision, it is crucial to comply with standardized examination protocols.[330] This also depends on the various sequences that can be used to measure diameter at defined anatomical points (▶ Fig. 4.189c), such as SSFP cine MRI sequences during systole (▶ Fig. 4.189a, ▶ Fig. 4.190b,c), angulated parasagittal black blood SE sequences (▶ Fig. 4.189b), and non-triggered, contrast-enhanced angiograms (▶ Fig. 4.189d).[331] It is necessary to use standardized protocols, particularly for follow-up examinations. The global and regional function of both ventricles (Marfan cardiomyopathy) and standardized phase contrast flow measurements (▶ Fig. 4.192l) should be a part of MRI examinations for evaluating heart valve function.

Invasive angiographic depiction using iodine-based contrast agent does not constitute an alternative purely for diagnosing Marfan syndrome due to the aforementioned benefits of tomographic procedures.

4.6.5 Williams–Beuren Syndrome

Heiner Latus, Gerald F. Greil

Definition

Williams–Beuren syndrome is a congenital neuropediatric disorder that most commonly affects the cardiovascular system. In terms of imaging diagnostics, Williams–Beuren syndrome is often associated with multiple stenoses near the great vessels, particularly supravalvular aortic stenosis (see Supravalvular Aortic Stenosis).[332] The syndrome was named after the first two physicians to describe it, British cardiologist Williams[333] and Goettingen cardiologist Beuren.[334]

Etiology

This syndrome occurs in approximately 1:10,000 live births[335] and is caused by submicroscopic deletion of multiple neighboring genes on chromosome 7, including the elastin gene.[336] The usually spontaneous mutation (family history is rare) affects multiple neighboring genes on one segment of the chromosome, meaning the phenotype of patients with Williams–Beuren syndrome can vary widely and may include craniofacial defects (such as elf face syndrome) or even cognitive impairments.[337]

Clinical Issues

Defects can occur in various organ systems (▶ Table 4.37). Most commonly, however, patients with Williams–Beuren syndrome suffer from cardiovascular defects (approximately 80% of patients), usually in the form of stenoses in the arterial vessels.[332] Since elastin constitutes an essential component of the extracellular matrix for arterial vessels and grants these vessels great elasticity and the corresponding favorable mechanical properties (Windkessel effect), a mutation in the *ELN* gene leads to histological changes in the vessels (media hypertrophy).[338] This causes generalized arteriopathy and increased vascular stiffness.

One characteristic finding is *supravalvular aortic stenosis*—defined as a narrowing in the ascending aorta superior to the aortic valve—which occurs in 45–75% of patients with Williams–Beuren syndrome[332] (▶ Fig. 4.193 and ▶ Fig. 4.194; ▶ Fig. 4.55c, ▶ Fig. 4.59, and ▶ Fig. 4.60).

The morphology and severity of supravalvular aortic stenosis is heterogeneous. More commonly (in 75% of cases), a ring-like, surrounded membranous narrowing near the aortic valve (with an hourglass shape) is located directly

Table 4.37 Summary of possible manifestations of Williams–Beuren syndrome, which possess variable incidence and varying degrees of severity.

Organ system	Characteristics
Facies	Facial deformities, typically elf face syndrome (sometimes called funny face or goblin face) with a broad forehead, short lid slits, deep nasal root, broad nostrils, prominent cheekbones, small chin, long philtrum, full lips, and edema of the eyelids
Ears, eyes, teeth	Hyperacusis, recurrent otitis media, spoke-like patterns in the iris (iris stellata), strabismus, bite anomalies with malformed teeth or wide gaps (known as mouse teeth)
Electrolytes/hormones	Hypercalcemia, vitamin D metabolic disorders, diabetes mellitus, osteopenia/osteoporosis, hypothyroidism, precocious puberty
Musculoskeletal	Delayed growth, dwarfism, muscular hypertonia, hyperreflexia, scoliosis, joint contraction
Gastrointestinal	Constipation, diverticulosis, lack of weight gain, rectal prolapse, celiac disease, gastroesophageal reflux
Urogenital	Displaced kidneys, renal agenesis, nephrocalcinosis, recurrent urinary tract infections, undescended testicles, umbilical/inguinal hernias
Neurology/development	Mental retardation (average IQ of 55), developmental delays, savant syndrome, microcephaly, friendly personality, anxiety disorders, phobias, impulsiveness, attention deficit disorders

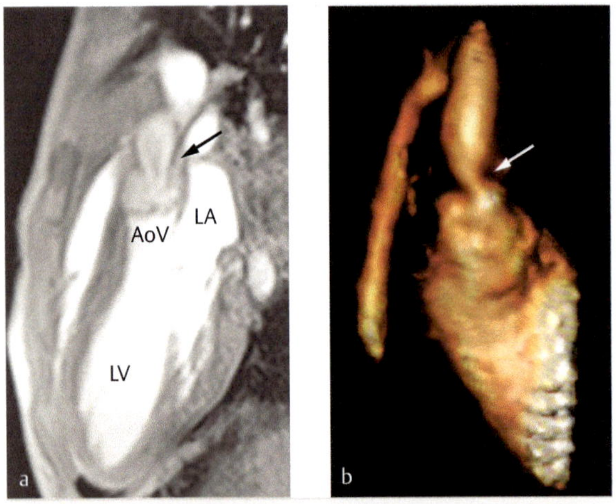

Fig. 4.193 Typical supravalvular aortic stenosis in a patient with Williams–Beuren syndrome. Six-year-old male patient. The arrows indicate the supravalvular aortic stenosis.
AoV = aortic valve
LA = left atrium
LV = left ventricle
a SSFP cine MRI, LVOT slice, through the LVOT.
b 3-D reconstruction of a contrast-enhanced MRA.

superior to the valsalva sinus (▸ Fig. 4.60). In these cases, the thickened intima may even extend to the margins of the aortic cusps. The rarer, diffuse, elongated lesions are characterized by a cylindrical thickening of the aortic wall that affects the ascending aorta, can extend to the aortic arch, and is often associated with stenoses of the effluent head and neck vessels.[339] Of all the types of congenital LVOT obstructions, supravalvular aortic stenosis comprises only 8–14%, and is thus a rather rare anomaly in early childhood.[340] Supravalvular aortic stenosis (see Supravalvular Aortic Stenosis) can occur in three different contexts:

- Sporadic and isolated, meaning with no concurrent vascular or cardiac defects (see ▸ Fig. 4.60; a mutation in the *ELN* gene can be verified in some of these defects, without any of the other surrounding genes being affected by a deletion[341])
- Autosomal-dominant inherited familial form[342]
- In association with Williams–Beuren syndrome (see ▸ Fig. 4.193 and ▸ Fig. 4.194)

Patients with Williams–Beuren syndrome may also have concurrent vascular defects in addition to supravalvular aortic stenosis. *Stenoses in the pulmonary arterial system*,[332] mostly near the main pulmonary trunk (▸ Fig. 4.195, ▸ Fig. 4.194) or more peripheral, likewise diffuse stenoses within a long segment are also present. Supravalvular pulmonary stenosis (▸ Fig. 4.194) occurs in only 12% of cases.[332] A hypoplastic pulmonary vascular bed may also be present.

To date, the prevalence of *coronary pathologies*[343] among patients with Williams–Beuren syndrome has most likely been underestimated. These pathologies may occur in the form of ostium stenosis, diffuse stenosis, or dilatation.

Stenoses of the aorta are an expression of high-grade artery disease, and may range in severity from a "simple" aortic coarctation to middle aortic syndrome with diffuse, extended *hypoplasia of the descending aorta* (▸ Fig. 4.196; ▸ Fig. 4.197c). The incidence of this defect is unclear, and ranges from 2% to 70%.[332]

The *renal arteries* are often also affected in up to 40% of patients with Williams–Beuren syndrome and systemic high arterial blood pressure, usually in the form of origin stenosis (▸ Fig. 4.196d).[344] The incidence of aortic valve abnormalities was listed as 50% in most surgical studies. They generally occur as adhesions of the leaflets to the sinotubular junction or as thickened bicuspid aortic valves. Furthermore, VSD (4–9% of patients, usually muscular; see the patient from ▸ Fig. 4.194 and ▸ Fig. 4.197), mitral valve prolapse, or stenoses of the mesenterial and intracranial vessels may occur.[332]

In addition to the described morphological abnormalities, further cardiac issues are associated with Williams–Beuren syndrome. An elevated risk of sudden cardiac death,[345] complications during anesthesia, and cardiac rhythm disorders in cases of increased QTc time have been described repeatedly.[346]

The most common cardiovascular defect, namely supravalvular stenosis, often remains clinically silent for a long period of time and is generally first noticed once it has become particularly pronounced. Patients report reduced exercise capacity with dyspnea and symptoms similar to angina pectoris, as well as syncopal episodes. From an auscultatory viewpoint, systolic noise with a pronounced aortic valve closing sound and click are apparent. If no supravalvular, but rather only peripheral stenosis are present in a case of Williams–Beuren syndrome, this disorder can remain clinically silent and may only manifest in the form of clinical symptoms of arterial hypertonia—for example, within the scope of a hypoplastic aorta (known as aorta angusta) or renal arterial stenosis (▸ Fig. 4.196). Left ventricular hypertrophy can be diagnosed in older children by means of ECG or imaging procedures due to the pressure overload. If additional pulmonary stenoses are present, then right ventricular hypertrophy can also be verified (▸ Fig. 4.194).

Hemodynamics, Natural Progression, and Indication for Treatment

The afterload in the left ventricle may be elevated based on the extent of supravalvular narrowing. Unlike valvular aortic stenosis, the coronary arteries are also subject to elevated perfusion pressure in cases of supravalvular aortic stenosis. This can lead to the development of atherosclerotic changes and dilatation more rapidly than is typical (▸ Fig. 4.194). The data pool regarding this disorder's natural progression is, to date, ambiguous.

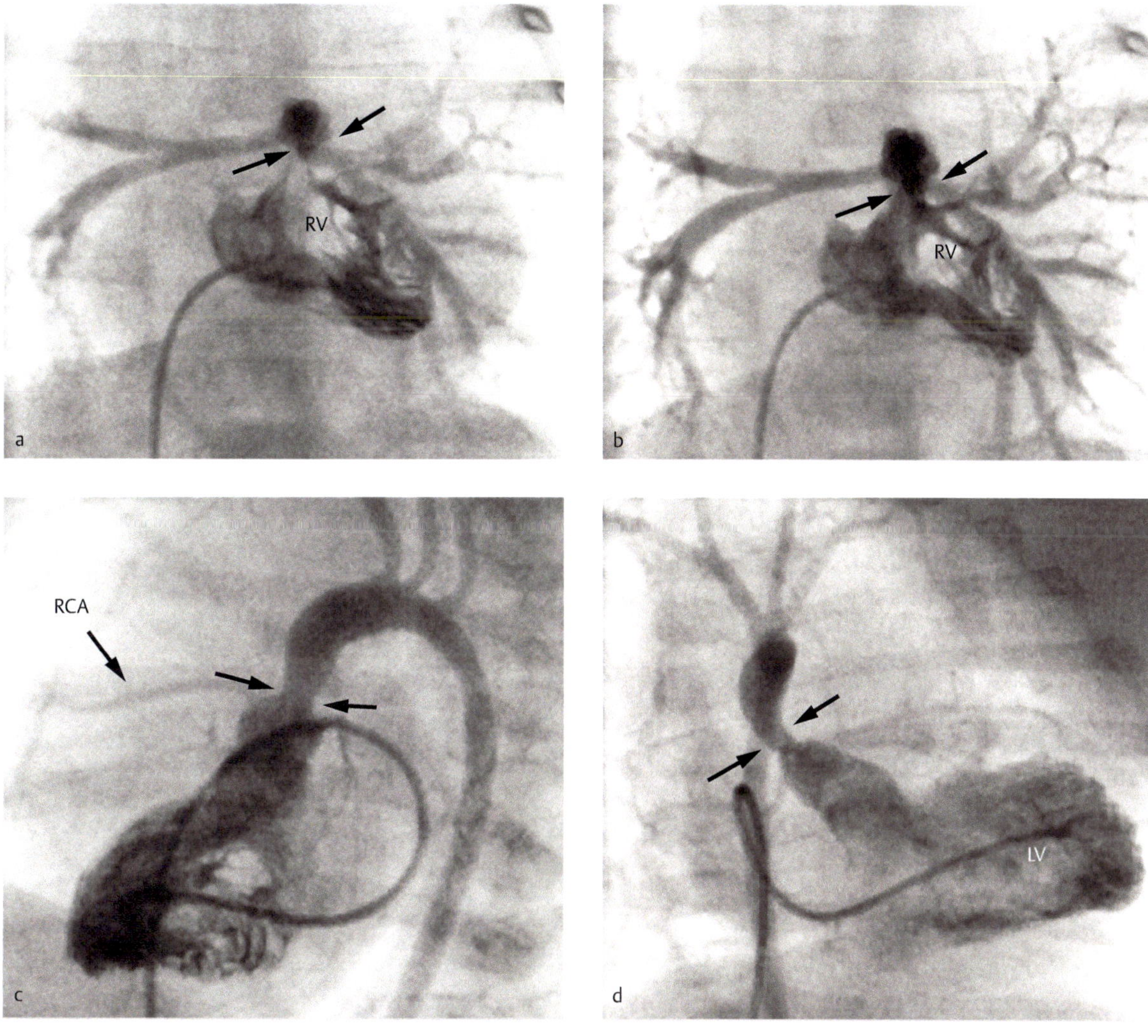

Fig. 4.194 Supravalvular aortic and pulmonary stenosis in a case of Williams–Beuren syndrome. One-year-old female patient with Williams–Beuren syndrome, small midventricular muscular VSD (▶ Fig. 4.197, same patient) and supravalvular aortic (c, d, arrows) and (a, b, arrows) pulmonary stenoses. Extensive hypoplasia of the right pulmonary artery is also present. Both the right and left ventricle demonstrate subsequent indications of ventricular hypertrophy. Angiography (c, d) also depicts the origins of the coronary arteries with no relevant stenosis or dilatation, particularly in the right coronary artery.

LV = left ventricle
RCA = right coronary artery
RV = right ventricle

- **a** Preoperative right ventricular catheter examination in an early phase of ventricular filling.
- **b** Preoperative right ventricular catheter examination depicting good contrast of the right ventricle and pulmonary arteries.
- **c** Preoperative left ventricular catheter examination and angiography, LAO projection.
- **d** Preoperative left ventricular catheter examination and angiography, RAO projection.

Generally speaking, minor supravalvular aortic stenosis (less than 20 mmHg) within the scope of Williams–Beuren syndrome does not tend to progress, but rather to regress. This means that interventions are generally unnecessary. Approximately 20% of patients with Williams–Beuren syndrome and minor supravalvular aortic stenosis do, however, require surgical or catheter interventional procedures (▶ Fig. 4.194 and ▶ Fig. 4.198) at a later date. At gradients in excess of 20 mmHg, progression was observed in virtually every case.[347]

Consequently, if minor supravalvular aortic stenosis occurs in isolation, with no clinical or echocardiographic indications of ventricular dysfunction during thorough follow-up examinations, it is recommended that clinicians adopt a wait-and-see approach. If symptoms of higher-grade stenosis (pressure gradient of at least 50 mmHg) are present, this constitutes a primary indication for surgical treatment. Timely intervention is necessary in the event that coronary obstruction is present.

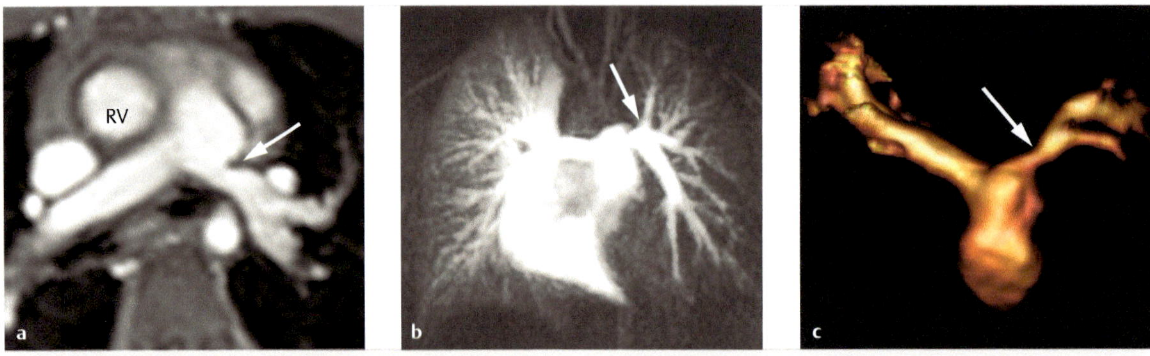

Fig. 4.195 Origin stenosis of the left pulmonary artery in a case of Williams–Beuren syndrome. Six-year-old male patient. The stenosis can be clearly visualized by means of MRI (a–c). Dynamic MRA (b) also depicts the pronounced pulmonary hypoperfusion on the left side due to the relevant stenosis of the left pulmonary artery (a–c, arrows).
a Transverse SSFP sequence.
b Dynamic, contrast-enhanced MRA with corresponding 3-D MIP reconstruction, RAO projection.
c 3-D reconstruction, volume rendering technique, of contrast-enhanced MRA.

Pulmonary stenoses generally recede spontaneously.[348] If an intervention is necessary, this intervention is used to attempt to treat the stenoses.

Treatment Options

Though performing simple surgical resection of supravalvular aortic stenosis with an end-to-end anastomosis is one treatment option, the *Doty technique* is generally used nowadays.[349] During this procedure, the ascending aorta is incised proximally in a Y shape toward the aortic root, the stenotic membrane is removed, and the aorta is then expanded and reconstructed using a patch.[350]

One alternative is *Brom's three-sinus technique*, in which the sinus is expanded using individual patches.[351] If a hypoplastic ascending aorta is present, then either an aortoplasty must be performed or a conduit from the left ventricle to the aortic arch must be implanted. Reconstruction or valvuloplasty of a bicuspid aortic valve can be performed in tandem.

Note

Due to the elastic vascular wall properties including recoil, as well as the proximity to the aortic valve and sinus, catheter interventional balloon angioplasty and stent implantation are not viable options.[350]

Higher-grade pulmonary stenoses are generally well tolerated clinically, meaning that regular follow-up examinations including right ventricular pressure gradient measurements are generally sufficient. Balloon angioplasty of stenoses of the central pulmonary arteries generally yields poor results. *Balloon angioplasty of peripheral stenoses* (intrapulmonary segments), on the other hand, achieves significantly better results. It can be helpful to perform regular, noninvasive imaging follow-up examinations by means of MRA (▶ Fig. 4.197) or CTA and to calculate ventricular parameters using echocardiography or MRI. *Stent implantation* can quickly lead to restenosis due to intima proliferation. Furthermore, aneurysms have been recorded as occurring after balloon dilatation.

The results after *resection of supravalvular aortic stenoses* are good. In the study conducted by Deo et al. 86% of all patients required no reoperation after 20 years.[352] Residual gradients between the left ventricle and aorta generally persisted (▶ Fig. 4.198).

Goals and Relative Value of Diagnostic Imaging

The variety of the aforementioned characteristics are the basis of suspected Williams–Beuren syndrome.

The heart appears to be normally sized in *thoracic X-ray images*. The sometimes-absent aortic shadows can make the superior mediastinum appear narrow (▶ Fig. 4.196a). If pronounced peripheral pulmonary stenosis is present, indications of an overloaded right ventricle and reduced pulmonary perfusion are recognizable (▶ Fig. 4.195b).

Echocardiography can be used to verify left ventricular hypertrophy or circumscribed (▶ Fig. 4.59c and d) or diffuse narrowing in the ascending aorta. These findings are supplemented by Doppler examination, which verifies accelerated flow via the narrowing (▶ Fig. 4.60d).

Peripheral pulmonary stenoses can rarely be depicted using echocardiography. Rather, *cardiac MRI* (▶ Fig. 4.195) and *cardiac multi-slice CT* are the methods of choice.[59] The hemodynamic relevance of the pulmonary stenosis can be evaluated either quantitatively using MRI flow measurements, or using a dynamic, contrast-enhanced MRA (▶ Fig. 4.195b). This has become also possible using dynamic

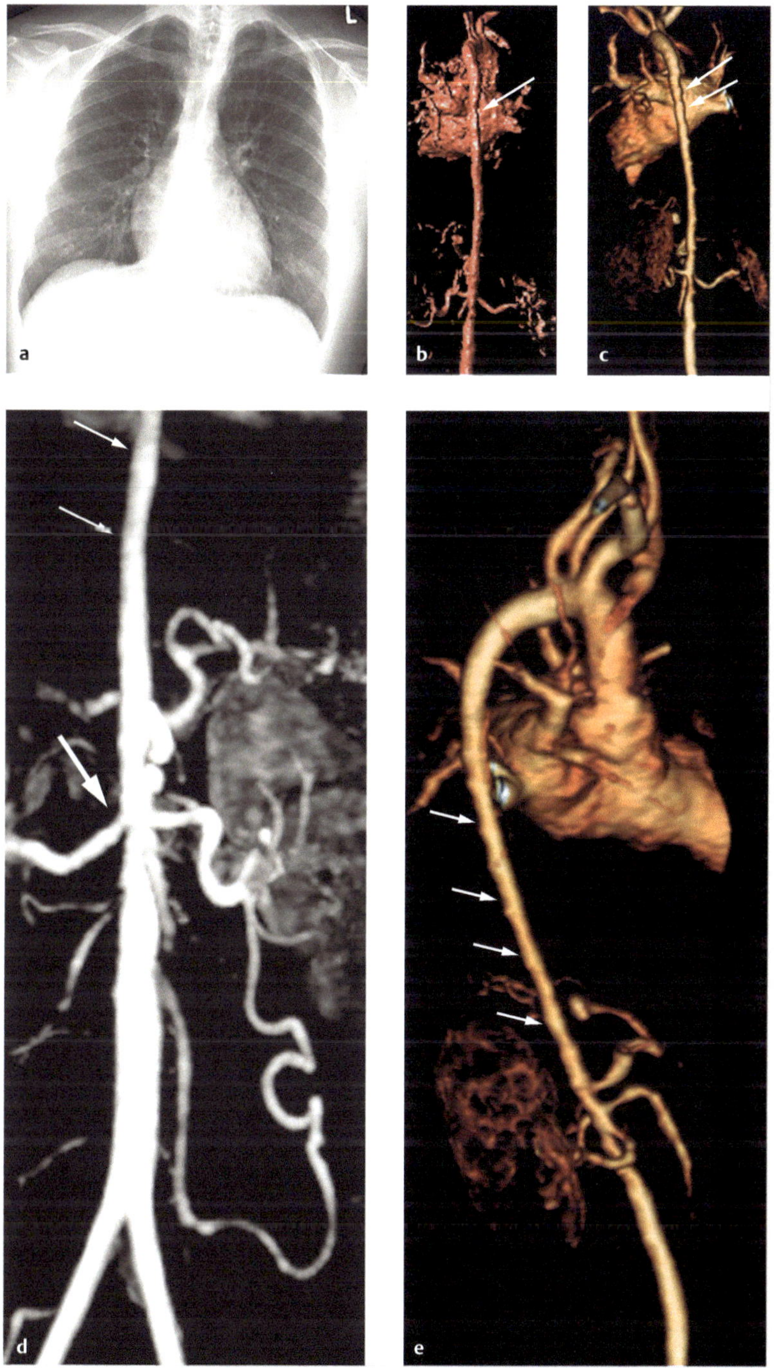

Fig. 4.196 Hypoplastic descending aorta in a case of Williams–Beuren syndrome. Nineteen-year-old male patient. The p.-a. thoracic X-ray (a) for initial diagnosis depicts a narrow superior mediastinum. The initial images using volume rendering technique and 3-D MIP reconstruction from a contrast-enhanced MRA depict several mid-grade renal origin stenoses, in addition to the extended hypoplastic descending aorta (b–d, arrows). The follow-up examination 4 years later (e) depicts primarily unchanged findings for the descending aorta and regression of the renal origin stenosis on the right side.

- **a** P.-a. thoracic X-ray.
- **b** Initial image, volume rendering technique, strictly dorsal view.
- **c** Initial image, volume rendering technique, dorsal view with minor left rotation, clearly depicting the hypoplastic descending aorta and right-side renal arterial origin stenosis.
- **d** 3-D MIP reconstruction from a contrast-enhanced MRA, with right renal origin stenosis (thick arrow).
- **e** Follow-up examination 4 years later, 3-D MRA in volume rendering technique, lateral projection.

CT, though this method is associated with higher radiation exposure. In addition, tomographic procedures can depict the ascending aorta and aortic arch precisely, and the extent of supravalvular aortic stenosis can be determined. On principle, purely morphological depiction of the aortic root, including the coronary origins, can be achieved using any noninvasive imaging procedure. A complete overview of stenoses in the potentially affected vessels can be achieved primarily using MRA or CTA, due to the nature of these procedures (▶ Fig. 4.196b-e). Potentially concurrent aortic insufficiency can be quantified precisely using echocardiography, primarily MR flow measurements.

Invasive cardiac catheter examinations are rarely necessary to depict the morphology of the RVOT and LVOT (▶ Fig. 4.194). Cardiac catheter examinations are performed to determine pressure gradients via stenoses and, above all, for interventional treatment.

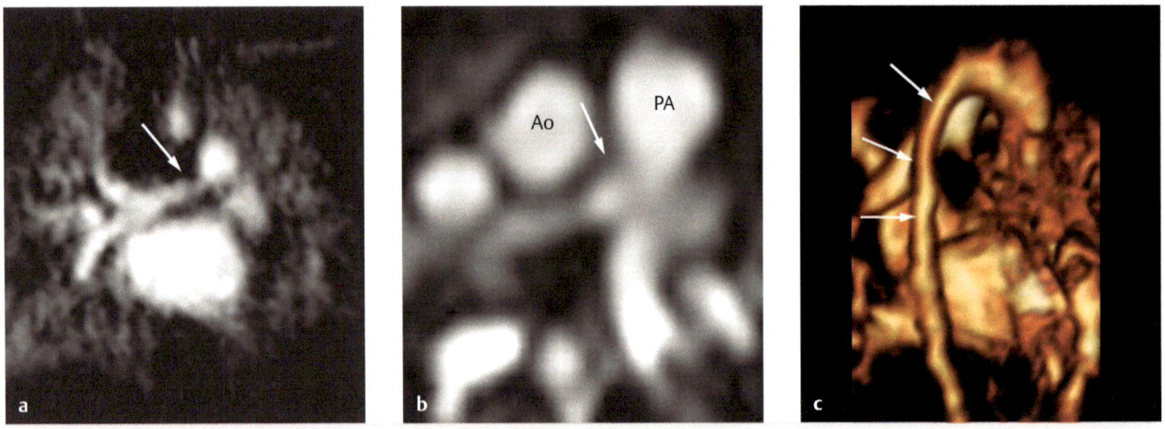

Fig. 4.197 Condition after surgical treatment for a supravalvular aortic and pulmonary stenosis in a patient with Williams–Beuren syndrome. An aortoplasty of the aortic root and patch enlargement of the supravalvular pulmonary stenosis was performed on the patient from ▶ Fig. 4.194. The time-resolved contrast-enhanced MRA images of the aorta acquired 3 years after the surgical procedure depict residual, extended hypoplasia of the right pulmonary artery and aorta.

Ao = aorta
PA = pulmonary artery

- **a** 3-D MIP reconstruction of a contrast-enhanced MRA, ventral view.
- **b** SSFP cine MRI, transverse section.
- **c** 3-D image, volume rendering technique, lateral projection.

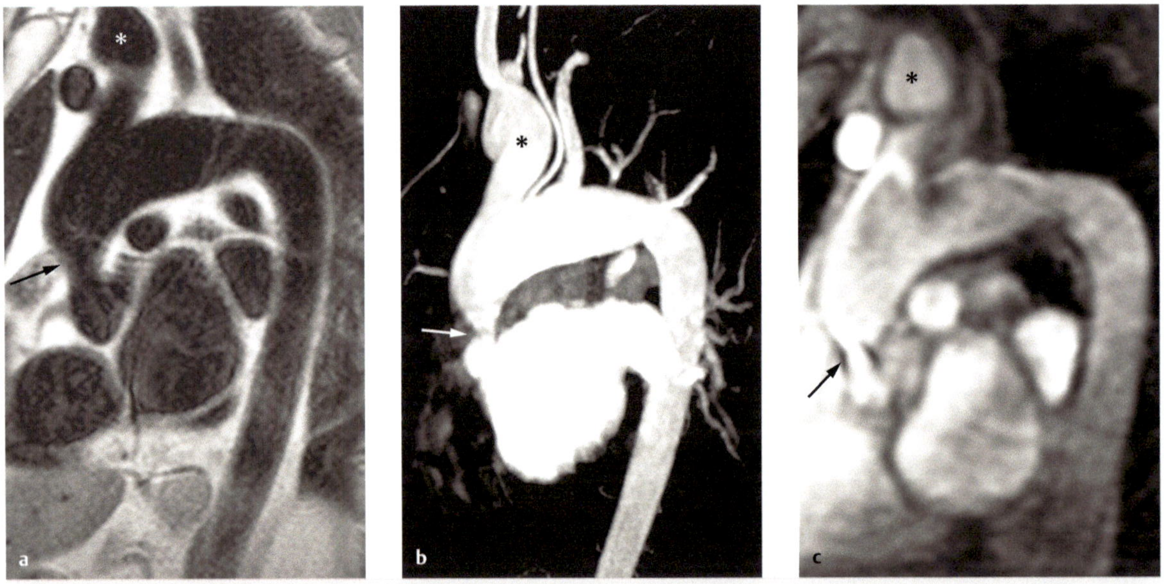

Fig. 4.198 Condition after correction of a supravalvular aortic stenosis using a patch enlargement procedure for a patient with Williams–Beuren syndrome. Postoperative MRIs of a 45-year-old male patient. All images depict a parasagittal orientation through the aortic arch with residual relative stenosis (a–c, arrows) near the ascending aorta and a maximum root diameter of 30 mm, a maximum dilatation of the ascending aorta of 36 mm, and a maximum stenosis diameter of 17 mm. Direct MR flow measurements resulted in a maximum flow acceleration of up to 2.5 m/s, corresponding to a residual maximum instantaneous pressure gradient of 25 mmHg. The residual stenosis is thus not relevant to treatment. The dilated brachiocephalic artery (a–c, asterisks) is clearly visible.

- **a** Black blood SE image.
- **b** Parasagittal MIP reconstruction of a contrast-enhanced MRA.
- **c** Magnitude image of an in-plane phase contrast flow measurement during systole, depicting minor dephasing via the relative stenosis as an indirect sign of flow acceleration.

4.6.6 Rhythm Disorders and Dyssynchrony

Jan Janoušek, Philipp Lurz

The individual imaging procedures are used in electrophysiology for pediatric patients with congenital heart defects, primarily for the following purposes:

- Prenatal echocardiography to detect and analyze cardiac rhythm disorders and assess the severity of fetal heart failure
- Assessing ventricular function and wall thickness
- Assessing ventricular mechanical dyssynchrony (indication for cardiac resynchronization treatment)
- 3-D reconstruction of the heart for imaging integration purposes in cases of catheter-based ablation therapy
- Assessing cardiac and vascular structure (obstructions, shunts) in terms of the possibility of transvenous pacemaker or ICD implantation

Prenatal Echocardiography

Prenatal cardiac ultrasound examinations have permitted clinicians to detect not just congenital heart defects, but also to diagnose, analyze, and treat rhythm disorders since the 1980s. In these applications, prenatal echocardiographic examinations have replaced the much more involved and not universally applicable fetal ECG or magnetocardiography. Diagnostics are based on the ability to analyze the connection between atrial and ventricular contraction and to increase their frequency. Either M-mode echocardiography or pulse Doppler is used to this end (▶ Fig. 4.199 and ▶ Fig. 4.200). Fetal tachyarrhythmia often leads to cardiac insufficiency, the severity of which can be assessed well using echocardiography.[353]

Assessing Ventricular Function and Wall Thickness

Generally well-known echocardiographic methods of measuring ventricular size (expressed as a *Z* value based on weight or body surface area), volume, and ejection fraction are used. In these cases, echocardiography can contribute to relatively accurate assessment of the left ventricle. The left ventricular shortening fraction and Simpson biplanar ejection fraction correlate to mortality in pediatric DCM patients. Quantitative examinations of the right ventricle, however, are less precise. This is true both of the right ventricle in a normal (subpulmonary) position and in a subaortic position in cases of ccTGA, or atrial switch in cases of TGA IVS. It is necessary to measure systemic ventricular function, particularly when assessing tachycardia-induced cardiomyopathy (▶ Fig. 4.201), determining indication for primary preventative ICD implantation,[354] and for cardiac resynchronization therapy for DCM patients.[355]

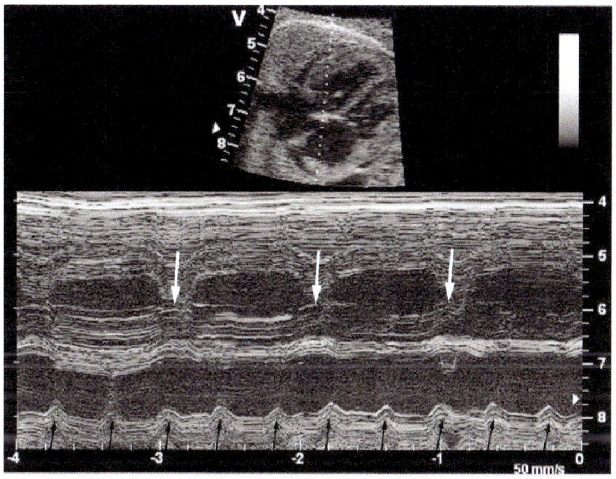

Fig. 4.199 Grade 3 fetal atrioventricular block. Exam during week 25 of pregnancy. Apical 4-chamber view, M-mode depiction of the right ventricle (top) and left atrium (bottom). Independent atrial (thin arrows) and ventricular contractions (thick arrows) with an atrial frequency of 150/minute and a ventricular frequency of 60/minute. (With the gracious approval of Dr. V. Tomek, Children's Heart Centre Prague, University Hospital in Motol, Czech Republic.)

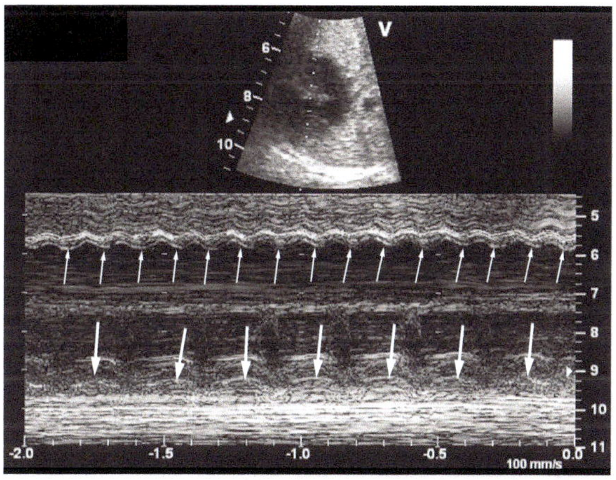

Fig. 4.200 Fetal atrial flutter. Examination during week 36 of pregnancy. Projection along the modified short axis, M-mode depiction of the right atrium (top) and left ventricle (bottom). Regular atrial contractions with a frequency of 480/minute (thin arrows) and a regular 2:1 transition with a ventricular frequency of 240/minute (thick arrows). (With the gracious approval of Dr. V. Tomek, Children's Heart Centre Prague, University Hospital in Motol, Czech Republic.)

The indication for cardiac resynchronization therapy for DCM patients is present if a left ventricular ejection fraction below 30–35% and simultaneous electromechanical dyssynchrony and left bundle branch block are present. If HCM (see Hypertrophic Cardiomyopathy) is present, left ventricular wall thickness above 30 mm is a main risk criterion for sudden cardiac death, and thus constitutes an indication for implanting a primary preventative ICD (▶ Fig. 4.202).[356]

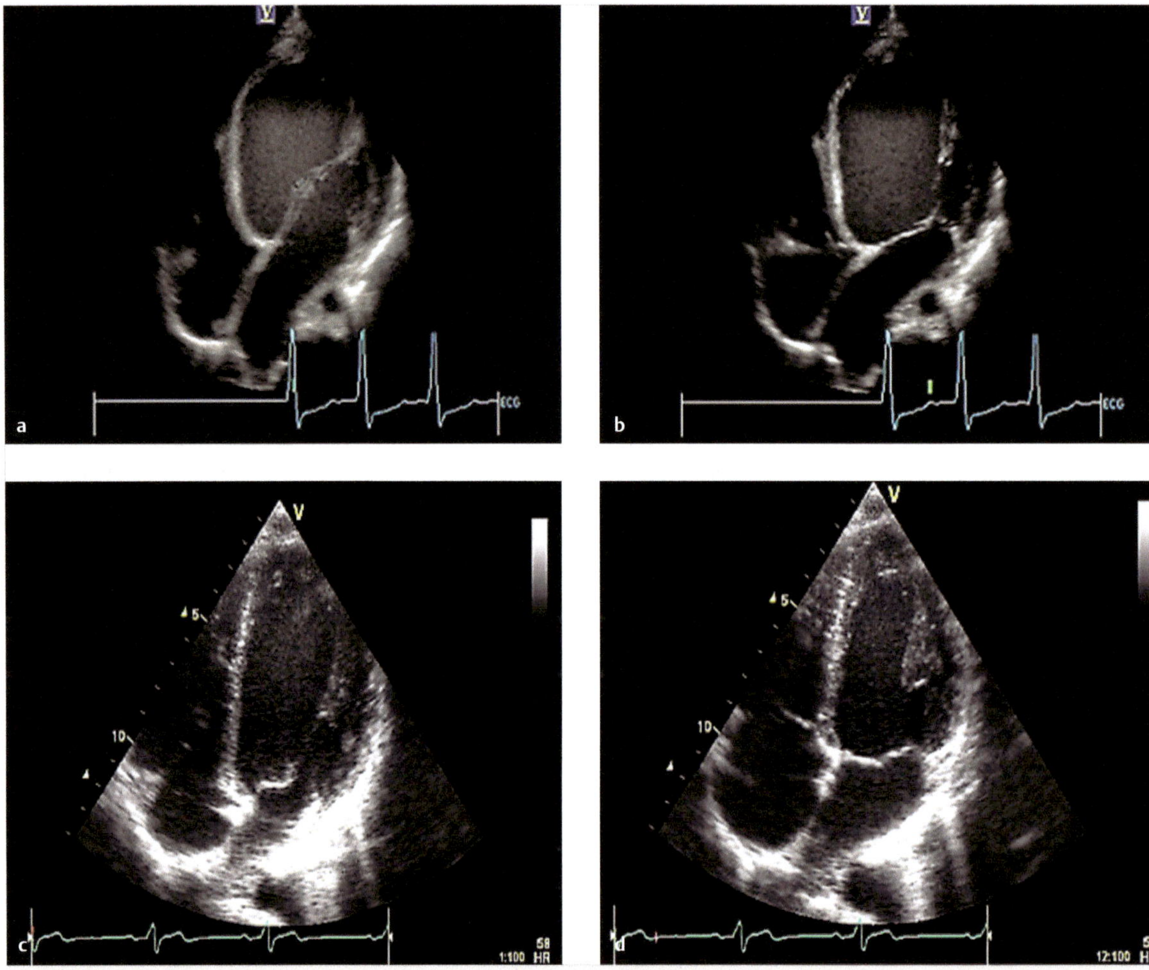

Fig. 4.201 Tachycardia-induced DCM with severe left ventricular dysfunction. Thirteen-year-old boy with ectopic atrial tachycardia. The left ventricular end diastolic diameter is 73 mm (+ 11.4 z), the shortening fraction is 11%, and the ejection fraction is 29%. Grade 2/4 mitral insufficiency is present (**a**, **b**). Complete reverse remodeling 1 year after successful catheter ablation, with normalization of end diastolic (**c**) and end systolic (**d**) size: the left ventricular end diastolic diameter is now 45.7 mm (−0.2 z), the shortening fraction is 34%, and the ejection fraction is 63%. Mitral insufficiency is no longer present.

a Apical 4-chamber view, end diastole.
b Apical 4-chamber view, end systole.
c Apical 4-chamber view, end diastole, after catheter ablation.
d Apical 4-chamber view, end systole, after catheter ablation.

Assessing Ventricular Mechanical Dyssynchrony

Both atrioventricular and intraventricular dyssynchrony can contribute to or intensify the development of heart failure. Intraventricular dyssynchrony of the systemic ventricle, in particular, is a significant factor for developing chronic cardiac insufficiency.[357] A left ventricular ejection fraction no higher than 35%, the presence of a left bundle branch block with a QRS interval of more than 150 ms, and functional NYHA classes II–IV are significant criteria for a class I indication for cardiac resynchronization therapy in adult patients. Since children and patients with congenital heart defects with an indication for cardiac resynchronization therapy may possess a broad spectrum of structural and functional substrates, assessing mechanical dyssynchrony using imaging procedures should be considered a supplement for determining indication. The following aspects are examined:

- Global timing of ejection and filling processes
- Identifying segments that contract early or late (with regard to segmental contraction in the systemic ventricle after closure of the aortic valve, and thus do not contribute to SV)
- Verifying the viability of segments that contract late (meaning ruling out scars) with regard to possible resynchronization potential, and thus the success of cardiac resynchronization therapy

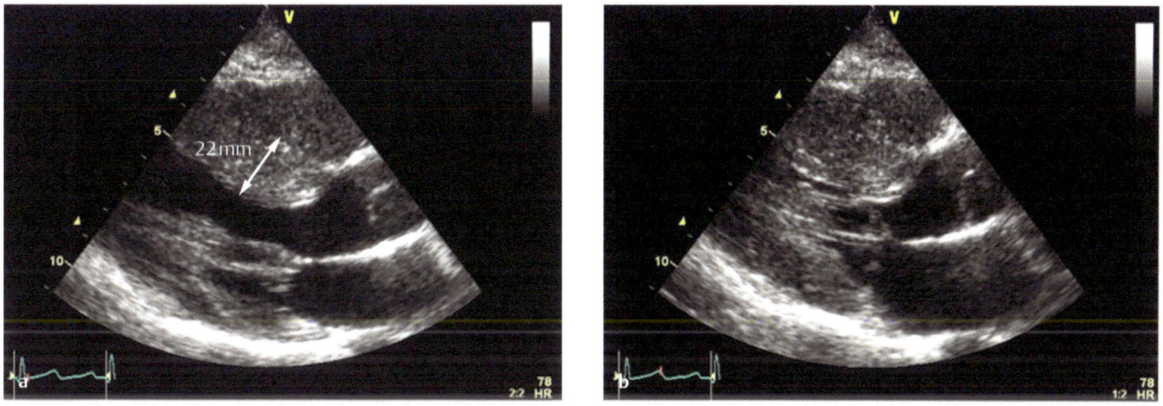

Fig. 4.202 **HOCM.** Seventeen-year-old female patient.

a 2-D TTE, parasternal long axis, depicting an open LVOT during end diastole.

b 2-D TTE, parasternal long axis, depicting complete closure of the LVOT during end systole and a peak gradient of 126 mmHg. Diastolic septum thickness, measured at 22 mm, remains below the threshold of a main risk criterion for sudden cardiac death in HCM patients. Nevertheless, surgical myectomy was recommended based on hemodynamic considerations.

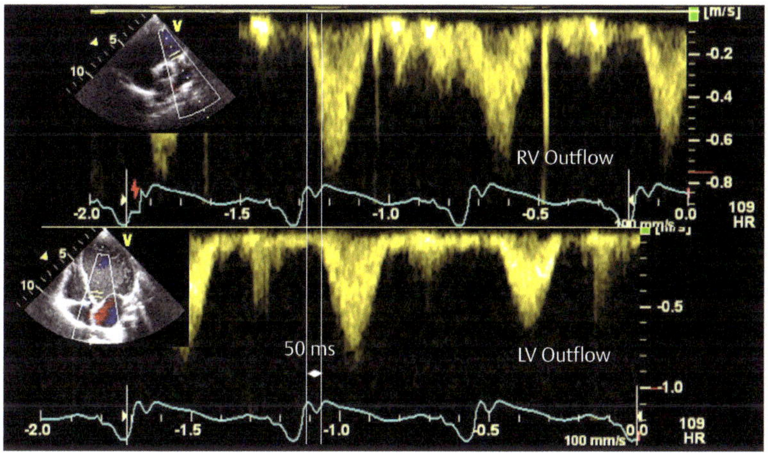

Fig. 4.203 **Interventricular mechanical delay.** The time lag between the start of right ventricular (top) and left ventricular ejection (bottom) is 50 ms in this case, and indicates delayed pressure increases in the left ventricle. Left ventricular dyssynchrony is often the culprit.

Primarily, echocardiography is used to asses mechanical dyssynchrony in clinical settings. Other imaging modalities, such as MRI or isotope methods, have played a secondary role to date due to their worse temporal resolution. The examination generally begins by assessing global timing using temporal marking for the opening and closing of the aortic and systemic atrioventricular valves. Valve motion, itself, can also be used. More commonly, however, the flow patterns via the mitral or tricuspid valves and in the systemic ventricular outflow tract (gleaned using pulse Doppler) are used. This temporal marking can be superimposed upon any other acquisitions in order to be able to assess the timing of the motion sequences. This allows clinicians to gain an overview of interventricular (▶ Fig. 4.203) and intraventricular dyssynchrony (▶ Fig. 4.204). Currently, the following three procedures are used to analyze segmental contraction and relaxation cycles:

- *Tissue Doppler:* this examination measures the time from the start of the QRS complex to the maximum local systolic velocity.[358]
- *Speckle tracking procedure:* this technique is based on detecting specific pixel combinations in a 2-D greyscale image (known as speckles), whose movement can be tracked throughout the entire cardiac cycle. This allows instantaneous local myocardial motion velocities to be determined. Segmental deformation during systole and diastole is then calculated as a velocity of deformation (2-D strain rate) and degree of deformation (2-D strain = segmental shortening or lengthening as a percent) using this data.[359]
- *3-D echocardiography:* as the third and newest method, 3-D has also been used in recent years to measure the time until the minimum segmental systolic volume is reached.

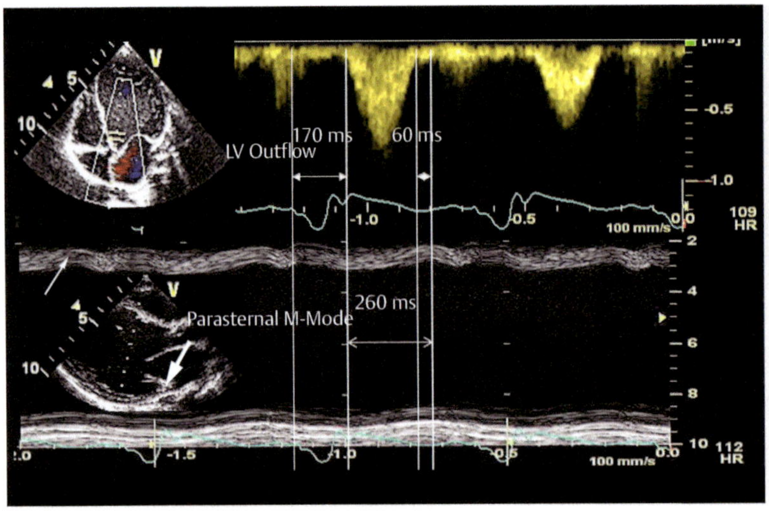

Fig. 4.204 Time course of left ventricular ejection in a case of pronounced dyssynchrony. Temporal compiled image of the pulse Doppler acquisition from the LVOT (top) and the parasternal M-mode depiction (bottom). Left ventricular ejection is delayed by pronounced dyssynchrony (left ventricular pre-ejection period of 170 ms) and begins once the septum contracts (thin arrow). The maximum contraction of the free wall of the left ventricle is delayed by 260 ms compared to the septum (known as septal to posterior wall motion delay; thick arrow) and first occurs 60 ms after closure of the aortic valve. Thus, a significant portion of left ventricular contraction no longer contributes to ejection.

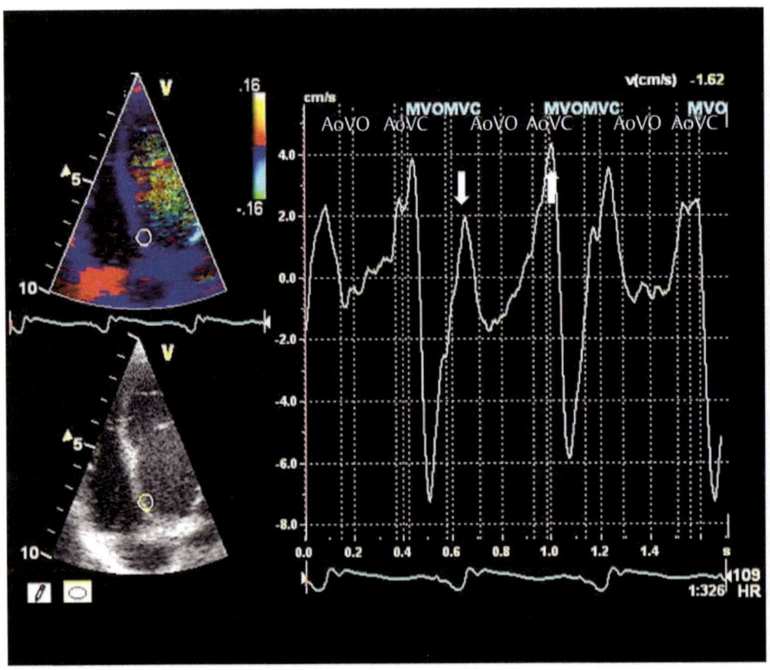

Fig. 4.205 Tissue Doppler examination for a patient with DCM and pronounced left ventricular dyssynchrony. Tissue Doppler from the basal septum of the left ventricle, depicting two peak velocities (arrows). Both occur outside the left ventricular ejection period. Identifying the actual peak systolic velocity is thus impossible without more thorough knowledge of the electrical and mechanical excitation processes. In these cases, the presystolic peak actually corresponded to contraction. This is a male patient with right ventricular pacing and corresponding dyssynchrony.
AoVC = aortic valve closure
AoVO = aortic valve opening
MVC = mitral valve closure
MVO = mitral valve opening

All three methods were able to assess mechanical dyssynchrony in studies of adults with idiopathic or ischemic DCM, and were able to anticipate the effects of cardiac resynchronization therapy. In a large, international, multicenter study,[360] the tissue Doppler method proved itself unable to yield adequately reproducible results. One reason for this may be the difficulty in identifying peak systolic velocities, which are associated with a high rate of interobserver variability. Based on our own experiences, this is often impossible to achieve without knowledge of the individual excitation processes, which is often the case during a blind study (▶ Fig. 4.205). The tissue Doppler method is also dependent upon angle, which can make it difficult to depict the entire dilated ventricle adequately.

The speckle tracking procedure has the advantage of being independent of angle and making it possible to distinguish between active motion processes (contractions) and passive ones (scar tissue being pulled by the surrounding myocardium). Strain and strain rate can be determined separately based on the projection for longitudinal (apical 4-chamber, 2-chamber, and 3-chamber views), radial, and circumferential contraction (parasternal short axis) (▶ Fig. 4.206). The time from the start

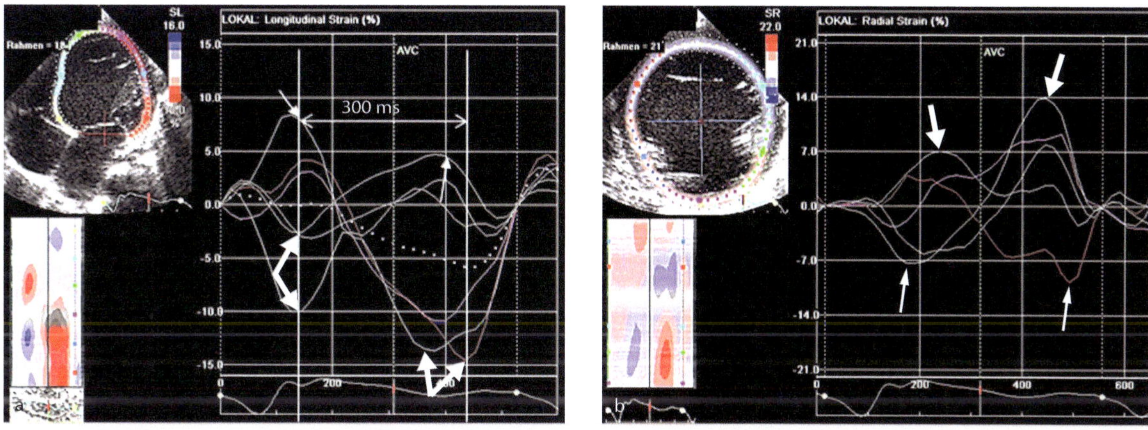

Fig. 4.206 Right ventricular pacing in a case of postsurgical complete atrioventricular block (after closure of a VSD). Two-year-old girl. Severe left ventricular dyssynchrony and dysfunction caused by right ventricular pacing. The color-coded curves reflect the deformation pattern in the corresponding segments of the left ventricle. Negative curves in the longitudinal and positive curves in the radial strain analysis correspond to systolic contraction. Early septal and late lateral contractions are visible in both images (**a**, **b**, thick arrows). The contralateral wall segments demonstrate strain (**a**, **b**, thin arrows). The maximum interventricular mechanical delay is 300 ms in this case. 2-D strain M-mode depictions (in **a** and **b**, bottom left) are a clearer alternative for depicting segmental curvature. This method color codes the strain value in the respective segment over time. The uncoordinated course of left ventricular contraction is clearly visible upon initial inspection of this image.

a Longitudinal strain depiction.

b Radial strain depiction.

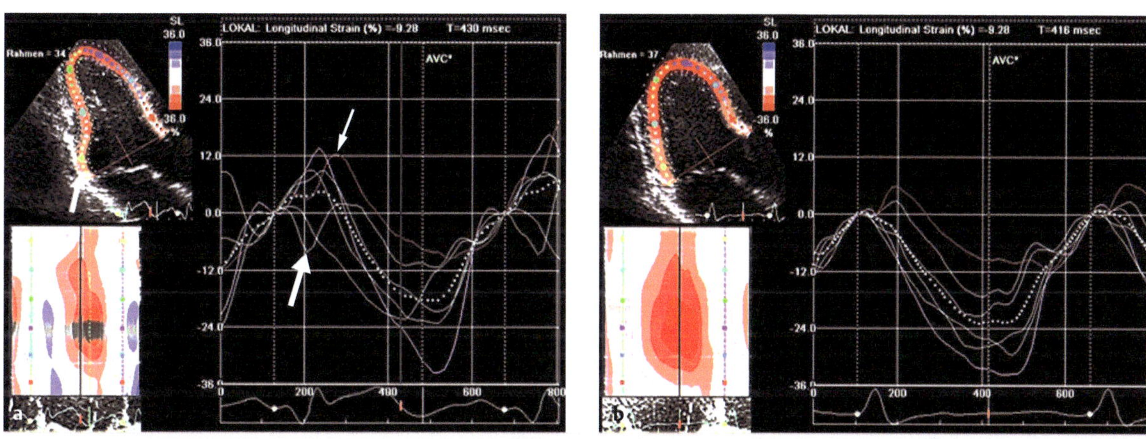

Fig. 4.207 Condition before and after ablation of a left inferior accessory pathway in a case of Wolff–Parkinson–White syndrome. Seven-year-old girl. The projection corresponds to the apical long axis.

a Longitudinal strain depiction prior to ablation. A very early contraction of the basal, inferior left ventricular segment located on the ventricular insertion site of the accessory pathway (thick arrow), beginning shortly after the delta wave, is clearly visible. At the same time, the not yet activated, removed left ventricular segments (thick arrow) deform.

b Longitudinal strain depiction after ablation. Successful ablation of the pathway leads to a synchronized contraction process.

of the QRS complex to the maximum segmental systolic strain is measured. The speckle tracking method allows good image quality and relatively precise mechanical myocardial activation mapping (▶ Fig. 4.207).

The measured time values can be used to calculate various indices, such as maximum intraventricular mechanical delay and standard deviation of the time until reaching maximum segmental velocity or strain. Published literature reports various indication thresholds for successfully implemented cardiac resynchronization therapy in adult patients.[361] To date, there have yet to be any specific values published for pediatric patients.

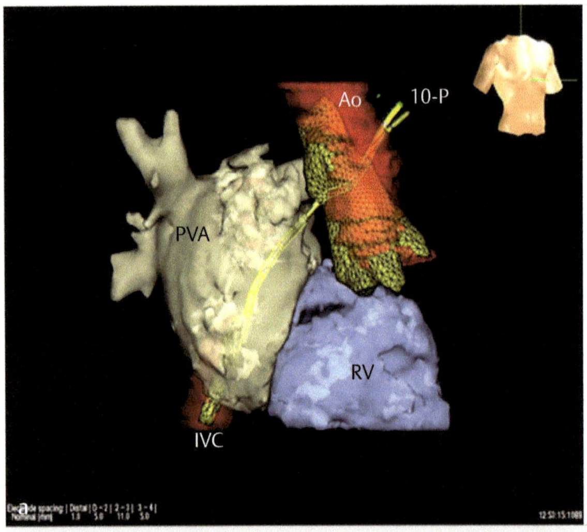

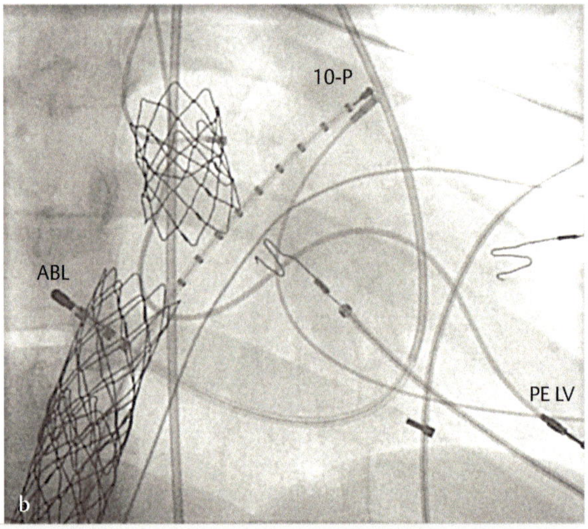

Fig. 4.208 Intraatrial reentry tachycardia after an atrial switch operation (Mustard procedure) in a case of TGA IVS. The position of a 10-pole electrophysiological catheter is visible in both images, introduced from the inferior vena cava into the anatomic left auricle. Imaging integration permits more precise catheter navigation and more exact activation mapping in 3-D space, and thus significantly simplifies the ablation procedure.

10-P = 10-pole electrophysiological catheter
ABL = catheter, inserted by means of retrograde introduction, in the pulmonary venous atrium
Ao = aorta
IVC = inferior vena cava
PVA = pulmonary venous atrium
RV = right ventricle
PE LV = left ventricular pacemaker electrode

a Image integration of the data from an electrophysiological navigation and mapping system (NavX) with the 3-D CT depiction of the heart.
b Corresponding fluoroscopic image, RAO projection, with stents in the tunnels of the superior and inferior vena cavas, the so-called venous baffle.

Three-Dimensional Reconstruction of the Heart for Imaging Integration in Catheter-Based Ablation Therapy

Electrophysiological mapping without additional imaging may be performed for the majority of traditional arrhythmogenic substrates, such as accessory pathways or atrioventricular node reentry tachycardia, with the exception of fluoroscopic or non-fluoroscopic navigation used during the examination. Ablation of post-incisional reentry tachycardia (after surgical treatment for congenital heart defects) in the atrium and ventricle, however, is hardly considered feasible nowadays without 3-D imaging integration. "3-D imaging integration" includes the integration of previously collected 3-D MRI or CT data with the data from an electrophysiological 3-D mapping system (such as CARTO or NavX) using defined anatomical orientation points.[362] More precise anatomical depictions by means of MRI or CT data enhance catheter navigation and activation mapping (▶ Fig. 4.208).

Imaging for Pacemaker Therapy and Treatment Using Implantable Cardioverter Defibrillators

The option to implant a transvenous pacemaker or ICD depends on the anatomical relationships of the vascular access points to the heart, and the presence of intracardiac shunts. After surgical treatment for congenital heart defects, the veins in the drainage area of the superior vena cava are often thrombosed due to central venous catheter or anatomical stenoses (such as after an atrial switch operation). In addition, intracardiac right–left shunts contraindicate transvenous probe implantation—at least without anticoagulation therapy—due to the danger of paradoxical embolisms. Echocardiography, angiography, MRI, and CT allow detailed morphological depictions for optimal surgical planning. After implanting a pacemaker or ICD, imaging is used to assess and reserve lead length while the patient grows, and to diagnose complications (▶ Fig. 4.209).

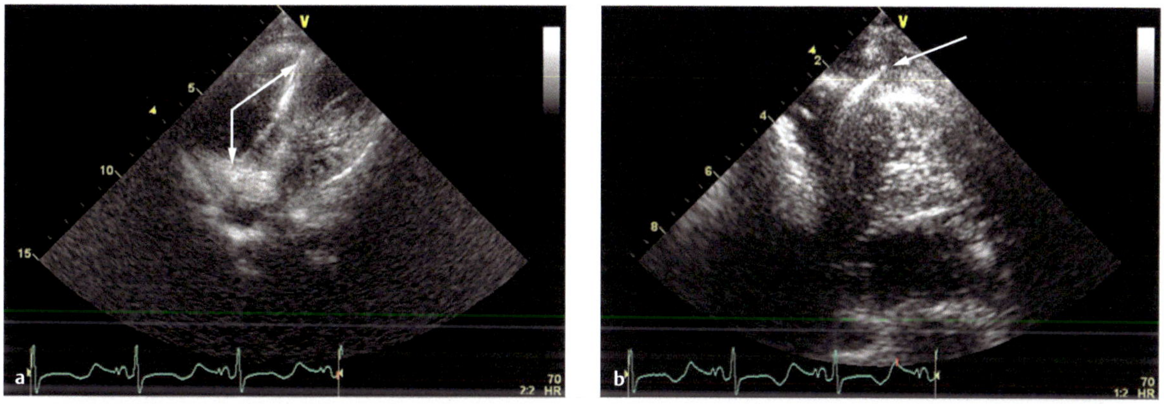

Fig. 4.209 Electrode perforation after implanting an ICD. Seven-year-old male patient with sudden chest pain 1 month after ICD implantation due to long QT syndrome.

a Overview image, modified apical 4-chamber projection. The arrows indicate the course of the right ventricular shock coil electrode, up to the apex.

b Electrode tip perforating the apical right ventricular wall, with subsequent pericardial effusion (arrow).

References

[1] Porter CJ, Edwards WD. Atrial septal defects. In: Allen HD, Driscoll DJ, Shaddy RE, Feltes TF, eds. Moss and Adams' heart disease in infants, children, and adolescents. Vol. 1. 7th ed. Philadelphia: Lippincott Williams & Wilkins; 2008: 632–645

[2] Erdmann E. Klinische Kardiologie. Berlin: Springer; 2008

[3] Schubert S, Peters B, Abdul-Khaliq H, Nagdyman N, Lange PE, Ewert P. Left ventricular conditioning in the elderly patient to prevent congestive heart failure after transcatheter closure of atrial septal defect. Catheter Cardiovasc Interv. 2005; 64(3):333–337

[4] Murphy JG, Gersh BJ, McGoon MD, et al. Long-term outcome after surgical repair of isolated atrial septal defect: follow-up at 27 to 32 years. N Engl J Med. 1990; 323(24):1645–1650

[5] Perloff JK. Ostium secundum atrial septal defect—survival for 87 and 94 years. Am J Cardiol. 1984; 53(2):388–389

[6] Baumgartner H, Bonhoeffer P, De Groot NM, et al. Task Force on the Management of Grown-up Congenital Heart Disease of the European Society of Cardiology (ESC), Association for European Paediatric Cardiology (AEPC), ESC Committee for Practice Guidelines (CPG). ESC Guidelines for the management of grown-up congenital heart disease (new version 2010). Eur Heart J. 2010; 31 (23):2915–2957

[7] Achenbach S, Barkhausen J, Beer M, et al. Konsensusempfehlungen der DRG/DGK/DGPK zum Einsatz der Herzbildgebung mit Computertomografie und Magnetresonanztomografie. RoFo Fortschr Geb Rontgenstr Nuklearmed. 2012; 184(4):345–368

[8] Beerbaum P, Körperich H, Barth P, Esdorn H, Gieseke J, Meyer H. Noninvasive quantification of left-to-right shunt in pediatric patients: phase-contrast cine magnetic resonance imaging compared with invasive oximetry. Circulation. 2001; 103(20):2476–2482

[9] Aliter H, El-Haddad A, Gallo R, Al-Halees Z. Atrial septal defect with drainage of the inferior vena cava into the left atrium. Eur J Cardiothorac Surg. 2011; 40(5):1256–1257

[10] Kharouf R, Luxenberg DM, Khalid O, Abdulla R. Atrial septal defect: spectrum of care. Pediatr Cardiol. 2008; 29(2):271–280

[11] Rigatelli G, Cardaioli P, Hijazi ZM. Contemporary clinical management of atrial septal defects in the adult. Expert Rev Cardiovasc Ther. 2007; 5(6):1135–1146

[12] Schmid C, Asfour B. Leitfaden Kinderherzchirurgie. 2. Aufl. Kiel: Steinkopf; 2009

[13] Schumacher G, Hess J, Bühlmeyer K. Klinische Kinderkardiologie. Berlin: Springer; 2007

[14] Soto B, Kassner EG, Baxley WA. Bildgebende Diagnostik in der Kardiologie. Weinheim: VCH; 1993

[15] Lai WW, Mertens LL, Geva T, Cohen MS. Echocardiography in pediatric and congenital heart disease. Hoboken: Wiley-Blackwell; 2009

[16] Lindinger A, Schwedler G, Hense HW. Prevalence of congenital heart defects in newborns in Germany: results of the first registration year of the PAN Study (July 2006 to June 2007). Klin Padiatr. 2010; 222 (5):321–326

[17] Harrild DM, Powell AJ, Tran TX, et al. Long-term pulmonary regurgitation following balloon valvuloplasty for pulmonary stenosis risk factors and relationship to exercise capacity and ventricular volume and function. J Am Coll Cardiol. 2010; 55(10):1041–1047

[18] Rao PS. Percutaneous balloon pulmonary valvuloplasty: state of the art. Catheter Cardiovasc Interv. 2007; 69(5):747–763

[19] Evans WN. "Tetralogy of Fallot" and Etienne-Louis Arthur Fallot. Pediatr Cardiol. 2008; 29(3):637–640

[20] Apitz C, Webb GD, Redington AN. Tetralogy of Fallot. Lancet. 2009; 374(9699):1462–1471

[21] Oosterhof T, van Straten A, Vliegen HW, et al. Preoperative thresholds for pulmonary valve replacement in patients with corrected tetralogy of Fallot using cardiovascular magnetic resonance. Circulation. 2007; 116(5):545–551

[22] Al Habib HF, Jacobs JP, Mavroudis C, et al. Contemporary patterns of management of tetralogy of Fallot: data from the Society of Thoracic Surgeons Database. Ann Thorac Surg. 2010; 90(3):813–819, discussion 819–820

[23] Kutty S, Kuehne T, Gribben P, et al. Ascending aortic and main pulmonary artery areas derived from cardiovascular magnetic resonance as reference values for normal subjects and repaired tetralogy of Fallot. Circ Cardiovasc Imaging. 2012; 5(5):644–651

[24] Sarikouch S, Koerperich H, Dubowy KO, et al. German Competence Network for Congenital Heart Defects Investigators. Impact of gender and age on cardiovascular function late after repair of tetralogy of Fallot: percentiles based on cardiac magnetic resonance. Circ Cardiovasc Imaging. 2011; 4(6):703–711

[25] Sarikouch S, Boethig D, Peters B, et al. Poorer right ventricular systolic function and exercise capacity in females after repair of tetralogy of Fallot: a gender comparison of standard deviation scores based on sex-specific reference values in healthy controls. Circ Cardiovasc Imaging. 2013; 6(6):924–933

[26] Cho JM, Puga FJ, Danielson GK, et al. Early and long-term results of the surgical treatment of tetralogy of Fallot with pulmonary atresia, with or without major aortopulmonary collateral arteries. J Thorac Cardiovasc Surg. 2002; 124(1):70–81

[27] El Louali F, Villacampa C, Aldebert P, Dragulescu A, Fraisse A. Pulmonary stenosis and atresia with intact ventricular septum. Arch Pediatr. 2011; 18(3):331–337
[28] Malhotra SP, Hanley FL. Surgical management of pulmonary atresia with ventricular septal defect and major aortopulmonary collaterals: a protocol-based approach. Semin Thorac Cardiovasc Surg Pediatr Card Surg Annu. 2009:145–151
[29] Wertaschnigg D, Jaeggi M, Chitayat D, et al. Prenatal diagnosis and outcome of absent pulmonary valve syndrome: contemporary single-center experience and review of the literature. Ultrasound Obstet Gynecol. 2013; 41(2):162–167
[30] Hraska V, Photiadis J, Schindler E, et al. A novel approach to the repair of tetralogy of Fallot with absent pulmonary valve and the reduction of airway compression by the pulmonary artery. Semin Thorac Cardiovasc Surg Pediatr Card Surg Annu. 2009:59–62
[31] Ebstein W. Über einen sehr seltenen Fall von Insuffizienz der Valvula tricuspidalis bedingt durch eine angeborene hochgradige Missbildung derselben. Arch Anat Physiol 1866; 238–254
[32] Freedom RM, Benson LN. Ebstein's malformation of the tricuspid valve. In: Freedom RM, Benson LN, Smallhorn JF, eds. Neonatal heart disease. London: Springer; 1991: 471–483
[33] Lev M, Liberthson RR, Joseph RH, et al. The pathologic anatomy of Ebstein's disease. Arch Pathol. 1970; 90(4):334–343
[34] Sharland GK, Chita SK, Allan LD. Tricuspid valve dysplasia or displacement in intrauterine life. J Am Coll Cardiol. 1991; 17 (4):944–949
[35] Seward JB, Tajik AJ, Feist DJ, Smith HC. Ebstein's anomaly in an 85-year-old man. Mayo Clin Proc. 1979; 54(3):193–196
[36] Watson H. Natural history of Ebstein's anomaly of tricuspid valve in childhood and adolescence. An international co-operative study of 505 cases. Br Heart J. 1974; 36(5):417–427
[37] Hebe J. Ebstein's anomaly in adults. Arrhythmias: diagnosis and therapeutic approach. Thorac Cardiovasc Surg. 2000; 48(4):214–219
[38] Celermajer DS, Bull C, Till JA, et al. Ebstein's anomaly: presentation and outcome from fetus to adult. J Am Coll Cardiol. 1994; 23 (1):170–176
[39] Carpentier A, Chauvaud S, Macé L, et al. A new reconstructive operation for Ebstein's anomaly of the tricuspid valve. J Thorac Cardiovasc Surg. 1988; 96(1):92–101
[40] Marcelletti C, Düren DR, Schuilenburg RM, et al. Fontan's operation for Ebstein's anomaly. Thorac Cardiovasc Surg. 1980; 79:63–66
[41] Danielson GK, Driscoll DJ, Mair DD, Warnes CA, Oliver WC, Jr. Operative treatment of Ebstein's anomaly. J Thorac Cardiovasc Surg. 1992; 104(5):1195–1202
[42] Hardy KL, Roe BB. Ebstein's anomaly: further experience with definitive repair. J Thorac Cardiovasc Surg. 1969; 58(4):553–561
[43] Schmidt-Habelmann P, Meisner H, Struck E, Sebening F. Results of valvuloplasty for Ebstein's anomaly. Thorac Cardiovasc Surg. 1981; 29(3):155–157
[44] Hetzer R, Nagdyman N, Ewert P, et al. A modified repair technique for tricuspid incompetence in Ebstein's anomaly. J Thorac Cardiovasc Surg. 1998; 115(4):857–868
[45] da Silva JP, Baumgratz JF, da Fonseca L, et al. The cone reconstruction of the tricuspid valve in Ebstein's anomaly. The operation: early and midterm results. J Thorac Cardiovasc Surg. 2007; 133(1):215–223
[46] Dearani JA, Danielson GK. Surgical management of Ebstein's anomaly in the adult. Semin Thorac Cardiovasc Surg. 2005; 17(2):148–154
[47] Celermajer DS, Cullen S, Sullivan ID, Spiegelhalter DJ, Wyse RK, Deanfield JE. Outcome in neonates with Ebstein's anomaly. J Am Coll Cardiol. 1992; 19(5):1041–1046
[48] Bhattacharyya S, West C, Kilner PJ, Senior R, Li W. Three-dimensional echocardiographic evaluation of quadricuspid systemic atrioventricular valve. Eur Heart J Cardiovasc Imaging. 2012; 13(12):1055
[49] Vettukattil JJ, Bharucha T, Anderson RH. Defining Ebstein's malformation using three-dimensional echocardiography. Interact Cardiovasc Thorac Surg. 2007; 6(6):685–690
[50] Mair DD. Ebstein's anomaly: natural history and management. J Am Coll Cardiol. 1992; 19(5):1047–1048
[51] Gutberlet M, Oellinger H, Ewert P, et al. Pre- and postoperative evaluation of ventricular function, muscle mass and valve morphology by magnetic resonance tomography in Ebstein's anomaly. RoFo Fortschr Geb Rontgenstr Nuklearmed. 2000; 172(5):436–442
[52] Kilner PJ. Imaging congenital heart disease in adults. Br J Radiol 2011; 84 (Spec. No. 3): S258–S268
[53] Lee CM, Sheehan FH, Bouzas B, Chen SS, Gatzoulis MA, Kilner PJ. The shape and function of the right ventricle in Ebstein's anomaly. Int J Cardiol. 2013; 167(3):704–710
[54] Tobler D, Yalonetsky S, Crean AM, et al. Right heart characteristics and exercise parameters in adults with Ebstein anomaly: new perspectives from cardiac magnetic resonance imaging studies. Int J Cardiol. 2013; 165(1):146–150
[55] Yalonetsky S, Tobler D, Greutmann M, et al. Cardiac magnetic resonance imaging and the assessment of Ebstein anomaly in adults. Am J Cardiol. 2011; 107(5):767–773
[56] Chauvaud SM, Hernigou AC, Mousseaux ER, Sidi D, Hébert JL. Ventricular volumes in Ebstein's anomaly: x-ray multislice computed tomography before and after repair. Ann Thorac Surg. 2006; 81 (4):1443–1449
[57] Sievers HH, Schmidtke C. A classification system for the bicuspid aortic valve from 304 surgical specimens. J Thorac Cardiovasc Surg. 2007; 133(5):1226–1233
[58] Jain D, Dietz HC, Oswald GL, Maleszewski JJ, Halushka MK. Causes and histopathology of ascending aortic disease in children and young adults. Cardiovasc Pathol. 2011; 20(1):15–25
[59] Aboulhosn J, Child JS. Left ventricular outflow obstruction: subaortic stenosis, bicuspid aortic valve, supravalvar aortic stenosis, and coarctation of the aorta. Circulation. 2006; 114(22):2412–2422
[60] Dähnert I, Dittrich S, Sreeram N, et al. Leitlinie Pädiatrische Kardiologie: subvalvuläre Aortenstenose bei Kindern und Jugendlichen. AWMF-Register Nr. 023/036; 2011. Im Internet: http://www.awmf.org/uploads/tx_szleitlinien/023-036l_S2k_Subvalvulaere_Aortenstenose_Kinder_Jugendliche_2014-06.pdf (Stand: 28.06.2015)
[61] Ewert P, Horke A, Haas N. Leitlinie Pädiatrische Kardiologie: Aortenklappenstenose im Kindes- und Jugendalter. AWMF-Register Nr. 023/008; 2011. Im Internet: http://www.awmf.org/uploads/tx_szleitlinien/023-008l_S2k__Aortenklappenstenose_Kinder_Jugendliche_2014-06.pdf (Stand: 28.06.2015)
[62] Haas NA, Kleideiter U. Kinderkardiologie. Stuttgart: Thieme; 2011
[63] Suri RM, Dearani JA, Schaff HV, Danielson GK, Puga FJ. Long-term results of the Konno procedure for complex left ventricular outflow tract obstruction. J Thorac Cardiovasc Surg. 2006; 132 (5):1064–1071
[64] Warnes CA, Williams RG, Bashore TM, et al. ACC/AHA 2008 Guidelines for the Management of Adults with Congenital Heart Disease: a report of the American College of Cardiology/American Heart Association Task Force on Practice Guidelines (writing committee to develop guidelines on the management of adults with congenital heart disease). Circulation. 2008; 118(23):e714–e833
[65] Suárez de Lezo J, Pan M, Medina A, et al. Immediate and follow-up results of transluminal balloon dilation for discrete subaortic stenosis. J Am Coll Cardiol. 1991; 18(5):1309–1315
[66] Ewert P, Bertram H, Breuer J, et al. Balloon valvuloplasty in the treatment of congenital aortic valve stenosis—a retrospective multicenter survey of more than 1000 patients. Int J Cardiol. 2011; 149(2):182–185
[67] Mavroudis C, Backer CL, Kaushal S. Aortic stenosis and aortic insufficiency in children: impact of valvuloplasty and modified Ross-Konno procedure. Semin Thorac Cardiovasc Surg Pediatr Card Surg Annu. 2009:76–86
[68] Baird CW, Myers PO, del Nido PJ. Aortic valve reconstruction in the young infants and children. Semin Thorac Cardiovasc Surg Pediatr Card Surg Annu. 2012; 15(1):9–19
[69] Gutberlet M, Abdul-Khaliq H, Stobbe H, et al. The use of cross-sectional imaging Modalitäten in the diagnosis of heart valve diseases. Z Kardiol. 2001; 90 Suppl. 6:2–12
[70] Tanous D, Benson LN, Horlick EM. Coarctation of the aorta: evaluation and management. Curr Opin Cardiol. 2009; 24(6):509–515

[71] Vriend JW, Oosterhof T, Hazekamp MG, Mulder BJ. Aortic arch morphology and hypertension in post-coarctectomy patients. Eur Heart J. 2005; 26(9):941

[72] Haas NA, Ewert P, Hager A, et al. Deutsche Gesellschaft für Pädiatrische Kardiologie. Leitlinie Pädiatrische Kardiologie: Aortenisthmusstenose. 2011. Im Internet: http://www.kinderkardiologie.org/Leitlinien/08%20LL%20AortenisthmusstenoseAS.pdf (Stand: 30.06.2015)

[73] Dodge-Khatami A, Backer CL, Mavroudis C. Risk factors for recoarctation and results of reoperation: a 40-year review. J Card Surg. 2000; 15(6):369–377

[74] Kaushal S, Backer CL, Patel JN, et al. Coarctation of the aorta: midterm outcomes of resection with extended end-to-end anastomosis. Ann Thorac Surg. 2009; 88(6):1932–1938

[75] von Kodolitsch Y, Aydin AM, Bernhardt AM, et al. Aortic aneurysms after correction of aortic coarctation: a systematic review. Vasa. 2010; 39(1):3–16

[76] Puranik R, Tsang VT, Puranik S, et al. Late magnetic resonance surveillance of repaired coarctation of the aorta. Eur J Cardiothorac Surg. 2009; 36(1):91–95, discussion 95

[77] Kenny D, Polson JW, Martin RP, Paton JF, Wolf AR. Hypertension and coarctation of the aorta: an inevitable consequence of developmental pathophysiology. Hypertens Res. 2011; 34(5):543–547

[78] Gutberlet M, Hosten N, Vogel M, et al. Quantification of morphologic and hemodynamic severity of coarctation of the aorta by magnetic resonance imaging. Cardiol Young. 2001; 11(5):512–520

[79] Hom JJ, Ordovas K, Reddy GP. Velocity-encoded cine MR imaging in aortic coarctation: functional assessment of hemodynamic events. Radiographics. 2008; 28(2):407–416

[80] Köhler B, Gasteiger R, Preim U, Theisel H, Gutberlet M, Preim B. Semi-automatic vortex extraction in 4D PC-MRI cardiac blood flow data using line predicates. IEEE Trans Vis Comput Graph. 2013; 19 (12):2773–2782

[81] Egan M, Holzer RJ. Comparing balloon angioplasty, stenting and surgery in the treatment of aortic coarctation. Expert Rev Cardiovasc Ther. 2009; 7(11):1401–1412

[82] Krueger JJ, Ewert P, Yilmaz S, et al. Magnetic resonance imaging-guided balloon angioplasty of coarctation of the aorta: a pilot study. Circulation. 2006; 113(8):1093–1100

[83] Schumacher G, Hess J, Bühlmeyer K. Klinische Kinderkardiologie. Berlin: Springer; 2001

[84] Dahiya A, Thamilarasan M, Arruda J, Bolen MA. New diagnosis of type A interrupted aortic arch at age 24 years. J Am Coll Cardiol. 2012; 60(20):2122

[85] Borgohain S, Gupta A, Grover V, Gupta VK. Isolated interrupted aortic arch in an 18-year-old man. Tex Heart Inst J. 2013; 40 (1):79–81

[86] Dong SZ, Zhu M, Li F. Preliminary experience with cardiovascular magnetic resonance in evaluation of fetal cardiovascular anomalies. J Cardiovasc Magn Reson. 2013; 15:40

[87] Kim AJ, Francis R, Liu X, et al. Microcomputed tomography provides high accuracy congenital heart disease diagnosis in neonatal and fetal mice. Circ Cardiovasc Imaging. 2013; 6(4):551–559

[88] Hirtler D, Geiger J, Jung B, Markl M, Arnold R. 4-D MRI flow analysis in the course of interrupted aortic arch reveals complex morphology and quantifies amount of collateral blood flow. Pediatr Radiol. 2013; 43(8):1037–1040

[89] Gutberlet M, Boeckel T, Hosten N, et al. Arterial switch procedure for D-transposition of the great arteries: quantitative midterm evaluation of hemodynamic changes with cine MR imaging and phase-shift velocity mapping-initial experience. Radiology. 2000; 214 (2):467–475

[90] Gutberlet M, Hoffmann J, Künzel E, et al. Preoperative and postoperative imaging in patients with transposition of the great arteries. Radiologe. 2011; 51(1):15–22

[91] Warnes CA. Transposition of the great arteries. Circulation. 2006; 114(24):2699–2709

[92] Rashkind WJ, Miller WW. Creation of an atrial septal defect without thoracotomy: a palliative approach to complete transposition of the great arteries. JAMA. 1966; 196(11):991–992

[93] Rastan AJ, Walther T, Alam NA, et al. Moderate versus deep hypothermia for the arterial switch operation—experience with 100 consecutive patients. Eur J Cardiothorac Surg. 2008; 33(4):619–625

[94] Hauser M, Bengel FM, Hager A, et al. Impaired myocardial blood flow and coronary flow reserve of the anatomical right systemic ventricle in patients with congenitally corrected transposition of the great arteries. Heart. 2003; 89(10):1231–1235

[95] Kozelj M, Prokselj K, Berden P, et al. The syndrome of cardiac failure in adults with congenitally corrected transposition. Cardiol Young. 2008; 18(6):599–607

[96] Mitropoulos FA, Kanakis M, Vlachos AP, et al. Congenitally corrected transposition of the great arteries: surgical repair in adulthood. Ann Thorac Surg. 2007; 83(2):672–674

[97] Zurick AO, III, Menon V. Dynamic outflow tract obstruction in congenitally corrected transposition of the great arteries. Int J Cardiovasc Imaging. 2010; 26(6):617–619

[98] Tulevski II, Zijta FM, Smeijers AS, Dodge-Khatami A, van der Wall EE, Mulder BJ. Regional and global right ventricular dysfunction in asymptomatic or minimally symptomatic patients with congenitally corrected transposition. Cardiol Young. 2004; 14(2):168–173

[99] Devaney EJ, Charpie JR, Ohye RG, Bove EL. Combined arterial switch and Senning operation for congenitally corrected transposition of the great arteries: patient selection and intermediate results. J Thorac Cardiovasc Surg. 2003; 125(3):500–507

[100] Reddy VM, McElhinney DB, Silverman NH, Hanley FL. The double switch procedure for anatomical repair of congenitally corrected transposition of the great arteries in infants and children. Eur Heart J. 1997; 18(9):1470–1477

[101] Mustard WT. Successful two-stage correction of transposition of the great vessels. Surgery. 1964; 55:469–472

[102] Winter MM, Bernink FJ, Groenink M, et al. Evaluating the systemic right ventricle by CMR: the importance of consistent and reproducible delineation of the cavity. J Cardiovasc Magn Reson. 2008; 10:40

[103] Janousek J, Paul T, Luhmer I, Wilken M, Hruda J, Kallfelz HC. Atrial baffle procedures for complete transposition of the great arteries: natural course of sinus node dysfunction and risk factors for dysrhythmias and sudden death. Z Kardiol. 1994; 83(12):933–938

[104] Jatene AD, Fontes VF, Paulista PP, et al. Successful anatomic correction of transposition of the great vessels: a preliminary report. Arq Bras Cardiol. 1975; 28(4):461–464

[105] Lecompte Y, Zannini L, Hazan E, et al. Anatomic correction of transposition of the great arteries. J Thorac Cardiovasc Surg. 1981; 82 (4):629–631

[106] Mussatto K, Wernovsky G. Challenges facing the child, adolescent, and young adult after the arterial switch operation. Cardiol Young. 2005; 15 Suppl 1:111–121

[107] Tzifa A, Tulloh RM. Coronary arterial complications before and after the arterial switch operation: is the future clear? Cardiol Young. 2002; 12(2):164–171

[108] Grotenhuis HB, Kroft LJ, van Elderen SG, et al. Right ventricular hypertrophy and diastolic dysfunction in arterial switch patients without pulmonary artery stenosis. Heart. 2007; 93(12):1604–1608

[109] Weiss F, Habermann CR, Lilje C, et al. MRI of pulmonary arteries in follow-up after arterial-switch-operation (ASO) for transposition of great arteries (d-TGA). RoFo Fortschr Geb Rontgenstr Nuklearmed. 2005; 177(6):849–855

[110] Taylor AM, Dymarkowski S, Hamaekers P, et al. MR coronary angiography and late-enhancement myocardial MR in children who underwent arterial switch surgery for transposition of great arteries. Radiology. 2005; 234(2):542–547

[111] Fratz S, Hager A, Busch R, et al. Patients after atrial switch operation for transposition of the great arteries can not increase stroke volume under dobutamine stress as opposed to patients with congenitally corrected transposition. Circ J. 2008; 72 (7):1130–1135

[112] Giardini A, Lovato L, Donti A, et al. Relation between right ventricular structural alterations and markers of adverse clinical outcome in adults with systemic right ventricle and either congenital complete

(after Senning operation) or congenitally corrected transposition of the great arteries. Am J Cardiol. 2006; 98(9):1277–1282
[113] Park JH, Han MC, Kim CW. MR imaging of congenitally corrected transposition of the great vessels in adults. AJR Am J Roentgenol. 1989; 153(3):491–494
[114] Rentzsch A, Abd El Rahman MY, Hui W, et al. Assessment of myocardial function of the systemic right ventricle in patients with D-transposition of the great arteries after atrial switch operation by tissue Doppler echocardiography. Z Kardiol. 2005; 94(8):524–531
[115] Takasugi JE, Godwin JD, Chen JT. CT in congenitally-corrected transposition of the great vessels. Comput Radiol. 1987; 11(5–6):215–221
[116] Voges I, Jerosch-Herold M, Helle M, Hart C, Kramer HH, Rickers C. 3 tesla magnetic resonance imaging in children and adults with congenital heart disease. Radiologe. 2010; 50(9):799–806, 808
[117] Chow PC, Liang XC, Cheung EW, Lam WW, Cheung YF. New two-dimensional global longitudinal strain and strain rate imaging for assessment of systemic right ventricular function. Heart. 2008; 94 (7):855–859
[118] Chow PC, Liang XC, Lam WW, Cheung EW, Wong KT, Cheung YF. Mechanical right ventricular dyssynchrony in patients after atrial switch operation for transposition of the great arteries. Am J Cardiol. 2008; 101(6):874–881
[119] Hornung TS, Kilner PJ, Davlouros PA, Grothues F, Li W, Gatzoulis MA. Excessive right ventricular hypertrophic response in adults with the mustard procedure for transposition of the great arteries. Am J Cardiol. 2002; 90(7):800–803
[120] Laffon E, Latrabe V, Jimenez M, Ducassou D, Laurent F, Marthan R. Quantitative MRI comparison of pulmonary hemodynamics in mustard/senning-repaired patients suffering from transposition of the great arteries and healthy volunteers at rest. Eur Radiol. 2006; 16 (7):1442–1448
[121] Ladouceur M, Bruneval P, Mousseaux E. Cardiovascular flashlight: magnetic resonance assessment of fibrosis in systemic right ventricle after atrial switch procedure. Eur Heart J. 2009; 30(21):2613
[122] Hardy CE, Helton GJ, Kondo C, Higgins SS, Young NJ, Higgins CB. Usefulness of magnetic resonance imaging for evaluating great-vessel anatomy after arterial switch operation for D-transposition of the great arteries. Am Heart J. 1994; 128(2):326–332
[123] Gutberlet M, Noeske R, Schwinge K, Freyhardt P, Felix R, Niendorf T. Comprehensive cardiac magnetic resonance imaging at 3.0 Tesla: feasibility and implications for clinical applications. Invest Radiol. 2006; 41(2):154–167
[124] Arnoldi E, Ramos-Duran I, Abro JA, et al. CT-Angiographie der Koronarien mit prospektivem EKG-Triggering: Hohe diagnostische Genauigkeit bei niedriger Strahlendosis. Radiologe. 2010; 50(6):500–506
[125] Chang DS, Barack BM, Lee MH, Lee HY. Congenitally corrected transposition of the great arteries: imaging with 16-MDCT. AJR Am J Roentgenol. 2007; 188(5):W428–30
[126] Lell MM, May M, Deak P, et al. High-pitch spiral computed tomography: effect on image quality and radiation dose in pediatric chest computed tomography. Invest Radiol. 2011; 46(2):116–123
[127] Lembcke A, Koch C, Dohmen PM, et al. Electrocardiographic-gated multislice computed tomography for visualization of cardiac morphology in congenitally corrected transposition of the great arteries. J Comput Assist Tomogr. 2005; 29(2):234–237
[128] Chen SJ, Lin MT, Lee WJ, et al. Coronary artery anatomy in children with congenital heart disease by computed tomography. Int J Cardiol. 2007; 120(3):363–370
[129] Kantarci M, Koplay M, Bayraktutan U, Gundogdu F, Ceviz N. Congenitally corrected transposition of the great arteries: MDCT angiography findings and interpretation of complex coronary anatomy. Int J Cardiovasc Imaging. 2007; 23(3):405–410
[130] Lehmkuhl L, Gosch D, Nagel HD, Stumpp P, Kahn T, Gutberlet M. Quantification of radiation dose savings in cardiac computed tomography using prospectively triggered mode and ECG pulsing: a phantom study. Eur Radiol. 2010; 20(9):2116–2125
[131] Cook SC, McCarthy M, Daniels CJ, Cheatham JP, Raman SV. Usefulness of multislice computed tomography angiography to evaluate intravascular stents and transcatheter occlusion devices in patients with d-transposition of the great arteries after mustard repair. Am J Cardiol. 2004; 94(7):967–969
[132] Kaemmerer H, Bahlmann M, Prokop M, Schirg E, Luhmer I, Kallfelz HC. Evaluation of congenital vena cava anomalies and acquired vena cava obstructions after atrial switch operation using spiral computerized tomography and 3-dimensional reconstruction. Z Kardiol. 1997; 86(9):669–675
[133] Ou P, Celermajer DS, Marini D, et al. Safety and accuracy of 64-slice computed tomography coronary angiography in children after the arterial switch operation for transposition of the great arteries. JACC Cardiovasc Imaging. 2008; 1(3):331–339
[134] Frank L, Dillman JR, Parish V, et al. Cardiovascular MR imaging of conotruncal anomalies. Radiographics. 2010; 30(4):1069–1094
[135] Van Praagh R, Van Praagh S. The anatomy of common aorticopulmonary trunk (truncus arteriosus communis) and its embryologic implications. A study of 57 necropsy cases. Am J Cardiol. 1965; 16 (3):406–425
[136] Calder L, Van Praagh R, Van Praagh S, et al. Truncus arteriosus communis. Clinical, angiocardiographic, and pathologic findings in 100 patients. Am Heart J. 1976; 92(1):23–38
[137] Walthers EM. Bildgebende Diagnostik in der Kardiologie. Weinheim: VCH; 1993
[138] Raisky O, Ali WB, Bajolle F, et al. Common arterial trunk repair: with conduit or without? Eur J Cardiothorac Surg. 2009; 36(4):675–682
[139] Johnson TR. Conotruncal cardiac defects: a clinical imaging perspective. Pediatr Cardiol. 2010; 31(3):430–437
[140] Fogel MA, Crawford M. Cardiac magnetic resonance of the common arterial trunk and transposition of the great arteries. Cardiol Young. 2012; 22(6):677–686
[141] Mahesh M. Advances in CT technology and application to pediatric imaging. Pediatr Radiol. 2011; 41 Suppl 2:493–497
[142] Matsumoto T, Miyakoshi K, Yoshimura Y. Prenatal images of the truncus arteriosus with an interrupted aortic arch. Pediatr Cardiol. 2013; 34(2):473–475
[143] Murugan MK, Gulati GS, Ramakrishnan S. Multidetector computed tomography for truncus arteriosus and associated complex arch anomaly. Pediatr Cardiol. 2013; 34(3):764–766
[144] Weidenbach M, Caffier P, Harnisch T, Daehnert I. Hypoplastic left heart syndrome with intact atrial septum—attempt of an interventional palliation by ductal and interatrial stent implantation. Clin Res Cardiol. 2006; 95(2):110–114
[145] Dähnert I, Riede FT, Razek V, et al. Catheter interventional treatment of Sano shunt obstruction in patients following modified Norwood palliation for hypoplastic left heart syndrome. Clin Res Cardiol. 2007; 96(10):719–722
[146] Barron DJ, Kilby MD, Davies B, Wright JG, Jones TJ, Brawn WJ. Hypoplastic left heart syndrome. Lancet. 2009; 374(9689):551–564
[147] Norwood WI, Kirklin JK, Sanders SP. Hypoplastic left heart syndrome: experience with palliative surgery. Am J Cardiol. 1980; 45 (1):87–91
[148] Murtuza B, Stumper O, Wall D, et al. The effect of morphologic subtype on outcomes following the Sano-Norwood procedure. Eur J Cardiothorac Surg. 2012; 42(5):787–793
[149] Cross RR, Harahsheh AS, McCarter R, et al. National Pediatric Cardiology Quality Improvement Collaborative (NPC-QIC). Identified mortality risk factors associated with presentation, initial hospitalisation, and interstage period for the Norwood operation in a multi-centre registry: a report from the National Pediatric Cardiology-Quality Improvement Collaborative. Cardiol Young. 2013:1–10
[150] Tabbutt S, Ghanayem N, Ravishankar C, et al. Pediatric Heart Network Investigators. Risk factors for hospital morbidity and mortality after the Norwood procedure: a report from the Pediatric Heart Network Single Ventricle Reconstruction trial. J Thorac Cardiovasc Surg. 2012; 144(4):882–895
[151] Egan MJ, Hill SL, Boettner BL, et al. Predictors of retrograde aortic arch obstruction after hybrid palliation of hypoplastic left heart syndrome. Pediatr Cardiol. 2011; 32(1):67–75

[152] Feinstein JA, Benson DW, Dubin AM, et al. Hypoplastic left heart syndrome: current considerations and expectations. J Am Coll Cardiol. 2012; 59(1) Suppl:S1–S42

[153] Fortuna RS, Ruzmetov M, Geiss DM. Outcomes of the modified norwood procedure: hypoplastic left heart syndrome versus other single-ventricle malformations. Pediatr Cardiol. 2014; 35(1):96–102

[154] Allen HD, Clark EB, Gutgesell HP, Driscoll DJ, Eds. Moss and Adams' heart disease in infants, children and adolescents. 6th ed. Philadelphia: Lippincott Williams & Wilkins; 2001

[155] Dos L, Pen V, Silversides C, et al. Images in cardiovascular medicine. Cardiac magnetic resonance imaging and multidetector computed tomography scan illustrating Damus-Kaye-Stansel operation. Circulation. 2007; 115(18):e440–e442

[156] Klimes K, Abdul-Khaliq H, Ovroutski S, et al. Pulmonary and caval blood flow patterns in patients with intracardiac and extracardiac Fontan: a magnetic resonance study. Clin Res Cardiol. 2007; 96 (3):160–167

[157] Gutberlet M, Hosten N, Abdul-Khaliq H, et al. The value of magnetic resonance tomography (MRT) for evaluating ventricular and anastomotic functions in patients with an extra- or intracardiac total cavopulmonary connection (TCPC)-modified Fontan operation. RoFo Fortschr Geb Rontgenstr Nuklearmed. 1999; 171(6):431–441

[158] Friedrich-Rust M, Koch C, Rentzsch A, et al. Noninvasive assessment of liver fibrosis in patients with Fontan circulation using transient elastography and biochemical fibrosis markers. J Thorac Cardiovasc Surg. 2008; 135(3):560–567

[159] Fratz S, Chung T, Greil GF, et al. Guidelines and protocols for cardiovascular magnetic resonance in children and adults with congenital heart disease: SCMR expert consensus group on congenital heart disease. J Cardiovasc Magn Reson. 2013; 15:51

[160] Klimes K, Ovroutski S, Abdul-Khaliq H, et al. Exercise capacity reflects ventricular function in patients having the Fontan circulation. Cardiol Young. 2009; 19(4):340–345

[161] Correa-Villaseñor A, Ferencz C, Boughman JA, Neill CA, The Baltimore-Washington Infant Study Group. Total anomalous pulmonary venous return: familial and environmental factors. Teratology. 1991; 44(4):415–428

[162] Craig JM, Darling RC, Rothney WB. Total pulmonary venous drainage into the right side of the heart; report of 17 autopsied cases not associated with other major cardiovascular anomalies. Lab Invest. 1957; 6(1):44–64

[163] Gathman GE, Nadas AS. Total anomalous pulmonary venous connection: clinical and physiologic observations of 75 pediatric patients. Circulation. 1970; 42(1):143–154

[164] Delisle G, Ando M, Calder AL, et al. Total anomalous pulmonary venous connection: report of 93 autopsied cases with emphasis on diagnostic and surgical considerations. Am Heart J. 1976; 91 (1):99–122

[165] Goswami KC, Shrivastava S, Saxena A, Dev V. Echocardiographic diagnosis of total anomalous pulmonary venous connection. Am Heart J. 1993; 126(2):433–440

[166] Lange R, Meisner FG, Haas F, et al. Total anomalous pulmonary venous connection (TAPVD): which factors influence the postoperative results? Thorac Cardiovasc Surg. 2001; 49 Suppl. 1:49

[167] Moss A. Heart disease in infants, children and adolescents. Including the fetus and young adult. Philadelphia: Lippincott Williams & Wilkins; 2001

[168] Dähnert W. Radiology review manual. Philadelphia: Lippincott Williams & Wilkins; 2011

[169] Edwin F. Left-sided partial anomalous pulmonary venous connection—should diagnosis lead to surgery? Interact Cardiovasc Thorac Surg. 2010; 11(6):847–848

[170] Majdalany DS, Phillips SD, Dearani JA, Connolly HM, Warnes CA. Isolated partial anomalous pulmonary venous connections in adults: twenty-year experience. Congenit Heart Dis. 2010; 5(6):537–545

[171] Knüppel M, Geipel A, Kohl T, et al. Die links persistierende obere Hohlvene als Marker fetaler kardialer und extrakardialer Fehlbildungen. Ultraschall Med. 2005:26

[172] Greil GF, Kuettner A, Sieverding L, et al. Multimedia articles. Images in cardiovascular medicine. Cervical origin of the subclavian artery: imaging of a rare but clinically relevant anomaly. Circulation. 2004; 109(14):e177–e178

[173] Kommerell B. Verlagerung des Ösophagus durch eine abnorm verlaufende A. subclavia dextra (A. lusoria). Fortschr Röntgenstr. 1936; 54:590–595

[174] Kopp R, Däbritz S, Weidenhagen R, et al. Extrathorakal zervikal-endovaskuläre Hybridoperationen zur Behandlung der symptomatischen und/oder aneurysmatischen A. lusoria. Gefasschirurgie. 2008; 13(3):179–188

[175] Greil GF, Kramer U, Dammann F, et al. Diagnosis of vascular rings and slings using an interleaved 3D double-slab FISP MR angiography technique. Pediatr Radiol. 2005; 35(4):396–401

[176] Fogel MA, Pawlowski TW, Harris MA, et al. Comparison and usefulness of cardiac magnetic resonance versus computed tomography in infants six months of age or younger with aortic arch anomalies without deep sedation or anesthesia. Am J Cardiol. 2011; 108 (1):120–125

[177] Dabizzi RP, Teodori G, Barletta GA, Caprioli G, Baldrighi G, Baldrighi V. Associated coronary and cardiac anomalies in the tetralogy of Fallot. An angiographic study. Eur Heart J. 1990; 11(8):692–704

[178] Hekmat M, Rafieyian S, Foroughi M, Majidi Tehrani MM, Beheshti Monfared M, Hassantash SA. Associated coronary anomalies in 135 Iranian patients with tetralogy of Fallot. Asian Cardiovasc Thorac Ann. 2005; 13(4):307–310

[179] Smith A, Arnold R, Wilkinson JL, Hamilton DI, McKay R, Anderson RH. An anatomical study of the patterns of the coronary arteries and sinus nodal artery in complete transposition. Int J Cardiol. 1986; 12 (3):295–307

[180] Angelini P. Coronary artery anomalies—current clinical issues: definitions, classification, incidence, clinical relevance, and treatment guidelines. Tex Heart Inst J. 2002; 29(4):271–278

[181] Levin DC, Fellows KE, Abrams HL. Hemodynamically significant primary anomalies of the coronary arteries. Angiographic aspects. Circulation. 1978; 58(1):25–34

[182] Bland E, White P, Garland J. Congenital anomalies of the coronary arteries. Am Heart J. 1933; 8:787–801

[183] Lücke C, Lurz P, Mangner N, et al. Komplett nichtinvasive präoperative Niedrigdosisevaluation eines Bland-White-Garland syndrome. Kardiologe. 2013; 7(3):209–211

[184] Friedman AH, Fogel MA, Stephens P, Jr, et al. Identification, imaging, functional assessment and management of congenital coronary arterial abnormalities in children. Cardiol Young. 2007; 17 Suppl 2:56–67

[185] Basso C, Maron BJ, Corrado D, Thiene G. Clinical profile of congenital coronary artery anomalies with origin from the wrong aortic sinus leading to sudden death in young competitive athletes. J Am Coll Cardiol. 2000; 35(6):1493–1501

[186] Vitiello R, McCrindle BW, Nykanen D, Freedom RM, Benson LN. Complications associated with pediatric cardiac catheterization. J Am Coll Cardiol. 1998; 32(5):1433–1440

[187] Geva T, Kreutzer J. Diagnostic pathways for evaluation of congenital heart disease. In: Crawford MH, DiMarco JP, eds. Cadiology. London: Mosby International; 2001: 7–41

[188] Tangcharoen T, Bell A, Hegde S, et al. Detection of coronary artery anomalies in infants and young children with congenital heart disease by using MR imaging. Radiology. 2011; 259(1):240–247

[189] Uribe S, Hussain T, Valverde I, et al. Congenital heart disease in children: coronary MR angiography during systole and diastole with dual cardiac phase whole-heart imaging. Radiology. 2011; 260(1):232–240

[190] Sorensen TS, Körperich H, Greil GF, et al. Operator-independent isotropic three-dimensional magnetic resonance imaging for morphology in congenital heart disease: a validation study. Circulation. 2004; 110(2):163–169

[191] Weber OM, Martin AJ, Higgins CB. Whole-heart steady-state free precession coronary artery magnetic resonance angiography. Magn Reson Med. 2003; 50(6):1223–1228

[192] Singh Nijjar P, Parameswaran A, Amanullah AM. Evaluation of anomalous aortic origins of the coronaries by 64-slice cardiac computed tomography. Rev Cardiovasc Med. 2007; 8(3):175–181

[193] Ghadri JR, Kazakauskaite E, Braunschweig S, et al. Congenital coronary anomalies detected by coronary computed tomography compared to invasive coronary angiography. BMC Cardiovasc Disord. 2014; 14:81

[194] Manso B, Castellote A, Dos L, Casaldáliga J. Myocardial perfusion magnetic resonance imaging for detecting coronary function anomalies in asymptomatic paediatric patients with a previous arterial switch operation for the transposition of great arteries. Cardiol Young. 2010; 20(4):410–417

[195] Castaneda AR, Jonas RA, Mayer JE, et al. Tetralogy of Fallot. In: Castaneda AR, Jonas RA, Mayer JE et al, eds. Cardiac surgery of the neonate and infant. Philadelphia: Saunders; 1994: 215–234

[196] Hofbeck M, Sunnegårdh JT, Burrows PE, et al. Analysis of survival in patients with pulmonic valve atresia and ventricular septal defect. Am J Cardiol. 1991; 67(8):737–743

[197] Haworth SG, Rees PG, Taylor JF, Macartney FJ, de Leval M, Stark J. Pulmonary atresia with ventricular septal defect and major aortopulmonary collateral arteries. Effect of systemic pulmonary anastomosis. Br Heart J. 1981; 45(2):133–141

[198] Marelli AJ, Perloff JK, Child JS, Laks H. Pulmonary atresia with ventricular septal defect in adults. Circulation. 1994; 89(1):243–251

[199] Seidel W, Kovacicek S, Klinner W. Operation for aplasia and atresia of the pulmonary artery. Thoraxchir Vask Chir. 1965; 13(6):436–445

[200] Lillehei CW, Cohen M, Warden HE, Varco RL. The direct-vision intracardiac correction of congenital anomalies by controlled cross circulation; results in thirty-two patients with ventricular septal defects, tetralogy of Fallot, and atrioventricularis communis defects. Surgery. 1955; 38(1):11–29

[201] Wallace RB, McGoon DC, Danielson GK. Complete correction of truncus arteriosus, pulmonary atresia, and transposition of the great arteries with ventricular septal defect and pulmonary stenosis. Adv Cardiol. 1974; 11(00):11–17

[202] Hessel EA, II, Boyden EA, Stamm SJ, Sauvage LR. High systemic origin of the sole artery to the basal segments of the left lung: findings, surgical treatment, and embryologic interpretation. Surgery. 1970; 67(4):624–632

[203] Maron BJ, Towbin JA, Thiene G, et al. Contemporary definitions and classification of the cardiomyopathies. An AHA scientific statement from the council on clinical cardiology, heart failure and transplantation committee; quality of care and outcomes research and functional genomics and translational biology interdisciplinary working groups; and council on epidemiology and prevention. Circulation. 2006; 113:1807–1816

[204] Elliott P, Andersson B, Arbustini E, et al. Classification of the cardiomyopathies: a position statement from the European society of cardiology working group on myocardial and pericardial diseases. Eur Heart J. 2008; 29(2):270–276

[205] Schmaltz AA. Hypertrophe Kardiomyopathie. In: Apitz J, Hrsg. Pädiatrische Kardiologie. Steinkopff: Darmstadt; 2002: 260–264

[206] Bos JM, Towbin JA, Ackerman MJ. Diagnostic, prognostic, and therapeutic implications of genetic testing for hypertrophic cardiomyopathy. J Am Coll Cardiol. 2009; 54(3):201–211

[207] Morrow AG, Fogarty TJ, Hannah H, III, Braunwald E. Operative treatment in idiopathic hypertrophic subaortic stenosis. Techniques, and the results of preoperative and postoperative clinical and hemodynamic assessments. Circulation. 1968; 37(4):589–596

[208] Ommen SR, Shah PM, Tajik AJ. Left ventricular outflow tract obstruction in hypertrophic cardiomyopathy: past, present and future. Heart. 2008; 94(10):1276–1281

[209] Sigwart U. Non-surgical myocardial reduction for hypertrophic obstructive cardiomyopathy. Lancet. 1995; 346(8969):211–214

[210] Nihoyannopoulos P, McKenna WJ. Hypertrophic cardiomyopathy. In: Roelandt JRTC, Sutherland GR, Iliceto S, eds. Cardiac ultrasound. Edinburgh: Churchill Livingstone; 1993: 371–389

[211] Shah JS, Esteban MTT, Thaman R, et al. Prevalence of exercise-induced left ventricular outflow tract obstruction in symptomatic patients with non-obstructive hypertrophic cardiomyopathy. Heart. 2008; 94(10):1288–1294

[212] Flachskampf FA, Breithardt OA, Daniel WG. Stellenwert des Gewebe-Dopplers in der Frühdiagnostik von Kardiomyopathien. Herz. 2007; 32(2):89–96

[213] Ho CY, Sweitzer NK, McDonough B, et al. Assessment of diastolic function with Doppler tissue imaging to predict genotype in preclinical hypertrophic cardiomyopathy. Circulation. 2002; 105 (25):2992–2997

[214] McMahon CJ, Nagueh SF, Pignatelli RH, et al. Characterization of left ventricular diastolic function by tissue Doppler imaging and clinical status in children with hypertrophic cardiomyopathy. Circulation. 2004; 109(14):1756–1762

[215] Alfakih K, Plein S, Thiele H, Jones T, Ridgway JP, Sivananthan MU. Normal human left and right ventricular dimensions for MRI as assessed by turbo gradient echo and steady-state free precession imaging sequences. J Magn Reson Imaging. 2003; 17(3):323–329

[216] Petersen SE, Selvanayagam JB, Francis JM, et al. Differentiation of athlete's heart from pathological forms of cardiac hypertrophy by means of geometric indices derived from cardiovascular magnetic resonance. J Cardiovasc Magn Reson. 2005; 7(3):551–558

[217] Olivotto I, Maron MS, Autore C, et al. Assessment and significance of left ventricular mass by cardiovascular magnetic resonance in hypertrophic cardiomyopathy. J Am Coll Cardiol. 2008; 52(7):559–566

[218] Rickers C, Wilke NM, Jerosch-Herold M, et al. Utility of cardiac magnetic resonance imaging in the diagnosis of hypertrophic cardiomyopathy. Circulation. 2005; 112(6):855–861

[219] Gutberlet M. Cardiac magnetic resonance imaging: from imaging to diagnosis. Radiologe. 2013; 53(11):1033–1052

[220] Hansen MW, Merchant N. MRI of hypertrophic cardiomyopathy: part I, MRI appearances. AJR Am J Roentgenol. 2007; 189(6):1335–1343

[221] Hansen MW, Merchant N. MRI of hypertrophic cardiomyopathy: part 2, Differential diagnosis, risk stratification, and posttreatment MRI appearances. AJR Am J Roentgenol. 2007; 189(6):1344–1352

[222] Chaowu Y, Shihua Z, Jian L, Li L, Wei F. Cardiovascular magnetic resonance characteristics in children with hypertrophic cardiomyopathy. Circ Heart Fail. 2013; 6(5):1013–1020

[223] Green JJ, Berger JS, Kramer CM, Salerno M. Prognostic value of late gadolinium enhancement in clinical outcomes for hypertrophic cardiomyopathy. JACC Cardiovasc Imaging. 2012; 5(4):370–377

[224] Puntmann VO, Voigt T, Chen Z, et al. Native T1 mapping in differentiation of normal myocardium from diffuse disease in hypertrophic and dilated cardiomyopathy. JACC Cardiovasc Imaging. 2013; 6(4):475–484

[225] Andrews RE, Fenton MJ, Ridout DA, Burch M, British Congenital Cardiac Association. New-onset heart failure due to heart muscle disease in childhood: a prospective study in the United kingdom and Ireland. Circulation. 2008; 117(1):79–84

[226] Towbin JA, Lowe AM, Colan SD, et al. Incidence, causes, and outcomes of dilated cardiomyopathy in children. JAMA. 2006; 296 (15):1867–1876

[227] Codd MB, Sugrue DD, Gersh BJ, Melton LJ, III. Epidemiology of idiopathic dilated and hypertrophic cardiomyopathy. A population-based study in Olmsted County, Minnesota, 1975–1984. Circulation. 1989; 80(3):564–572

[228] Malhotra R, Mason PK. Lamin A/C deficiency as a cause of familial dilated cardiomyopathy. Curr Opin Cardiol. 2009; 24(3):203–208

[229] Pasotti M, Klersy C, Pilotto A, et al. Long-term outcome and risk stratification in dilated cardiolaminopathies. J Am Coll Cardiol. 2008; 52(15):1250–1260

[230] Felker GM, Thompson RE, Hare JM, et al. Underlying causes and long-term survival in patients with initially unexplained cardiomyopathy. N Engl J Med. 2000; 342(15):1077–1084

[231] Shaddy RE, Boucek MM, Hsu DT, et al. Pediatric Carvedilol Study Group. Carvedilol for children and adolescents with heart failure: a randomized controlled trial. JAMA. 2007; 298(10):1171–1179

[232] McMahon CJ, Nagueh SF, Eapen RS, et al. Echocardiographic predictors of adverse clinical events in children with dilated cardiomyopathy: a prospective clinical study. Heart. 2004; 90(8):908–915

[233] Koikkalainen JR, Antila M, Lötjönen JM, et al. Early familial dilated cardiomyopathy: identification with determination of disease state parameter from cine MR image data. Radiology. 2008; 249(1):88–96

[234] Wu KC, Weiss RG, Thiemann DR, et al. Late gadolinium enhancement by cardiovascular magnetic resonance heralds an adverse prognosis in nonischemic cardiomyopathy. J Am Coll Cardiol. 2008; 51 (25):2414–2421

[235] Lurz P, Luecke C, Eitel I, et al. Comprehensive cardiac magnetic resonance imaging in patients with suspected myocarditis: The MyoRacer-Trial. J Am Coll Cardiol. 2016; 67(15):1800–1811

[236] Mogensen J, Arbustini E. Restrictive cardiomyopathy. Curr Opin Cardiol. 2009; 24(3):214–220

[237] Calkins H. Arrhythmogenic right-ventricular dysplasia/cardiomyopathy. Curr Opin Cardiol. 2006; 21(1):55–63

[238] Marcus FI, McKenna WJ, Sherrill D, et al. Diagnosis of arrhythmogenic right ventricular cardiomyopathy/dysplasia: proposed modification of the task force criteria. Circulation. 2010; 121 (13):1533–1541

[239] Bomma C, Rutberg J, Tandri H, et al. Misdiagnosis of arrhythmogenic right ventricular dysplasia/cardiomyopathy. J Cardiovasc Electrophysiol. 2004; 15(3):300–306

[240] Grothoff M, Pachowsky M, Hoffmann J, et al. Value of cardiovascular MR in diagnosing left ventricular non-compaction cardiomyopathy and in discriminating between other cardiomyopathies. Eur Radiol. 2012; 22(12):2699–2709

[241] Lilje C, Rázek V, Joyce JJ, et al. Complications of non-compaction of the left ventricular myocardium in a paediatric population: a prospective study. Eur Heart J. 2006; 27(15):1855–1860

[242] Sasse-Klaassen S, Probst S, Gerull B, et al. Novel gene locus for autosomal dominant left ventricular noncompaction maps to chromosome 11p15. Circulation. 2004; 109(22):2720–2723

[243] Jenni R, Oechslin E, Schneider J, Attenhofer Jost C, Kaufmann PA. Echocardiographic and pathoanatomical characteristics of isolated left ventricular non-compaction: a step towards classification as a distinct cardiomyopathy. Heart. 2001; 86(6):666–671

[244] Petersen SE, Selvanayagam JB, Wiesmann F, et al. Left ventricular non-compaction: insights from cardiovascular magnetic resonance imaging. J Am Coll Cardiol. 2005; 46(1):101–105

[245] Myokarditis-Diagnostik KR. Dtsch Med Wochenschr. 2011; 136:829–835

[246] Klingel K, Sauter M, Bock CT, Szalay G, Schnorr JJ, Kandolf R. Molecular pathology of inflammatory cardiomyopathy. Med Microbiol Immunol (Berl). 2004; 193(2–3):101–107

[247] Badorff C, Lee GH, Lamphear BJ, et al. Enteroviral protease 2A cleaves dystrophin: evidence of cytoskeletal disruption in an acquired cardiomyopathy. Nat Med. 1999; 5(3):320–326

[248] Stiller B, Dähnert I, Weng YG, Hennig E, Hetzer R, Lange PE. Children may survive severe myocarditis with prolonged use of biventricular assist devices. Heart. 1999; 82(2):237–240

[249] Bowles NE, Ni J, Kearney DL, et al. Detection of viruses in myocardial tissues by polymerase chain reaction. evidence of adenovirus as a common cause of myocarditis in children and adults. J Am Coll Cardiol. 2003; 42(3):466–472

[250] Wang JN, Tsai YC, Lee WL, Lin CS, Wu JM. Complete atrioventricular block following myocarditis in children. Pediatr Cardiol. 2002; 23 (5):518–521

[251] Kececioglu D, Gehrmann J, Mugler M, et al. Myokarditis simuliert akuten Myokardinfarkt im Säuglingsalter. Herz Kreislauf. 1993; 25:353–355

[252] Ghelani SJ, Spaeder MC, Pastor W, Spurney CF, Klugman D. Demographics, trends, and outcomes in pediatric acute myocarditis in the United States, 2006 to 2011. Circ Cardiovasc Qual Outcomes. 2012; 5 (5):622–627

[253] Friedrich MG, Sechtem U, Schulz-Menger J, et al. International Consensus Group on Cardiovascular Magnetic Resonance in Myocarditis. Cardiovascular magnetic resonance in myocarditis: A JACC White Paper. J Am Coll Cardiol. 2009; 53(17):1475–1487

[254] Gutberlet M, Lücke C, Krieghoff C, et al. MRI for myocarditis. Radiologe. 2013; 53(1):30–37

[255] Gutberlet M, Spors B, Thoma T, et al. Suspected chronic myocarditis at cardiac MR: diagnostic accuracy and association with immunohistologically detected inflammation and viral persistence. Radiology. 2008; 246(2):401–409

[256] Lauer B, Niederau C, Kühl U, et al. Cardiac troponin T in patients with clinically suspected myocarditis. J Am Coll Cardiol. 1997; 30 (5):1354–1359

[257] Liu PP, Yan AT. Cardiovascular magnetic resonance for the diagnosis of acute myocarditis: prospects for detecting myocardial inflammation. J Am Coll Cardiol. 2005; 45(11):1823–1825

[258] Felker GM, Boehmer JP, Hruban RH, et al. Echocardiographic findings in fulminant and acute myocarditis. J Am Coll Cardiol. 2000; 36 (1):227–232

[259] Lurz P, Eitel I, Klieme B, et al. The potential additional diagnostic value of assessing for pericardial effusion on cardiac magnetic resonance imaging in patients with suspected myocarditis. Eur Heart J Cardiovasc Imaging. 2014; 15(6):643–650

[260] Mendes LA, Dec GW, Picard MH, Palacios IF, Newell J, Davidoff R. Right ventricular dysfunction: an independent predictor of adverse outcome in patients with myocarditis. Am Heart J. 1994; 128(2):301–307

[261] Cooper LT, Baughman KL, Feldman AM, et al. American Heart Association, American College of Cardiology, European Society of Cardiology, Heart Failure Society of America, Heart Failure Association of the European Society of Cardiology, Endorsed by the Heart Failure Society of America and the Heart Failure Association of the European Society of Cardiology. The role of endomyocardial biopsy in the management of cardiovascular disease: a scientific statement from the American Heart Association, the American College of Cardiology, and the European Society of Cardiology. J Am Coll Cardiol. 2007; 50 (19):1914–1931

[262] Gagliardi MG, Bevilacqua M, Di Renzi P, Picardo S, Passariello R, Marcelletti C. Usefulness of magnetic resonance imaging for diagnosis of acute myocarditis in infants and children, and comparison with endomyocardial biopsy. Am J Cardiol. 1991; 68(10):1089–1091

[263] Lurz P, Eitel I, Adam J, et al. Diagnostic performance of CMR imaging compared with EMB in patients with suspected myocarditis. JACC Cardiovasc Imaging. 2012; 5(5):513–524

[264] Drucker NA, Colan SD, Lewis AB, et al. γ-globulin treatment of acute myocarditis in the pediatric population. Circulation. 1994; 89 (1):252–257

[265] Frustaci A, Chimenti C, Calabrese F, Pieroni M, Thiene G, Maseri A. Immunosuppressive therapy for active lymphocytic myocarditis: virological and immunologic profile of responders versus nonresponders. Circulation. 2003; 107(6):857–863

[266] Maisch B, Hufnagel G, Schönian U, Hengstenberg C. The European study of epidemiology and treatment of cardiac inflammatory disease (ESETCID). Eur Heart J. 1995; 16 Suppl O:173–175

[267] Mason JW, O'Connell JB, Herskowitz A, et al. The Myocarditis Treatment Trial Investigators. A clinical trial of immunosuppressive therapy for myocarditis. N Engl J Med. 1995; 333(5):269–275

[268] Kühl U, Pauschinger M, Schwimmbeck PL, et al. Interferon-β treatment eliminates cardiotropic viruses and improves left ventricular function in patients with myocardial persistence of viral genomes and left ventricular dysfunction. Circulation. 2003; 107(22):2793–2798

[269] Wojnicz R, Nowalany-Kozielska E, Wojciechowska C, et al. Randomized, placebo-controlled study for immunosuppressive treatment of inflammatory dilated cardiomyopathy: two-year follow-up results. Circulation. 2001; 104(1):39–45

[270] Schmaltz AA, Demel KP, Kallenberg R, et al. Immunosuppressive therapy of chronic myocarditis in children: three cases and the design of a randomized prospective trial of therapy. Pediatr Cardiol. 1998; 19(3):235–239

[271] Felix SB, Staudt A, Baumann G. Immunoadsorption as a new therapeutic principle for treatment of dilated cardiomyopathy. Eur Heart J. 2002 Suppl. 4:163–168

[272] Canter CE, Simpson KE. Diagnosis and treatment of myocarditis in children in the current era. Circulation. 2014; 129(1):115–128

[273] Newburger JW, Fulton DR. Kawasaki disease. Curr Opin Pediatr. 2004; 16(5):508–514

[274] Newburger JW, Takahashi M, Gerber MA, et al. Committee on Rheumatic Fever, Endocarditis, and Kawasaki Disease, Council on Cardiovascular Disease in the Young, American Heart Association. Diagnosis, treatment, and long-term management of Kawasaki disease: a statement for health professionals from the Committee on Rheumatic Fever, Endocarditis, and Kawasaki Disease, Council on Cardiovascular Disease in the Young, American Heart Association. Pediatrics. 2004; 114(6):1708–1733

[275] Kawasaki T. [Acute febrile mucocutaneous syndrome with lymphoid involvement with specific desquamation of the fingers and toes in children]. Arerugi. 1967; 16(3):178–222

[276] Taubert KA, Rowley AH, Shulman ST. Seven-year national survey of Kawasaki disease and acute rheumatic fever. Pediatr Infect Dis J. 1994; 13(8):704–708

[277] Dajani AS, Taubert KA, Gerber MA, et al. Diagnosis and therapy of Kawasaki disease in children. Circulation. 1993; 87(5):1776–1780

[278] Newburger JW, Takahashi M, Gerber MA, et al. Committee on Rheumatic Fever, Endocarditis and Kawasaki Disease, Council on Cardiovascular Disease in the Young, American Heart Association, American Academy of Pediatrics. Diagnosis, treatment, and long-term management of Kawasaki disease: a statement for health professionals from the Committee on Rheumatic Fever, Endocarditis and Kawasaki Disease, Council on Cardiovascular Disease in the Young, American Heart Association. Circulation. 2004; 110(17):2747–2771

[279] Council on Cardiovascular Disease in the Young, Committee on Rheumatic Fever, Endocarditis, and Kawasaki Disease, American Heart Association. Diagnostic guidelines for Kawasaki disease. Circulation. 2001; 103(2):335–336

[280] Kato H, Inoue O, Kawasaki T, Fujiwara H, Watanabe T, Toshima H. Adult coronary artery disease probably due to childhood Kawasaki disease. Lancet. 1992; 340(8828):1127–1129

[281] Mavrogeni S, Papadopoulos G, Hussain T, Chiribiri A, Botnar R, Greil GF. The emerging role of cardiovascular magnetic resonance in the evaluation of Kawasaki disease. Int J Cardiovasc Imaging. 2013; 29 (8):1787–1798

[282] Yoshikawa H, Nomura Y, Masuda K, et al. Four cases of Kawasaki syndrome complicated with myocarditis. Circ J. 2006; 70(2):202–205

[283] Kato H, Sugimura T, Akagi T, et al. Long-term consequences of Kawasaki disease. A 10- to 21-year follow-up study of 594 patients. Circulation. 1996; 94(6):1379–1385

[284] Newburger JW, Takahashi M, Beiser AS, et al. A single intravenous infusion of gamma globulin as compared with four infusions in the treatment of acute Kawasaki syndrome. N Engl J Med. 1991; 324 (23):1633–1639

[285] Newburger JW, Takahashi M, Burns JC, et al. The treatment of Kawasaki syndrome with intravenous gamma globulin. N Engl J Med. 1986; 315(6):341–347

[286] Dajani AS, Taubert KA, Takahashi M, et al. Guidelines for long-term management of patients with Kawasaki disease. Report from the Committee on Rheumatic Fever, Endocarditis, and Kawasaki Disease, Council on Cardiovascular Disease in the Young, American Heart Association. Circulation. 1994; 89(2):916–922

[287] Baer AZ, Rubin LG, Shapiro CA, et al. Prevalence of coronary artery lesions on the initial echocardiogram in Kawasaki syndrome. Arch Pediatr Adolesc Med. 2006; 160(7):686–690

[288] Geva T, Kreutzer J, Crawford MH, et al. Diagnostic pathways for evaluation of congenital heart disease. Cardiology. 2001:7–41

[289] Hiraishi S, Misawa H, Takeda N, et al. Transthoracic ultrasonic visualisation of coronary aneurysm, stenosis, and occlusion in Kawasaki disease. Heart. 2000; 83(4):400–405

[290] Greil GF, Stuber M, Botnar RM, et al. Coronary magnetic resonance angiography in adolescents and young adults with kawasaki disease. Circulation. 2002; 105(8):908–911

[291] Greil GF, Seeger A, Miller S, et al. Coronary magnetic resonance angiography and vessel wall imaging in children with Kawasaki disease. Pediatr Radiol. 2007; 37(7):666–673

[292] Sohn S, Kim HS, Lee SW. Multidetector row computed tomography for follow-up of patients with coronary artery aneurysms due to Kawasaki disease. Pediatr Cardiol. 2004; 25(1):35–39

[293] Chu WC, Mok GC, Lam WW, Yam MC, Sung RY. Assessment of coronary artery aneurysms in paediatric patients with Kawasaki disease by multidetector row CT angiography: feasibility and comparison with 2D echocardiography. Pediatr Radiol. 2006; 36 (11):1148–1153

[294] Jan SL, Hwang B, Fu YC, et al. Comparison of 201Tl SPET and treadmill exercise testing in patients with Kawasaki disease. Nucl Med Commun. 2000; 21(5):431–435

[295] Ho NC, Tran JR, Bektas A. Marfan's syndrome. Lancet. 2005; 366 (9501):1978–1981

[296] Pyeritz RE, McKusick VA. The Marfan syndrome: diagnosis and management. N Engl J Med. 1979; 300(14):772–777

[297] Kainulainen K, Pulkkinen L, Savolainen A, Kaitila I, Peltonen L. Location on chromosome 15 of the gene defect causing Marfan syndrome. N Engl J Med. 1990; 323(14):935–939

[298] Robinson PN, Godfrey M. The molecular genetics of Marfan syndrome and related microfibrillopathies. J Med Genet. 2000; 37(1):9–25

[299] Jondeau G, Michel JB, Boileau C. The translational science of Marfan syndrome. Heart. 2011; 97(15):1206–1214

[300] McKUSICK VA. The cardiovascular aspects of Marfan's syndrome: a heritable disorder of connective tissue. Circulation. 1955; 11 (3):321–342

[301] Kaiser T, Kellenberger CJ, Albisetti M, Bergsträsser E, Valsangiacomo Buechel ER. Normal values for aortic diameters in children and adolescents—assessment in vivo by contrast-enhanced CMR-angiography. J Cardiovasc Magn Reson. 2008; 10:56

[302] De Paepe A, Devereux RB, Dietz HC, Hennekam RC, Pyeritz RE. Revised diagnostic criteria for the Marfan syndrome. Am J Med Genet. 1996; 62(4):417–426

[303] Loeys BL, Dietz HC, Braverman AC, et al. The revised Ghent nosology for the Marfan syndrome. J Med Genet. 2010; 47(7):476–485

[304] Keane MG, Pyeritz RE. Medical management of Marfan syndrome. Circulation. 2008; 117(21):2802–2813

[305] Détaint D, Faivre L, Collod-Beroud G, et al. Cardiovascular manifestations in men and women carrying a FBN1 mutation. Eur Heart J. 2010; 31(18):2223–2229

[306] Bhudia SK, Troughton R, Lam BK, et al. Mitral valve surgery in the adult Marfan syndrome patient. Ann Thorac Surg. 2006; 81 (3):843–848

[307] Underwood MJ, El Khoury G, Deronck D, Glineur D, Dion R. The aortic root: structure, function, and surgical reconstruction. Heart. 2000; 83(4):376–380

[308] Fujiseki Y, Okuno K, Tanaka M, Shimada M, Takahashi M, Kawanishi K. Myocardial involvement in the Marfan syndrome. Jpn Heart J. 1985; 26(6):1043–1050

[309] De Backer JF, Devos D, Segers P, et al. Primary impairment of left ventricular function in Marfan syndrome. Int J Cardiol. 2006; 112 (3):353–358

[310] Kiotsekoglou A, Sutherland GR, Moggridge JC, et al. Impaired right ventricular systolic function demonstrated by reduced atrioventricular plane displacement in adults with Marfan syndrome. Eur J Echocardiogr. 2009; 10(2):295–302

[311] Yetman AT, Bornemeier RA, McCrindle BW. Long-term outcome in patients with Marfan syndrome: is aortic dissection the only cause of sudden death? J Am Coll Cardiol. 2003; 41(2):329–332

[312] Alpendurada F, Wong J, Kiotsekoglou A, et al. Evidence for Marfan cardiomyopathy. Eur J Heart Fail. 2010; 12(10):1085–1091

[313] Saleh RS, Finn JP, Fenchel M, et al. Cardiovascular magnetic resonance in patients with pectus excavatum compared with normal controls. J Cardiovasc Magn Reson. 2010; 12:73

[314] Shores J, Berger KR, Murphy EA, Pyeritz RE. Progression of aortic dilatation and the benefit of long-term beta-adrenergic blockade in Marfan's syndrome. N Engl J Med. 1994; 330(19):1335–1341

[315] Danyi P, Elefteriades JA, Jovin IS. Medical therapy of thoracic aortic aneurysms: are we there yet? Circulation. 2011; 124 (13):1469–1476

[316] Brooke BS, Habashi JP, Judge DP, Patel N, Loeys B, Dietz HC, III. Angiotensin II blockade and aortic-root dilation in Marfan's syndrome. N Engl J Med. 2008; 358(26):2787–2795

[317] Ahimastos AA, Aggarwal A, D'Orsa KM, et al. Effect of perindopril on large artery stiffness and aortic root diameter in patients with Marfan syndrome: a randomized controlled trial. JAMA. 2007; 298 (13):1539–1547

[318] Gott VL, Greene PS, Alejo DE, et al. Replacement of the aortic root in patients with Marfan's syndrome. N Engl J Med. 1999; 340 (17):1307–1313

[319] Bentall H, De Bono A. A technique for complete replacement of the ascending aorta. Thorax. 1968; 23(4):338–339

[320] Treasure T. Elective replacement of the aortic root in Marfan's syndrome. Br Heart J. 1993; 69(2):101–103

[321] Treasure T. The evolution of aortic root surgery for Marfan syndrome. Interact Cardiovasc Thorac Surg. 2010; 10(3):353–355

[322] Benedetto U, Melina G, Takkenberg JJ, Roscitano A, Angeloni E, Sinatra R. Surgical management of aortic root disease in Marfan syndrome: a systematic review and meta-analysis. Heart. 2011; 97(12):955–958

[323] Sievers HH, Misfeld M. Erworbene Vitien der Aortenklappe. In: Ziemer G, Haverich A, Hrsg. Herzchirurgie. Berlin: Springer; 2009

[324] Murdoch JL, Walker BA, Halpern BL, Kuzma JW, McKusick VA. Life expectancy and causes of death in the Marfan syndrome. N Engl J Med. 1972; 286(15):804–808

[325] Krause KJ. Marfan syndrome: literature review of mortality studies. J Insur Med. 2000; 32(2):79–88

[326] Silverman DI, Gray J, Roman MJ, et al. Family history of severe cardiovascular disease in Marfan syndrome is associated with increased aortic diameter and decreased survival. J Am Coll Cardiol. 1995; 26 (4):1062–1067

[327] Li H, Tanaka K, Anzai H, et al. Influence of pre-existing donor atherosclerosis on the development of cardiac allograft vasculopathy and outcomes in heart transplant recipients. J Am Coll Cardiol. 2006; 47 (12):2470–2476

[328] Shiga T, Wajima Z, Apfel CC, Inoue T, Ohe Y. Diagnostic accuracy of transesophageal echocardiography, helical computed tomography, and magnetic resonance imaging for suspected thoracic aortic dissection: systematic review and meta-analysis. Arch Intern Med. 2006; 166(13):1350–1356

[329] Meijboom LJ, Groenink M, van der Wall EE, Romkes H, Stoker J, Mulder BJ. Aortic root asymmetry in marfan patients; evaluation by magnetic resonance imaging and comparison with standard echocardiography. Int J Card Imaging. 2000; 16(3):161–168

[330] Dormand H, Mohiaddin RH. Cardiovascular magnetic resonance in Marfan syndrome. J Cardiovasc Magn Reson. 2013; 15:33

[331] Potthast S, Mitsumori L, Stanescu LA, et al. Measuring aortic diameter with different MR techniques: comparison of three-dimensional (3D) navigated steady-state free-precession (SSFP), 3D contrast-enhanced magnetic resonance angiography (CE-MRA), 2D T2 black blood, and 2D cine SSFP. J Magn Reson Imaging. 2010; 31(1):177–184

[332] Collins RT, II, Kaplan P, Somes GW, Rome JJ. Cardiovascular abnormalities, interventions, and long-term outcomes in infantile Williams syndrome. J Pediatr. 2010; 156(2):253–8.e1

[333] Williams JC, Barratt-Boyes BG, Lowe JB. Supravalvular aortic stenosis. Circulation. 1961; 24:1311–1318

[334] Beuren AJ, Apitz J, Harmjanz D. Supravalvular aortic stenosis in association with mental retardation and a certain facial appearance. Circulation. 1962; 26:1235–1240

[335] Stromme P, Bjornstad PG, Ramstad K. Prevalence estimation of Williams syndrome. J Child Neurol. 2002; 17(4):269–271

[336] Adams GN, Schmaier AH. The Williams–Beuren syndrome—a window into genetic variants leading to the development of cardiovascular disease. PLoS Genet. 2012; 8(2):e1002479

[337] Pober BR. Williams–Beuren syndrome. N Engl J Med. 2010; 362 (3):239–252

[338] Karnik SK, Brooke BS, Bayes-Genis A, et al. A critical role for elastin signaling in vascular morphogenesis and disease. Development. 2003; 130(2):411–423

[339] Hickey EJ, Jung G, Williams WG et al. Congenital supravalvular aortic stenosis: defining surgical and nonsurgical outcomes. Ann Thorac Surg 2008; 86(6): 1919–1927; discussion 1927

[340] Kitchiner D, Jackson M, Malaiya N, Walsh K, Peart I, Arnold R. Incidence and prognosis of obstruction of the left ventricular outflow tract in Liverpool (1960–91): a study of 313 patients. Br Heart J. 1994; 71(6):588–595

[341] Ewart AK, Jin W, Atkinson D, Morris CA, Keating MT. Supravalvular aortic stenosis associated with a deletion disrupting the elastin gene. J Clin Invest. 1994; 93(3):1071–1077

[342] Kumar A, Stalker HJ, Williams CA. Concurrence of supravalvular aortic stenosis and peripheral pulmonary stenosis in three generations of a family: a form of arterial dysplasia. Am J Med Genet. 1993; 45(6):739–742

[343] Yilmaz AT, Arslan M, Ozal E, Býngöl H, Tatar H, Oztürk OY. Coronary artery aneurysm associated with adult supravalvular aortic stenosis. Ann Thorac Surg. 1996; 62(4):1205–1207

[344] Bouchireb K, Boyer O, Bonnet D, et al. Clinical features and management of arterial hypertension in children with Williams–Beuren syndrome. Nephrol Dial Transplant. 2010; 25(2):434–438

[345] Wessel A, Gravenhorst V, Buchhorn R, Gosch A, Partsch CJ, Pankau R. Risk of sudden death in the Williams–Beuren syndrome. Am J Med Genet A. 2004; 127A(3):234–237

[346] Collins RT, II, Aziz PF, Swearingen CJ, Kaplan PB. Relation of ventricular ectopic complexes to QTc interval on ambulatory electrocardiograms in Williams syndrome. Am J Cardiol. 2012; 100(11):1671–1676

[347] Collins RT, II. Cardiovascular disease in Williams syndrome. Circulation. 2013; 127(21):2125–2134

[348] Wren C, Oslizlok P, Bull C. Natural history of supravalvular aortic stenosis and pulmonary artery stenosis. J Am Coll Cardiol. 1990; 15 (7):1625–1630

[349] Brown JW, Ruzmetov M, Vijay P, Turrentine MW. Surgical repair of congenital supravalvular aortic stenosis in children. Eur J Cardiothorac Surg. 2002; 21(1):50–56

[350] Del Pasqua A, Rinelli G, Toscano A, et al. New findings concerning cardiovascular manifestations emerging from long-term follow-up of 150 patients with the Williams–Beuren syndrome. Cardiol Young. 2009; 19(6):563–567

[351] Kaushal S, Backer CL, Patel S, Gossett JG, Mavroudis C. Midterm outcomes in supravalvular aortic stenosis demonstrate the superiority of multisinus aortoplasty. Ann Thorac Surg. 2010; 89(5):1371–1377

[352] Deo SV, Burkhart HM, Schaff HV, et al. Late outcomes for surgical repair of supravalvar aortic stenosis. Ann Thorac Surg. 2012; 94(3):854–859

[353] Falkensammer CB, Paul J, Huhta JC. Fetal congestive heart failure: correlation of Tei-index and Cardiovascular-score. J Perinat Med. 2001; 29(5):390–398

[354] Epstein AE, DiMarco JP, Ellenbogen KA, et al. American College of, Cardiology/American Heart Association Task Force on Practice Guidelines (Writing Committee to Revise the ACC/AHA/NASPE 2002 Guideline Update for Implantation of Cardiac Pacemakers and Antiarrhythmia Devices), American Association for Thoracic Surgery, Society of Thoracic Surgeons. ACC/AHA/HRS 2008 Guidelines for Device-Based Therapy of Cardiac Rhythm Abnormalities: a report of the American College of Cardiology/American Heart Association Task Force on Practice Guidelines (Writing Committee to Revise the ACC/AHA/NASPE 2002 Guideline Update for Implantation of Cardiac Pacemakers and Antiarrhythmia Devices) developed in collaboration with the American Association for Thoracic Surgery and Society of Thoracic Surgeons. J Am Coll Cardiol. 2008; 51(21):e1–e62

[355] Swedberg K, Cleland J, Dargie H, et al. Task Force for the Diagnosis and Treatment of Chronic Heart Failure of the European Society of Cardiology. Guidelines for the diagnosis and treatment of chronic heart failure: executive summary (update 2005): The Task Force for the Diagnosis and Treatment of Chronic Heart Failure of the European Society of Cardiology. Eur Heart J. 2005; 26(11):1115–1140

[356] Maron BJ, McKenna WJ, Danielson GK, et al. Task Force on Clinical Expert Consensus Documents. American College of Cardiology, Committee for Practice Guidelines. European Society of Cardiology. American College of Cardiology/European Society of Cardiology clinical expert consensus document on hypertrophic cardiomyopathy. A report of the American College of Cardiology Foundation Task Force on Clinical Expert Consensus Documents and the European Society

of Cardiology Committee for Practice Guidelines. J Am Coll Cardiol. 2003; 42(9):1687–1713

[357] Kass DA. An epidemic of dyssynchrony: but what does it mean? J Am Coll Cardiol. 2008; 51(1):12–17

[358] Yu CM, Zhang Q, Fung JW, et al. A novel tool to assess systolic asynchrony and identify responders of cardiac resynchronization therapy by tissue synchronization imaging. J Am Coll Cardiol. 2005; 45 (5):677–684

[359] Suffoletto MS, Dohi K, Cannesson M, Saba S, Gorcsan J, III. Novel speckle-tracking radial strain from routine black-and-white echocardiographic images to quantify dyssynchrony and predict response to cardiac resynchronization therapy. Circulation. 2006; 113(7):960–968

[360] Chung ES, Leon AR, Tavazzi L, et al. Results of the predictors of response to CRT (PROSPECT) trial. Circulation. 2008; 117(20):2608–2616

[361] Hawkins NM, Petrie MC, MacDonald MR, Hogg KJ, McMurray JJ. Selecting patients for cardiac resynchronization therapy: electrical or mechanical dyssynchrony? Eur Heart J. 2006; 27(11):1270–1281

[362] Wu J, Pflaumer A, Deisenhofer I, et al. Mapping of intraatrial reentrant tachycardias by remote magnetic navigation in patients with d-transposition of the great arteries after mustard or senning procedure. J Cardiovasc Electrophysiol. 2008; 19(11):1153–1159

Suggested Readings

Bass JE, Redwine MD, Kramer LA, Huynh PT, Harris JH, Jr. Spectrum of congenital anomalies of the inferior vena cava: cross-sectional imaging findings. Radiographics. 2000; 20(3):639–652

Bell A, Rawlins D, Bellsham-Revell H, Miller O, Razavi R, Simpson J. Assessment of right ventricular volumes in hypoplastic left heart syndrome by real-time three-dimensional echocardiography: comparison with cardiac magnetic resonance imaging. Eur Heart J Cardiovasc Imaging. 2014; 15(3):257–266

Cincinnati Children's. Total anomalous pulmonary venous return (TAPVR). Im Internet: http://www.cincinnatichildrens.org/health/heart-encyclopedia/anomalies/tapvr.htm#symptoms (Stand: 01.07.2015)

Cissarek T, Kröger K, Santosa F, Zeller T, Eds. Gefäßmedizin—Therapie und Praxis. Berlin: ABW Wissenschaftsverlag; 2009: 412

Dittrich S, Klassen S, Kandolf R et al. DGPK-Leitlinie—Primäre Kardiomyopathien (S2). 2016; S. 237–250

Elliot PM, Anastakis A, Borger MA, et al. ESC Guideline on diagnosis and management of hypertrophic cardiomyopathy. Eur Heart J. 2014; 35: 2733–2779

Ginaldi S, Chuang VP, Wallace S. Absence of hepatic segment of the inferior vena cava with azygous continuation. J Comput Assist Tomogr. 1980; 4(1):112–114

Kim HJ, Goo HW, Park SH, Yun TJ. Left ventricle volume measured by cardiac CT in an infant with a small left ventricle: a new and accurate method in determining uni- or biventricular repair. Pediatr Radiol. 2013; 43(2):243–246

Kinderkardiochirurgie online. Im Internet: http://www.kinderkardiochirurgie.de/as.html; Stand: 27.06.2015

cardiacmorphology.com. Im Internet: http://www.cardiacmorphology.com (Stand: 30.06.2015)

Medscape. Total anomalous pulmonary venous connection. Im Internet: http://emedicine.medscape.com/article/899491-overview (Stand: 01.07.2015)

Müther S, Dähnert I. Das Heterotaxiesyndrom. Z Herz Thorax Gefäßchir. 2000; 14(3):134–136

Nationwide Children's. Coarctation of the aorta. Im Internet: http://www.nationwidechildrens.org/coarctation-of-the-aorta (Stand: 30.06.2015)

Paul T, Tschöpe C, Kandolf R. DGPK-Leitlinie—Myokarditis im Kindesalter (S2). 2016; S. 219–226

Therrien J, Provost Y, Merchant N, Williams W, Colman J, Webb G. Optimal timing for pulmonary valve replacement in adults after tetralogy of Fallot repair. Am J Cardiol. 2005; 95(6):779–782

Wilkenshoff U, Kruck I, Eds. Handbuch der Echokardiographie. 3. Aufl. Berlin: Blackwell; 2002

5 Standard Values and Formulas

Hashim Abdul-Khaliq, Petra Böttler, Samir Sarikouch

5.1 Preliminary Remarks

This chapter is intended only to provide a brief overview of common standard values tables. The fundamental issue of standard values—which are subject to numerous factors dependent upon patients, devices, or examiners—is something that any user should always keep in mind. In general, standard values for children and adolescents are rarer than for adults. In some cases, such as for new MRI methods including T1 and T2 mapping and determining extracellular volume fraction, no values exist for pediatric patients. Refer to the literature for information regarding adult patients.[1]

Regardless of the selected method and the applied algorithm, absolute values should not be applied. Rather, indicated standards (which are generally based on body surface area) should be used. Furthermore, the same methods and protocols should be used for follow-up examinations. The DuBois formula for calculating body surface area has been tried and tested in pediatric patients.[2,3] Furthermore, it should be noted that the trabecula and papillary muscles are considered part of muscle mass for volumetric data, yet are excluded from the volume calculations.[1] In addition to the guidelines for quality assurance and standard values published by societies such as the DGPK,[4,5] web-based, continually updated large databases (such as the *Z*-Scores of Cardiac Structures, Detroit,[6,7] which uses data from 782 patients from the Children's Hospital of Michigan) will be available for use in standard values tables. Body size and weight are entered on an input screen in order to calculate standard values using the Z-Scores of Cardiac Structures website. The user can then select which of the five various calculation algorithms (Boyd, DuBois, Gehan & George, Haycock, or Mosteller) should be used to determine body surface area (BSA), or whether it should be calculated using only body weight. The measured values can then be entered for various parameters, which the website subsequently uses to calculate *Z*-scores. Certain authors prefer using the Mosteller formula to calculate body surface area in pediatric patients.[2,3] Large registries, such as the Competence Network for Congenital Heart Defects, are another source of standard values.[8–11] This chapter will make reference to both sources.

> **Note**
>
> The *Z*-score is a measure of the number of standard deviations a particular measured value deviates from the mean value of the sample (here, a group of standards). (Freely accessible website for pediatric cardiology CMR *Z*-scores: http://cmr.pedz.de)

The *Z*-score is calculated using the following formula[2]:

$$Z = \frac{X - \mu}{\sigma}$$

where

- Z = standardized random variable
- X = random variable
- μ = mean or "expected" value of the sample (or group of standards)
- σ = standard deviation of the sample (or group of standards)

A negative *Z*-value indicates that the measured value is smaller than the mean, while a positive *Z*-value indicates the opposite.

5.2 Standard Values and Formulas for Echocardiography

5.2.1 Standard Values

Cardiovascular parameters for transthoracic echocardiography, M-mode (▶ Table 5.1,▶ Table 5.2 and ▶ Table 5.3).

Table 5.1 Diameter reference values based on body surface area. Diameter value as mean value ± 2 standard deviations.[4,5]

Body surface area (m^2)	RVWd (mm)	RVDd (mm)	IVSd (mm)	LVDd (mm)	LVWd (mm)	AOd (mm)	LADs (mm)
0.25	2.6 ± 1.2	8.7 ± 4.5	3.8 ± 1.4	20.0 ± 3.6	3.6 ± 1.0	10.4 ± 2.4	14.0 ± 3.5
0.30	2.7 ± 1.1	8.7 ± 4.4	3.9 ± 1.4	22.9 ± 3.9	4.1 ± 1.3	11.3 ± 2.3	15.3 ± 3.8
0.40	2.7 ± 1.1	8.9 ± 4.5	4.1 ± 1.5	26.0 ± 5.0	4.2 ± 1.3	12.9 ± 2.0	16.8 ± 3.8
0.50	2.8 ± 1.1	9.3 ± 4.5	4.3 ± 1.6	29.0 ± 5.6	4.6 ± 1.5	14.9 ± 2.7	18.7 ± 4.2
0.60	2.8 ± 1.1	9.6 ± 4.4	4.8 ± 1.5	31.6 ± 5.6	4.8 ± 1.5	15.6 ± 2.8	20.1 ± 4.0
0.70	2.8 ± 1.1	10.1 ± 4.4	5.0 ± 1.5	33.9 ± 6.5	5.2 ± 1.7	16.9 ± 3.4	21.2 ± 5.0
0.80	2.8 ± 1.1	10.5 ± 4.7	5.2 ± 1.6	35.8 ± 6.2	5.7 ± 2.1	17.9 ± 3.4	22.5 ± 6.0
0.90	2.8 ± 1.1	11.0 ± 4.6	5.6 ± 1.8	37.1 ± 6.1	5.9 ± 2.2	18.7 ± 3.6	23.2 ± 6.2
1.00	2.8 ± 1.1	11.2 ± 4.8	5.8 ± 1.8	38.5 ± 6.8	5.9 ± 2.2	19.9 ± 3.6	25.0 ± 5.8
1.10	2.9 ± 1.1	11.8 ± 4.4	6.2 ± 1.9	39.4 ± 6.9	6.3 ± 2.4	20.9 ± 3.4	25.2 ± 5.7
1.20	2.9 ± 1.1	12.4 ± 4.8	6.5 ± 1.8	41.7 ± 6.2	6.6 ± 2.5	21.0 ± 3.5	26.0 ± 5.1
1.30	3.0 ± 1.1	13.5 ± 5.0	6.6 ± 1.8	42.4 ± 6.6	6.9 ± 2.6	21.7 ± 4.2	27.3 ± 5.6
1.40	3.0 ± 1.1	14.0 ± 5.0	6.7 ± 1.8	43.3 ± 6.0	6.9 ± 2.6	22.7 ± 4.8	28.2 ± 5.4
1.50	3.1 ± 1.2	15.6 ± 5.6	7.4 ± 2.2	45.4 ± 6.4	7.7 ± 2.8	23.6 ± 5.4	29.9 ± 6.2
1.75	3.1 ± 1.2	16.5 ± 6.2	8.0 ± 2.4	46.8 ± 6.0	8.1 ± 3.0	24.4 ± 6.2	30.4 ± 6.6
2.00	3.1 ± 1.2	17.5 ± 6.0	8.3 ± 2.5	53.4 ± 8.0	8.1 ± 3.0	27.4 ± 4.4	32.5 ± 8.8

AOd, aorta, diastolic; IVSd, interventricular septum, diastolic; LADs, left atrial diameter, systolic; LVDd, left ventricular diameter, diastolic; LVWd, left ventricular posterior wall, diastolic; RVDd, right ventricular diameter, diastolic; RVWd, right ventricular posterior wall, diastolic.

Table 5.2 2-D echocardiography standard values for certain ventricular, atrial, and vascular parameters based on transducer position (indicating 5th–95th percentile).[5]

Body surface area (m^2)	Apical		Parasternal/suprasternal			Subcostal	
	LVd (mm)	TV/MV diff. (mm)	PAd (mm)	AoAd (mm)	IVCd (mm)	RVd (mm)	RAd (mm)
0.20	33–50	2.5–5.6	7–12	6–12	3–6	12–25	12–22
0.40	43–63	3.0–7.0	9–16	8–14	5–9	17–32	16–29
0.60	51–77	3.5–7.7	11–19	10–16	6–12	21–42	19–36
0.80	60–90	3.8–8.5	12–22	11–18	8–14	25–48	22–41
1.00	67–98	4.1–9.0	13–25	12–20	9–16	27–53	25–46
1.20	73–105	4.3–9.5	15–27	13–22	10–18	29–58	27–49
1.40	78–112	4.4–10.1	16–29	14–23	11–21	31–63	29–52
1.60	82–119	4.5–10.5	17–31	14–24	12–22	33–67	31–55

AoAd, aortic arch diameter; LVd, left ventricular diameter; PAd, pulmonary arterial diameter; RAd, right atrial diameter; RVd, right ventricular diameter; TV/MV diff., tricuspid/mitral valve distance from the septal insertion; IVCd, inferior vena cava diameter.

Table 5.3 Standard flow velocity values for Doppler echocardiography in pediatric patients.[5]

Vessel/valve	Diastolic filling parameter		V_{max} (m/s)
Publications[12,13]			
Aortic valve		1.20–1.80	1.52 (1.20–1.70)
Pulmonary valve		0.70–1.20	0.84 (0.60–1.20)
Mitral valve	E wave	0.70–1.10	1.00 (0.70–1.40)
	A wave	0.30–0.70	
	E/A ratio	1.10–2.70	
Tricuspid valve	E wave	0.40–0.80	0.62 (0.50–0.90)
	A wave	0.20–0.60	
	E/A ratio	0.60–2.60	
Proximal descending aorta		0.80–1.80	
LVOT		0.70–1.20	
Caval vein		0.50–1.50*	

*Extremely dependent upon respiration

V_{max}, maximum velocity; E, maximum velocity in the early filling phase; A, maximum velocity in the late (atrial) filling phase; LVOT, left ventricular outflow tract.

5.2.2 Formulas with Standard Values

Modified in accordance with Wilkenshoff and Kruck (2002).[13]

General Quantification of Valve Stenoses

Note

The following formulas can, in part, also be used analogously in MRI flow measurements.

Stenosis Quantification Using the Modified Bernoulli Equation and Flow Velocity Before a Stenosis ($V_1 < 1$ m/s)

$$\Delta p_{max} = 4 \times V_{max}^2$$

$$\Delta p_{max} = 4 \times V_{mean}^2$$

where

V_1 = maximum flow velocity before the stenosis in m/s
Δp_{max} = maximum pressure in mmHg
V_{max} = maximum velocity in the stenosis in m/s
Δp_{mean} = median pressure in mmHg
V_{mean} = median flow velocity in m/s

Stenosis Quantification Based on the Original Bernoulli Equation with Elevated Flow Velocity Before the Stenosis ($V_1 > 1$ m/s)

$$\Delta p_{max} = 4 \times (V_{max}^2 - V_1^2)$$

where

V_1 = maximum flow velocity before the stenosis in m/s
Δp_{max} = maximum pressure in mmHg
V_{max} = maximum velocity in the stenosis in m/s

Calculating Valve Orifice Area Using the Continuity Equation

$$BSA = \pi \times \left(\frac{d}{2}\right)^2 \times \frac{V_1}{V_{max}}$$

where

BSA = body surface area in cm^2
d = maximum diameter of the left or right ventricular outflow tract in cm
V_1 = maximum flow velocity before the stenosis in m/s
V_{max} = maximum velocity in the stenosis in m/s

Quantifying Orifice Area of the Atrioventricular Valve Using Pressure Half-Time

$$BSA = \frac{220}{PHT}$$

$$PHT = \frac{V_{max}}{\sqrt{2}}$$

where
BSA = body surface area in cm^2
PHT = pressure half-time in s
V_{max} = maximum velocity in m/s

Calculating Stroke, Cardiac Output, and Shunt Volumes

Calculating Stroke Volume

$$SV = \int V \times \text{cross} - \text{sectional area}$$

where
SV = stroke volume in ml
∫V = flow velocity integral via the cardiac valve

Calculating Cardiac Minute Volume

$$CMV = \text{cross} - \text{sectional area} \times \int V \times HF$$

where
CMV = cardiac minute volume in l/min

$$\text{cross} - \text{sectional area} = \pi \times \left[\left(\frac{d}{2}\right)^2\right]$$

∫V = flow velocity integral via the cardiac valve
CF = heart rate (beats/minute)
d = maximum diameter of the valve ring or outflow tract

Standard value for cardiac minute volume, determined using the thermodilution method[13]: 6.99 (4.00–10.20) l/min.

Estimating Shunt Size

$$\frac{Q_p}{Q_s} = \frac{SV_{Pulmonary\ artery}}{SV_{Aorta}}$$

where
Q_p = pulmonary flow
Q_s = systemic flow
$SV_{pulmonary\ artery}$ = stroke volume of the pulmonary artery
SV_{aorta} = stroke volume of the aorta
Standard value: 1.

> **Note**
> If an open ductus arteriosus Botalli, MAPCAs, and extracardiac collaterals are present, flow volume should be determined via the atrioventricular valves.

Estimating Left Ventricular Function and Volume Using 2-D Echocardiography

Determining Regional Shortening Fraction Using M-Mode

$$FS = \frac{LVEDD - LVESD}{LVEDD} \times 100$$

where
FS = fractional shortening in %
LVEDD = left ventricular end diastolic diameter
LVESD = left ventricular end systolic diameter
Standard value: 25–45%.

Estimating Left Ventricular Volume Using 2-D Echocardiography (Surface-Length Method)

Modified in accordance with Hahn et al. (1982),[14] Wilkenshoff and Kruck (2002).[13]

Monoplanar (4-chamber view)

$$LVV = \frac{\pi}{6} \times D^2 \times L = \frac{8}{3}\pi \times \frac{A^2}{L}$$

where
LVV = left ventricular volume in ml
D = diameter
L = ventricular length (length of both axes)
A = area perpendicular to the long axis

Biplanar (2-chamber and 4-chamber views)

$$LVV = \frac{\pi}{6} \times D_1 \times D_2 \times L = \frac{8}{3}\pi \times \left(\frac{A_1 \times A_2}{L}\right)$$

where
LVV = left ventricular volume in ml
$D_{1/2}$ = diameter 1/2
L = ventricular length (length of both axes)
$A_{1/2}$ = area 1/2 perpendicular to the long axis

5.2.3 Regional Functional Analysis Using Echocardiography

Echocardiography permits fast, noninvasive, user-friendly analysis of cardiac function. Regional myocardial function can be quantified via echocardiography using various methods:

- *Pulsed tissue Doppler:* Analysis includes the basal, median, and apical segments of a myocardial wall and is performed on both the left and right ventricles. In addition, radial myocardial motion of the left ventricular posterior wall is examined. This method is used to determine the velocity of myocardial motion at various measurement points.[15] In principle, the values can be collected either along the short axis or in 4-chamber view. Examples of values from a 4-chamber view are listed in ▸ Table 5.4.
- *Tissue Doppler:* The development of tissue Doppler analysis permits segmental examination of the myocardium. Using this method, the individual myocardial segments can be analyzed within the same cardiac cycle, meaning that the temporal sequences of myocardial contraction can be compared to one another (prerequisite for synchronization measurement).[16]
- *Myocardial deformation (strain/strain rate) based on tissue Doppler:* The regional functional parameters *strain* and *strain rate* can be calculated using the data from tissue Doppler analysis. This method's applicability is limited, however, due to the time-intensive data acquisition and post-processing, it is only used for special diagnostic tasks in pediatric cardiology. A further development of this method, known as 2-D strain analysis, is easy to use and permits the analysis of conventionally acquired imaging data. The analysis method and standard values listed here[17–20] thus apply exclusively to 2-D strain analyses.

5.3 Standard Values for Magnetic Resonance Imaging

5.3.1 Children with Healthy Hearts

It is well-known that the ratio of heart size to body size is "allometric," meaning that it changes between infancy, early childhood, and adulthood.[21] Naturally, it is also dependent upon body size, body weight, and thus body surface area. For this reason, absolute volumetric values should not be used, particularly for children. Instead, standardized reference values based on body surface area (▸ Table 5.5 and ▸ Table 5.6), body weight (▸ Table 5.7), or body size (▸ Table 5.8 and ▸ Table 5.9) should be used. In addition to age, sex also plays a large role. Thus, standard cardiac values should always be used based on sex and age. There are, however, study results that indicate that, in addition to the standardization based on body surface area most commonly used in pediatric cardiology, simple standardized values based on body weight and independent of sex[9] could be adequate, at least for volumetric data, particularly when used in the form of percentages. Certain MRI standard values for children and adolescents based on body surface area are explained below. The segmented trabecula and papillary muscles were included in muscle mass in the studies cited here,[9,10] and were then subtracted from ventricular volume calculations.

Table 5.4 Myocardial velocity in healthy children (n = 160) during systole, early diastole, and late diastole for the interventricular septum and left and right ventricles, 4-chamber view.[15,16]

Localization	Systole/ Diastole	Maximum velocity (cm/s)					
		Intraventricular septum		Left ventricle		Right ventricle	
		Median	5th–95th percentile	Median	5th–95th percentile	Median	5th–95th percentile
Basal	S	8.1	6.8–9.8	9.7	6.3–13.5	12.8	10.7–16.5
	E	14.3	11.2–18.5	17.6	13.0–23.0	16.2	12.6–21.1
	A	5.8	4.4–7.9	5.5	3.8–8.0	8.6	5.5–12.1
Central	S	6.1	4.7–7.5	9.5	6.2–13.3	10.9	8.6–13.7
	E	13.0	9.2–16.2	15.9	10.0–21.0	13.9	9.4–17.7
	A	4.9	3.5–6.5	4.6	3.2–7.1	7.1	4.7–10.0
Apical	S	4.6	3.1–6.4	8.7	5.0–12.4	8.0	5.7–10.8
	E	9.0	5.9–12.7	10.7	6.5–15.3	10.8	7.0–14.3
	A	3.7	2.4–5.0	3.9	1.9–5.8	5.3	3.6–7.8

A, late diastole; E, early diastole; S, systole.

Table 5.5 Volumetric and functional MRI standard values (mean values with standard deviation from an axial acquisition of SSFP sequences) for children and adolescents with healthy hearts (age: 8–20 years, n = 114, with 55 boys and 59 girls) for the right and left ventricle,[9] based on body surface area in m^2. All volumetric parameters are standardized based on body surface area in ml/m^2 or g/m^2 as index "i."

Parameter (unit)	Male		Female	
	Mean	Standard deviation	Mean	Standard deviation
RV-EDV$_i$ (ml/m^2)	84.5	12.7	76.9	12.7
RV-ESV$_i$ (ml/m^2)	32.5	6.4	28.6	5.4
RV-MM$_i$ (g/m^2)	20.5	7.5	17.6	4.8
RV-SV$_i$ (ml/m^2)	52.0	8.4	48.2	6.8
RV-EF (%)	61.6	4.5	62.8	4.3
LV-EDV$_i$ (ml/m^2)	85.1	13.8	77.9	10.8
LV-ESV$_i$ (ml/m^2)	30.5	7.6	28.5	6.2
LV-MM$_i$ (g/m^2)	55.9	12.3	47.6	8.2
LV-SV$_i$ (ml/m^2)	54.6	8.2	49.3	8.1
LV-EF (%)	64.4	4.9	63.4	6.1

EDV, end diastolic volume; EF, ejection fraction; ESV, end systolic volume; LV, left ventricle; MM, muscle mass; RV, right ventricle; SV, Stroke volume.

Table 5.6 Standard MRI values for vascular diameter of the great vessels (median value with standard deviation from the magnitude images of an MRI phase contrast flow measurement) of children and adolescents with healthy hearts (age: 4–20 years, n = 105, with 55 boys and 50 girls),[8] as absolute values and based on body surface area in m^2.

Parameter (unit)		Mean (unisex)		Standard deviation		Range
		Male	Female	Male	Female	
Aortic diameter	(cm)	2.20		0.40		1.40–3.10
	(cm/m^2)	1.62	1.70	0.28	0.28	
Aortic cross-sectional area	(cm^2)	4.00		1.40		1.60–7.30
	(cm^2/m^2)	2.91	2.86	0.50	0.61	
Pulmonary artery diameter	(cm)	2.30		0.40		1.20–3.30
	(cm/m^2)	1.61	1.67	0.40	0.46	
Pulmonary artery cross-sectional area	(cm^2)	4.40		1.60		1.10–8.70
	(cm^2/m^2)	3.15	3.17	0.58	0.67	

Table 5.7 Volumetric standard MRI values (mean value with standard deviation) for the right and left ventricle of children and adolescents with healthy hearts (age: 8–20 years, n = 114, with 55 boys and 59 girls) from an axial acquisition of SSFP sequences[9] based on body weight in kg. All volumetric parameters are standardized based on body weight in ml/g or g/kg as index "G."

Parameter (unit)	Male		Female	
	Mean	Standard deviation	Mean	Standard deviation
RV-EDV$_G$ (ml/kg)	2.59	0.45	2.52	0.37
RV-EDV$_G$ (ml/kg)	0.99	0.20	0.94	0.17
RV-MM$_G$ (g/kg)	0.61	0.17	0.58	0.15
LV-EDV$_G$ (ml/kg)	2.60	0.45	2.55	0.39
LV-ESV$_G$ (ml/kg)	0.93	0.21	0.94	0.23
LV-MM$_G$ (g/kg)	1.69	0.30	1.56	0.30

EDV, end diastolic volume; ESV, end systolic volume; LV, left ventricle; MM, muscle mass; RV, right ventricle.

Table 5.8 Volumetric standard MRI values (mean value with standard deviation) for the right and left ventricles of children and adolescents with healthy hearts (age: 8–20 years, n = 114, with 55 boys and 59 girls) from an axial acquisition of SSFP sequences[9] based on body size in cm. All volumetric parameters are standardized based on body size in ml/cm or g/cm as index "H."

Parameter (unit)	Male		Female	
	Mean	Standard deviation	Mean	Standard deviation
RV-EDV$_H$ (ml/cm)	0.79	0.20	0.67	0.15
RV-ESV$_H$ (ml/cm)	0.31	0.09	0.25	0.07
RV-MM$_H$ (g/cm)	0.19	0.09	0.15	0.05
LV-EDV$_H$ (ml/cm)	0.80	0.22	0.68	0.16
LV-ESV$_H$ (ml/cm)	0.29	0.01	0.25	0.07
LV-MM$_H$ (g/cm)	0.53	0.20	0.42	0.10

EDV, end diastolic volume; ESV, end systolic volume; LV, left ventricle; MM, muscle mass; RV, right ventricle.

Table 5.9 Volumetric and functional standard MRI values (mean value with standard deviation) of the atria of children and adolescents with healthy hearts (age: 8–20 years, n = 115) from an axial acquisition of SSFP sequences[10] (absolute values and values based on body surface area in m^2).

Parameter (unit)		Right atrium		Left atrium	
		Male	Female	Male	Female
Maximum volume	(ml)	89.2 ± 43.3	71.0 ± 25.3	71.2 ± 30.4	58.6 ± 19.5
	(ml/BSA)	58.1 ± 15.7	53.3 ± 11.8	46.7 ± 10.1	44.2 ± 8.7
Minimum volume	(ml)	41.8 ± 21.3	31.3 ± 12.8	32.9 ± 15.1	25.6 ± 8.9
	(ml/BSA)	27.0 ± 7.9	23.2 ± 6.2	21.5 ± 5.1	19.2 ± 3.9
Stroke volume	(ml)	47.4 ± 24.3	39.8 ± 14.7	38.2 ± 16.3	33.0 ± 11.6
Ejection fraction	(%)	53.2 ± 7.4	56.3 ± 8.0	53.7 ± 6.3	56.2 ± 5.5

BSA, body surface area.

5.3.2 Patients with Valve Stenoses

See ▶ Table 5.10.

Table 5.10 Reference values for valve stenoses, adapted for MRI.[1]

Valve disease	Parameter (unit)	Degree of severity		
		Mild	Moderate	Severe
Aortic valve stenosis	Peak velocity (m/s)	< 3.0	3.0–4.0	> 4.0
	Valve orifice area (cm^2)	> 1.50	1.00–1.50	< 1.00
	Valve orifice area index (cm^2/m^2)			< 0.60
Aortic valve insufficiency	Regurgitation fraction (%)	< 30	30–49	≥ 50
	Regurgitant orifice area (cm^2)	< 0.10	0.10–0.29	≥ 0.30
Mitral valve stenosis	Peak velocity (m/s)	< 1.2	1.2–2.2	> 2.2
	Valve orifice area (cm^2)	> 1.50	1.00–1.50	< 1.00
Mitral valve insufficiency	Regurgitation fraction (%)	< 30	30–49	≥ 50
	Regurgitant orifice area (cm^2)	< 0.20	0.20–0.39	≥ 0.30
Pulmonary valve stenosis	Peak velocity (m/s)	< 3.0	3.0–4.0	> 4.0
	Valve orifice area (cm^2)			< 1.00
Pulmonary valve insufficiency	Regurgitation fraction (%)	< 30	30–40	> 40
	Regurgitant orifice area (cm^2)	< 25.00	20.00–35.00	> 35.00
Tricuspid valve stenosis	Valve orifice area (cm^2)			< 1.00

References

[1] Kawel-Boehm N, Maceira A, Valsangiacomo-Buechel ER, et al. Normal values for cardiovascular magnetic resonance in adults and children. J Cardiovasc Magn Reson. 2015; 17(7):29

[2] Kaiser T, Kellenberger CJ, Albisetti M, Bergsträsser E, Valsangiacomo Buechel ER. Normal values for aortic diameters in children and adolescents–assessment in vivo by contrast-enhanced CMR-angiography. J Cardiovasc Magn Reson. 2008; 10:56

[3] Mosteller RD. Simplified calculation of body-surface area. N Engl J Med. 1987; 317(17):1098

[4] Kampmann C, Wiethoff CM, Wenzel A, et al. Normal values of M mode echocardiographic measurements of more than 2000 healthy infants and children in central Europe. Heart. 2000; 83 (6):667–672

[5] Schmidt KG, Beyer C, Häusler HJ, et al. Reports by the German Society of Pediatric Cardiology. Quality Standards for echocardiography in children and adolescents. Recommendations by the German Society of Pediatric Cardiology for echocardiography studies in childhood and adolescence. Z Kardiol. 1999; 88(9):699–707

[6] Parameter(z) Echo Z-Score Calculators. Im Internet: http://www.parameterz.blogspot.com/2008/09/z-scores-of-cardiac-structures.html (Stand: 06.04.2016)

[7] Pettersen MD, Du W, Skeens ME, Humes RA. Regression equations for calculation of z scores of cardiac structures in a large cohort of healthy infants, children, and adolescents: an echocardiographic study. J Am Soc Echocardiogr. 2008; 21(8):922–934

[8] Kutty S, Kuehne T, Gribben P, et al. Ascending aortic and main pulmonary artery areas derived from cardiovascular magnetic resonance as reference values for normal subjects and repaired tetralogy of Fallot. Circ Cardiovasc Imaging. 2012; 5(5):644–651

[9] Sarikouch S, Peters B, Gutberlet M, et al. Sex-specific pediatric percentiles for ventricular size and mass as reference values for cardiac MRI: assessment by steady-state free-precession and phase-contrast MRI flow. Circ Cardiovasc Imaging. 2010; 3(1):65–76

[10] Sarikouch S, Koerperich H, Boethig D, et al. Reference values for atrial size and function in children and young adults by cardiac MR: a study of the German competence network congenital heart defects. J Magn Reson Imaging. 2011; 33(5):1028–1039

[11] Sarikouch S, Koerperich H, Dubowy KO, et al. German Competence Network for Congenital Heart Defects Investigators. Impact of gender and age on cardiovascular function late after repair of tetralogy of Fallot: percentiles based on cardiac magnetic resonance. Circ Cardiovasc Imaging. 2011; 4(6):703–711

[12] Snider AR, Serwer GA, Ritter SB. Echocardiography in pediatric heart disease. 2nd ed. St. Louis: Mosby; 1997

[13] Wilkenshoff U, Kruck I. Handbuch der Echokardiographie. 3. Aufl. Berlin: Blackwell; 2002

[14] Hahn B, Bohn I, Strauer BE. Functional evaluation of left ventricular dynamics by use of 2-dimensional echocardiography: comparison with left ventriculography and assessment of normal 2-dimensional echocardiographical values. Z Kardiol. 1982; 71(7):445–451

[15] Mori K, Hayabuchi Y, Kuroda Y, Nii M, Manabe T. Left ventricular wall motion velocities in healthy children measured by pulsed wave Doppler tissue echocardiography: normal values and relation to age and heart rate. J Am Soc Echocardiogr. 2000; 13(11):1002–1011

[16] Kapusta L, Thijssen JM, Cuypers MH, Peer PG, Daniëls O. Assessment of myocardial velocities in healthy children using tissue Doppler imaging. Ultrasound Med Biol. 2000; 26(2):229–237

[17] Boettler P, Hartmann M, Watzl K, et al. Heart rate effects on strain and strain rate in healthy children. J Am Soc Echocardiogr. 2005; 18 (11):1121–1130

[18] Bussadori C, Moreo A, Di Donato M, et al. A new 2D-based method for myocardial velocity strain and strain rate quantification in a normal adult and paediatric population: assessment of reference values. Cardiovasc Ultrasound. 2009; 7(7):8

[19] Bussadori C, Oliveira P, Arcidiacono C, et al. Right and left ventricular strain and strain rate in young adults before and after percutaneous atrial septal defect closure. Echocardiography. 2011; 28(7):730–737

[20] Marcus KA, Mavinkurve-Groothuis AM, Barends M, et al. Reference values for myocardial two-dimensional strain echocardiography in a healthy pediatric and young adult cohort. J Am Soc Echocardiogr. 2011; 24(6):625–636

[21] Dewey FE, Rosenthal D, Murphy DJ, Jr, Froelicher VF, Ashley EA. Does size matter? Clinical applications of scaling cardiac size and function for body size. Circulation. 2008; 117(17):2279–2287

Suggested Reading

Wessel A. Normal values of two-dimensional echocardiographic evaluation of left and right ventricular geometry in children. Herz. 1985; 10(4):248–254

Index

Note: Page numbers set in **bold** or *italic* indicate headings or figures, respectively.

D

E

F

G

H

I

J

K

L